Next-Gen Healthcare

Nour Eldeen M. Khalifa •
Mohamed Hamed N. Taha
Editors

Next-Gen Healthcare

AI-Powered Medical Innovations

Springer

Editors
Nour Eldeen M. Khalifa
Cairo University
Giza, Egypt

Mohamed Hamed N. Taha
Cairo University
Giza, Egypt

ISBN 978-3-032-07266-5 ISBN 978-3-032-07267-2 (eBook)
https://doi.org/10.1007/978-3-032-07267-2

This Springer imprint is published by the registered company Springer Nature Switzerland AG
The registered company address is: Gewerbestrasse 11, 6330 Cham, Switzerland

Dedicated to the memory of my father (Mahmoud Khalifa Ali)

Nour Eldeen M. Khalifa

Dedicated to my father, mother, sister, and my children's (Abdelrahman, Nelly)

Mohamed Hamed

Preface

The landscape of healthcare is undergoing a transformation that few could have expected even a decade ago. Artificial Intelligence (AI) has transitioned from promising prototypes to real-world clinical solutions, redefining the limits of diagnostics, treatment planning, and personalized medicine. However, as these technologies mature, they bring both unprecedented opportunities and new responsibilities. "*Next-Gen Healthcare: AI-Powered Medical Innovations*" sets out to capture this duality by showcasing the scientific rigor behind medical AI advancements while foregrounding the ethical and safety considerations necessary for responsible adoption. This book is structured into two main parts, reflecting the dual imperatives of methodology and translation. The chapters included covered the following parts:

- Part I: Methodologies, Robustness, and LLM Safety in Medical AI
- Part II: Translational Applications and Disease-Focused Studies using AI

Part I establishes the technical, ethical, and safety foundations. We open with a comprehensive exploration of adversarial threats in healthcare, framing the security vulnerabilities that permeate AI-driven medical practice. From there, readers are taken on a progression: first toward generalizable methods for cross-population analysis, then into the automatic tones of optimized fine-tuning of deep learning models, and further still into frontier approaches such as quantum neural networks. The section then pins interpretability, highlighting the importance of explainable learning approaches in cardiovascular disease detection. Finally, it anchors today's most urgent discourse by examining the rise of large language models in error detection, data privacy, and medical safety. Together, these chapters not only map today's research landscape but also illuminate the gaps where future inquiry must lie.

Part II, "Translational Applications and Disease-Focused Studies," shifts from methodology to application. It begins with high-impact areas of modern medicine early Alzheimer's and dementia diagnosis, before expanding into oncology through predictive models for lymphoma treatment response. Chronic conditions then take the spotlight, as innovations in AI-assisted diabetes stratification and retinopathy detection illustrate how deep learning augments day-to-day clinical workflows. The section also spans dermatology, obesity, and mental health, underscoring the breadth of AI's reach from the surface of the skin to the complexities of the mind. By interlacing disease-specific studies with explainability and domain-specific concerns, this part of the book demonstrates how theory translates into life-improving reality.

Across both sections, the sequencing of chapters has been carefully maintained. We chose to begin with high-level vulnerabilities and safety challenges, ensuring the reader appreciates that technological power must always be met with resilience and responsibility. Only then do we dive into generalizable and frontier methodologies, before closing with the translational realities of disease-focused studies. This order reflects a planned philosophy: safety sets the stage, innovation drives advancement, and clinical translation defines true impact.

We extend our sincere gratitude and acknowledgement to everyone involved in the publication of this book—authors, reviewers, and the publishing team. Their dedication and support have been influential in bringing "Next-Gen Healthcare: AI-Powered Medical Innovations" to realization. We hope that readers will find the chapters insightful and appreciate the effort invested in this collective work.

Giza, Egypt Nour Eldeen M. Khalifa
Giza, Egypt Mohamed Hamed N. Taha

Contents

Editors and Contributors

About the Editors

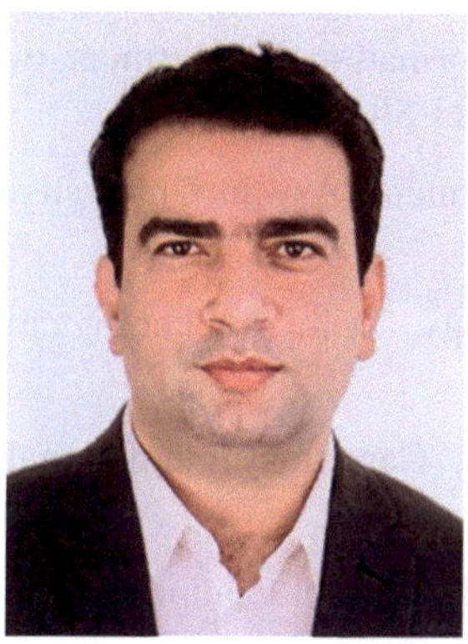

Nour Eldeen M. Khalifa received his B.Sc., M.Sc., and Ph.D. degree in 2006, 2009 and 2013 respectively, all from Cairo University, Faculty of Computers and Artificial Intelligence, Cairo, Egypt. He also had a Professional M.Sc. Degree in Cloud Computing in 2018. He authored/coauthored more than 50 publications and 4 edited books. He had more than 4000 citations. His name had been consecutively listed among Stanford University's top 2% of global scholars (2022–2023–2024). He has the Encouraging State Award (Egypt) in the Field of Engineering Science in 2024. He maintained significant editorial responsibilities as a board member for the Journal of World Science, Medical Data Mining, Academic Editor for PLOS One Journal, and reviewer for multiple international journals. Currently, he is an associate professor at Faculty of Computers and Artificial Intelligence, Cairo University. His research interests include wireless sensor networks, cryptography, multimedia, network security, machine, and deep learning. https://scholar.cu.edu.eg/nourmahmoud

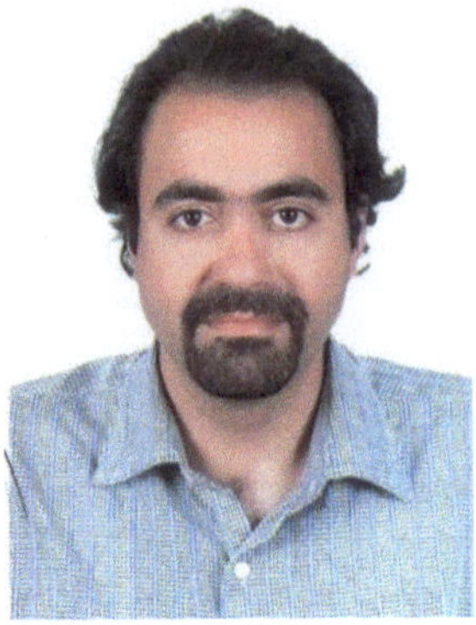

Mohamed Hamed N. Taha received the B.Sc., M.Sc., and Ph.D. degrees from the Faculty of Computers and Artificial Intelligence, Cairo University, in 2006, 2009, and 2013, respectively. He has been an Associate Professor with the Information Technology Department, Faculty of Computers and Artificial Intelligence, Cairo University, since 2016. He is a Reviewer of the IEEE internet of things journal. Deep learning, machine learning, the Internet of Things, wireless sensor networks, and blockchain are his research interests.

Contributors

Atrab A. Abd El-Aziz Faculty of Computers and Information, Department of Information Technology, Kafr El Sheikh University, Kafr el-Sheikh, Egypt

Mohamed Abdel-Nasser Electrical Engineering Department, Aswan University, Tingar, Egypt

Aman Ahlawat Department of Information Technology, Delhi Technological University, New Delhi, India

Hamza Kamel Ahmed School of Computer Science, Canadian International College (CIC), Cairo, Egypt

Walid Al-Dhabyani Department of Computer Science, Faculty of Computers and Artificial Intelligence, Cairo University, Cairo, Egypt

G. Aramvalartha Nayaki School of Chemical and Biotechnology, SASTRA University, Thanjavur, Tamil Nadu, India

Sohaib Asif Taizhou Key Laboratory of Minimally Invasive Interventional Therapy and Artificial Intelligence, Taizhou Campus of Zhejiang Cancer Hospital (Taizhou Cancer Hospital), Taizhou, Zhejiang, China

Center of Intelligent Diagnosis and Therapy (Taizhou), Hangzhou Institute of Medicine (HIM), Chinese Academy of Sciences, Taizhou, Zhejiang, China

Wenling Institute of Big Data and Artificial Intelligence in Medicine, Taizhou, Zhejiang, China

Hasret Irmak Baran Faculty of Engineering and Architecture, Department of Software Engineering, Istanbul Beykent University, Istanbul, Turkey

Dipendra Bhattrai School of Science and Technology, University of New England, Armidale, NSW, Australia

Roshan Chandru Dundalk Institute of Technology, Dundalk, Ireland

Youqin Chen Department of Respiratory Medicine, Taizhou Campus of Zhejiang Cancer Hospital (Taizhou Cancer Hospital), Taizhou, Zhejiang, China

Raymond Chiong School of Science and Technology, University of New England, Parramatta, NSW, Australia

School of Medicine and Public Health, University of Newcastle, Callaghan, NSW, Australia

Gulay Cicek Faculty of Engineering and Architecture, Department of Biomedical Engineering, Istanbul Beykent University, Istanbul, Turkey

Siyuan Dai Department of Electrical and Computer Engineering, University of Pittsburgh, Pittsburgh, PA, USA

Fareed Ud Din School of Science and Technology, University of New England, Armidale, NSW, Australia

Samar Elbedwehy Faculty of Artificial Intelligence, Kafr El Sheikh University, Kafr El-Sheikh, Egypt

University of Science and Technology, Zewail City of Science and Technology, Giza, Egypt

Reda A. El-Khoribi Department of Information Technology, Faculty of Computers and Artificial Intelligence, Cairo University, Cairo, Egypt

Eman K. Elsayed Faculty of Science, Al-Azhar University (Girls Branch), Cairo, Egypt

College of Information Technology, Misr University for Science and Technology (MUST), Giza, Egypt

Randa Hamada Faculty of Artificial Intelligence, Kafr El Sheikh University, Kafr El-Sheikh, Egypt

Mariam M. Hassan Department of Computer Engineering and Mathematics, Universitat Rovira i Virgili, Tarragona, Spain

Institute of National Planning, Cairo, Egypt

Yunus Emre Hos Faculty of Engineering and Architecture, Department of Software Engineering, Istanbul Beykent University, Istanbul, Turkey

Provia Kadusabe Dundalk Institute of Technology, Dundalk, Ireland

Hemalatha Karnan School of Chemical and Biotechnology, SASTRA University, Thanjavur, Tamil Nadu, India

Abhishek Kaushik Dundalk Institute of Technology, Dundalk, Ireland

Youssef Khalaf Faculty of Artificial Intelligence, Kafr El Sheikh University, Kafr El-Sheikh, Egypt

Nour Eldeen M. Khalifa Department of Information Technology, Faculty of Computers and Artificial Intelligence, Cairo University, Cairo, Egypt

Mahmoud Khalil School of Medicine, University of Pittsburgh, Pittsburgh, PA, USA

Andrew Macaulay School of Science and Technology, University of New England, Armidale, NSW, Australia

Malak Magdy School of Computer Science, Canadian International College (CIC), Cairo, Egypt

School of Information Technology and Computer Science, Nile University, Giza, Egypt

Asifa Mehmood Qureshi Dundalk Institute of Technology, Dundalk, Ireland

Alina Georgiana Mihăescu National Institute for Research and Development in Informatics, Bucharest, Romania

Faculty of Automatic Control and Computers, National University of Science and Technology Politehnica Bucharest, Bucharest, Romania

Phuong Anh Nguyen School of Science and Technology, University of New England, Armidale, NSW, Australia

Domenec Puig Department of Computer Engineering and Mathematics, Universitat Rovira i Virgili, Tarragona, Spain

Mohamed Ragab Institute for Infocomm Research, A*STAR, Singapore, Singapore

Nisa Sahinoglu Faculty of Engineering and Architecture, Department of Software Engineering, Istanbul Beykent University, Istanbul, Turkey

Gehad Ismail Sayed Faculty of Informatics and Computer Science, The British University in Egypt (BUE), Cairo, Egypt

Niusha Shafiabady Department of IT, Peter Faber Business School, Australian Catholic University, North Sydney, NSW, Australia

Faculty of Science and Technology, Charles Darwin University (Sydney Campus), Haymarket, NSW, Australia

Shubham Sharma Technological University Dublin, Dublin, Ireland

K. Srinika School of Chemical and Biotechnology, Sastra University, Thanjavur, Tamil Nadu, India

Seba Susan Department of Information Technology, Delhi Technological University, New Delhi, India

Irina Andra Tache Department of Automatic Control and Systems Engineering, National University of Science and Technology Politehnica Bucharest, Bucharest, Romania

Department of Image Fusion and Analysis - Artificial Intelligence, Siemens srl, Braşov, Romania

Baraa Tantawi School of Computer Science, Canadian International College (CIC), Cairo, Egypt

Sultan Tazefidan Software Engineering Department, Faculty of Engineering and Architecture, Istanbul Beykent University, Istanbul, Turkey

Phillip J. Tully Centre for Men's Wellbeing, University of Adelaide, Adelaide, SA, Australia

School of Psychology, Deakin University, Burwood, VIC, Australia

Enyu Wang Taizhou Key Laboratory of Minimally Invasive Interventional Therapy and Artificial Intelligence, Taizhou Campus of Zhejiang Cancer Hospital (Taizhou Cancer Hospital), Taizhou, Zhejiang, China

Department of Radiology Imaging, Taizhou Campus of Zhejiang Cancer Hospital (Taizhou Cancer Hospital), Taizhou, Zhejiang, China

Dong Xu Taizhou Key Laboratory of Minimally Invasive Interventional Therapy and Artificial Intelligence, Taizhou Campus of Zhejiang Cancer Hospital (Taizhou Cancer Hospital), Taizhou, Zhejiang, China

Center of Intelligent Diagnosis and Therapy (Taizhou), Hangzhou Institute of Medicine (HIM), Chinese Academy of Sciences, Taizhou, Zhejiang, China

Department of Radiology Imaging, Taizhou Campus of Zhejiang Cancer Hospital (Taizhou Cancer Hospital), Taizhou, Zhejiang, China

Fuguo Xue Department of Respiratory Medicine, Taizhou Campus of Zhejiang Cancer Hospital (Taizhou Cancer Hospital), Taizhou, Zhejiang, China

Aman Yadav Department of Information Technology, Delhi Technological University, New Delhi, India

Ruxuan Yan Department of Radiology Imaging, Taizhou Campus of Zhejiang Cancer Hospital (Taizhou Cancer Hospital), Taizhou, Zhejiang, China

Liang Zhan Department of Electrical and Computer Engineering, University of Pittsburgh, Pittsburgh, PA, USA

Lingying Zhu Department of Radiology Imaging, Taizhou Campus of Zhejiang Cancer Hospital (Taizhou Cancer Hospital), Taizhou, Zhejiang, China

Part I
Methodologies, Robustness, and LLM Safety in Medical AI

Adversarial Threats in Health Care: A Comprehensive Analysis of Vulnerabilities, Defense Mechanisms, and Recent Research

Atrab A. Abd El-Aziz, Reda A. El-Khoribi, and Nour Eldeen M. Khalifa

Abstract Recently, medical adversarial attacks had grave repercussions for both patients and healthcare providers. The resistance of deep learning-based medical models to adversarial attacks in dynamic situations is a topic of great interest since they are easily fooled using simple imperceptible perturbations called adversarial attacks. These attacks can exploit vulnerabilities in medical systems and can take various forms such as manipulating medical images, medical question answering (MQA), or compromising electronic health records. These attacks resulted from some limitations in medical images such as the scarcity of high-quality imaging datasets and image labeling. Medical systems are very challenging because their safety and accuracy are vital considerations. Although several defense techniques have been introduced to defend against these attacks, there is still a significant demand for more robust defense solutions. Notably, the domain of MQA and medical text is significantly under-researched, with virtually no established defense methods to counter adversarial threats in these areas. This chapter contributes to the field by bridging the gap between adversarial attacks in medical images and medical text special MQA. It ensures that the review offers valuable insights and practical recommendations for researchers and practitioners in healthcare and cybersecurity. This chapter covers various aspects of medical adversarial attack techniques, sources of vulnerabilities, defense strategies, and provides insights into the motivations and tactics of medical attacks. Finally, we provide recommendations for enhancing the resistance of medical systems to adversarial attacks. This review serves as a valuable resource for a diverse audience includes researchers and practitioners for healthcare and cybersecurity providers. It contributes to the

A. A. Abd El-Aziz (✉)
Faculty of Computers and Information, Department of Information Technology, Kafr El Sheikh University, Kafr El-Sheikh, Egypt
e-mail: Atrab_ahmed@fci.kfs.edu.eg

R. A. El-Khoribi · N. E. M. Khalifa
Faculty of Computers and Artificial Intelligence, Department of Information Technology, Cairo University, Cairo, Egypt
e-mail: r.abdelwahab@fci-cu.edu.eg; nourmahmoud@cu.edu.eg

N. E. M. Khalifa, M. H. N. Taha (eds.), *Next-Gen Healthcare*,
https://doi.org/10.1007/978-3-032-07267-2_1

collective knowledge base and offers practical recommendations for safeguarding medical systems against adversarial threats, particularly in the understudied areas of MQA and medical text.

Keywords Adversarial attacks · Deep learning · Defense methods · Medical images · Medical question answering (MQA) · Security

1 Introduction

There has been a notable surge of interest regarding the application of artificial intelligence (AI) technology in the field of medical imaging for the purposes of disease diagnosis. A branch of AI known as deep learning (DL) enables computational models to learn from experience. DL is composed of many processing layers and uses the backpropagation technique to derive the data representation of each layer from the representation in the preceding layer. Convolutional neural network (CNN) is a DL technique used for the processing of image and analysis [1].

DL has gained popularity for medical imaging tasks such as diabetic identification and cancer diagnosis due to its current success in natural imaging. Medical images are frequently used in patient care as prognostic and diagnostic imaging modalities [2]. Manual evaluations of medical images by human professionals are labor-intensive in practice. Therefore, automated DL systems have been suggested to aid in clinical decision-making and assist with human diagnosis [3]. Recently, several DL models have demonstrated performance better than the human specialist level in a variety of medical imaging jobs [4].

Recent research has shown that despite the increased performance of DL techniques, they are susceptible to a new type of attack called adversary attacks. The vulnerability of high-performance DL techniques to adversarial attacks was initially identified by Szegedy et al. [5]. DL models can be tricked into making inaccurate predictions with a high degree of confidence if their input examples are slightly perturbated [6]. The explanation: this type of attack was caused by the high nonlinearity of DL networks coupled with the regularization of the supervised learning techniques. Medical DL classification and segmentation models have proven susceptible to rapidly enhanced and updated adversarial attacks due to the features of medical images and the sparse number of annotated images. Many techniques are developed to generate these attacks such as Carlini and Wagner (C&W) [7], projected gradient descent (PGD) [8], and fast gradient sign method (FGSM) [9].

DL models have been implemented in safety-critical applications that raise safety concerns. A variety of detection and mitigation strategies have been offered to defend against these attacks. Adversarial training is among the most frequently defended strategies. By augmenting the training dataset by adding adversarial samples. This technique increases the robustness of neural networks against these attacks. It has been shown that one of the main causes of these limitations is the scarcity of a sufficient number of high-quality tagged photos and data [10].

Main contributions of this chapter:

1. Comprehensive coverage: This chapter is the first to examine adversarial attacks and defense mechanisms across both medical imaging and medical text. It provides a holistic understanding of the vulnerabilities present in DL-based medical systems.
2. Addressing research gaps: The chapter identifies and discusses the significant research gaps particularly in the defenses for MQA systems. It highlights the urgent need for robust strategies in this area.
3. Holistic analysis: It offers an in-depth exploration of the goals and motivations of adversarial attackers. It shades light on the various tactics employed against medical systems.
4. Taxonomy and variability: The chapter presents a detailed overview of the different branches of adversarial attacks. It includes their taxonomy, current examples, and implications for both medical imaging and text.
5. Visual representation of trends: This chapter provides valuable insights into trends and advancements in the field. It provides an analyses and visualization for the state of current research publications.
6. Future research directions: The chapter outlines potential avenues for future research. It includes exploring more defense and detection techniques specifically tailored for medical text.
7. Addressing limitations: It critically examines the limitations of existing approaches and emphasizes the need for collaborative efforts to enhance the resilience of medical systems against adversarial threats.

In this chapter, a complete review of the recently developed adversary attacks and defensive techniques on DL-based medical system diagnosis is introduced. Section 2 explains the motivation to investigate this chapter. Section 3 discusses the research gap concerning the defenses for MQA systems and highlights the lack of existing strategies. Section 4 examines the goals of adversarial attackers by providing insight into their underlying motivations and tactics. Section 5 offers an overview of the various branches of adversarial attacks by focusing on their application in medical systems. This section delves into the variability, taxonomy, and current examples of attacks as well as the existing defense and detection strategies for DL-based medical imaging and text. Section 6 analyzes and visualizes the current state of research publications in this field by providing a clear representation of trends and advancements. Section 7 explores potential future research directions and outlines the limitations of current approaches. Finally, Sect. 8 concludes the chapter, summarizing the key findings and implications of the chapter.

2 Research Motivations

According to a recent industry report reported by Cearley [11], 30% of all attacks on artificial intelligence (AI) systems would use adversarial attacks, poisoning of training data, or stolen models. Given that, the healthcare sector is expected to experience two to three times more cyberattacks than the other sectors. Therefore, adversarial attacks could be a serious threat to the medical industry. Adversarial attacks can lead to fraudulent behavior in fee-for-service healthcare systems such as healthcare professionals and insurance companies falsifying patient diagnosis codes to influence diagnostic decisions. The security of the medical-based deep learning models against adversarial attacks is an important open research area. According to Fig. 1, the main objective of the attacker is to significantly reduce the performance of the medical images system and make changes invisible to the human eye [12].

The motivations behind adversarial attacks on MQA systems are varied but generally align with the broader goals of malicious exploitation in healthcare settings. One primary motivation could be to create miscommunication between patients and healthcare providers. By manipulating responses in MQA systems, attackers can degrade the quality of care that potentially led to patient mistrust or legal liabilities for healthcare providers. In other cases, adversaries may seek to introduce errors into automated diagnoses to cause reputational damage to a healthcare provider or institution. Financial gain could also be a driver as attackers might exploit

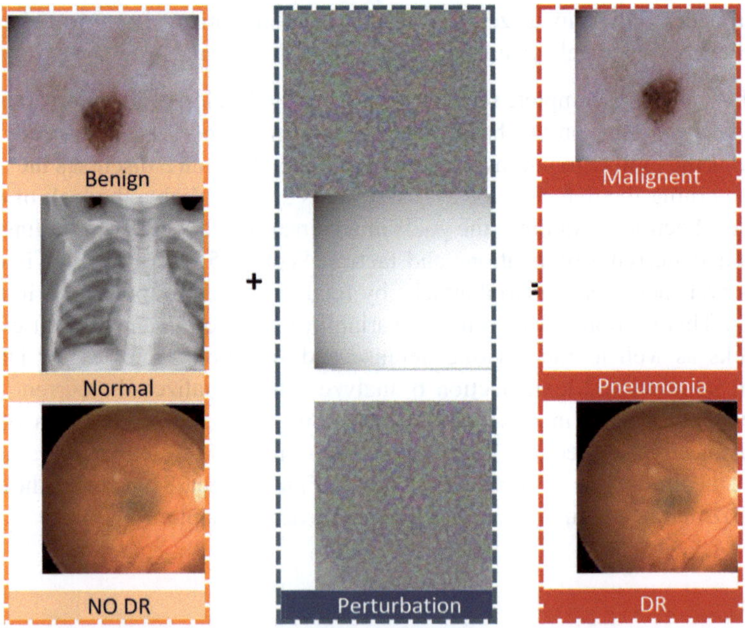

Fig. 1 Example of adversarial attacks developed to fool trained medical models

system vulnerabilities to disrupt billing systems, alter medical records or commit fraud. Additionally, state-sponsored attacks or hacktivists may target MQA systems to sabotage healthcare operations or compromise sensitive patient information, leveraging these adversarial tactics for political or ideological purposes.

This chapter allows researchers to choose their field of study within the field of medical deep learning-based adversarial attack methods.

3 The Research Gap in Defending Medical Question Answering Systems

The field of adversarial defense for medical systems has made significant strides in recent years, particularly in the context of medical imaging. However, one area that remains notably under-researched is adversarial defense in MQA systems and medical text-based systems. MQA systems, which rely on natural language processing (NLP) models to provide responses to patient and clinician inquiries, are especially vulnerable to adversarial attacks. These attacks can subtly manipulate textual inputs, causing the system to generate inaccurate or even dangerous answers, thereby compromising clinical decision-making and patient safety.

Despite the critical role of MQA systems in clinical environments, there is a conspicuous absence of research focused on defending these systems against adversarial text perturbations. Unlike adversarial attacks on medical images which have been the subject of extensive research and development of defense strategies, the domain of medical text remains largely unprotected. This gap poses a significant risk as text-based adversarial attacks can be as detrimental as image-based ones, leading to misdiagnoses, incorrect treatment recommendations, or compromised patient data.

Current defense mechanisms for general question-answering (QA) systems, such as synonym replacement or adversarial training, have not been sufficiently adapted or optimized for the medical domain. Medical text often contains highly specific terminology and complex syntactic structures. This makes it particularly susceptible to adversarial modifications. Moreover, the lack of large, well-labeled medical text datasets hampers the development of robust adversarial defense models, further contributing to the research gap.

The absence of tailored defenses for MQA systems suggests a pressing need for novel approaches that can effectively safeguard these systems. Future research should prioritize the development of advanced defense mechanisms that are specifically designed to address the unique challenges of medical text including word-level and character-level attacks. Additionally, interdisciplinary collaborations between NLP, cybersecurity, and healthcare researchers could drive the innovation required to create more resilient MQA systems.

The limited focus on adversarial defense in medical text-based systems presents a significant vulnerability in health care. Addressing this research gap is essential to ensuring the safety, accuracy, and reliability of MQA systems, which are increasingly integrated into clinical practice.

4 Goals of Adversarial Attackers

An attacker attempts to feed the target DL model with an input x,* which misleads the result to an incorrect class. The attacker's goal is deduced from the misclassification of the model. The attacker objectives can be categorized based on their influence on the accuracy of the classifier output, as shown in Fig. 2 [13]:

1. Confidence reduction: The attacker attempts to decrease the target's confidence model's prediction. For illustration, the "stop" sign image can be predicted with less confidence and a lower probability of belonging to the actual class.
2. Targeted misclassification: The attacker tries to manipulate the inputs so that the model generates the results of a specific target label. For example, the model of classification can classify that any input belongs to a category of photos with a label "go" sign.
3. Misclassification: The attacker attempts to modify the output classification of an input instance so that it is assigned to a different class. For example, a real image of represent "stop" image can be classified to any class other than the actual class of the stop sign.
4. Misclassification of source and target: The attacker attempts to assign a specific input source to a target class that has already been established. For example, the classification model will classify the input sign as "go" while it is actually a "stop" sign.

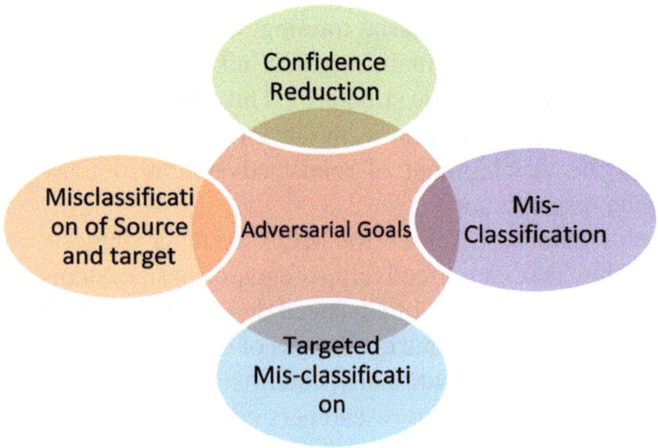

Fig. 2 Main goals of adversarial attacks

5 Adversarial Attacks in Medical Systems: Forms and Motivations

Adversarial attacks in medical systems pose significant threats to patient safety and the integrity of healthcare practices. This section provides an overview of the various forms of adversarial attacks, adversarial attacks on medical images, and adversarial attacks on medical text.

5.1 *Taxonomy of Image-Based Adversarial Attacks*

Adversarial samples are inputs that have been generated and modified by adding a small perturbation to the actual input to force the model to classify something incorrectly in DL systems. By creating these samples, the adversaries' primary goal is to significantly alter system performance and make the changes invisible to the human eye. As shown in Fig. 3, there are three main classification branches of adversarial attacks [14].

5.1.1 Adversarial Knowledge-Based Attacks

There are three different forms of attacks that can be used, depending on the attacker's knowledge of the target model [15]. Figure 4 shows the most common techniques applied in each category.

1. White-box attacks: The attacker understands the target model's parameters and architecture in detail. This is the simplest plan of attack and has the potential to

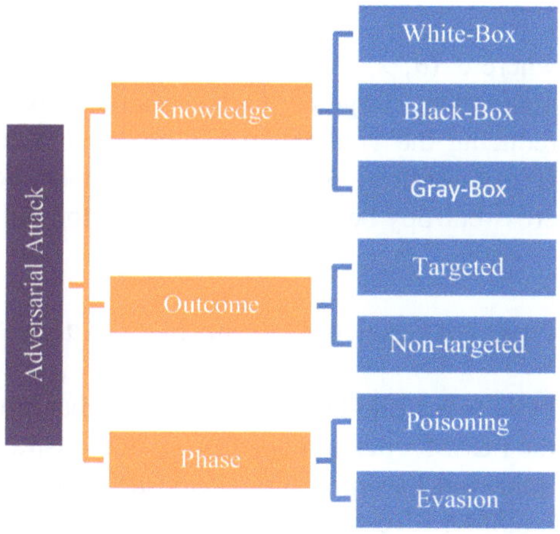

Fig. 3 Taxonomy of adversarial attacks

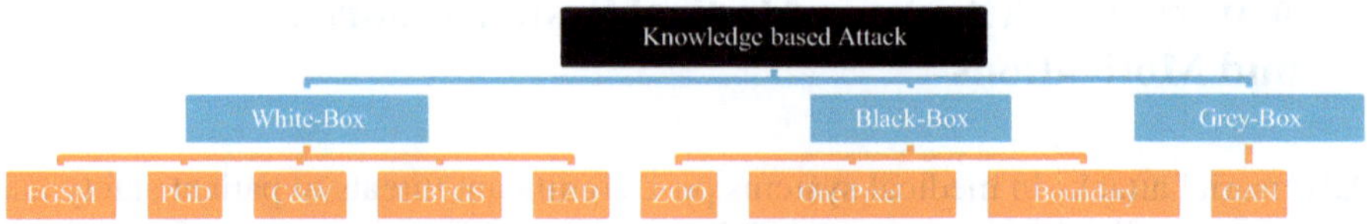

Fig. 4 Examples of knowledge-based attack techniques

cause the most damage. The attacker may be the model developer or an insider who can consider the worst-case situation of the model being attacked. The most common techniques of this category are the C&W, PGD, and FGSM attacks.

Fast Gradient Sign Method (FGSM) Attack

FGSM was first introduced by Goodfellow et al. It is one of the famous white-box, evasion, and a one-step technique. FGSM is used to create adversarial samples by adding a significant amount of perceivable noise (perturbations) in one or more pixels of an image. These perturbations result in model misclassification. This noise is calculated by multiplying the image-related parameters based on gradient signs. Epsilon functions as a minor constant; the model is fooled when epsilon rises. FGSM raises the loss in the most vertical direction by performing the one-step update along the gradient of the opposite loss. Formally, the adversarial sample produced by the untargeted FGSM is formulated by Eq. (1), while Eq. (2) serves as the targeted FGSM update rule, as follows:

$$x' = x + \in . \operatorname{sign} \lfloor \nabla_x J(\theta, x, y) \rfloor \tag{1}$$

$$x' = x - \in . \operatorname{sign} \left\lfloor \nabla_x J\left(\theta, x, y'\right) \right\rfloor \tag{2}$$

where $J(\theta, x, y)$ represents the gradient loss and $\in$ represents the perturbation magnitude. Targeted FGSM can be extended from the untargeted FGSM by reducing the gradient loss $J(\theta, x, y)$. Where y' is the target adversarial sample. If cross-entropy is used as the adversary loss, this update process can reduce the cross-entropy between the target vector and the predicted vector.

Projected Gradient Descent (PGD) Attack

PGD is a white-box evasion attack that was presented by Madry et al. to enhance the FGSM's performance. They demonstrate how the performance of FGSM can be improved by repeatedly executing a better iterative optimizer. The BIM trims the modified adversarial sample to a suitable range for T iterations using a reduced step size, with the following update rule at the t_{th} iteration:

$$x'_{t+1} = \text{Clip}\left\{x'_t + \propto . \,\text{sign}\left[\nabla_x J\left(\theta, x'_{t,}, y\right)\right]\right\} \tag{3}$$

where x'_t is the perturbated sample at iteration t. The iteration number is represented by t, and α is the perturbation magnitude.

Limited-Memory Broyden-Fletcher-Goldfarb-Shanno (L-BFGS) Attack

L-BFGS is a limited memory, nonlinear gradient-based numerical optimization methodology. L-BFGS white-box attack is used to discover adversarial perturbations with the minimum L_p norm. L-BFGS is used in an effort to lessen the amount of image disturbances. These images mislead the model output. Adversarial samples are produced that are conceptually identical to the original input.

$$\min_x \left\|x - x'\right\| p \text{ subject to } f\left(x'\right) \neq y' \tag{4}$$

where $\|x - x' \|p$ represents the L_p norm perturbations and y' represents the adversarial output. Hybrid loss is minimized by $C\|x - x' \|p + J(\theta, x', y')$, where the hyper parameters are represented by C. Grid search could identify the ideal value of C.

Carlini and Wagner (C&W) Attack

C&W is an optimization-based white-box attack that was introduced by Carlini and Wagner. The L-BFGS attack served as the model for this one. It does away with multiple objective functions and box constraints. Unlike adversarial training and defensive distillation, it more effectively generates adversarial cases to overcome the most recent defenses. It can produce adversarial samples measured according to the norm L0, L2, and L1, or CW0, CW2, and CW∞. The optimization objective is formulated as follows:

$$\min_\delta D\left(x, x + \delta\right) + c.f\left(x + \delta\right) \text{ subject to } x + \delta \epsilon \left[0, 1\right] \tag{5}$$

where the adversarial perturbation is represented by δ, the L0, L2, or L1 metric is represented by $D(x, x + \delta)$, and $f(x + \delta)$ represents the adversarial loss.

Elastic-Net Attack (EAD)

EAD was introduced by Chen et al. [16]. It is an adversary technique in which the adversarial sample production process is considered a regularized optimization problem. The overall goal of EAD is to create adversarial samples that can mislead the DL models and cause the least amount of disturbance in terms of L1 and L2 distance metrics. Consequently, this is how the optimization problem is defined:

$$\min_{x'} cJ\left(\theta, x', y'\right) + \beta \left\|x' - x\right\| 1 - \left\|x' - x\right\| 2^2 \text{ subject to } x' \in [0, 1]^d \quad (6)$$

where $J(\theta, x', y')$ is the targeted adversarial loss, β and c are hyperparameters, and $\left\|x' - x\right\| 1 - \left\|x' - x\right\| 2^2$ is used to penalize the $L1$ and $L2$ distances between the adversarial samples x' and the benign sample x.

2. Black-box attacks: The attacker has no knowledge of the target model's design or parameters, but they can provide input and track model output. This is the most plausible and difficult attack scenario. If two machine learning models are used to solve the same problem, the adversarial example of one machine learning model can successfully fool the other model with a high success rate. Therefore, in black-box attacks, the attacker can create adversarial examples from DL models and then attack the original target model by repeatedly querying the target model to create a training set.

Zero-Order Optimization (ZOO) Attack

ZOO is a black-box attack that was first introduced by Chen et al. [17]. ZOO performs an attack against the destination DNN by sending numerous queries and evaluating the output trust values in response. ZOO computes the network gradient through zero-order optimization while improving attack efficiency with hierarchical attack, dimensionality reduction, and importance sampling techniques. ZOO's optimization strategy is comparable to C&W's algorithm; however, because it uses a black-box approach, it cannot acquire the gradient of the model. ZOO computes the estimated gradient using the symmetric difference ratio. The best perturbation is created using the ADAM and stochastic coordinate descent approach to increase the efficiency of convergence.

3. Gray-box attacks: this is a partial knowledge attack in which the attacker only knows part of the training data used to modify the target model. In this approach, attackers can compute parameters and scores based on gradients and can only use probability distribution methods to grant access rights to the output labels assigned to them. In most cases, defending against an adversary attack is evaluated in a gray-box environment.

Generative Adversarial Networks (GAN)

GAN is an adversarial attack where two different types of neural networks, such as the discriminator and generator are competing together. It was first introduced by Xiao et al. [18] to create adversarial samples. By optimizing both target adversary loss and GAN loss, a generator is specifically trained to learn the adversary's distribution. The generator creates instances that the discriminator classifies incorrectly. The discriminator tries to distinguish between the genuine samples and the fraudulent ones produced by the generator itself in the meantime. Unrestrained adversarial instances are those that are generated because there are no benign samples adjacent to them. This approach doesn't follow the typical constraints set for adversarial samples, making it more successful when attacking models that have been trained through adversarial means using attacks that comply with those constraints.

5.1.2 Adversarial Outcome-Based Attacks

Depending on the outcome of the attack, there are two classifications of attacks called targeted and non-targeted attacks [19]. Figure 5 presents outcome-based adversary attack techniques.

1. Targeted attacks: These attacks cause a model to classify particular samples or a specific area of feature space to a particular (often incorrect) class. For illustration, assume that the class labels in a 3-Class classification problem are A, B, and C. In a targeted attack, the input can be forced into Class A, regardless of its actual class. Jacobian-based saliency map (JSMA) is a famous technique for a targeted attack. Gradient approaches (FGSM and PGD) can also be designed as targeted white-box attacks in case of the perturbation noise that has been added seeks to reduce the loss function of the image for a certain target class.

Jacobian-Based Saliency Map (JSMA) Attack

JSMA is a targeted white-box attack proposed by Piperno et al. [20]. It is based on the feature selection technique to decrease the number of features that need to be

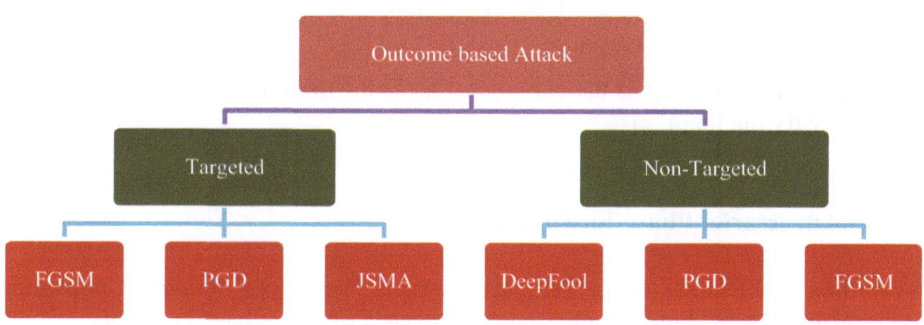

Fig. 5 Outcome-based adversary attack techniques

updated during adversarial sample construction. Perturbations are iteratively added to features in an increasingly prominent manner.

$$\nabla l(x) = \frac{\partial l(x)}{\partial x} = \left[\frac{\partial l_i(x)}{\partial x_y} \right]_{y \in 1,..m_{in}, i \in 1,...,m_{out}} \quad (7)$$

where x is the input, $l(x)$ is the Jacobian matrix, m_{in} and m_{out} are the neutrons' number in both the input and output layers sequentially. The Jacobian matrix shows how the logit outputs of various classes are affected by the components of the input x. The Jacobian matrix is used to build an adversarial salience map, which selects the features or pixels that need to be modified to produce the necessary changes in the logit outputs.

2. Non-targeted attacks: These attacks cause a DL model to incorrectly predict a subset of instances or parts of the feature space and don't specify which class they should be assigned to. From the previous example, a non-targeted attack does not stipulate that the input must be Class B or Class C. Exampled of the untargeted attack techniques are DeepFool (DF) attack, FGSM and PGD attacks. While, FGSM and PGD attacks can be implemented as untargeted attacks when maximizing the loss function of the model.

DeepFool (DF) Attack

DeepFool is an untargeted white-box attack introduced by Moosavi-Dezfooli et al. [21]. DF is based on gradient iteration. This attack initially computes the perturbations, then continuously and iteratively moves the normal instances toward the decision boundary until adversarial examples are obtained after passing the decision boundary. Reducing the Euclidean distance between the real and perturbed samples is the basis of this method. Iteratively add perturbations while evaluating the decision boundary between classes.

$$\underset{\delta t}{\text{argmin}} \, \|\delta_t\| \, 2 \text{ subjected to } f\left(x_t'\right) + \nabla f\left(x_t'\right)^t \delta_t = 0 \quad (8)$$

where x is the input and f is the classifier, $\|\delta_t\|$ is the minimal perturbation required to misclassify the input.

5.1.3 Adversarial Phase-Based Attacks

According to the attack execution phase, there are two types of attacks: poisoning and evasion attacks. Figure 6 presents an overview of phase-based attacks.

1. Poisoning attacks [22]: This attack takes place during the training phase by constructing backdoors in the target model. These backdoors include poising

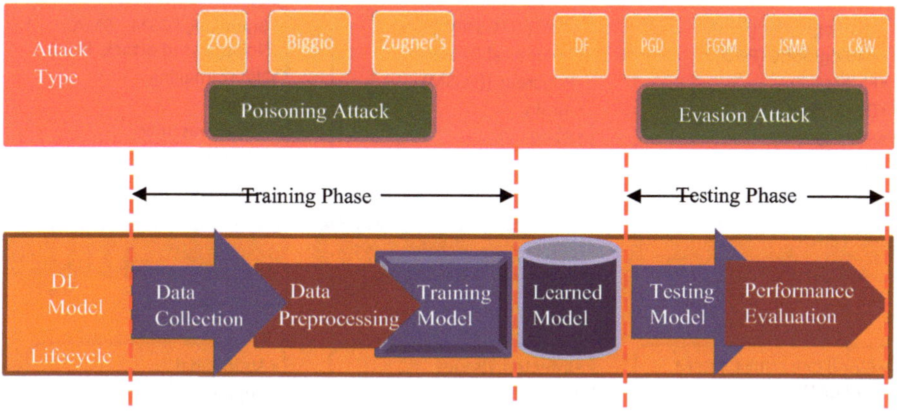

Fig. 6 Overview of phase-based attacks. The current attack threat in DL is shown at the top of the image. The DL life cycle is shown in the second section

adversarial examples in the training set. These attacks are usually white-box attacks or gray-box attacks, carried out by data modification or data injection. The Zoo, Biggio, and zugner's are examples of poising attacks.

Evasion attacks [23]: These attacks take place during the testing phase and involve adding small perturbations to benign test samples to fool the target model. This attack occurs when the model network has some perturbated inputs. These adversary inputs fool the model's classifier. These attacks may be black-box attacks or white-box attacks. The common techniques as mentioned before are the DF, FGSM, JSMA, PGD, and C&W attacks.

5.2 *Adversarial Attacks on Medical Images*

The lack of robustness in DL models is demonstrated by the ability of adversarial samples to alter the behavior of classifiers and segmentation tasks. A weakness during segmentation could result in an inaccurate description of reality throughout the later phases of diagnosis. Another problem that creates a potential attack vector is the irregular and poorly understood boundaries of the classification. Although much research has been investigated on adversarial attacks for nature images, there is far less for medical imaging. According to many academics, adversarial scenarios are too challenging to occur in medical imaging. This section illustrates in detail the analysis of medical images, current adversarial attacks on medical images, the detection techniques, and the defenses model that have been applied in the medical domain using various imaging modalities.

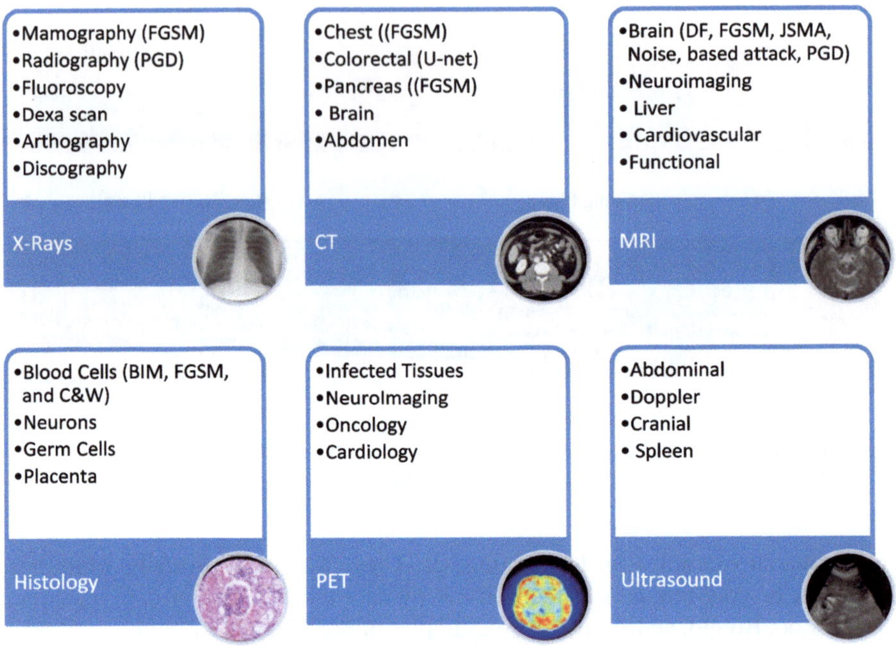

Fig. 7 Sources of medical images modalities with existing applied adversarial attacks

5.2.1 Taxonomy of Medical Images

DL techniques are used in medical images to effectively extract information obtained from medical images captured utilizing a variety of imaging modalities. These modalities include ultrasound, computed tomography (CT), magnetic resonance imaging (MRI), etc. These techniques are vital for the identification, location, and diagnosis processes of abnormalities because they provide anatomical data regarding several human organs. Figure 7 shows a taxonomy of different medical imaging modalities and the existing applied adversarial attacks against each modality. The primary goal of medical image analysis is to help radiologists and physicians effectively diagnose and predict disease. The primary tasks of DL-based medical systems analysis, include image segmentation, retrieval, detection, classification, and reconstruction.

5.2.2 Sources of Medical Vulnerabilities

As mentioned before, researchers have already shown that DL-based medical systems are susceptible to adversarial attacks. To ensure the security and integrity of DL-based models and health data [24], it is crucial to address the following points, as shown in Fig. 8.

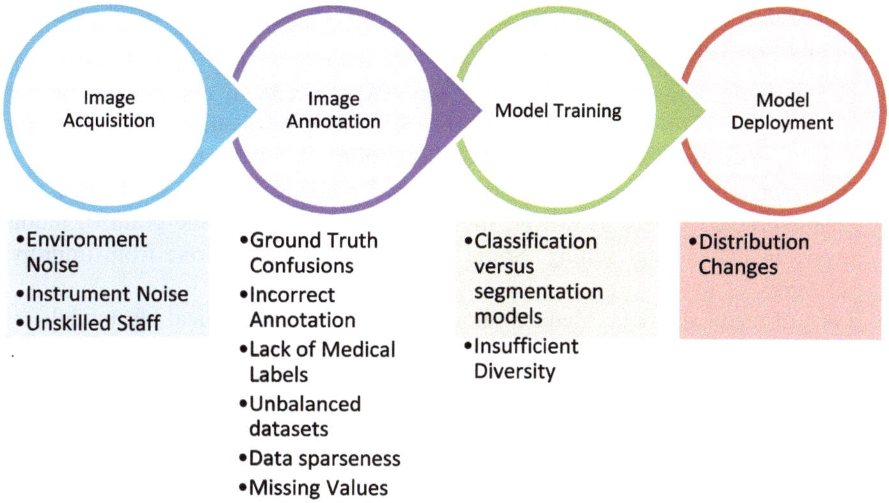

Fig. 8 Vulnerabilities of medical deep learning pipeline

Image Acquisition Vulnerabilities

Some of the vulnerabilities that can affect the performance of the DL systems are discussed below, even if in practice medical images are carefully collected to ensure diagnostic accuracy.

- Environmental and instrumental noise: Medical imaging properties can be exploited by attackers. Camera direction can change benign retinal fundus pictures into adversarial samples. Similarities between the medical pictures' foreground and background make it challenging for the network to identify clean and perturbed samples. This is due to high-quality, consistent photo exposure. Noise can produce data artifacts. Due to the roughness of medical photos, DL models might focus on nonessential elements. Medical pictures are more vulnerable to assault than real-world images due to their nature.
- Unskilled staff: Healthcare systems include both technical and nontechnical staff, and are so interdisciplinary. Therefore, they often struggle to find qualified individuals who can build and manage DL systems.

Medical Annotation Vulnerabilities

Medical annotation is the process of labeling each sample. Ideally, qualified physicians should handle most of this duty (radiologists or physicians) to provide domain-enriched data sets, which are necessary for effective DL modeling in healthcare systems. According to research, it could be dangerous to train DL models without a firm understanding of the domain. This section discusses particular vulnerabilities based on image annotations:

- Ground truth confusions: Malicious users who intend to manipulate the data worsen this problem by making its effects difficult to diagnose and impossible to recognize, even with expert human evaluation.
- Incorrect annotation: Most commonly used medical images are tagged with coarse-grained labels. However, the true utility of DL is fine-grained, hidden layers in the clinical setting. Some efficiency issues can arise from improper labeling.
- Lack of medical labels: Medical photos are rare to train medical DL models due to a lack of legal regulations to communicate medical data, privacy issues, and time-consuming labeling. Even doctors and radiologists occasionally misinterpret medical pictures. All of these causes generate overfitting and memorization in medical DL models, which lowers generalizability and makes the network vulnerable to assaults.
- Unbalanced and limited datasets: The number of datasets used to train DL models is insufficient. The lack of large-scale datasets is a major barrier to the effective implementation of DL techniques, as medical data is often modest in size.
- Data sparseness (missing values): This is a typical occurrence in real-world data and can occur from several different causes. The effectiveness of DL models is substantially affected by the missing observations.

Model Training Vulnerabilities

Model training vulnerabilities include privacy, ineffective or insufficient training, model tampering, and theft. When the DL models are trained with the wrong parameters, this is called incomplete or inappropriate training. Therefore, such critical applications must ensure the security and integrity of DL systems.

- Classification versus segmentation models: Due to these factors, segmentation is more prone to attacks than classification models. Unlike classification, which assigns a label to the entire image, semantic segmentation assigns a label to each pixel. Second, it is not easy to determine the success rate of attacks in segmentation models. Third, these models typically don't include high-quality image samples, which causes overfitting. Fourth, a segmentation image can easily be fooled by a minor change in image intensity.
- Insufficient diversity: The architecture is uniform across nearly all medical machine vision tasks, although few learning models are similar. Since the design of transferable or global adversarial attacks has simplified attacking any medical system, the lack of a widespread variety of architectures and datasets makes it easier to compromise the security of neural networks.
- Deployment vulnerabilities: Ensuring the robustness of the system throughout the deployment phase is crucial.

Distribution changes: occur when DL models that have been trained on images from one domain are subsequently operated on data from another domain. The performance of the model suffers greatly under these conditions. Additionally, these models used in health care are typically tested on new patients after being built using data from previous patients, raising concerns regarding the accuracy of DL predictions.

5.2.3 Existing Adversarial Attacks on Medical Images

Recent research studies have proved that the most sophisticated medical DL systems are considerably susceptible to adversarial attacks in three phases including the medical images classification phase, segmentation phase, and regression phase [25]. Figure 9 presents a review of some existing attacks on different DL medical images phases.

Classification Phase Attacks

Classification is a significant use of DL in medical image analysis. Images are used as inputs, and deep learning models sort them into several categories. Models often indicate whether or not a patient has a disease. Many studies have been investigated in the area of DL medical classification attacks. For example, three adversarial attacks that are successfully used against many DL medical models (skin lesions classification and brain tumor segmentation) are first studied by Paschali et al. [26]. They used adversarial samples to investigate the vulnerabilities of these medical DL models. These adversarial samples are used to compare model performance on clean, crafted, and noisy data. The authors applied many DL models for skin lesions

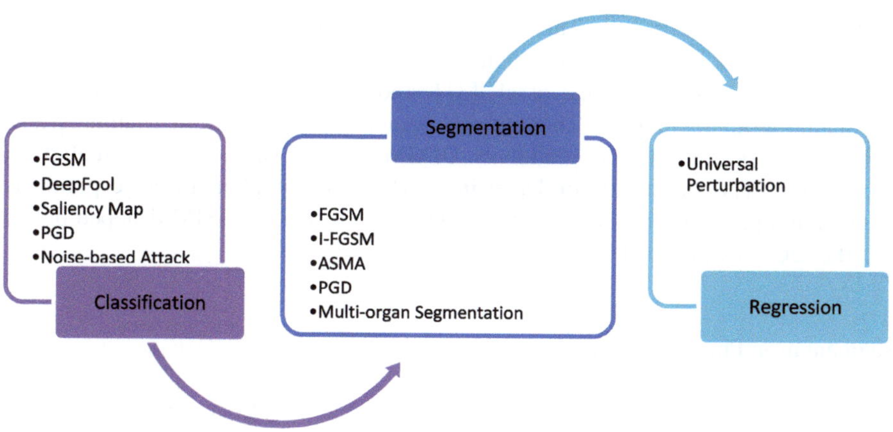

Fig. 9 Review of some existing attacks on different DL medical images phases

classifications including Inception (IV3), (IV4), and MobileNet (MN). While U-Net, SegNet, and DenseNet models have been utilized for the segmentation of the whole-brain. Many attack techniques have been used to create perturbated samples such as FGSM, DeepFool (DF) methods, and saliency map attacks (SMA). Finally, despite variations in accuracy when applying different attacks, the authors conclude that IV4 is recommended due to its equivalent generalization ability and resilience, among others. The scientists showed that for classification, the model's robustness is related to its depth, while for dense blocks, segmentation, and jump connections improve the model's effectiveness. As the adversary perturbation was from 0.97 to 0.99 was imperceptible. Finlayson et al. [27] demonstrated how the white and black-box attacks weaken the medical DL models. The pretrained ResNet50 model was used for diabetic retinopathy that is classified via retinal fundoscopy, dermoscopic, and pneumothorax from chest radiography. The black-and-white-box PGD attacks are applied against this model. The findings demonstrated that in both cases, the accuracy was significantly reduced. Kotia et al. [28] analyzed the impact of virtual adversarial training (VAT), FGSM, and noise-based adversarial attacks on brain tumor classification. The most successful attack was the FGSM, which reduced accuracy by 69%, At the same time, noise-based attacks and VAT only reduced accuracy by 34% and 24%, respectively. An adversarial training technique was used to increase the robustness of the model against noise-based and FGSM and produced excellent results. The training accuracy on the perturbated images was nearly identical to the test accuracy. In contrast, VAT adversary training was ineffective because it resulted in a 14% reduction in accuracy compared to training.

Huq et al. [29] examined the impact of adversary attacks on the classification of skin cancer. VGG16 and MobileNet models were used to classify seven types of skin cancer. Two white-box attacks were used to create perturbated samples including the FGSM and PGD. Accuracy dropped drastically after using those attacks. To increase the robustness, they recommended applying the adversarial training technique. Pal et al. [30] studied the impact of the FGSM attack on the CT and X-ray of COVID images. The VGG-16 and InceptionV3 models were used for the classification process. The results proved that these models are vulnerable to adversarial attack because the model accuracy decreased up to 63% in InceptionV3 and 90% in VGG-16. Yilmaz et al. [31] studied the impact of FGSM attacks on mammographic images. The Digital Database for Screening Mammograms (DDSM) has been used for experiments. DDSM includes two categories: malignant and normal. The structural similarity index (SSIM) is applied to correspond the original and perturbated images. They showed that when the SSIM dropped below 0.2, the accuracy dropped by as much as 30%.

Segmentation Phase Attacks

In medical imaging, segmentation refers to the extraction of particular components of the medical image, such as organs, cells, and tumors. In addition, clinical factors can be examined such as shape and volume. Li et al. [32] presented a custom attack against DL medical model called a query-based black box (QBB). QBB within a limited query budget could change the foreground pixel classes. This attack used a more accurate gradient loss estimate and changed the fixed variance of the adaptive distribution to a learnable one. Experiments proved the efficiency of the suggested attack in deconstructing medical imaging segmentation models. Another contribution by Li et al. [33] applied FGSM and I-FGSM against pancreas segmentation. The pancreas is extremely hard to segment because of its small size, irregularities, texture, and location. They suggested a deep coarse-to-fine 3D model to address this issue. Datasets from JHMI and NIH were used in experiments. The framework is susceptible to the two types of attacks since they have significantly lower accuracy (85.83%). To address this issue, the authors suggested adversarial training for this model. Another segmentation attack called the adaptive segmentation mask attack (ASMA) was introduced by Ozbulak et al. [34].

ASMA is a targeted approach for medical image segmentation. U-Net model is used for the segmentation of two medical datasets for ISIC skin lesion segmentation and glaucoma optic disc. They proved that DL-based medical segmentation models are vulnerable to adversarial attacks. Cheng et al. [35] applied the universal random perturbation attack against the DL segmentation of brain tumors. The U-Net model has been used for segmentation. The MICCAI BraTS 2019 dataset was used in all experiments. The results indicated that concurrent perturbation significantly decreases model accuracy, while single-modal perturbation minimally reduces accuracy. Yao et al. [36] proposed an add-on to a white-box attack called hierarchical feature constraint (HFC). HFC can be incorporated into any attack by hiding the adversarial perturbation in the original feature distribution. Adversary attacks are more easily identified on medical domain images than on natural domain images. The goal of HFC is to hide adversary features so that they are not easily detectable. The technique is applied to chest X-ray and fundoscopy datasets. ResNet50 and VGG16 models were used. The results proved that HFC can be applied to avoid adversarial samples from being detected. Another study by Anand et al. [37] applied the FGSM and PGD attacks against the segmentation of two medical datasets called MRI RVSC cardiac segmentation and chest radiography for pneumonia detection. Self-supervised learning (SSL), VGG11, and the U-Net segmentation model were used for experiments. The experimental results demonstrated that SSL produced better results as it learns more important features. Chen et al. [38] applied another adversarial attack against organ segmentation from CT scans. The intensity variations and geometrical deformations are used to create adversarial samples. The U-Net model was used for experiments. The results showed that the Dice score metric is significantly lowered in all organs.

Regression Phase Attacks

Regression models are used in the medical field. Examining the resistance of the regression models to attacks can be applicable for the reliability and security of medical systems. Li, Zhang et al. [39] published the first study on the effect of adversarial attacks against medical regression-based prediction models. They used 3D MRI brain samples to predict an individual's age. The experiments were performed using the hybrid DL and CNNs models. The adversarial samples were created with limited magnitude perturbation of l_0, l_2, and l_∞. A universal perturbation, as well as image-specific perturbation, are very successful in reducing the accuracy of the age prediction model. Since a single perturbation can inject considerable bias into the predictions, there is still serious concern about how resistant DL is to adversarial attacks. Table 1 lists the details and comparison between the abovementioned attacks.

5.2.4 Defenses Against Medical Adversarial Attacks

This section discusses both the defense and detection techniques for DL-based medical imaging against adversarial attacks, as shown in Fig. 10.

Adversarial Training Defense Technique

Adversarial training (ADVT) is an adversarial defense technique in which DL models create adversarial examples and embed those examples in the training data. It is a natural defense mechanism against adversarial examples that increases the robustness of a neural network while the model is being trained. Biggio et al. [63] reported that a neural network can be trained on adversarial examples to be resistant to first-order attack strategies. For example, Huang et al. [64] advocated robust adversarial training techniques to solve the limited-angle tomography (LAT) problem. This problem can cause problems with CT reconstruction. Since poisonous noise is frequently found on CT scans, they used it as a disturbance in the images for training. The U-Net model was utilized for experiments with the dataset of low-dose CT scans. The poison noise retraining is quite substantial for angle-limited reconstruction, but insufficient for nonlocal adversarial instances. Another contribution proposed by Vatian et al. [65] is on natural adversary attacks. They used the CNN model for brain MRI and CT scans for lung cancer classification. They showed that a noise that behaves like a "natural" adversarial example can exist in sophisticated medical imaging systems. To protect against these attacks, three defense strategies were applied. The ADVT with FGSM and JSMA achieved the best defense strategy compared with the other two strategies, while layer activation function switching with bounded ReLU and data augmentation with gaussian noise were the other two strategies. Liu et al. [66] studied the robustness of the ADVT defense technique in the classification of lung nodules using CT images. Three 3DResUNets models were used for model training and data were obtained from the NLST and LUNA datasets. They applied the PGD attack to confidently identify patterns that result in misclassification before training the network. The authors suggest using ADVT for nodule classification to increase model resistance to

Table 1 Comparison of current adversarial attack techniques against medical images

References	Advs. attacks	DL model	Task	Performance reduction	Dataset	Advantages	Limitation
[26]	DF, FGSM, JSMA	MobileNet, inception, U-net, SegNet, DenseNet	Segmentation, classification	Accuracy 19–40% 6–24%	Brain OASIS [40], skin dermofit [41]	• Studied both the classification and segmentation tasks • Applied five DL models against three attacks	• Studied only the effect of white-box attacks • Tested on only two medical modalities
[27]	PGD	ResNet50	Classification	50–100%	Diabetic [42], chest X-Ray [43]	• Outlined why adversarial examples provide disproportionately large threats in the medical realm	• Study the effect of a single attack against a single model • Tested on only two medical modalities
[28]	VAT, FGSM, noise-based attack	CNN	Classification	Reduction rate 34%, 69%, 24%	Brain MRI [44]	• Tested against three different attacks • Achieved a high reduction rate with some attacks	• Tested with only a single DL model and single medical modality
[29]	FGSM, PGD	MobileNet, VGG16	Classification	Reduction rate up to 75%	HAM10000 [45]	• Tested two different attacks against two DL models • Achieved high-performance reduction rate	• Dataset lacks a sufficient number of training samples • Tested on only two medical modalities
[30]	FGSM	VGG-16, Incep-tionV3	Classification	Reduction rate up to 90%	CT images [46, 47]	• Tested against two different DL models • Achieved high-performance reduction rate	• Tested against single white-box attack • Ignored the effect of black-box attacks

(continued)

Table 1 (continued)

References	Advs. attacks	DL model	Task	Performance reduction	Dataset	Advantages	Limitation
[31]	FGSM	Custom CNN	Classification	Reduction rate up to 30%	Breast mammography [48]	• The first study was on mammography attacks • Discussed the telemedicine application	• The reduction rate was not high enough • Ignored the effect of black-box attacks
[32]	QBB	UNet, attention-UNet, COPLENet	Segmentation	Reduction rate 80%	Chest X-ray JSRT [49]	• Enhanced the adaptive square attack • Achieved a high reduction rate	• Ignored the 3D images datasets
[33]	FGSM, I-FGSM	ResDSN coarse	Segmentation	Reduction rate 84.5%	JHMI [50] and NIH [50]	• Achieved a high success rate • It also provides a defense technique to increase the 3D model robustness	• They ignored the reasons that lead to inaccurate segmentation • Tested only the impact of two white-box attacks
[34]	ASMA	U-net	Segmentation	Reduction rate 98%	Glaucoma optic [51], ISIC skin [52]	• The first technique for producing targeted samples for image segmentation • Achieved a high success rate	• Experiment applied on only a single DL model structure
[35]	UAP	U-net	Segmentation	Reduction rate up to 65%	BraTS 2019 [53]	• Studied the effect of the attack on MRI single and four modalities • Achieved a high success rate	• Experiments should study more attacks against many medical modalities

[36]	HFC on (PGD and FGSM)	ResNet50, VGG16	Segmentation	Reduction rate by 20%	Chest X-ray [54], diabetic	• Developed an add-on to white-box techniques to increase the imperceptibility of attack • Tested with two different models	• Low reduction rate compared with other attacks
[37]	FGSM, PGD	VGG11, U-net	Classification, segmentation	Reduction rate up to 100%	X-ray [55], MRI [56]	• Tested with different models and tasks against two medical modalities • Achieved a high success rate	• Experiments should study more black-box attacks
[38]	Multiorgan segmenta-tion	U-net	Segmentation	Reduction rate up to 85%	CT [57]	• Achieved a high success rate	• Experiments should study more attacks against many medical modalities
[39]	UAP	CNN, hybrid CNN	Regression	Reduction rate up to 50%	MRI ABIDE 1 [59], IXI [58], FCON-1000 [59], OASIS1 [60], NDAR [61], ADHD200 [62], NKI Rockland [63]	• Experiment with multiple medical datasets	• The reduction rate is low compared with another attack impact

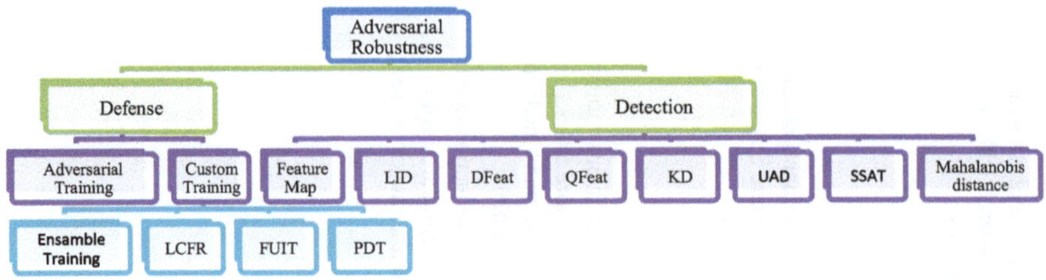

Fig. 10 Medical DL-based adversarial robustness techniques

unexpected noise. Wu et al. [67] applied the adversarial training defense technique to increase the robustness of the diabetic retinopathy-based DL classification model. The PGD attack was combined with ResNet32 to create the perturbated samples. They proved that the effectiveness of the model under attack was greatly enhanced using the adversary training defense technique.

Custom Defense Techniques

Rao et al. [68] applied many attacks to diagnose X-ray thorax disease. As well, the authors investigate two different forms of protection techniques, the transformation of pixel deviation (PDT) and adversary PGD training. PDT chooses a random pixel from adverse instances and changes it with a different pixel chosen from a small square region. They concluded that their novel method solved the problem of poor performance of existing defense strategies for large disturbances. Mani et al. [69] proposed a custom adversarial defense model named a fuzzy unique image transformation (FUIT) to protect the COVID-19 classification model. Before feeding the training samples to the model, the image's pixels are modeled into an interval. The results proved that this technique is successful against six untargeted attacks. Although this approach does not change the design of the model, it requires additional time to transform the images during testing. Liu et al. [70] suggested another successful defense strategy for medical image segmentation using low-cost frequency refinement (LCFR). ASMA attack was applied against fundoscopy and skin photographs classification models. Since only frequency refinement of the images is required, this method does not effect on the model's complexity. Raul et al. [71] introduced an ensemble training defense technique on adversarial attacks using CT scans of the NLST dataset to predict the malignancy of lung nodules. The one-pixel black-box and FGSM white-box attacks were used to create the adversarial samples. The attacks lead to a 28–36% decrease in accuracy. Each CNN architecture of the proposed ensemble model was initialized with seven different parameters to drastically reduce the accuracy of the attack.

Detection Techniques

The detection of DL adversarial attacks is another essential technique to defend the medical classifiers. These techniques determine whether the input is benign or perturbated before feeding into the classification model input.

The medical DL model refuses to predict the input sample if it can determine that it is perturbated. However, DL models used for medical imaging are more susceptible to adversary attacks than in the real world, instances of medical adversaries are easier to detect. Li et al. [72] implemented a detection technique for adversarial attack based on the feature map. Where adversarial samples have different feature maps compared with the original samples. The detection model rejects adversarial instances before the classification process. The PGD, FGSM, and BIM attacks were applied. The DenseNet121 model was used for the classification of chest X-rays. This technique does not require any change in the model architecture. Also, this technique does not need knowledge of the target model. Ma et al. [6] studied the performance of four adversarial detection techniques for medical DL models. The four detection techniques include the local intrinsic dimensionality (LID), deep features (DFeat), kernel density (KD), and quantized features (QFeat) applied against four attacks. Four attack strategies including PGD, FGSM, C&W, and BIM are applied against the ResNet50 model. Three medical datasets were used for experiments including fundoscopy, chest X-ray, and ISIC. The results demonstrated that the detection techniques against the four attacks offer highly robust performance. KD achieved the maximum AUC of 99% compared with other attacks for all three datasets.

Since these methods rely on guessing the density of the adversary's samples, even if the performance is quite good, the method's applicability is restricted to a few common attack types. Li et al. [73] introduced a hybrid adversarial detection technique based on unsupervised adversarial detection (UAD) and semi-supervised adversarial training (SSAT). The system is proposed to deliver a robust DL medical imaging framework. The ResNet18 model was used to classify the OCT images. The results proved that the semi-supervised training greatly reduces the vulnerability of the model. This approach increases the complexity of the model by finding robust features. The authors also suggested a new risk metric for the adversarial attack that would depend on the classification scenario and the acceptance or rejection of unsupervised adversarial detection. Uwimana et al. [74] proposed another medical adversarial detection technique. The Mahalanobis distance is applied to detect the out-of-distribution (OOD) data and the adversarial samples of the malaria classification model. The DeepFool, BIM, FGSM, and C&W attacks were applied. This technique offers a detection accuracy of up to 99.95%. Table 2 shows a detailed comparison of these defense and detection techniques against DL-based medical adversarial attacks.

Table 2 Comparison of existing defense and detection techniques against adversarial medical attacks

References	Advs. attacks	DL model	Defense technique	Performance improvement	Dataset	Advantages	Limitation
[64]	LAT	U-net	ADVT	More resistance to poison noise	CT [75]	• The U-net can reduce most artifacts	• The model is still vulnerable to nonlocal attack
[65]	FGSM, JSMA	CNN	ADVT, bounded ReLU and Gaussian noise	Improves up to 2%	LIDCIDRI [76], BRATS 2015 [77]	• Studied the impact of three defense techniques	• Defend against only two types of white-box attacks
[66]	PGD	3D ResNets	ADVT	Improves up to 10% and 35%	LUNA [78], NLST [79]	• Model robustness against three types of image noise • The model can be applied to other similar models if the data and the model are fully differentiable	• The model did not synthesize all types of nodules • Motion distortion and metal artifacts noise not investigated
[67]	PGD	ResNet32	ADVT	Accuracy enhanced by 40%	APTOS [80]	• Achieved a high defense rate	• Tested against a single model structure with a single medical modality against a single attack
[68]	FGSM, DII-FGSM, PGD, MIFGSM	DenseNet, Res-50 and VGG16	PDT and ADVT	AUC up to 85%	CheXpert [81]	• Solve the limitation of excessive iterations • High success rate. • Experiment against many attacks with different dl model structures	• More enhancement is required to handle the large and different values of perturbations • The performance of the PDT was tested against a single medical modality
[69]	FGSM, C&W, BIM, DF, PGD, PGD-r	CNN	FUIT	The accuracy increased by up to 40%	COVID-19 chest X-ray [46], CT scans [82]	• Six attacks are studied against binary and multi-class data • Achieved a high robustness rate	• The experiments are performed using small datasets with fewer images

[70]	ASMA	ResNet-50, U-net, DenseNet	LCFR	The accuracy increased by up to 40%	Glaucoma optic [83], ISIC skin [84]	• Authors evaluate both segmentation and classification robustness • High defense rate	• Many attacks should be studied
[71]	FGSM, one-pixel	CNN	Ensemble training	Accuracy increased up to 34%	NLST [85]	• High defense rate • Seven CNN architectures with different seed points are trained to verify the stability	• Defense against 3D slices should be studied • Segmentation is performed based on a semiautomatic technique
[72]	FGSM, BIM, PGD	DenseNet121	Detection-based feature map (FM)	F1 detection score up to 0.97	NIH ChestX-ray14 [86]	• Defend against white and black-box attacks • Can be embedded in any DL medical system	• Multimodal distributions of complex datasets are required to be studied • A new dimension reduction technique is required to be investigated
[6]	FGSM, BIM, PGD, C&W	ResNet50	Detection techniques (DFeat, LID, QFeat, KD)	Detection accuracy up to 98%	Diabetic retinopathy [87], chest X-ray [88], melanoma [89]	• Four detection methods against four attacks are studied • Binary and multi-class datasets are tested	• Experiments ignored the effect of black-box attacks
[73]	FGSM, PGD, C&W	ResNet18	Detection UAD, SSAT	Detection accuracy up to 0.97	OCT [90]	• Two detection methods against three white-box attacks are studied • High-detection rate	• Experiments ignored the binary classification results and the detection of black-box attacks
[74]	BIM, FGSM, and C&W	VGG-19, ResNet-18	Detection using Mahalanobis distance	Detection accuracy of up to 99.95%	Malaria cells [91]	• The system handles both the adversarial and out-of-distribution samples against three attacks	• Experiments ignored multi-class datasets and the detection of black-box attacks

5.3 *Adversarial Attacks on Medical Text (MQA Systems)*

5.3.1 Nature of Text Attacks

Adversarial attacks on MQA systems typically involve subtle manipulations of text that exploit the vulnerabilities of natural language processing (NLP) models. These attacks can take various forms including word-level, character-level, sentence-level, and multilevel manipulations.

- Word-level attacks: Attackers replace or substitute key medical terms with semantically similar or dissimilar words to confuse the system. For example, a term like "malignant" could be replaced with "benign." This leads to incorrect or misleading medical advice.
- Character-level attacks: Involve altering individual letters within a word such as changing "cancer" to "cqncer," which can fool the model while remaining unnoticed by human users.
- Sentence-based attacks: involve reordering words or altering sentence structure to distort the meaning without significantly changing the overall content. This disrupt the MQA system's ability to accurately process and respond to medical queries.
- Multilevel attacks: Involve many types of attacks such as character-, word-, and sentence-level attacks.

5.3.2 Impact on MQA

The consequences of these adversarial text attacks can be severe. Since MQA systems are often used to provide critical health information or assist in clinical decision-making, an adversarial perturbation could lead to dangerous misinterpretations of medical advice. For instance, an altered query might cause the system to recommend inappropriate treatments or incorrect diagnoses. This could result in real-world harm to patients. Misleading medical responses could undermine the trust between healthcare providers and patients. Also, this could lead to delays in diagnosis, inappropriate medication prescriptions, or even life-threatening decisions in clinical settings. The subtle nature of these attacks makes them particularly insidious as the erroneous output may not be immediately recognized as incorrect by users.

Adversarial attacks on medical text and MQA systems represent a critical and underexplored threat to the integrity of healthcare delivery. With the growing reliance on NLP-driven systems for clinical decision support and patient interaction, it is essential to develop robust defenses to mitigate the impact of these sophisticated attacks.

6 The Importance of Medical Adversarial Attacks in the Research Field

This section discusses the analysis of the importance of adversarial attacks based on the Scopus database [92] articles as a base with keywords "Adversarial attacks, defense of Medical images, healthcare" from 2018 to 2022. The following sections will illustrate how articles are distributed based on time and funding institutions, respectively. The overall evolution of the adversarial attack field can be understood intuitively and efficiently by gaining a broad perspective from field publications.

6.1 Distribution of Articles Related to Medical Adversarial Attacks Over Time

After 2018, medical adversarial attack research started a new era of development, as evidenced by a significant increase in research interest. Research in this sector has grown rapidly and has not quite gained its peak yet. The published research in this field is expected to exceed 2000 by 2023. Research of medical adversarial attacks remains a major research focus at this time.

6.1.1 Top Funding Sponsors Entities Related to Medical Adversarial Attacks

Figure 11 demonstrates how institutions have supported researchers over the past 5 years in the area of adversarial attacks against DL medical models. It also indicates that China's National Natural Science Foundation funded more than 700 research publications in the area of adversarial attacks, which is related to the field of computer science, according to the Scopus database.

The institutions are listed in order by the number of researches as follows: "National Natural Science Foundation of China, National Science Foundation, National Institutes of Health, National Key Research and Development Program of China, National Research Foundation of Korea, Fundamental Research Funds for the Central Universities, Horizon 2020 Framework Programme, Engineering, and Physical Sciences Research Council, European Regional Development Fund, Ministry of Science, and ICT and Future Planning." Based on financing, China has the most publications in this discipline. Also, adversarial attacks have been the subject of extensive research in all of the world's major nations and areas. This indicates that security research on adversarial attacks and related topics is highly regarded worldwide. As this topic is multidisciplinary, research in it has not become more difficult across national boundaries.

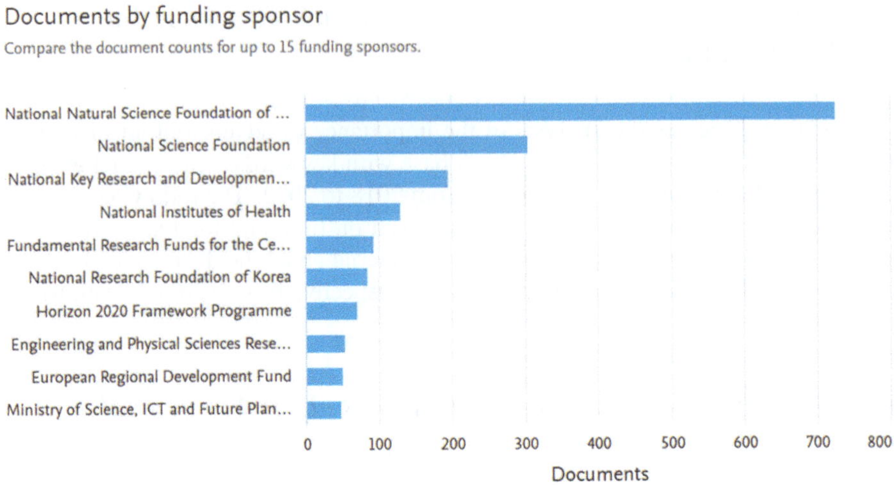

Fig. 11 Medical adversarial attack research numbers funded by institutions from 2018 to 2022

7 Discussion and Future Directions of Medical Adversarial Attacks

The integration of DL technologies in the healthcare sector is progressing rapidly. Below, we discuss the potential, limitations, and future directions for research on medical adversarial attacks.

7.1 Potential Vulnerabilities of Deep Learning in Health Care

The applications of DL technologies in the healthcare industry are expanding rapidly. DL models are a branch of AI that have shown the potential to aid in diagnostics, analysis, and constitute an inexpensive tool to support human decision-making. DL medical models are susceptible to cyberattacks, which have the potential to be seriously damaging. DL systems can be tricked by adversarial attacks into making inaccurate predictions. However, it is crucial to ensure that these systems are resilient to artifacts interference throughout this future widespread deployment of AI systems. In this chapter, many research contributions proved that DL models for medical imaging are more susceptible to adversary attacks than natural images. Furthermore, adversarial training techniques are often partially effective against adversarial attacks on medical imaging. The perturbation size of adversarial attacks against medical imaging modalities is substantially less than what is used for natural imaging in a different study.

7.2 Importance of Understanding Adversarial Attacks

1. Mechanisms of exploitation: Understanding how adversarial attacks manipulate DL models is critical for developing robust solutions. The transformation of AI in healthcare is not a simple task.
2. Collaborative efforts: Multiple stakeholders must collaborate to address ethical and legal considerations in AI deployment. These ethics include:
   (a) Legal rules: For data governance usage of patient data and regulations.
   (b) Data governance: Covers a variety of topics, such as how data is secured and stored, maintained, kept, and who has the privilege to access the medical database.
   (c) Policies and procedures: To ensure the protection of patient data. Regulations were published to ensure that medical data is used correctly. It is commonly recognized that good labeling and image quality are essential for the development of medical systems.

7.3 Limitations of Current Research

It has become clear that adversary attacks are essential to assessing the vulnerability of DL networks. The improvement of adversarial attack techniques could help researchers address problems and develop more secure and effective medical learning systems. The main issues shortly will continue to be the visibility of the perturbation and the transferability of attack methods while having a significant impact on network predictions. Current research faces many limitations such as:

- Complexity of medical data: The variability and complexity of medical data can hinder the application of adversarial defense strategies.
- Challenges in data annotation: The high costs and privacy concerns associated with extensive labeled data can be a barrier to training robust models.
- Computational overhead: Adversarial training may introduce additional computational demands that are impractical in resource-constrained clinical settings.

More techniques of adversarial attacks aimed at weakening the robustness of targeting segmentation models will also be considered. Another direction could be investigating new methods to maintain larger datasets and quickly produce images with medical annotations to create more reliable medical learning systems. Altering the neural network architecture which hasn't yet been examined is another method that can decrease network vulnerability.

7.4 Future Directions

The deployment of AI technologies in healthcare presents significant opportunities for improving clinical outcomes. However, addressing the vulnerabilities posed by adversarial attacks is essential for ensuring patient safety and maintaining the integrity of healthcare systems. Continued research in this domain is crucial for developing effective defenses and establishing a framework for the responsible and ethical use of AI in medical applications.

- Advancing adversarial attack techniques: Researchers should explore more sophisticated techniques to better understand vulnerabilities in medical systems.
- Focus on key issues: Future investigations should prioritize the visibility of perturbations and the transferability of attack methods impacting network predictions.
- Improving medical datasets: Developing methods for maintaining larger datasets and rapidly generating annotated medical images will enhance the reliability of medical learning systems.
- Exploring neural network architectures: Investigating alternative neural network architectures could potentially reduce vulnerabilities and enhance resilience against adversarial threats.
- Developing defense and detection techniques for medical text: There is a need to explore robust defense mechanisms and detection techniques specifically for adversarial attacks on medical question answering (MQA) systems and medical text. To ensure that text-based applications are equally protected against manipulation.

8 Conclusion

The adversarial attacks phenomenon against deep learning models has become a major barrier when DL-based applications are used in security-critical contexts. This presents serious security threats and challenges for DL-based medical models. Therefore, it has become urgently necessary to investigate robust techniques that are more resistant to these attacks. This chapter provides an extensive and in-depth overview of adversarial attacks in the area of medical diagnosis-based DL models. It provides a taxonomy that summarized the different strategies of adversarial attacks. It also discusses and evaluates many published attack, detection, and defense techniques that have been published in the area of DL-based medical adversarial attacks field. This chapter introduces an in-depth discussion for the root sources of medical vulnerabilities and the potential impact of these vulnerabilities on the robustness of healthcare systems. The state of art research direction is also visualized to better understand the development of medical adversarial attacks over the last 5 years. Based on the extensive field of research from multiple aspects such as model improvement, new research areas with significant and practical relevance are suggested. New proposed medical adversarial attacks in other areas such as medical visual question answering, clinical data, etc. have not been reviewed, which would require further future work to accomplish.

References

1. M. Avanzo, M. Porzio, L. Lorenzon, L. Milan, R. Sghedoni, G. Russo, R. Massafra, et al., Artificial intelligence applications in medical imaging: A review of the medical physics research in Italy. Phys. Med. **83**, 221–241 (2021)
2. Z. Harofte, M.S. Samaneh, S. Siavashy, K. Raahemifar, Recent advances of utilizing artificial intelligence in lab on a Chip for diagnosis and treatment. Small **18**(42), 2203169 (2022)
3. S. Wang, G. Cao, Y. Wang, S. Liao, Q. Wang, J. Shi, C. Li, D. Shen, Review and prospect: Artificial intelligence in advanced medical imaging. Front. Radiol. **1**, 781868 (2021)
4. T.N. Arvanitis, Informatics opportunities and challenges in medical imaging: A journey, in *Achievements, Milestones and Challenges in Biomedical and Health Informatics*, (IOS Press, Amsterdam, 2022), pp. 19–29
5. C. Szegedy, W. Zaremba, I. Sutskever, J. Bruna, D. Erhan, I. Goodfellow, R. Fergus, Intriguing properties of neural networks (2013). arXiv preprint arXiv:1312.6199, from http://arxiv.org/abs/1312.6199. Accessed 30 November 2022
6. X. Ma, Y. Niu, G. Lin, Y. Wang, Y. Zhao, J. Bailey, L. Feng, Understanding adversarial attacks on deep learning based medical image analysis systems. Pattern Recogn. **110**, 107332 (2021)
7. N. Carlini, D. Wagner, Towards evaluating the robustness of neural networks, in *2017 IEEE Symposium on Security and Privacy (sp)*, (IEEE, New York, 2017), pp. 39–57
8. A. Madry, A. Makelov, L. Schmidt, D. Tsipras, A. Vladu, Towards deep learning models resistant to adversarial attacks (2017). arXiv preprint arXiv:1706.06083
9. I.J. Goodfellow, J. Shlens, C. Szegedy, Explaining and harnessing adversarial examples (2014). arXiv preprint arXiv:1412.6572
10. A. Kurakin, I.J. Goodfellow, S. Bengio, Adversarial examples in the physical world, in *Artificial Intelligence Safety and Security*, (Chapman and Hall, Boca Raton, 2018), pp. 99–112
11. Cearley, Top 10 strategic technology trends for 2020: a Gartner special report (2019), https://www.gartner.com/en/doc/432920-top-10-strategic-technology-trends-for-2020. Accessed 5 December 2022
12. L. Boone, M. Biparva, P.M. Forooshani, J. Ramirez, M. Masellis, R. Bartha, S. Symons, et al., ROOD-MRI: Benchmarking the robustness of deep learning segmentation models to out-of-distribution and corrupted data in MRI (2022). arXiv preprint arXiv:2203.06060
13. D. Bhusal, N. Rastogi, Adversarial patterns: Building robust android malware classifiers (2022). arXiv preprint arXiv:2203.02121
14. D.J. Miller, Z. Xiang, G. Kesidis, Adversarial learning targeting deep neural network classification: A comprehensive review of defenses against attacks. Proc. IEEE **108**(3), 402–433 (2020)
15. X. Zhang, W. Dongrui, On the vulnerability of CNN classifiers in EEG-based BCIs. IEEE Trans. Neural Syst. Rehabil. Eng. **27**(5), 814–825 (2019)
16. P.-Y. Chen, Y. Sharma, H. Zhang, J. Yi, C.-J. Hsieh, Ead: elastic-net attacks to deep neural networks via adversarial examples. Proc. AAAI Conf. Artif. Intell. **32**, 1 (2018)
17. P.-Y. Chen, H. Zhang, Y. Sharma, J. Yi, C.-J. Hsieh, Zoo: Zeroth order optimization based black-box attacks to deep neural networks without training substitute models, in *Proceedings of the 10th ACM Workshop on Artificial Intelligence and Security*, (ACM, New York, 2017), pp. 15–26

18. C. Xiao, B. Li, J.-Y. Zhu, W. He, M. Liu, D. Song, Generating adversarial examples with adversarial networks (2018). arXiv preprint arXiv:1801.02610
19. S. Qiu, Q. Liu, S. Zhou, W. Chunjiang, Review of artificial intelligence adversarial attack and defense technologies. Appl. Sci. **9**(5), 909 (2019)
20. N. Papernot, P. McDaniel, S. Jha, M. Fredrikson, Z.B. Celik, A. Swami, The limitations of deep learning in adversarial settings, in *Proceedings of the 2016 IEEE European Symposium on Security and Privacy*, (IEEE, New York, 2016), pp. 372–387
21. S.-M. Moosavi-Dezfooli, A. Fawzi, P. Frossard, Deepfool: A simple and accurate method to fool deep neural networks, in *Proceedings of the IEEE Conference on Computer Vision and Pattern Recognition*, (IEEE, New York, 2016), pp. 2574–2582
22. Y. Hu, W. Kuang, Z. Qin, K. Li, J. Zhang, Y. Gao, W. Li, K. Li, Artificial intelligence security: Threats and countermeasures. ACM Comput. Surv. **55**(1), 1–36 (2021)
23. U. Ahmed, J.C.-W. Lin, G. Srivastava, Mitigating adversarial evasion attacks of ransomware using ensemble learning. Comput. Electr. Eng. **100**, 107903 (2022)
24. G.A. Kaissis, M.R. Makowski, D. Rückert, R.F. Braren, Secure, privacy-preserving and federated machine learning in medical imaging. Nat. Machine Intell. **2**(6), 305–311 (2020)
25. L. Qu, N. Balachandar, M. Zhang, D. Rubin, Handling data heterogeneity with generative replay in collaborative learning for medical imaging. Med. Image Anal. **78**, 102424 (2022)
26. M. Paschali, S. Conjeti, F. Navarro, N. Navab, Generalizability vs. robustness: Investigating medical imaging networks using adversarial examples, in *International Conference on Medical Image Computing and Computer-Assisted Intervention*, (Springer, Cham, 2018), pp. 493–501
27. S.G. Finlayson, H.W. Chung, I.S. Kohane, & A. L. Beam, Adversarial attacks against medical deep learning systems (2018). arXiv preprint arXiv:1804.05296.
28. J. Kotia, A. Kotwal, R. Bharti, Risk susceptibility of brain tumor classification to adversarial attacks, in *International Conference on Man–Machine Interactions*, (Springer, Cham, 2019), pp. 181–187
29. A. Huq, T. Pervin, Analysis of adversarial attacks on skin cancer recognition, in *2020 International Conference on Data science and Its Applications (ICoDSA)*, (IEEE, New York, 2020), pp. 1–4
30. B. Pal, D. Gupta, Rashed-Al-Mahfuz, S.A. Alyami, M.A. Moni, Vulnerability in deep transfer learning models to adversarial fast gradient sign attack for covid-19 prediction from chest radiography images. Appl. Sci. **11**(9), 4233 (2021)
31. I. Yilmaz, M. Baza, R. Amer, A. Rasheed, F. Amsaad, R. Morsi, On the assessment of robustness of telemedicine applications against adversarial machine learning attacks, in *International Conference on Industrial, Engineering and Other Applications of Applied Intelligent Systems*, (Springer, Cham, 2021), pp. 519–529
32. S. Li, G. Huang, X. Xing, L. Huimin, Query-based black-box attack against medical image segmentation model. Futur. Gener. Comput. Syst. **133**, 331–337 (2022)
33. Y. Li, Z. Zhu, Y. Zhou, Y. Xia, W. Shen, E.K. Fishman, A.L. Yuille, Volumetric medical image segmentation: A 3D deep coarse-to-fine framework and its adversarial examples, in *Deep Learning and Convolutional Neural Networks for Medical Imaging and Clinical Informatics*, (Springer, Cham, 2019), pp. 69–91
34. U. Ozbulak, A. Van Messem, W. De Neve, Impact of adversarial examples on deep learning models for biomedical image segmentation, in *International Conference on Medical Image Computing and Computer-Assisted Intervention*, (Springer, Cham, 2019), pp. 300–308
35. G. Cheng, H. Ji, Adversarial perturbation on MRI modalities in brain tumor segmentation. IEEE Access **8**, 206009–206015 (2020)
36. Q. Yao, Z. He, Y. Lin, K. Ma, Y. Zheng, S. Kevin Zhou, A hierarchical feature constraint to camouflage medical adversarial attacks, in *International Conference on Medical Image Computing and Computer-Assisted Intervention*, (Springer, Cham, 2021), pp. 36–47
37. D. Anand, D. Tank, H. Tibrewal, A. Sethi, Self-supervision vs. transfer learning: Robust biomedical image analysis against adversarial attacks, in *2020 IEEE 17th International Symposium on Biomedical Imaging (ISBI)*, (IEEE, New York, 2020), pp. 1159–1163

38. L. Chen, P. Bentley, K. Mori, K. Misawa, M. Fujiwara, D. Rueckert, Intelligent image synthesis to attack a segmentation CNN using adversarial learning, in *International Workshop on Simulation and Synthesis in Medical Imaging*, (Springer, Cham, 2019), pp. 90–99
39. Y. Li, H. Zhang, C. Bermudez, Y. Chen, B.A. Landman, Y. Vorobeychik, Anatomical context protects deep learning from adversarial perturbations in medical imaging. Neurocomputing **379**, 370–378 (2020)
40. D.S. Marcus, T.H. Wang, J. Parker, J.G. Csernansky, J.C. Morris, R.L. Buckner, Open access series of imaging studies (OASIS): Cross-sectional MRI data in young, middle aged, nondemented, and demented older adults. J. Cogn. Neurosci. **19**(9), 1498–1507 (2007)
41. L. Ballerini, R.B. Fisher, R.B. Aldridge, J. Rees, A color and texture based hierarchical K-NN approach to the classification of non-melanoma skin lesions, in *Color Medical Image Analysis*, (Springer, Cham, 2013)
42. Diabetic Retinopathy Detection. (Available Online), https://www.kaggle.com/c/diabetic-retinopathy-detection/data. Accessed 22 December 2022
43. X. Wang, Y. Peng, L. Le, L. Zhiyong, M. Bagheri, R.M. Summers, Chestx-ray8: Hospital-scale chest X-ray database and benchmarks on weakly-supervised classification and localization of common thorax diseases, in *2017 IEEE Conference on Computer Vision and Pattern Recognition (CVPR)*, (IEEE, New York, 2017), pp. 3462–3471
44. J. Cheng, Brain tumor dataset. Figshare. Dataset (2017). https://doi.org/10.6084/m9.figshare.1512427.v5
45. P. Tschandl, C. Rosendahl, H. Kittler, The HAM10000 dataset, a large collection of multi-source dermatoscopic images of common pigmented skin lesions. Sci. Data **5**, 180161 (2018)
46. J.P. Cohen, P. Morrison, L. Dao, K. Roth, T.Q. Duong, M. Ghassemi, Covid-19 image data collection: Prospective predictions are the future. arXiv 2020, arXiv:2006.11988, https://arxiv.org/pdf/2006.11988.pdf. Accessed 15 April 2021
47. X. Yang, X. He, J. Zhao, Y. Zhang, S. Zhang, P. Xie, COVID-CT-Dataset: A CT Scan Dataset about COVID-19 (2020). arXiv 2020, arXiv:2003.13865
48. Breast database., http://marathon.csee.usf.edu/Mammography/Database.html Accessed 22 December 2022
49. J. Shiraishi, S. Katsuragawa, J. Ikezoe, T. Matsumoto, T. Kobayashi, K.-i. Komatsu, M. Matsui, H. Fujita, Y. Kodera, K. Doi, Development of a digital image database for chest radiographs with and without a lung nodule: Receiver operating characteristic analysis of radiologists' detection of pulmonary nodules. Am. J. Roentgenol. **174**(1), 71–74 (2000)
50. Roth, H. R., Lu, L., Farag, A., Shin, H.-C., Liu, J., Turkbey, E., Summers, R. M. (2021). DeepOrgan: Multi-level deep convolutional networks for automated pancreas segmentation. arXiv 2015, arXiv:1506.06448. http://arxiv.org/abs/1506.064. Accessed 4 June 2021
51. C. Pena-Betancor et al., Estimation of the relative amount of hemoglobin in the cup and neuroretinal rim using stereoscopic color fundus images. Invest. Ophthalmol. Vis. Sci. **56**(3), 1562–1568 (2015)
52. Gutman, D., et al., Skin lesion analysis toward melanoma detection: A challenge at the international symposium on biomedical imaging (ISBI) 2016, hosted by the international skin imaging collaboration (ISIC). CoRR. abs:1605.01397 (2016)
53. B.H. Menze, A. Jakab, S. Bauer, J. Kalpathy-Cramer, K. Farahani, J. Kirby, Y. Burren, N. Porz, J. Slotboom, R. Wiest, et al., The multimodal brain tumor image segmentation benchmark (BRATS). IEEE Trans. Med. Imaging **34**, 1993–2024 (2015)
54. Kaggle: Chest X-ray images (pneumonia) (2019), https://www.kaggle.com/paultimothymooney/chest-xray-pneumonia. Accessed 25 December 2022
55. Mendeley data—labeled optical coherence tomography (OCT) and chest X-ray images for classification, https://data.mendeley.com/datasets/rscbjbr9sj/2. Accessed 5 June 2021
56. D. Kermany, K. Zhang, M. Goldbaum, Labeled optical coherence tomography (oct) and chest X-ray images for classification. Mendeley Data **2**, 9 (2018)
57. T. Tong et al., Discriminative dictionary learning for abdominal multi-organ segmentation. Med. Image Anal. **23**(1), 92–104 (2015)
58. IXI, http://brain-development.org/ixi-dataset/. Accessed 25 December 2022

59. FCON-1000. Accessed 25 December 2022
60. OASIS1, https://www.oasis-brains.org/. Accessed 25 December 2022
61. NDAR, https://ndar.nih.gov/study.html?id=318. Accessed 25 December 2022
62. ADHD200. Accessed 25 December 2022
63. NKI Rockland. Accessed 25 December 2022
64. Y. Huang, T. Würfl, K. Breininger, L. Liu, G. Lauritsch, A. Maier, Some investigations on robustness of deep learning in limited angle tomography, in *International Conference on Medical Image Computing and Computer-Assisted Intervention*, (Springer, Cham, 2018), pp. 145–153
65. A. Vatian, N. Gusarova, N. Dobrenko, S. Dudorov, N. Nigmatullin, A. Shalyto, A. Lobantsev, Impact of adversarial examples on the efficiency of interpretation and use of information from high-tech medical images, in *2019 24th Conference of Open Innovations Association (FRUCT)*, (IEEE, New York, 2019), pp. 472–478
66. S. Liu, A.A.A. Setio, F.C. Ghesu, E. Gibson, S. Grbic, B. Georgescu, D. Comaniciu, No surprises: Training robust lung nodule detection for low-dose CT scans by augmenting with adversarial attacks. IEEE Trans. Med. Imaging **40**(1), 335–345 (2020)
67. D. Wu, S. Liu, J. Ban, Classification of diabetic retinopathy using adversarial training. IOP Conf. Ser. Mater. Sci. Eng. **806**(1), 012050 (2020)
68. C. Rao, J. Cao, R. Zeng, Q. Chen, H. Fu, Y. Xu, & M. Tan, A thorough comparison study on adversarial attacks and defenses for common thorax disease classification in chest X-rays (2020). arXiv preprint arXiv:2003.13969
69. A. Mani Tripathi, & A. Mishra, Fuzzy unique image transformation: Defense against adversarial attacks on deep COVID-19 models (2020). arXiv e-prints: arXiv-2009
70. Q. Liu, H. Jiang, T. Liu, Z. Liu, S. Li, W. Wen, Y. Shi, Defending deep learning-based biomedical image segmentation from adversarial attacks: A low-cost frequency refinement approach, in *International Conference on Medical Image Computing and Computer-Assisted Intervention*, (Springer, Cham, 2020), pp. 342–351
71. R. Paul, M. Schabath, R. Gillies, L. Hall, D. Goldgof, Mitigating adversarial attacks on medical image understanding systems, in *2020 IEEE 17th International Symposium on Biomedical Imaging (ISBI)*, (IEEE, New York, 2020), pp. 1517–1521
72. X. Li, D. Zhu, Robust detection of adversarial attacks on medical images, in *2020 IEEE 17th International Symposium on Biomedical Imaging (ISBI)*, (IEEE, New York, 2020), pp. 1154–1158
73. X. Li, D. Pan, D. Zhu, Defending against adversarial attacks on medical imaging AI system, classification or detection? in *2021 IEEE 18th International Symposium on Biomedical Imaging (ISBI)*, (IEEE, New York, 2021), pp. 1677–1681
74. A. Uwimana, R. Senanayake, Out of distribution detection and adversarial attacks on deep neural networks for robust medical image analysis (2021). arXiv preprint arXiv:2107.04882
75. AAPM low-dose CT grand challenge, https://www.aapm.org/grandchallenge/lowdosect/. Accessed 22 December 2022
76. lidc-dataset, Web, https://github.com/topics/lidc-dataset. Accessed 22 December 2022
77. How to join BRATS 2015: Brain tumor image segmentation challenge, https://www.virtualskeleton.ch/BRATS/Start2015. Accessed 22 December 2022
78. A.A.A. Setio et al., Validation, comparison, and combination of algorithms for automatic detection of pulmonary nodules in computed tomography images: The LUNA16 challenge. Med. Image Anal. **42**, 1–13 (2017)
79. N. Lung Screening Trial Research Team, The national lung screening trial: Overview and study design. Radiology **258**(1), 243–253 (2011)
80. APTOS 2019 blindness detection, https://www.kaggle.com/c/aptos2019-blindness-detection. Accessed 22 December 2022
81. J. Irvin, P. Rajpurkar, M. Ko, Y. Yu, S. Ciurea-Ilcus, C. Chute, H. Marklund, B. Haghgoo, R. Ball, K. Shpanskaya, et al., *Chexpert: A Large Chest Radiograph Dataset with Uncertainty Labels and Expert Comparison* (AAAI, Philadelphia, 2019)

82. J. Zhao, Y. Zhang, X. He, P. Xie, Covid-CT-dataset: Act scan dataset about covid-19 (2020). arXiv preprint arXiv:2003.13865
83. J. Sivaswamy, S. Krishnadas, A. Chakravarty, G. Joshi, A.S. Tabish, et al., A comprehensive retinal image dataset for the assessment of glaucoma from the optic nerve head analysis. JSM Clin. Med. Imaging Cases Rev. **2**(1), 1004 (2015)
84. N.C. Codella et al., Skin lesion analysis toward melanoma detection: A challenge at the 2017 international symposium on biomedical imaging (ISBI), hosted by the international skin imaging collaboration (ISIC), in *2018 IEEE 15th International Symposium on Biomedical Imaging (ISBI 2018)*, (IEEE, New York, 2018), pp. 168–172
85. N. L. S. T. R. Team, Reduced lung-cancer mortality with low-dose computed tomographic screening. N. Engl. J. Med. **365**(5), 395–409 (2011)
86. X. Wang et al., Chest X-ray8: Hospital-scale chest X-ray database and benchmarks on weakly-supervised classification and localization of common thorax diseases. CVPR **2017**, 2097–2106 (2017)
87. Kaggle, Kaggle diabetic retinopathy detection challenge (2015), https://www.kaggle.com/c/diabetic-retinopathy-detection. Accessed 22 December 2022
88. X. Wang, Y. Peng, L. Lu, Z. Lu, M. Bagheri, R. Summers, ChestX-ray8: Hospital-scale chest X-ray database and benchmarks on weakly-supervised classification and localization of common thorax diseases, in *IEEE Conference on Computer Vision and Pattern Recognition*, (IEEE, New York, 2017), pp. 3462–3471
89. ISIC, The international skin imaging collaboration (2019), https://www.isic-archive.com/. Accessed 23 December 2022
90. D.S. Kermany, M. Goldbaum, W. Cai, C.C.S. Valentim, H. Liang, S.L. Baxter, A. McKeown, G. Yang, W. Xiaokang, F. Yan, et al., Identifying medical diagnoses and treatable diseases by image-based deep learning. Cell **172**(5), 1122–1131 (2018)
91. NLM, Malaria data. (2022), https://lhncbc.nlm.nih.gov/LHC-research/LHC-projects/image-processing/malaria-datasheet.html. Accessed 22 December 2022
92. Scopus database, https://www.scopus.com/sources.uri. Accessed 2 January 2023

Masked Autoencoder-Based Domain Adaptation for Cross-Population Breast-Lesion Classification in Mammograms

Mariam M. Hassan, Mahmoud Khalil, Siyuan Dai, Liang Zhan, Mohamed Ragab, Mohamed Abdel-Nasser, and Domenec Puig

Abstract Domain shifts between mammography datasets driven by variations in imaging equipment, clinical protocols, and patient populations present a major challenge to the generalizability of artificial intelligence (AI)-based breast cancer diagnostic tools. Recent unsupervised domain adaptation (UDA) frameworks have introduced contrastive learning to mitigate these discrepancies. This chapter investigates domain shifts across four publicly available mammography datasets from different geographic and clinical settings: VinDr-Mammo (Vietnam), INbreast (Portugal), CDD-CESM (Egypt), and KAU-BCMD (Saudi Arabia). We employ a ConvNeXt V2-based masked autoencoder to extract robust and representative features

M. M. Hassan (✉)
Department of Computer Engineering and Mathematics, Universitat Rovira i Virgili, Tarragona, Spain

Institute of National Planning, Cairo, Egypt
e-mail: mariam.moustafa@urv.cat

M. Khalil
School of Medicine, University of Pittsburgh, Pittsburgh, PA, USA
e-mail: mak429@pitt.edu

S. Dai · L. Zhan
Department of Electrical and Computer Engineering, University of Pittsburgh, Pittsburgh, PA, USA
e-mail: siyuan.dai@pitt.edu; liang.zhan@pitt.edu

M. Ragab
Institute for Infocomm Research, A*STAR, Singapore, Singapore
e-mail: mohamedr002@e.ntu.edu.sg

M. Abdel-Nasser
Electrical Engineering Department, Aswan University, Aswan, Egypt
e-mail: mohamed.abdelnasser@aswu.edu.eg

D. Puig
Department of Computer Engineering and Mathematics, Universitat Rovira i Virgili, Tarragona, Spain
e-mail: domenec.puig@urv.cat

N. E. M. Khalifa, M. H. N. Taha (eds.), *Next-Gen Healthcare*,
https://doi.org/10.1007/978-3-032-07267-2_2

from the mammography images. For UDA, we adapt the CoTMix framework, originally designed for time-series data. Unlike conventional UDA approaches based on adversarial training or statistical alignment, CoTMix introduces a novel contrastive mix-up strategy. It generates intermediate augmented representations from both source and target domains and aligns them by maximizing feature similarity with their original views. This enables effective alignment of diverse domain distributions in a shared latent space. Experimental evaluation shows that the proposed framework improves generalization across domains, achieving higher precision, F1 scores, and AUC compared to baseline adaptation methods. These findings demonstrate the potential of combining masked autoencoders with contrastive mix-up techniques for reliable AI-based diagnostics in heterogeneous clinical environments.

Keywords Mammography · Domain adaptation · Contrastive learning · Masked autoencoder · cross-population · Breast cancer · Generalization

Acronyms

AUC	Area under the curve
BI-RADS	Breast imaging reporting and data system
CAD	Computer-aided diagnosis
CLAHE	Contrast limited adaptive histogram equalization
CMMD	Chinese mammography medical data
DANN	Domain-adversarial neural network
DICOM	Digital imaging and communications in medicine
FFDM	Full-field digital mammography
KAU-BCMD	King Abdulaziz University Breast Cancer Mammogram Dataset
ROI	Region of interest
SimCLR	Simple framework for contrastive learning
SMOTE	Synthetic minority over-sampling technique
UDA	Unsupervised domain adaptation
VinDr	Vietnamese imaging dataset for radiology

1 Introduction

In 2022, 2.3 million women were diagnosed with breast cancer, and 670,000 died from the disease [27, 62]. In nearly half of all countries, incidence rates have increased by 1–5% annually. If these trends continue, global breast cancer cases are projected to rise by 38% and deaths by 68% by 2050 [27]. High-income countries have reduced mortality through widespread screening and advances in treatment.

In contrast, low-income regions continue to experience rising death rates, primarily due to limited access to early detection and adequate care [63].

Early detection through routine screening significantly improves survival rates and quality of life in breast cancer patients [5]. Mammography remains the primary screening tool, capable of detecting early signs of malignancy such as microcalcifications, architectural distortions, and suspicious masses [53]. Despite its clinical value, mammographic interpretation is complex and requires specialized expertise. Radiologists must distinguish subtle pathological signs from normal anatomical structures. This challenge intensifies in dense breast tissue, particularly among populations with higher breast density, such as Japanese and Korean women, where mammography sensitivity is reduced [55].

Recent studies suggest that integrating radiologists' gaze behavior with image features can help predict diagnostic errors, with improved performance among experienced readers [57]. The study in [52] analyzed interpretation errors in dense mammograms using a radiomics-based AI model involving 36 radiologists from China and Australia. Radiomic features were extracted from both false-positive and false-negative regions. Random forest models were then trained to identify patterns associated with diagnostic mistakes. The results showed higher AUCs for the Chinese cohort. Key features such as texture and intensity variations were strongly linked to misinterpretations. These findings highlight the combined influence of image complexity and reader experience on diagnostic performance.

Insights into human diagnostic error have increased interest in AI-driven tools to support clinical decision-making. AI-based systems show strong potential to improve mammography screening by reducing interpretation time, minimizing errors, and ensuring consistent performance across patient populations [13]. The PRAIM study [15] demonstrated that AI-assisted double reading increases cancer detection rates without raising recall rates in real-world settings. However, the generalizability of these systems remains a key limitation. Variability in imaging equipment, patient demographics, and screening protocols can lead to significant performance drops. The VAIB study [46], for example, reported differences of up to $\pm 33\%$ in cancer detection rates and substantial shifts in false-positive rates due to calibration mismatches across clinical sites. These results highlight the need for robust, standardized AI systems capable of adapting to diverse clinical environments, while maintaining stable diagnostic performance.

These findings emphasize the need for robust, standardized AI tools that can operate reliably across diverse clinical settings. However, developing such systems is challenging due to domain shifts, performance degradation that occurs when models trained on one dataset are applied to different populations, imaging devices, or clinical environments [25].

Deep learning models, while effective in mammogram analysis, often show limited generalization under these conditions [20, 28]. To address domain shift in mammography, researchers have explored various unsupervised domain adaptation (UDA) approaches, including adversarial training, decision boundary refinement, image-to-image translation with cycle GANs, and transformer-based architectures [4, 58, 65]. Although these methods improve adaptation in many cases, they often

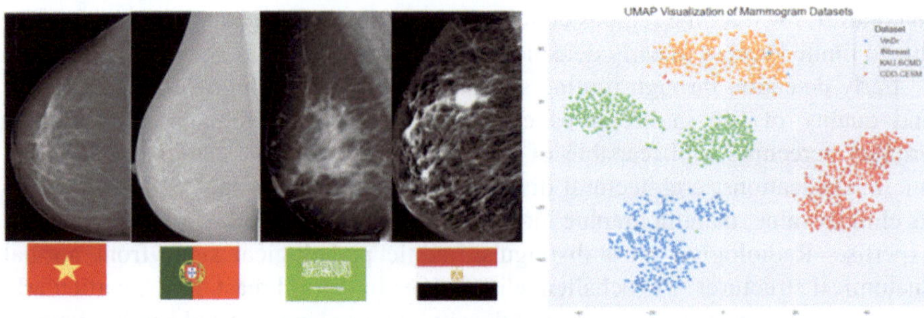

Fig. 1 Representative mammograms from each dataset: VinDr (Vietnam), INbreast (Portugal), KAU-BCMD (Saudi Arabia), and CDD-CESM (Egypt), illustrating population and imaging differences. The UMAP plot on the right visualizes the distribution of image features from each dataset, revealing clear inter-dataset separation due to domain shift

encounter limitations such as unstable training, overfitting, visual artifacts, or high computational demands.

Recent research has expanded domain adaptation strategies beyond conventional methods. Wang et al. [60] proposed a dynamic extension network that reduces domain shift by manipulating decision boundaries without requiring labeled target data. Chen et al. [11] developed a discriminative adversarial framework tailored for mammography, achieving better domain alignment. Liu et al. [33] applied contrastive learning to improve cross-domain generalization in 2D mammography by enhancing feature space separability. Other studies explored semi-supervised learning to improve model calibration and uncertainty estimation [36], and data augmentation to reduce vendor-specific biases [26]. Lightweight models have also been proposed for small-scale datasets with limited annotations [1]. Additional advances include multi-style contrastive learning to enable style-invariant generalization [66], and deployment studies demonstrating the clinical feasibility of adapted models in resource-constrained environments [50].

Figure 1 shows a representative mammogram image from each of the four datasets used in this study: VinDr (Vietnam), INbreast (Portugal), KAU-BCMD (Saudi Arabia), and CDD-CESM (Egypt). These examples highlight visual differences that arise from variations in population demographics and imaging protocols across countries. The UMAP plot further illustrates the domain shift between datasets by projecting their image features into a shared low-dimensional space, where distinct clusters indicate substantial distribution gaps across domains. Figure 2 outlines two potential experimental settings for domain adaptation in mammography: cross-population (adapting across countries) and cross-scanner (adapting across imaging devices). In this chapter, we focus on the cross-population setting to examine how demographic and acquisition differences affect performance. Each dataset corresponds to a different country and is acquired using a specific mammography scanner, which contributes to both interpopulation and inter-device

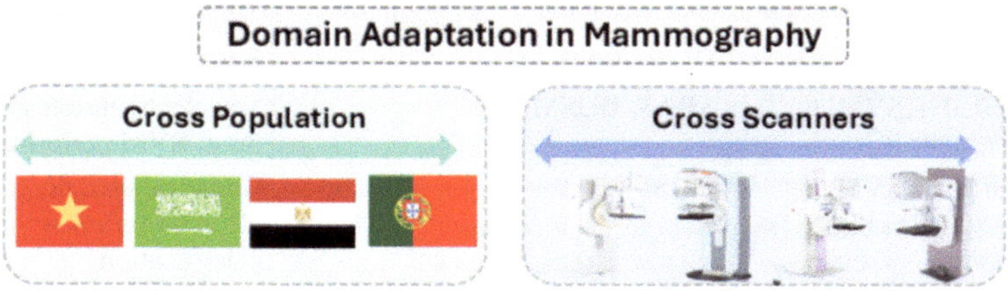

Fig. 2 Experimental setup for domain adaptation, including cross-population (between countries) and cross-scanner (between imaging devices) adaptation

variability. The cross-scanner scenario is included for context but is not explored in this work.

Contribution To address domain shift challenges, we present a UDA framework that combines a ConvNeXtV2-based masked autoencoder with CoTMix, a contrastive learning strategy originally developed for time-series data. Unlike conventional UDA methods that depend on adversarial training or statistical matching, CoTMix aligns source and target domains through contrastive learning. We introduce a temporal mix-up mechanism that generates intermediate augmented views for both domains. These views are optimized to retain semantic consistency, while integrating temporal dynamics. A contrastive loss function then maximizes similarity between each domain and its corresponding augmented view, progressively aligning both domains in a shared latent space. In our approach, we extend CoTMix to mammography. The masked autoencoder extracts robust feature representations, while CoTMix bridges interdomain shifts caused by variations in populations, imaging devices, and clinical practices.

2 Literature Review

2.1 Mammogram Classification: Benchmarks and Challenges

Before the deep learning era, computer-aided diagnosis (CAD) systems for mammogram analysis predominantly relied on handcrafted feature extraction techniques combined with traditional machine learning classifiers (e.g., support vector machines (SVM), decision trees, K-nearest neighbors, etc.). A typical workflow in these approaches starts with image preprocessing, involving noise removal, contrast enhancement, pectoral muscle suppression, etc., to ensure the clarity and usability of mammogram images. Regions of interest (ROIs) are then identified either manually or through semiautomatic methods, providing focused areas for detailed analysis. With these ROIs or entire images, various descriptive features

Table 1 Comparison of traditional and domain adaptation methods in mammogram classification

Approach	Dataset(s)	Key contribution
Handcrafted + SVM + wavelet (2018) [6]	MIAS, DDSM	Wavelet texture features boost SVM performance
Handcrafted + SVM + contours (2017) [32]	DDSM	Contour-based descriptors effective for mass classification
Handcrafted + LBP (2020) [17]	MIAS	Texture descriptors achieve high sensitivity
DANN (2020) [47]	DDSM, INbreast, private	Unsupervised adversarial adaptation improves detection
DADA (2021) [59]	DDSM, West-China	Dual-classifier adversarial method boosts AUC
Flavorizing (2023) [30]	Danish, Dutch	Style transfer reduces vendor gap
Contrastive + CMMD (2024) [42]	FFDM w/wo LUT	Contrastive loss improves generalization
D-Master (2024) [4]	INbreast, DDSM, RSNA-BSD1K	Transformer learns domain-invariant features
Histogram matching + fine-tuning (2020) [49]	FFDM, MIP, HM, DBT	Simple fine-tuning improves cross-modality adaptation

are extracted. Common features include texture descriptors like Haralick's gray-level co-occurrence matrix (GLCM) statistics and run-length matrices, shape-based descriptors such as compactness and measures of spiculation, and multiscale representation methods, including wavelets and contourlets. These handcrafted features are subsequently fed into the above conventional machine learning classifiers or ensemble methods [40]. Traditional machine learning frameworks that employ these feature extraction methods have dominated mammogram classification tasks for decades and continue to serve as comparative baselines in contemporary studies.

Several significant studies demonstrate the effectiveness of this classical pipeline. For example, Berbar et al. [6] extracted seven texture features using a hybrid wavelet-based method, achieving an impressive accuracy of 97–98% in distinguishing benign from malignant lesions using SVM classifiers on the MIAS and DDSM [7] datasets. Meanwhile, Li et al. [32] combined local contour feature descriptors with SVM classifiers and reported a classification accuracy of 99.6% on mass classification using the DDSM dataset. Additionally, Farhan et al. [17] utilized local binary patterns (LBPs), another popular texture-based feature descriptor, achieving a sensitivity of approximately 99.6% and a specificity of about 99.2% on the MIAS benchmark. Moreover, more studies conducted diverse feature extraction strategies with similar success. For example, Oliver et al. [40] reviewed various techniques, including wavelets, fractal analyses, and intensity-based methods, underscoring their potential in mammogram classification tasks. These studies collectively underscore the substantial capabilities of handcrafted features processed with traditional classifiers, providing impressive performance benchmarks and valuable insights for contemporary deep learning approaches. Table 1 summarizes representative traditional methods alongside domain-adaptation approaches and the datasets they use, providing a compact map of benchmarks and ideas we refer to below.

Differences in dataset properties, such as imaging modality, dataset size, annotation protocols, and file formats, significantly impact the generalizability of traditional CAD models. For instance, MIAS and DDSM involve digitized film mammograms, while INbreast [38] is captured entirely digitally. Even within film-based datasets, variations in scanning devices and image resolution exist. Moreover, each public dataset tends to be "skewed towards a particular clinical use-case," reflecting unique class imbalances and annotation criteria [34].

The lack of standardization implies that a model trained in one dataset may not perform well on another without explicit adaptation [8]. Empirical studies have confirmed that the application of a CAD classifier outside of its training domain easily leads to substantial performance degradation. Junior et al. [8] proposed a novel method combining diversity metrics, geostatistical modeling, and alpha-shape concave geometry, evaluated with an SVM across MIAS and DDSM. They reported high accuracy within each dataset but also noted domain-specific performance discrepancies. Similarly, another breast cancer detection model posted an accuracy drop when tested across datasets among the MIAS, DDSM, INbreast, and BCDR datasets. These performance gaps are largely caused by the discrepancies in image quality and content: MIAS images are relatively clean and homogeneous. By contrast, DDSM is a large, public scanned-film dataset ($\sim$2,620 screening exams) and therefore shows greater heterogeneity from variable breast densities and digitization artifacts. In DDSM, some normal/benign labels rely on radiologist assessment or follow-up rather than biopsy, which can introduce label noise that affects CAD training.

The technical variation adds another layer of challenge: older datasets used formats such as LJPEG or PGM, requiring custom decompression and preprocessing that may unintentionally alter extracted features. Taken together, these factors underscore that traditional CAD models are inherently domain-specific, often overfitting to the specific distribution they are trained on, and consequently struggling to generalize to other hospitals or imaging environments.

Despite notable successes in controlled studies, traditional mammogram classification approaches face several clinical and technical limitations:

- Traditional classification approaches generally have limited generalization ability outside their training domain [34]. A classifier may perform well on a specific public dataset, but the performance is easily degraded when applied to data from a different institution or other imaging devices, signifying poor robustness when used across hospitals. This stems from dataset biases, and also because handcrafted features only capture specific image characteristics, subtle differences in acquisition (e.g., film vs. digital, machine calibrations), or variations in patient populations can shift data distributions in ways these models cannot accommodate.

- Most traditional pipelines are not end-to-end models, as they rely heavily on manual or semiautomatic steps, such as ROI selection, careful tuning of preprocessing parameters, or deciding which features to extract. This continual dependence on expert input makes the workflow time-consuming, less scalable, and prone to device-related variability [64].
- Handcrafted feature design demands extensive domain expertise, for instance, that texture entropy or spicule sharpness differentiates malignancy. Such models may overlook complex, higher-order patterns that emerge only when integrating numerous low-level features. Clinically, these engineered features rarely align with radiologists' interpretative criteria, reducing their transparency, interpretability, and trustworthiness.
- Additional issues result from the small sample sizes of many datasets (e.g., MIAS or INbreast) [24]. While augmentation and cross-validation alleviate overfitting to some extent, they cannot fully compensate. Those high accuracies reported in limited datasets may be hard to generalize to real-world, large-scale screening environments.
- Reproducibility suffers from cross-dataset differences: file formats (film vs digital, PGM vs LJPEG), annotation protocols (label unit and BI-RADS field availability), and evaluation metrics are not aligned, making comparisons across studies or deployment in diverse institutions challenging [3, 31].

These limitations highlight a key challenge: building mammography CAD models that remain robust across diverse domains. This has driven a shift toward domain adaptation methods [19], aiming to bridge dataset gaps and reduce performance losses when traditional models encounter new institutions or imaging devices. Recognizing the constraints of feature extraction modules, limited generalizability, scalability, and fragility to a domain shift problem, researchers increasingly explore learning-based and adaptive pipelines [42], as more details will be discussed in the next section.

2.2 Deep Learning-Based Domain Adaptation

Deep learning models have demonstrated remarkable success in mammogram classification, particularly when trained and evaluated on large, well-annotated datasets from a single source. However, these models often face substantial performance degradation when deployed on data from different clinical sites, imaging devices, protocols, or distinct imaging modalities. This phenomenon, the so-called domain shift, arises due to variations in imaging settings, patient demographics, and modality types (such as conventional 2D mammography versus 3D digital breast tomosynthesis). To address this challenge, recent research has increasingly focused on deep learning-based domain adaptation methods, aiming to effectively transfer or adapt existing models across diverse data distributions while preserving classification performance.

2.2.1 Modality-Oriented Domain Adaptation

The most obvious domain shift comes from modality variety. Computed tomography, X-ray, and mammogram images arise from different imaging principles. Handling modality-oriented domain shifts is crucial for mammogram-based cancer detection. A popular solution is adversarial domain adaptation, which aims to learn domain-invariant feature representations through adversarial training. Domain-adversarial neural networks (DANN), proposed by Ganin et al. [18], utilize a gradient reversal layer to confuse a domain classifier, aligning source and target feature distributions. In mammography, Shen et al. [47] proposed an unsupervised adversarial domain adaptation method with a domain discriminator and adversarial loss, achieving improved breast mass detection sensitivity on private clinical mammograms. Similarly, Wang et al. [58] developed DADA (dual-classifier adversarial adaptation). Using CBIS-DDSM as the source and hospital data from West China Hospital as the target, they demonstrated notable AUC improvements in breast cancer detection.

By encouraging indistinguishable feature representations, Wang et al.'s method substantially boosted cancer classification performance relative to baselines. Despite their effectiveness, these methods can face training instabilities due to bi-level optimization dynamics, necessitating careful hyperparameter tuning [54]. Image-level adaptation using generative models, such as CycleGAN-based style transfer to harmonize source and target modality appearances, also shows great potential [56], though explicit mammography examples are limited. Properly executed adversarial methods have demonstrated substantial performance improvements.

2.2.2 Discrepance-Driven Domain Adaptation

A prominent strategy for domain adaptation is to directly minimize the distance between the source and target feature distributions. For example, deep adaptation networks explicitly minimize feature distribution discrepancies using measures such as maximum mean discrepancy (MMD) to align the source and target domains [35].

Although direct applications in mammography remain limited, this concept shows great promise. Lauritzen et al. [30] introduced an augmentation-based approach, termed "flavorizing," that stylistically transforms images from source to target domain, reducing the inter-vendor feature gap. This novel technique maintained consistent performance (AUC around 0.65–0.71) across different vendor images. Contrastive representation learning offers another powerful discrepancy-driven adaptation method. Specifically, supervised contrastive learning enforces feature proximity for similarly labeled samples from distinct domains, while separating differently labeled instances [23]. Quintana et al. [42] employed supervised contrastive learning to train on heterogeneous mammography datasets. They improved AUC from 0.745 to 0.816 on an independent unseen dataset, outperforming standard cross-entropy training.

Quintana et al. [43] provide theoretical grounding that supervised contrastive loss reduction approximates minimizing class-wise MMD (CMMD), thus explicitly shrinking distribution gaps between domains. Unlike adversarial methods, discrepancy and contrastive adaptation frameworks avoid unstable generator-discriminator dynamics, providing a more stable training process. Recent unsupervised techniques continuously exploit clustering losses combined with entropy minimization, refining decision boundaries. One such boundary-refinement strategy significantly outperformed standard adversarial domain adaptation approaches in mammography classification, highlighting the effectiveness of careful discrepancy-driven feature alignment to overcome substantial domain shift.

2.2.3 Attention-Based Domain Adaptation

In addition to adversarial and discrepancy-driven approaches, transformer-based architectures have recently emerged as promising domain adaptation methods in mammography. Vision transformers (ViTs) [21], by capturing global context effectively, can inherently generalize better in diverse imaging domains, guiding several works for effective domain adaptation methods. For example, Ashraf et al. [4] proposed the D-MASTER model, which embeds a transformer-based masked autoencoder into an unsupervised adaptation pipeline. The reconstructing masked multiscale features approach which they utilized was able to learn domain-invariant representations and effectively reduce label noise in the target domain. As a result, this approach had significantly improved lesion detection sensitivity on public mammogram datasets (INbreast and DDSM) that typically cause severe domain shifts in other models.

Furthermore, transformer-based hybrid models, such as the CNN-Transformer architecture by Hamzehei et al. [45], have demonstrated high classification accuracy (AUC 0.93) by jointly modeling current and prior mammograms. Although not explicitly designed for domain adaptation, their powerful representational capabilities suggest strong potential for adaptation via fine-tuning or leveraging attention mechanisms to highlight domain-invariant features. A critical application area of these emerging methods is cross-modality domain adaptation, such as transferring models between full-field digital mammography (FFDM) and digital breast tomosynthesis (DBT) or between traditional and synthetic mammograms. Differences in dimensionality and tissue contrast typically degrade the performance of the FFDM-trained model when directly applied to DBT.

Singh et al. [49] demonstrated a successful cross-modality approach by adapting an FFDM-trained malignancy detection model to DBT data through histogram matching and fine-tuning on limited DBT examples. This straightforward adaptation considerably improved DBT performance (AUC 0.85) considerably over direct FFDM-to-DBT transfer (AUC 0.75). Synthetic mammograms generated from DBT scans further facilitate adaptation, enabling effective model transfer between conventional and synthetic 2D images with minimal recalibration. Similarly, domain adaptation between contrast-enhanced spectral mammography (CESM) and standard mammography is increasingly viable, especially with the availability of annotated datasets such as CDD-CESM [37].

Although explicit CESM adaptation studies are emerging, feature alignment and style-transfer techniques promise effective domain transfer despite contrast-agent-induced intensity differences, representing an active and expanding research direction.

2.2.4 Benchmarks and Performance Metrics

To assess domain adaptation in mammography, researchers rely on standardized datasets and established metrics. Common benchmarks include INbreast (410 digital mammograms with lesion annotations) [38], CBIS-DDSM (a curated film-based dataset) [67], and the large-scale RSNA Screening Mammography dataset (240,000+ U.S. exams) [9]. Cross-population evaluation is also supported by datasets like the Chinese Mammography Database (CMMD) [12], containing 3,712 biopsy-confirmed digital mammograms, and VinDr-Mammo from Vietnam (5,000 exams with BI-RADS and lesion labels) [39]. Typically, models are trained on one dataset (e.g., CBIS-DDSM or VinDr-Mammo) and evaluated or fine-tuned on another (e.g., INbreast or CMMD) to measure generalization and adaptation efficacy. Evaluation metrics include AUC, accuracy, sensitivity, and specificity for classification, and Free-ROC curves or sensitivity at fixed false positives per image (FPI) for detection tasks.

Adaptation is successful when the performance on the target-domain approaches that of the source. For instance, Lauritzen et al. [30] showed that their cross-vendor model preserved AUCs (0.65–0.71) across vendors, avoiding large performance drops seen without adaptation. Quintana et al. [41] reported gains in both AUC and specificity using contrastive adaptation. In the D-MASTER study [4], unsupervised adaptation improved the sensitivity to lesion detection by 11–17% at 0.3 FPI in target datasets. Together, these benchmarks and metrics highlight that domain adaptation can restore and even enhance model performance under domain shifts. Achieving high AUC (often > 0.85) and balanced sensitivity/specificity on unseen data supports the clinical reliability of the adapted models.

3 Proposed Method

3.1 Backbone Network

We employ a masked autoencoder (MAE) architecture based on ConvNeXt V2-B [61] as the backbone network. Mammogram images are resized to 224×224 pixels and partitioned into nonoverlapping 16×16 patches. A masking ratio of 0.6 is applied, and the remaining visible patches are processed by a ConvNeXt V2 encoder employing sparse convolutions enabled via MinkowskiEngine. Sparse convolutions efficiently handle sparse masked inputs, significantly reducing computational and memory demands. The ConvNeXt V2-B encoder is pretrained on the ImageNet-22K dataset (resolution: 224 × 224, parameters: 89M, FLOPs: 15.4G) and further fine-tuned using labeled images from the VinDr-Mammo dataset with a self-supervised reconstruction loss.

3.2 Proposed Method

Our proposed method addresses UDA in mammogram classification by leveraging the pretrained ConvNeXt V2 encoder $F(\cdot)$ within the CoTMix framework [16]. VinDr-Mammo serves as the labeled source domain, with INbreast, CDD-CESM, and KAU-BCMD acting as unlabeled target domains. Fine-tuning involves training $F(\cdot)$ alongside a lightweight linear classifier $C(\cdot)$ using temporal mix-up augmentation and contrastive losses to create a domain-invariant representation space, as illustrated in Fig. 3.

Cross-Domain Temporal Mix-Up To generate intermediate representations that blend domain-specific styles while preserving semantic consistency, we apply a temporal mix-up strategy to paired inputs from source and target domains. Specifically, we generate two intermediate domains: (1) source-dominant domain and (2) target-dominant domain. We fix a mixing coefficient λ in the range $0.5 < \lambda < 1$, ensuring the dominant domain retains the larger contribution. Each time step in the dominant domain is mixed with an averaged temporal window of T time

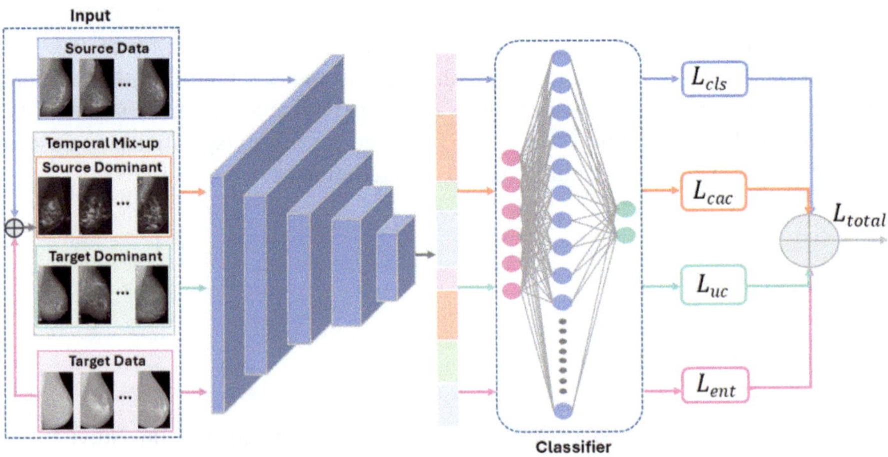

Fig. 3 Methodology overview: Inputs undergo temporal mix-up and then pass through the encoder and classifier. Four complementary losses are optimized jointly

steps from the complementary domain. Using a moving average smooths short-term fluctuations and mitigates extreme values. Given source samples $x^s = (x_1^s, \ldots, x_L^s)$ and target samples $x^t = (x_1^t, \ldots, x_L^t)$, the source-dominant samples are generated as

$$x\_i^{sd} = \lambda x\_i^s + (1-\lambda)\frac{1}{T}\sum\_j = i - \frac{T}{2}^{i+\frac{T}{2}} x\_j^t. \tag{1}$$

Similarly, the target-dominant samples are

$$x\_i^{td} = \lambda x\_i^t + (1-\lambda)\frac{1}{T}\sum\_j = i - \frac{T}{2}^{i+\frac{T}{2}} x\_j^s. \tag{2}$$

The resulting sequences x^{sd} and x^{td} preserve characteristics from their dominant domains, while incorporating smoothed temporal context from the complementary domain. We obtain four distinct views $\{x^s, x^t, x^{sd}, x^{td}\}$, which are processed through the encoder and classifier to produce predictive vectors for subsequent joint loss computations.

Loss Functions Four complementary losses guide the fine-tuning process:

1. **Source Cross-Entropy Loss** ($\mathcal{L}_{\text{cls}}$): This loss ensures that the classifier makes accurate predictions on labeled data from the source domain. It is calculated by taking the expectation over source-domain samples and computing the negative log likelihood of the true labels. By doing so, it encourages the model to learn discriminative and meaningful features directly tied to the diagnostic task in mammography.

$$\mathcal{L}_{\text{cls}} = -\mathbb{E}_{(x_s, y_s)\sim P_s} \sum_{k=1}^{K} \mathbb{1}_{[y_s=k]} \log p_s(k). \tag{3}$$

2. **Class-Aware Contrastive Loss** ($\mathcal{L}_{\text{cac}}$): This loss function enhances intraclass similarity in the source domain by pulling together feature embeddings of samples with identical labels. It computes the similarity between pairs of embeddings in the latent space, weighted by temperature scaling τ. This mechanism ensures tightly clustered feature distributions within each class, improving classification robustness and accuracy.

$$\mathcal{L}_{\text{CAC}} = \sum_{k\in I} \frac{-1}{|U(k)|} \sum_{u\in U(k)} \log \frac{\exp(\mathbf{p}_{so}^k \cdot \mathbf{p}_{so}^u/\tau)}{\sum_{a\in A(k)} \exp(\mathbf{p}_{so}^k \cdot \mathbf{p}_{so}^a/\tau)}. \tag{4}$$

3. **Unsupervised Contrastive Loss** ($\mathcal{L}_{\text{UC}}$): Given n_t target-domain samples and their corresponding n_t target-dominant mixed domain samples, we obtain $2n_t$ total samples. Let the prediction vectors be $\mathbf{p}_t = C(\mathcal{F}(x_t))$ and $\mathbf{p}_{td} = C(\mathcal{F}(x_{td}))$.

The combined set is denoted as $\mathbf{p}_{to} = (\mathbf{p}_t^1, \ldots, \mathbf{p}_t^{n_t}, \mathbf{p}_{td}^1, \ldots, \mathbf{p}_{td}^{n_t})$. Each $\mathbf{p}_{to}^k$ forms a positive pair with $\mathbf{p}_{to}^{f(k)}$, where $f(k) = k+n_t$ if $k \leq n_t$, and $f(k) = k-n_t$ otherwise. The loss is defined as

$$\mathcal{L}_{\text{UC}} = -\frac{1}{2n_t} \sum_{k \in I} \log \frac{\exp\left(\mathbf{p}_{to}^k \cdot \mathbf{p}_{to}^{f(k)} / \tau\right)}{\sum_{a \in A(k)} \exp\left(\mathbf{p}_{to}^k \cdot \mathbf{p}_{to}^a / \tau\right)}. \tag{5}$$

4. **Conditional-Entropy Minimization** ($\mathcal{L}_{\text{ent}}$): To encourage confident predictions on the unlabeled target data, we minimize the entropy of their predicted class distributions:

$$\mathcal{L}_{\text{ent}} = -\mathbb{E}_{x_t \sim P_t} \left[\mathbf{p}_t^\top \log \mathbf{p}_t\right]. \tag{6}$$

Overall Optimization The proposed method optimizes all loss components in a joint end-to-end manner. The total training objective is a weighted sum of the four losses:

$$\mathcal{L}\text{total} = \beta 1 \mathcal{L}\text{cls} + \beta 2 \mathcal{L}\text{cac} + \beta 3 \mathcal{L}\text{uc} + \beta 4 \mathcal{L}_{\text{ent}}. \tag{7}$$

The weights β_i balance the contribution of source supervision and target adaptation objectives. This unified optimization leads to features that are both discriminative and transferable across diverse mammogram datasets and imaging conditions.

4 Experimental Settings

4.1 Datasets and Settings

Mammography datasets vary significantly due to differences in imaging equipment, clinical protocols, patient demographics, and diagnostic criteria. These variations, collectively known as domain shift, pose critical challenges in building robust and fair artificial intelligence models. This section examines several publicly available mammography datasets, each originating from distinct geographic regions and healthcare systems, including VinDr-Mammo (Vietnam), INbreast (Portugal), CDD-CESM (Egypt), and KAU-BCMD (Saudi Arabia). Understanding these datasets' characteristics and domain differences is crucial for developing domain adaptation techniques that ensure fairness, minimize bias, and improve model generalization across diverse patient populations and clinical settings. A summary of these datasets and their key attributes is provided in Table 2.

VinDr-Mammo [39] is a Vietnamese full-field digital mammography dataset assembled to support the development and evaluation of computer-aided detection and diagnosis tools. It comprises 5,000 four-view exams, for a total of 20,000

Table 2 Comparison of selected public mammography datasets

Attribute	VinDr	INbreast	CDD-CESM	KAU-BCMD
Country	Vietnam	Portugal	Egypt	Saudi Arabia
Year	2018–20	2008–2010	2019–21	2022
Access	PhysioNet	Req.	TCIA	Kaggle
Format	DICOM	DICOM	JPG	JPG
Patients	5000	115	326	1416
Images	20,000	410	2,006	5662
Views	CC, MLO	CC, MLO	CC, MLO	CC, MLO
Laterality	L, R	L, R	L, R	L, R
Vendors	Siemens+	Siemens	IMS Giotto	GE/Hologic
Sex	Female	Female	Female	Female
Density	Yes (A–D)	Yes (1–4)	Yes (1–4)	Percentage
BI-RADS	Yes (1–5)	Yes (0–6)	Yes (1–6)	Yes (1–5)
Split	Yes (4k/1k)	No	No	No

DICOM images. The dataset fills a regional gap in large-scale mammography resources and provides both breast-level assessments and detailed lesion-level annotations to enable more robust and interpretable AI systems. All exams were drawn retrospectively from the Hospital 108 and Hanoi Medical University Hospital, covering routine screening and diagnostic workflows between 2018 and 2020. Images originate from four manufacturers: Siemens (15,244 images), Planmed (3,796), IMS s.r.l. (736), and IMS Giotto S.p.A. (224). Three experienced radiologists (mean 19 years of mammography practice) independently double-read every exam using the VinDr Lab annotation platform. They assigned a BI-RADS category and breast density level to each breast and marked all non-benign findings mass, calcification, asymmetry, architectural distortion, and associated features with bounding rectangles. Any discordant annotations were resolved by a third, senior reader, ensuring consensus ground truth for both breast-level and lesion-level labels. To support reproducibility, the dataset provides a default split into 4,000 training exams (15,210 benign, 790 malignant images) and 1,000 test exams, as detailed in Table 3. All images and annotations are publicly available on PhysioNet under a credentialed health-data license, with breast-level and finding-level labels provided in CSV format alongside the DICOM images.

INbreast [38], introduced in 2011, was the first publicly available high-quality digital mammography dataset, containing 410 images from 115 subjects. The dataset was collected at the Breast Centre of CHSJ, Porto, with approvals from both the hospital's Ethics Committee and the National Data Protection Authority. Mammograms were acquired from April 2008 to July 2010 using a MammoNovation Siemens FFDM system. This system uses an amorphous selenium detector with a pixel size of 70 microns and 14-bit contrast resolution. Images were saved in DICOM format, with dimensions of either 3328×4084 or 2560×3328 pixels, depending on the compression plate used. All patient-identifying data was removed in line with DICOM Supplement 55. Unique IDs allow tracking of images from the same patient without exposing identities. INbreast includes FFDM scans from screening, diagnostic, and follow-up exams. Screening follows national and regional protocols; diagnostic scans are taken after identifying abnormalities; follow-up scans track patients with a history of breast cancer. A total of 115 cases were collected. Of these, 90 contain MLO and CC views for both breasts, while the remaining 25 involve patients who had a mastectomy and thus only one breast was imaged. This results in 410 total images. The dataset covers a range of mammographic findings, including normal cases, masses, calcifications, architectural distortions, asymmetries, and combinations of these.

CDD-CESM [22], collected between 2019 and 2021, contains 2006 images with CC and MLO views (1003 low-energy images and 1003 subtracted CESM images) from 326 Egyptian women aged 18 to 90 years. The dataset was gathered from the Radiology Department of the National Cancer Institute, Cairo University, Egypt. The images are high resolution, averaging 2355×1315 pixels, and include CC and MLO views. Two mammography systems were used for image acquisition: GE Healthcare Senographe DS and Hologic Selenia Dimensions Mammography Systems. Expert radiologists manually annotated the images according to the BI-RADS assessments, providing detailed descriptors of breast composition, mass characteristics, and calcifications. The dataset includes both follow-up and pathological results, along with full medical reports for each case. For our study, we used only the low-energy images from the CDD-CESM dataset.

KAU-BCMD [2] King Abdulaziz University Breast Cancer Mammogram Dataset is the first publicly available mammography dataset from Saudi Arabia, created to address the lack of localized breast cancer datasets to develop robust computer-aided diagnosis (CAD) systems. Collected from Sheikh Mohammed Hussein Al-Amoudi Center of Excellence in Breast Cancer at King Abdulaziz University, Jeddah, between April 2019 and March 2020, the dataset includes 1,416 cases resulting in 5,662 mammogram images. Each patient case contains CC and MLO views, categorized according to the BI-RADS (0–5). Radiologists manually annotated suspicious areas, validated through majority voting. The screening was performed using a breast imaging system from IMS Giotto, part of the GMM Group. The device delivers high-resolution images with a very low signal-to-noise ratio (SNR). The dataset also includes supplementary ultrasound images corresponding to select mammography cases, enhancing its utility for multimodal breast cancer diagnosis. The KAU-BCMD dataset uniquely represents demographic characteristics and clinical practices specific to Saudi Arabia, aiding researchers in building accurate, fair, and culturally relevant AI models.

In this chapter, relevant patient data was collected, including age and breast density. A retrospective analysis of mammogram images was performed using BI-RADS mammography descriptors. The images were classified into two clinical categories: non-cancer (BI-RADS 1, 2 and 3) and cancer (BI-RADS 4, 5, and 6) [14]. The distribution of BI-RADS categories in the four datasets is illustrated in

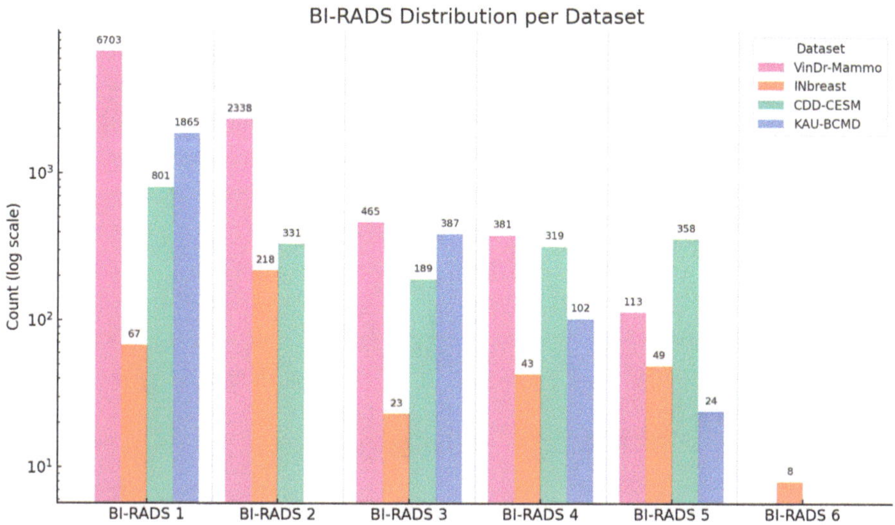

Fig. 4 BI-RADS category distribution across four mammogram datasets

Fig. 4. The dataset was divided into training and testing subsets with a 70/30 split per class and dataset, as detailed in Table 3. The dataset incorporated images from multiple mammography scanners, including Siemens, Planmed, IMS Giotto, and IMS s.r.l., summarized in Fig. 5.

4.2 Data Preprocessing

We implemented a structured, three-step preprocessing and augmentation pipeline to unify imaging characteristics across datasets, extract diagnostic regions, and enhance model generalization. Each stage was implemented using efficient Python scripts and GPU-accelerated tools.

Step 1: Metadata Structuring and Dataset Preparation
Raw mammogram datasets often in DICOM format were parsed using pydicom and dicomsdl. Key metadata such as WindowCenter, WindowWidth, RescaleSlope, and RescaleIntercept were extracted to guide image normalization. These were merged with external CSV or Excel files containing labels (e.g., BIRADS, pathology reports). A new directory named step1 was created per dataset, where images were symlinked or copied using patient and image ID naming conventions. For ROI detection training, a subset of RSNA images was manually annotated with bounding boxes in the YOLOv5 format. These were converted into the COCO format using

Table 3 Dataset-level train/test split by binary class (70% train and 30% test)

Class	Training data				Testing data			
	VinDr-Mammo	INbreast	CDD-CESM	KAU-BCMD	VinDr-Mammo	INbreast	CDD-CESM	KAU-BCMD
Non-cancer	15,210	245	532	1,576	3 802	65	140	676
Cancer	790	83	270	86	198	17	61	38
Total	16,000	328	802	1,662	4,000	82	201	714

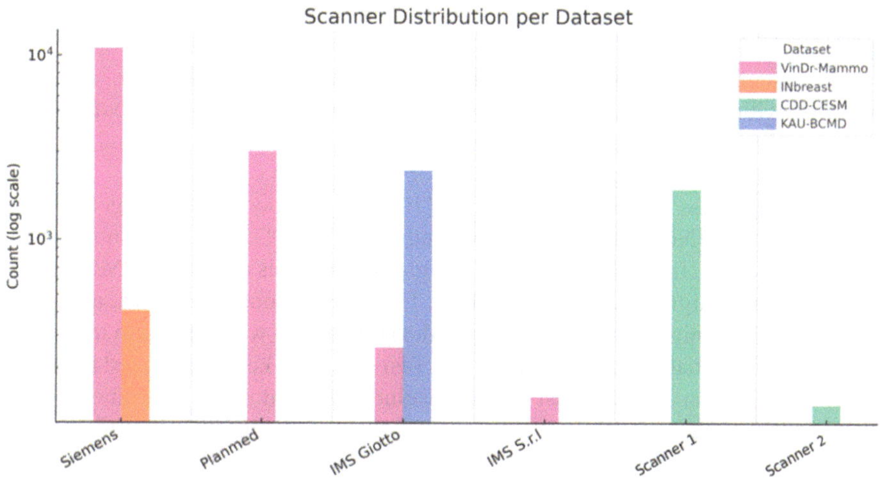

Fig. 5 Distribution of mammography scanner types used in the four datasets Note: The CDD-CESM collection contains images from two machines named Machine 1 and Machine 2 in the metadata. Their manufacturer identities (GE Senographe DS vs. Hologic) are not provided

the YOLO2COCO toolkit.[1] DICOMs were decoded to 8-bit PNGs using parallel workers and saved in the format expected by YOLOX.

Step 2: Breast ROI Detection and Windowing

We trained a YOLOX-nano model on the annotated dataset to localize the breast regions. The model was converted from PyTorch to TensorRT format using `torch2trt` for optimized inference on GPU. For each input image, the ROI was extracted using the highest-confidence bounding box. If no box met the threshold ($\geq$0.5), fallback options included Otsu-thresholded segmentation or the full image. ROI patches were then normalized using DICOM windowing. If windowing parameters were unavailable, we applied percentile-based scaling. For inverted images (as flagged in metadata), the pixel values were reversed. The final outputs were saved as padded 224 $\times$ 224 grayscale PNG images with consistent naming.

Step 3: Contrast Enhancement and Augmentation

The denoising was applied via a median filter (3 $\times$ 3). Local contrast was enhanced using CLAHE (clip limit $=$0.02, kernel size $=$ 8 $\times$ 8), implemented by `skimage.exposure`. Each image was resized and padded to 224 $\times$ 224 using `PIL.ImageOps.pad()`. For training data, we applied a fixed set of geometric

[1] https://github.com/RapidAI/YOLO2COCO

augmentations to each image: (1) horizontal flip, (2) rotate 90°, and (3) vertical flip.

All augmented images were saved with unique suffixes. The test sets were processed with denoising, CLAHE, and resizing, to preserve the distribution used during model evaluation. This pipeline ensured uniform resolution and contrast across domains, improving generalization for downstream classification.

To address class imbalance, SMOTE [10] was applied to the target-domain training datasets (INbreast, CDD-CESM, and KAU-BCMD), balancing non-cancer and cancer classes. In target datasets where malignant cases dominate, SMOTE was applied to the benign class to prevent bias. For VinDr (source domain), a random subset of 2,000 benign samples was selected, and SMOTE was applied to malignant cases to achieve a balanced 1:1 training set. Test sets were kept unchanged to ensure unbiased evaluation. VinDr's test set was excluded from domain adaptation experiments because the evaluation focused on testing model generalization to external target datasets (INbreast, CDD-CESM, and KAU-BCMD). Including VinDr's test set would assess performance within the same domain, which does not reflect the objective of cross-domain adaptation. To accurately measure the model's ability to handle domain shifts, only the target datasets were used for testing.

4.3 Implementation Details

Training followed two phases:

- **Phase 1:** Masked autoencoder pretraining. A ConvNeXt V2-B encoder was trained as the MAE backbone for 100 epochs with a batch size of 64. We used AdamW (base learning rate 5×10^{-4}, weight decay 0.05) and introduced a 20-epoch warm-up followed by cosine decay. For each image, 60% of the 16×16 patches were randomly masked, forcing the network to reconstruct the hidden content.
- **Phase 2:** CoTMix fine-tuning. The pretrained encoder was then adapted jointly with a single linear classifier on the source-target pairs for a further 100 epochs. Fine-tuning employed Adam (lr $= 1 \times 10^{-3}$) with a step scheduler that reduced the learning rate ten-fold every 20 epochs; the batch size was 32. Mix-up used a coefficient λ drawn from (0.5, 1) and a temporal shift window of 14. Loss weights were set to 0.78 for the source cross-entropy, 0.10 for the supervised contrastive term, 0.10 for the unsupervised contrastive term, and 0.05 for conditional-entropy minimization. We adopted all hyperparameters from the original CoTMix implementation reported by Eldele et al. [16].

All experiments were run on a single NVIDIA GeForce RTX 3080 GPU.

5 Results and Analysis

We evaluated our method using VinDr-Mammo as the labeled source domain and three target domains representing distinct populations: INbreast, CDD-CESM, and KAU-BCMD. Tables 4, 5, and 6 summarize the classification performance in various baseline and state-of-the-art domain adaptation methods. The metrics reported include accuracy, F1 score, and area under the ROC curve (AUC) for each dataset. Our proposed method consistently outperforms all baselines and domain adaptation approaches across the evaluated datasets.

For the INbreast dataset (Table 4), our method achieves the highest accuracy (85.0%), F1 score (0.76), and AUC (0.80), indicating strong predictive capacity and balanced classification performance. This contrasts with the baseline without adaptation, which attains only 75.0% accuracy and substantially lower F1 score and AUC, underscoring the benefits of domain adaptation. On the CDD-CESM dataset, our approach yields an accuracy of 72.0%, an F1 score of 0.72, and an AUC

Table 4 Classification performance on INbreast using VinDr-Mammo as source

Method	Accuracy	F1 score	Precision	Recall	AUC
Supervised	0.92	0.86	1.0	0.76	0.89
No adaptation	0.75	0.50	1.00	0.09	0.68
DANN [18]	0.72	0.69	0.50	**0.73**	0.73
Deep CORAL [51]	0.65	0.60	0.40	0.55	0.68
MMDA [44]	0.75	0.60	0.60	0.27	0.70
DSAN [68]	0.67	0.63	0.44	0.64	0.79
DIRT [48]	0.75	0.64	0.57	0.36	0.72
DAMS [29]	0.82	0.71	1.0	0.36	0.72
Ours	**0.85**	**0.76**	**1.00**	0.45	**0.80**

Note. Bold denotes the best value in each column

Table 5 Classification performance on CDD-CESM using VinDr-Mammo as source

Method	Accuracy	F1 score	Precision	Recall	AUC
Supervised	0.85	0.84	0.95	0.73	0.90
No adaptation	0.44	0.51	0.43	0.60	0.42
DANN [18]	0.63	0.58	0.83	0.28	0.78
Deep CORAL [51]	0.64	0.64	0.60	0.74	0.72
MMDA [44]	0.69	0.68	0.62	0.85	0.81
DSAN [68]	0.62	0.57	0.55	**0.97**	**0.85**
DIRT [48]	0.70	0.68	**0.85**	0.45	0.80
DAMS [29]	0.71	0.64	0.80	0.54	0.81
Ours	**0.72**	**0.72**	0.73	0.66	0.83

Note. Bold denotes the best value in each column

Table 6 Classification performance on KAU-BCMD using VinDr-Mammo as source

Method	Accuracy	F1 score	Precision	Recall	AUC
Supervised	0.93	0.70	0.98	0.54	1.00
No adaptation	0.60	0.08	0.04	0.34	0.47
DANN [18]	0.92	0.36	0.34	0.39	0.89
Deep CORAL [51]	0.95	0.34	0.60	0.23	0.84
MMDA [44]	0.92	**0.42**	0.36	**0.50**	0.92
DSAN [68]	0.94	0.27	0.38	0.21	0.70
DIRT [48]	0.92	0.33	0.30	0.36	0.92
DAMS [29]	0.95	0.34	**0.88**	0.21	0.91
Ours	**0.95**	0.40	0.48	0.34	**0.92**

Note. Bold denotes the best value in each column

of 0.83, surpassing all competing algorithms in accuracy and F1 score. Although DSAN achieves the highest AUC (0.85), and DIRT shows competitive accuracy (70.0%) and F1 score (0.68), these methods exhibit trade-offs between sensitivity and specificity. Our method effectively balances these metrics, resulting in the best overall classification performance.

For the KAU-BCMD dataset, our method leads with an accuracy of 95.0%, an F1 score of 0.40, and an AUC of 0.92, significantly outperforming the baseline without adaptation and traditional domain adaptation methods such as DANN, Deep CORAL, and DIRT. It is important to note that the original dataset excludes BI-RADS 2 cases, and there exists a pronounced class imbalance: non-cancer cases (BI-RADS 1 and 2 combined) total approximately 2,252, while cancer cases (BI-RADS 4 and 5 combined) are 126. This results in an approximate 17.9:1 ratio favoring non-cancer samples, which likely influences classification outcomes and should be considered when interpreting these results.

Figures 6, 7, and 8 present the ROC curves for each domain adaptation scenario: VinDr to CDD-CESM, VinDr to INbreast, and VinDr to KAU-BCMD, respectively. The curves corroborate our quantitative findings and the proposed method, achieving higher true-positive rates at lower false-positive rates compared to baselines. In general, these findings demonstrate that integrating masked autoencoders with the CoTMix contrastive domain adaptation strategy effectively addresses cross-population domain shifts in mammogram classification. Balanced improvements across accuracy, F1 score, and AUC highlight the practical potential of our approach for reliable clinical application.

Figure 9 visualizes the learned feature distributions using UMAP for both the baseline ConvNeXt V2 model without domain adaptation (left) and our proposed method with domain adaptation (right). In the baseline setting, features from each dataset form distinct and well-separated clusters, indicating strong domain shifts between VinDr, INbreast, KAU-BCMD, and CDD-CESM. In contrast, our method produces a more continuous and overlapping feature space, where data points from different domains are more intermixed. This reflects improved domain alignment and suggests that the model learns a domain-invariant representation.

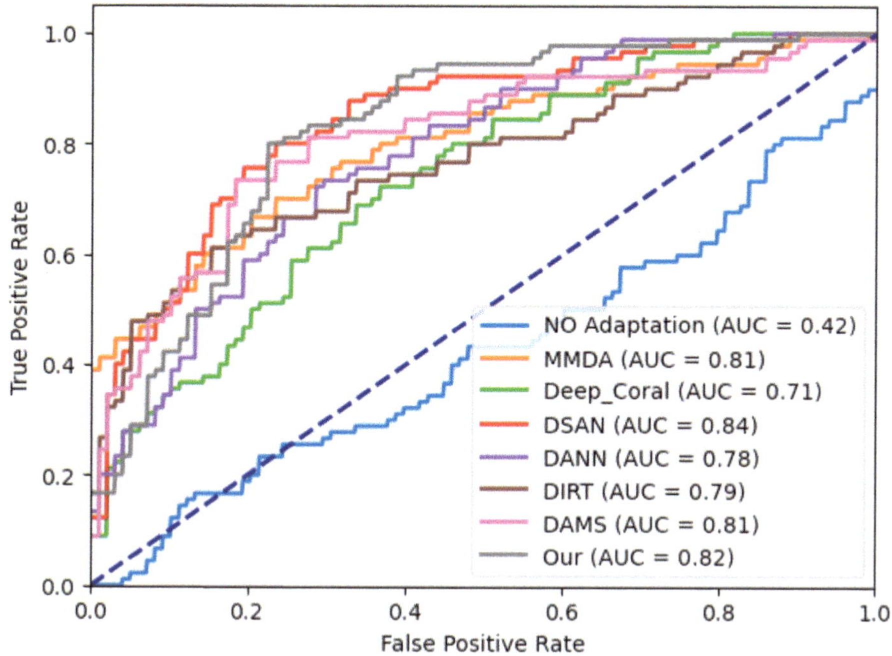

Fig. 6 ROC curve for domain adaptation from VinDr to CDD-CESM

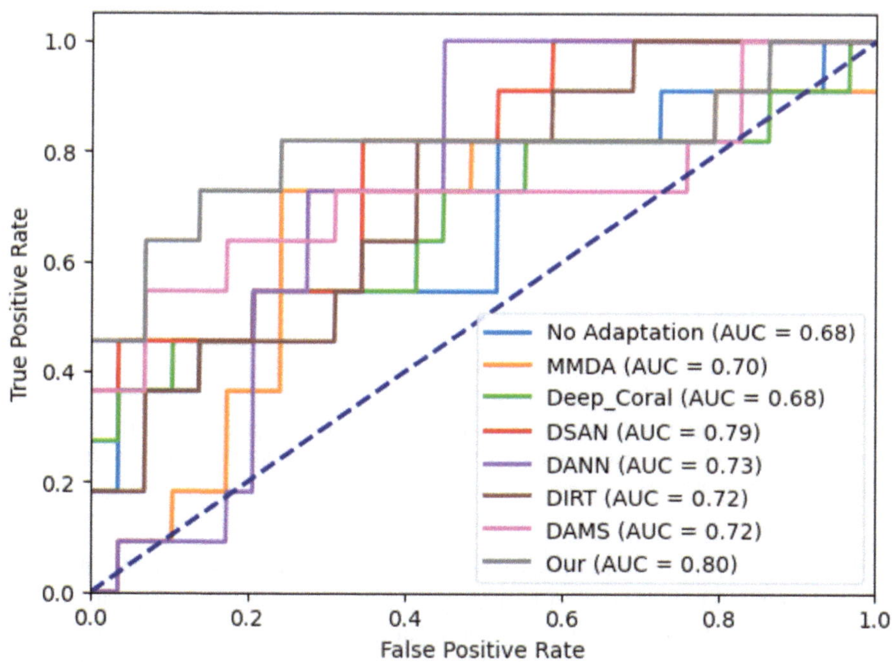

Fig. 7 ROC curve for domain adaptation from VinDr to INbreast

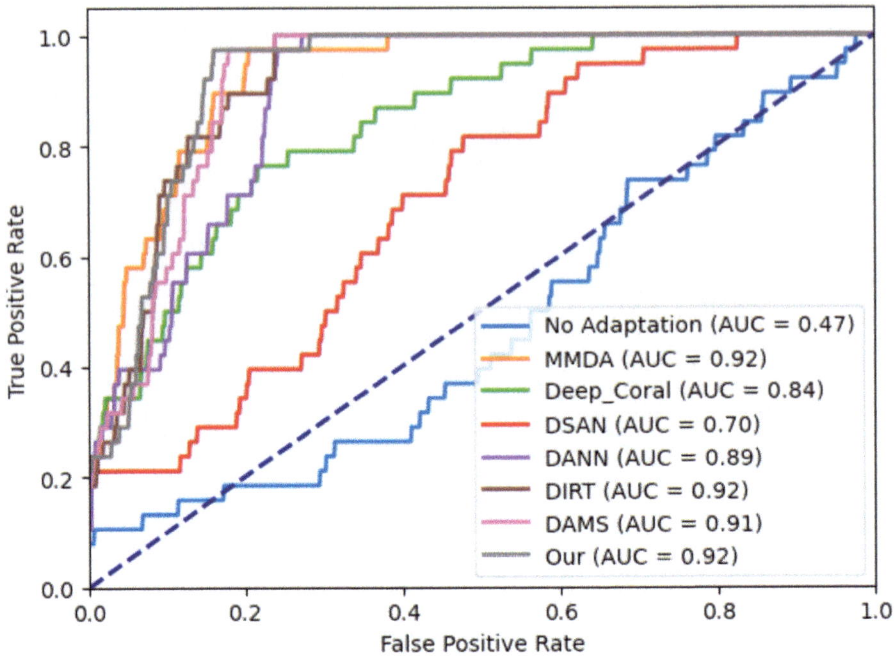

Fig. 8 ROC curve for domain adaptation from VinDr to KAU-BCMD

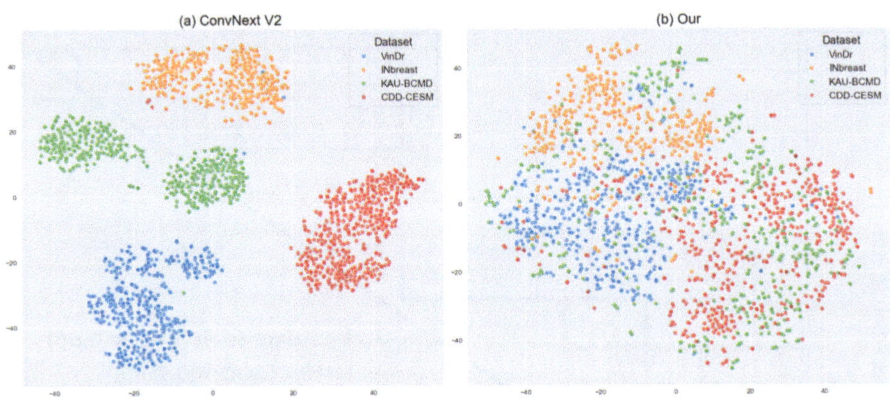

Fig. 9 UMAP visualization for extracted features from mammographic images: (left) Features learned by ConvNeXt V2 trained only on the source domain, (right) Features after domain adaptation using our method

Such alignment is critical for cross-population generalization, as it enables the classifier to apply a shared decision boundary across diverse datasets. The qualitative improvement in feature overlap supports our quantitative results and highlights the effectiveness of integrating masked autoencoders with contrastive domain adaptation in mitigating dataset-specific biases.

6 Discussion

This chapter examined how artificial intelligence models trained to detect breast cancer in mammograms perform when tested across different imaging sources, specifically focusing on domain adaptation between populations and imaging technologies. When trained solely on VinDr-Mammo data without domain adaptation (no adaptation), the model showed significant performance degradation across all target datasets. For example, the accuracy dropped to 0.44 in the CDD-CESM dataset, accompanied by a low AUC of 0.42. Although accuracy on INbreast reached 0.75, the extremely low recall of 0.09 indicated severe under-diagnosis, suggesting the model was primarily classifying cases as benign due to domain shifts. Likewise, the KAU-BCMD dataset revealed an accuracy of 0.60 yet an alarmingly low F1 score of 0.08, highlighting how severe class imbalance masked true model limitations.

Adversarial domain adaptation methods, such as DANN and DIRT, aimed to align feature distributions by encouraging domain-invariant representations. However, these approaches showed mixed results between datasets. In INbreast, DANN significantly improved recall to 0.73 but reduced precision to 0.50, indicating a trade-off where subtle malignant features were recognized, but false positives increased markedly. In contrast, on CDD-CESM, adversarial training methods such as DANN and DIRT improved precision (up to 0.85) but led to substantial drops in recall (0.28 and 0.45, respectively). This behavior suggests that the adversarial approach inadvertently suppressed critical textural features, essential for recognizing subtle cancer patterns specific to contrast-enhanced mammography. A similar pattern emerged for KAU-BCMD, where adversarial methods maintained high accuracy (approximately 0.92) but failed to improve detection of minority malignant classes, reflected by low F1 scores ($\leq$0.36). These results underscore the potential for adversarial alignment to unintentionally eliminate diagnostically important features.

Statistical matching techniques, specifically Deep CORAL, performed in varying degrees across the evaluated datasets. Deep CORAL attempted to align second-order statistics between domains, which effectively addressed basic intensity and contrast variations on CDD-CESM, raising the F1 score to 0.64 compared to no adaptation (0.51). However, Deep CORAL showed limited effectiveness on INbreast, with accuracy decreasing to 0.65 and recall remaining relatively low (0.55). Such limitations can be attributed to the distinctive visual characteristics of INbreast's digital mammograms, whose subtle textural variations and detailed features were inadequately captured by the covariance alignment approach. Furthermore, in the KAU-BCMD dataset, Deep CORAL improved accuracy to 0.95 but significantly compromised recall (0.23), reinforcing the notion that second-order alignment alone is insufficient in highly imbalanced and complex domains.

The minimum mean discrepancy-based approach (MMDA) demonstrated more consistent performance, particularly on datasets exhibiting complex statistical variability. For CDD-CESM, MMDA achieved significantly higher recall (0.85),

F1 score (0.68), and AUC (0.81), demonstrating its strength in addressing the challenging contrast-enhanced imaging domain. Similarly, MMDA achieved the highest F1 score on KAU-BCMD (0.42) and exhibited balanced sensitivity and specificity, suggesting robustness against heterogeneous scanner characteristics and imaging protocols. However, MMDA produced a relatively poor recall (0.27) in INbreast, properly due to the absence of explicit class-aware mechanisms that could better capture subtle malignant features distinct from this digitized dataset.

Class-aware adaptation methods like DSAN specifically aligned cancerous and noncancerous features separately, aiming to optimize sensitivity. This approach delivered the highest recall (0.97) and AUC (0.85) in CDD-CESM but at the cost of low precision (0.55), leading to excessive false positives. In INbreast, DSAN improved recall moderately (0.64), but precision remained low (0.44), reflecting the persistent challenge of overclassification of benign regions. However, the low recall (0.21) and poor F1 score (0.27) observed in KAU-BCMD highlighted that class-aware alignment alone could not adequately compensate for severe domain shifts and dataset-specific complexities.

The DAMS method, combining Deep CORAL with maximum mean discrepancy (MMD), consistently emphasized precision, achieving near-perfect specificity but relatively low recall across all datasets. For example, DAMS obtained a precision of 1.00 in INbreast but had recall limited to 0.45, and similar behavior was evident in KAU-BCMD, with precision at 0.88 and recall at 0.21. This conservative behavior indicates DAMS favors certainty in classification, identifying fewer cases but ensuring high confidence in those identified. Our proposed method, which integrates cross-domain mix-up and contrastive learning with reconstruction-based alignment, provided the most balanced and robust results across the datasets. In INbreast, it delivered the highest overall accuracy (0.85), F1 score (0.76), and competitive AUC (0.80), successfully balancing precision (1.00) and recall (0.45). For CDD-CESM, our method reached the highest balanced performance (an F1 score of 0.72 and an AUC of 0.83), effectively capturing subtle lesion features within contrast-enhanced images. On KAU-BCMD, our method maintained high accuracy (0.95), improved F1 score (0.40), and delivered robust AUC (0.92), reflecting effective handling of both global domain shifts and minority-class challenges.

Several critical observations emerged from this study. First, accuracy alone is insufficient for evaluating domain adaptation performance due to sensitivity to class imbalance; metrics, such as F1 score and recall, provide more meaningful insights. Second, adversarial training risks suppressing subtle but diagnostically critical image features, demonstrating the importance of careful feature preservation during domain alignment. Third, methods aligning second-order statistics like Deep CORAL perform best on simple intensity shifts but falter on complex or subtle texture variations. Finally, explicitly modeling and combining global, local, and class-specific adaptation strategies, as in our proposed method, yields superior overall robustness.

Despite its promising performance, our study exposes several constraints that must be addressed before any domain-adapted mammography system can be safely deployed in routine screening. First, severe class imbalance significantly impacts model robustness. Although our contrastive mix-up strategy mitigates some bias toward the majority class, substantial class imbalance remains. VinDr-Mammo exhibits a non-cancer-to-cancer ratio of 19:1 (19,012 non-cancer vs. 988 cancer images), while KAU-BCMD has a similar imbalance at 18:1 (2,252 vs. 124). Even INbreast and CDD-CESM, although less skewed, maintain noticeable imbalances (approximately 3:1 and 2:1, respectively). This imbalance artificially inflates accuracy and precision, masking gaps in recall for minority malignant classes. For instance, the residual gap between accuracy and F1 score on KAU-BCMD demonstrates that rare cancers continue to be missed. Second, our evaluation spans only three external cohorts and a limited selection of scanner vendors; broader validation, particularly on low-resource sites with analog-to-digital conversions, is required to confirm robustness. Third, the current models optimize generic losses that treat all errors symmetrically, yet in clinical practice a missed cancer carries far greater cost than an additional recall. Finally, we compare single algorithm baselines in isolation, whereas radiologists often benefit from complementary second reads; our methodology does not yet exploit such ensemble effects.

Therefore, progress hinges on explicitly encoding clinical priorities into the learning objective. Cost-sensitive or focal formulations that weight malignant misclassifications more heavily than benign ones are a natural extension and should be coupled with calibrated decision thresholds tuned to each screening program's recall capacity. Hybrid or ensemble approaches also deserve investigation: For example, a cascade in which a high-recall sub-domain aligner (e.g., DSAN) flags suspect studies that are then scrutinized by a high-specificity contrastive model could preserve sensitivity, while containing false-positive workload. Moreover, adaptation techniques must be tested across a wider spectrum of hospitals, acquisition protocols, and population demographics to ensure equitable performance. Finally, integrating rich meta-data, compression force, patients' age into the adaptation pipeline may allow fine-grained, context-aware normalization, pushing the field closer to truly reliable, cross-site AI support for breast cancer screening.

7 Conclusion and Future Work

This research demonstrated that cross-domain mix-up with contrastive alignment provided superior and balanced performance, significantly improving model generalization across diverse mammography datasets. Despite notable advancements, critical challenges persist, particularly severe class imbalance and limited external validation. Future efforts must prioritize integrating cost-sensitive and focal-loss techniques to enhance detection of rare malignant cases. Expanding validation efforts to include more exams from multiple institutions, covering more imaging modalities, and additional imaging vendors, will ensure robustness and clinical reliability. Additionally, incorporating clinical metadata directly into domain adaptation frameworks could yield context-aware normalization and further enhance generalizability. Additionally, developing ensemble strategies that combine high-recall and high-specificity models may effectively balance clinical workload and accuracy, paving the way for reliable and equitable AI-supported breast cancer screening. Finally, combining federated learning with domain adaptation can enable collaborative model training across institutions without data sharing, preserving patient privacy while improving model robustness, adaptability, and fairness across geographically and demographically diverse populations.

Acknowledgments This research is funded by the Agency for Management of University and Research Grants (AGAUR), grant number 2022 FI_B 00557, cofinanced by the European Union, and project TED2021-130081B-C21.

References

1. A.P. Adedigba, S.A. Adeshina, A.M. Aibinu, Performance evaluation of deep learning models on mammogram classification using small dataset. Bioengineering **9**(4), 161 (2022)
2. A.S. Alsolami, W. Shalash, W. Alsaggaf, S. Ashoor, H. Refaat, M. Elmogy, King Abdulaziz University breast cancer mammogram dataset (KAU-BCMD). Data **6**(11), 111 (2021)
3. S. Arun Kumar, S. Sasikala, Review on deep learning-based CAD systems for breast cancer diagnosis. Tech. Cancer Res. Treat. **22**, 15330338231177977 (2023)
4. T. Ashraf, K. Rangarajan, M. Gambhir, R. Gauba, C. Arora, D-master: mask annealed transformer for unsupervised domain adaptation in breast cancer detection from mammograms, in *International Conference on Medical Image Computing and Computer-Assisted Intervention* (Springer, Berlin, 2024), pp. 189–199
5. A. Bennett, N. Shaver, N. Vyas, F. Almoli, R. Pap, A. Douglas, T. Kibret, B. Skidmore, M. Yaffe, A. Wilkinson et al., Screening for breast cancer: a systematic review update to inform the Canadian task force on preventive health care guideline. Syst. Rev. **13**(1), 304 (2024)
6. M.A. Berbar, Hybrid methods for feature extraction for breast masses classification. Egypt. Inf. J. **19**(1), 63–73 (2018)
7. K. Bowyer, D. Kopans, R. Moore, P. Kegelmeyer, The digital database for screening mammography, in *Proceedings of the Third International Workshop on Digital Mammography, Chicago* (1996), pp. 9–12
8. G. Braz Junior, S.V. da Rocha, J.D.S. de Almeida, A.C. de Paiva, A.C. Silva, M. Gattass, Breast cancer detection in mammography using spatial diversity, geostatistics, and concave geometry. Multimed. Tools Appl. **78**(10), 13005–13031 (2019)
9. C. Carr, G. Partridge, J. Kalpathy-Cramer, J. Mongan, K. Andriole, L.M. Vazirabad, M. Riopel, R. Ball, S. Dane, Y. Chen, RSNA screening mammography breast cancer detection. https://kaggle.com/competitions/rsna-breast-cancer-detection (2022). Kaggle
10. N.V. Chawla, K.W. Bowyer, L.O. Hall, W. Philip Kegelmeyer, SMOTE: synthetic minority over-sampling technique. J. Artif. Intell. Res. **16**, 321–357 (2002)
11. Y. Chen, A. Singh, X. Liu, Deep adversarial domain adaptation for breast cancer screening from mammograms. Med. Image Anal. **84**, 102711 (2021)
12. H. Cai, J. Wang, T. Dan, J. Li, Z. Fan, W. Yi, C. Cui, X. Jiang, L. Li, An online mammography database with biopsy confirmed types. Sci. Data. **10**(1), 123 (2023)
13. K. Dembrower, A. Crippa, E. Colón, M. Eklund, F. Strand, Artificial intelligence for breast cancer detection in screening mammography in Sweden: a prospective, population-based, paired-reader, non-inferiority study. Lancet Digit. Health **5**(10), e703–e711 (2023)
14. C.J. D'Orsi, E.A. Sickles, E.B. Mendelson, E.A. Morris, *2013 ACR BI-RADS Atlas: Breast Imaging Reporting and Data System* (American College of Radiology, Reston, 2014)

15. N. Eisemann, S. Bunk, T. Mukama, H. Baltus, S.A. Elsner, T. Gomille, G. Hecht, S. Heywang-Köbrunner, R. Rathmann, K. Siegmann-Luz et al., Nationwide real-world implementation of AI for cancer detection in population-based mammography screening. Nat. Med. **31**(3), 917–924 (2025)
16. E. Eldele, M. Ragab, Z. Chen, M. Wu, C.-K. Kwoh, X. Li, Contrastive domain adaptation for time-series via temporal mixup. IEEE Trans. Artif. Intell. **5**(3), 1185–1194 (2023)
17. A.H. Farhan, M.Y. Kamil, Texture analysis of mammogram using local binary pattern method, in *Journal of Physics: Conference Series*, vol. 1530 (IOP Publishing, Bristol, 2020), p. 012091
18. Y. Ganin, E. Ustinova, H. Ajakan, P. Germain, H. Larochelle, F. Laviolette, M. March, V. Lempitsky, Domain-adversarial training of neural networks. J. Mach. Learn. Res. **17**(59), 1–35 (2016)
19. L. Garrucho, K. Kushibar, S. Jouide, O. Diaz, L. Igual, K. Lekadir, Domain generalization in deep learning based mass detection in mammography: a large-scale multi-center study. Artif. Intell. Med. **132**, 102386 (2022)
20. H. Guan, M. Liu, Domain adaptation for medical image analysis: a survey. IEEE Trans. Biomed. Eng. **69**(3), 1173–1185 (2021)
21. K. Han, Y. Wang, H. Chen, X. Chen, J. Guo, Z. Liu, Y. Tang, A. Xiao, C. Xu, Y. Xu et al., A survey on vision transformer. IEEE Trans. Pattern Anal. Mach. Intell. **45**(1), 87–110 (2022)
22. R. Khaled, M. Helal, O. Alfarghaly, O. Mokhtar, A. Elkorany, H. El Kassas, A. Fahmy, Categorized contrast enhanced mammography dataset for diagnostic and artificial intelligence research. Sci. Data **9**(1), 122 (2022)
23. P. Khosla, P. Teterwak, C. Wang, A. Sarna, Y. Tian, P. Isola, A. Maschinot, C. Liu, D. Krishnan, Supervised contrastive learning. Adv. Neural Inform. Proces. Syst. **33**, 18661–18673 (2020)
24. Y. Khourdifi, A. El Alami, M. Zaydi, Y. Maleh, O. Er-Remyly, Early breast cancer detection based on deep learning: an ensemble approach applied to mammograms. BioMedInformatics **4**(4), 2338–2373 (2024)
25. O. Kilim, A. Olar, T. Joó, T. Palicz, P. Pollner, I. Csabai, Physical imaging parameter variation drives domain shift. Sci. Rep. **12**(1), 21302 (2022)
26. H. Kim, S. Park, E. Choi, Robust cross-vendor mammographic texture models using augmentation-based domain adaptation for long-term breast cancer risk. NPJ Breast Cancer **9**, 18 (2023)
27. J. Kim, A. Harper, V. McCormack et al., Global patterns and trends in breast cancer incidence and mortality across 185 countries. Nat. Med. **31**, 1154–1162 (2025). https://doi.org/10.1038/s41591-025-03502-3
28. D. Kollias, A. Arsenos, S. Kollias, Domain adaptation explainability & fairness in AI for medical image analysis: diagnosis of covid-19 based on 3-d chest CT-scans, in *Proceedings of the IEEE/CVF Conference on Computer Vision and Pattern Recognition* (2024), pp. 4907–4914
29. R. Kushol, R. Frayne, S.J. Graham, A.H. Wilman, S. Kalra, Y.-H. Yang, Domain adaptation of MRI scanners as an alternative to MRI harmonization, in *MICCAI Workshop on Domain Adaptation and Representation Transfer* (Springer, Berlin, 2023), pp. 1–11
30. A.D. Lauritzen, M.C. von Euler-Chelpin, E. Lynge, I. Vejborg, M. Nielsen, N. Karssemeijer, M. Lillholm, Robust cross-vendor mammographic texture models using augmentation-based domain adaptation for long-term breast cancer risk. J. Med. Imaging **10**(5), 054003 (2023)
31. S.-H. Lee, H. Park, E.S. Ko, Radiomics in breast imaging from techniques to clinical applications: a review. Korean J. Radiol. **21**(7), 779 (2020)
32. H. Li, X. Meng, T. Wang, Y. Tang, Y. Yin, Breast masses in mammography classification with local contour features. Biomed. Eng. Online **16**, 1–12 (2017)
33. R. Liu, S. Ahmed, J. Kim, Contrastive learning: an efficient domain adaptation strategy for 2D mammography image classification, in *Proceedings of the IEEE/CVF Conference on Computer Vision and Pattern Recognition (CVPR)* (2024), pp. 5678–5687
34. J. Logan, P.J. Kennedy, D. Catchpoole, A review of the machine learning datasets in mammography, their adherence to the fair principles and the outlook for the future. Sci. Data **10**(1), 595 (2023)

35. M. Long, Y. Cao, J. Wang, M. Jordan, Learning transferable features with deep adaptation networks, in *International Conference on Machine Learning* (PMLR, 2015), pp. 97–105
36. L. Martinez, D. Reyes, C. Chang, Improving uncertainty estimations for mammogram classification using semi-supervised learning. Artif. Intell. Med. **145**, 102540 (2024)
37. T.P. Matthews, S. Singh, B. Mombourquette, J. Su, M.P. Shah, S. Pedemonte, A. Long, D. Maffit, J. Gurney, R.M. Hoil et al., A multisite study of a breast density deep learning model for full-field digital mammography and synthetic mammography. Radiol. Artif. Intell. **3**(1), e200015 (2020)
38. I.C. Moreira, I. Amaral, I. Domingues, A. Cardoso, M.J. Cardoso, J.S. Cardoso, Inbreast: toward a full-field digital mammographic database. Acad. Radiol. **19**(2), 236–248 (2012)
39. H.T. Nguyen, H.Q. Nguyen, H.H. Pham, K. Lam, L.T. Le, M. Dao, V. Vu, VinDr-Mammo: a large-scale benchmark dataset for computer-aided diagnosis in full-field digital mammography. Sci. Data **10**(1), 277 (2023)
40. P. Oza, P. Sharma, S. Patel, A. Bruno, A bottom-up review of image analysis methods for suspicious region detection in mammograms. J. Imaging **7**(9), 190 (2021)
41. G.I. Quintana, *Leveraging domain adaptation methods for federated learning applied to 2D mammography image classification*. PhD thesis, École normale supérieure Paris-Saclay (2024)
42. G.I. Quintana, V. Jugnon, L. Vancamberg, A. Desolneux, M. Mougeot, Contrastive learning: an efficient domain adaptation strategy for 2D mammography image classification, in *2024 IEEE International Symposium on Biomedical Imaging (ISBI)* (IEEE, Piscataway, 2024), pp. 1–5
43. G.I. Quintana, L. Vancamberg, V. Jugnon, A. Desolneux, M. Mougeot, Bridging contrastive learning and domain adaptation: theoretical perspective and practical application. Preprint. arXiv:2502.00052 (2025)
44. M.M. Rahman, C. Fookes, M. Baktashmotlagh, S. Sridharan, On minimum discrepancy estimation for deep domain adaptation, in *Domain Adaptation for Visual Understanding* (2020), pp. 81–94
45. K.u. Rehman, J. Li, Y. Pei, A. Yasin, S. Ali, Y. Saeed, Architectural distortion-based digital mammograms classification using depth wise convolutional neural network. Biology **11**(1), 15 (2021)
46. H. Schurz, K. Solander, D. Åström, F. Cossío, T. Choi, M. Dustler, C. Lundström, H. Gustafsson, S. Zackrisson, F. Strand, Simulating mismatch between calibration and target population in AI for mammography the retrospective VAIB study. NPJ Digit. Med. **8**(1), 1–12 (2025)
47. R. Shen, J. Yao, K. Yan, K. Tian, C. Jiang, K. Zhou, Unsupervised domain adaptation with adversarial learning for mass detection in mammogram. Neurocomputing **393**, 27–37 (2020)
48. R. Shu, H.H. Bui, H. Narui, S. Ermon, A dirt-t approach to unsupervised domain adaptation. Preprint. arXiv:1802.08735 (2018)
49. S. Singh, T.P. Matthews, M. Shah, B. Mombourquette, T. Tsue, A. Long, R. Almohsen, S. Pedemonte, J. Su, Adaptation of a deep learning malignancy model from full-field digital mammography to digital breast tomosynthesis, in *Medical Imaging 2020: Computer-Aided Diagnosis*, vol. 11314 (SPIE, Bellingham, 2020), pp. 25–32
50. A. Solano, M. Ramirez, L. Gutierrez, A real use case of semi-supervised learning for mammogram classification in a local clinic of Costa Rica. J. Biomed. Inf. **141**, 104362 (2023)
51. B. Sun, K. Saenko, Deep coral: correlation alignment for deep domain adaptation, in *Computer Vision–ECCV 2016 Workshops: Amsterdam, October 8–10 and 15–16, 2016, Proceedings, Part III 14* (Springer, Berlin, 2016), pp. 443–450
52. X. Tao, Z. Gandomkar, T. Li, P.C. Brennan, W.M. Reed, Radiomic analysis of cohort-specific diagnostic errors in reading dense mammograms using artificial intelligence. Br. J. Radiol. **98**(1165), 75–88 (2025)
53. A. Trentham-Dietz, C.H. Chapman, J. Jayasekera, K.P. Lowry, B. Heckman-Stoddard, J.M. Hampton, J. Caswell-Jin, Y. Lu, R.E. Gangnon, L. Sun et al., Breast cancer screening with mammography: an updated decision analysis for the US Preventive Services Task Force (2024)

54. E. Tzeng, J. Hoffman, K. Saenko, T. Darrell, Adversarial discriminative domain adaptation, in *Proceedings of the IEEE Conference on Computer Vision and Pattern Recognition* (2017), pp. 7167–7176
55. T. Uematsu, A. Izumori, W.K. Moon, Overcoming the limitations of screening mammography in Japan and Korea: a paradigm shift to personalized breast cancer screening based on ultrasonography. Ultrasonography **42**(4), 508 (2023)
56. A.A. Valliani, F.F. Gulamali, Y.J. Kwon, M.L. Martini, C. Wang, D. Kondziolka, V.J. Chen, W. Wang, A.B. Costa, E.K. Oermann, Deploying deep learning models on unseen medical imaging using adversarial domain adaptation. PloS One **17**(10), e0273262 (2022)
57. S. Voisin, F. Pinto, G. Morin-Ducote, K.B. Hudson, G.D. Tourassi, Predicting diagnostic error in radiology via eye-tracking and image analytics: preliminary investigation in mammography. Med. Phys. **40**(10), 101906 (2013)
58. Y. Wang, Y. Feng, L. Zhang, Z. Wang, Q. Lv, Z. Yi, Deep adversarial domain adaptation for breast cancer screening from mammograms. Med. Image Anal. **73**, 102147 (2021)
59. Y. Wang, Y. Feng, L. Zhang, Z. Wang, Q. Lv, Y. Zhang, Deep adversarial domain adaptation for breast cancer screening from mammograms. Med. Image Anal. **73**, 102147 (2021)
60. J. Wang, T. Zhao, H. Lin, Unsupervised domain adaptation of dynamic extension networks based on class decision boundaries. IEEE Trans. Med. Imaging **42**(5), 1234–1246 (2023)
61. S. Woo, S. Debnath, R. Hu, X. Chen, Z. Liu, I.S. Kweon, S. Xie, ConvNeXt V2: co-designing and scaling ConvNets with masked autoencoders, in *Proceedings of the IEEE/CVF Conference on Computer Vision and Pattern Recognition* (2023), pp. 16133–16142
62. World Health Organization (WHO). Breast cancer. https://www.who.int/news-room/fact-sheets/detail/breast-cancer (2024). Accessed 17 Jun 2024
63. Y. Xu, M. Gong, Y. Wang, Y. Yang, S. Liu, Q. Zeng, Global trends and forecasts of breast cancer incidence and deaths. Sci. Data **10**(1), 334 (2023)
64. J.R. Zech, M.A. Badgeley, M. Liu, A.B. Costa, J.J. Titano, E.K. Oermann, Confounding variables can degrade generalization performance of radiological deep learning models. Preprint. arXiv:1807.00431 (2018)
65. Y. Zhang, G. Liang, N. Jacobs, X. Wang, Unsupervised domain adaptation for mammogram image classification: a promising tool for model generalization. Preprint. arXiv:2003.01111 (2020)
66. Z. Li, et al., in *Domain Generalization for Mammography Detection via Multi-style and Multi-view Contrastive Learning*, vol. 12907, ed. by M. de Bruijne, et al. Medical Image Computing and Computer Assisted Intervention - MICCAI 2021. MICCAI 2021. Lecture Notes in Computer Science (Springer, Cham, 2021). https://doi.org/10.1007/978-3-030-87234-2_10
67. Y. Zhou, J. Wei, D. Wu, Y. Zhang, Generating full-field digital mammogram from digitized screen-film mammogram for breast cancer screening with high-resolution generative adversarial network. Front. Oncol. **12**, 868257 (2022)
68. Y. Zhu, F. Zhuang, J. Wang, G. Ke, J. Chen, J. Bian, H. Xiong, Q. He, Deep subdomain adaptation network for image classification. IEEE Trans. Neural Netw. Learn. Syst. **32**(4), 1713–1722 (2020)

Optimized Block-Wise Fine-Tuning of VGG Models for Accurate and Explainable Detection of Chest Infectious Diseases Using Chest X-rays

Sohaib Asif, Fuguo Xue, Youqin Chen, Ruxuan Yan, Lingying Zhu, Enyu Wang, and Dong Xu

Abstract The recent outbreak of coronavirus disease 2019 (COVID-19) has proven to be a dangerous virus, causing thousands of deaths and showing catastrophic effects on a large global population. Artificial intelligence (AI)-driven tools, particularly those leveraging chest X-ray (CXR) images, have emerged as effective solutions for early screening and diagnosis. However, upon inspection, many new methods are being developed and focus primarily on accuracy, but most lack explanation of the classification process. Training a model from scratch requires large amounts of annotated data, which is a tedious and time-consuming task, especially in medical imaging. In this chapter, we address a critical question

S. Asif
Taizhou Key Laboratory of Minimally Invasive Interventional Therapy and Artificial Intelligence, Taizhou Campus of Zhejiang Cancer Hospital (Taizhou Cancer Hospital), Taizhou, Zhejiang, China

Center of Intelligent Diagnosis and Therapy (Taizhou), Hangzhou Institute of Medicine (HIM), Chinese Academy of Sciences, Taizhou, Zhejiang, China

Wenling Institute of Big Data and Artificial Intelligence in Medicine, Taizhou, Zhejiang, China
e-mail: songhb@zjcc.org.cn

F. Xue · Y. Chen
Department of Respiratory Medicine, Taizhou Campus of Zhejiang Cancer Hospital (Taizhou Cancer Hospital), Taizhou, Zhejiang, China

R. Yan · L. Zhu
Department of Radiology Imaging, Taizhou Campus of Zhejiang Cancer Hospital (Taizhou Cancer Hospital), Taizhou, Zhejiang, China

E. Wang
Taizhou Key Laboratory of Minimally Invasive Interventional Therapy and Artificial Intelligence, Taizhou Campus of Zhejiang Cancer Hospital (Taizhou Cancer Hospital), Taizhou, Zhejiang, China

Department of Radiology Imaging, Taizhou Campus of Zhejiang Cancer Hospital (Taizhou Cancer Hospital), Taizhou, Zhejiang, China
e-mail: wangey@zjcc.org.cn

N. E. M. Khalifa, M. H. N. Taha (eds.), *Next-Gen Healthcare*,
https://doi.org/10.1007/978-3-032-07267-2_3

in the accurate diagnosis of COVID-19: Can fine-tuning (FT) pretrained models improve performance and eliminate the need for training models from scratch? To answer this, we shift the focus beyond accuracy and aim to comprehensively evaluate four distinct training strategies using the widely recognized VGG16 and VGG19 architectures for early COVID-19 detection with CXR images. The four training strategies explored are training from scratch, using pretrained models as off-the-shelf feature extractors, model truncation, and block-wise fine-tuning. The dataset used in this work contains a mixture of 4055 chest radiographs with COVID-19, healthy, and pneumonia cases. We also provide a visual interpretation of the different training strategies using Grad-CAM to highlight the areas of interest the model focuses on when making its diagnosis. Extensive experiments demonstrate that (1) our block-wise fine-tuning (FT) strategy significantly enhances classification performance compared to the other three strategies; (2) a moderate level of FT strikes the optimal balance and proves to be more robust than both shallow and deep FT; and (3) the best fine-tuned VGG16 and VGG19 models achieve impressive classification accuracies of 98.73% and 98.44%, respectively, with Grad-CAM visualizations focusing on the infected regions. These findings suggest that block-wise FT yields the highest accuracy and outperforms other existing studies in COVID-19 detection.

Keywords Block-wise fine-tuning · COVID-19 · Deep learning · Chest radiographs · Transfer learning

1 Introduction

In recent years, the rapid spread of COVID-19 has brought enormous pressure to the world, affecting the normal life of all people. This is a highly contagious disease, spreading mainly from person to person, that emerged in December 2019 and affected more than 200 countries of the world, officially declared a pandemic by the World Health Organization (WHO) on March 11, 2020 [1]. Patients infected with COVID-19 may take about 2 days to 2 weeks to show full symptoms. Some common signs and symptoms of infection include coughing, chest pain, shortness of breath,

D. Xu
Taizhou Key Laboratory of Minimally Invasive Interventional Therapy and Artificial Intelligence, Taizhou Campus of Zhejiang Cancer Hospital (Taizhou Cancer Hospital), Taizhou, Zhejiang, China

Center of Intelligent Diagnosis and Therapy (Taizhou), Hangzhou Institute of Medicine (HIM), Chinese Academy of Sciences, Taizhou, Zhejiang, China

Wenling Institute of Big Data and Artificial Intelligence in Medicine, Taizhou, Zhejiang, China

Department of Diagnostic Ultrasound Imaging and Interventional Therapy, Zhejiang Cancer Hospital, Hangzhou Institute of Medicine (HIM), Chinese Academy of Sciences, Hangzhou, Zhejiang, China
e-mail: xudong@zjcc.org.cn

and myalgia. In severe cases, these signs of infection can turn into serious health complications, such as blue lips, alveolar damage, and chest pain [2, 3]. With the number of cases increasing rapidly each day, accurate detection of infected patients is an urgent need to control the spread of the virus. Effective screening of patients is the most accurate way to control this epidemic. The most common application for the diagnosis COVID-19 is the reverse transcription polymerase chain reaction (RT-PCR) [4, 5], which is prone to misdiagnoses. However, this testing method is manual, costly and time-consuming, as it requires multiple executions for assurance. Therefore, given the unprecedented speed of the spread of the virus around the world and the lack of availability of test kits, a faster screening tool is needed to monitor the spread of the disease in a timely manner [6]. Medical image analysis [7] that plays an important role in analyzing the effects of COVID-19 infection on the human body. Therefore, the use of medical images for the diagnosis of COVID-19 cases may be a key tool for screening in infected areas. Recently, a combination of chest scans and artificial intelligence (AI) [8] has been found to help explain the complications of COVID-19. Researchers [9] have found that chest abnormalities are caused by COVID-19, so CXR [10] and CT [9] have become an effective and alternative tool than RT-PCR screening method. Both methods show visual markers like ground glass opacity, which can be further used to detect COVID-19. CXR and CT images have been used globally, but there is still a shortage of skilled radiologists. These imaging modalities require a skilled radiologist to visualize the final interpretations. Therefore, there is an urgent need for effective and rapid diagnostic systems to help radiologists make accurate decisions.

Recently, the role of deep learning (DL)-based AI systems has been shown to be an effective cutting-edge solution for diagnosing COVID-19 patients. Many researchers have used radiological images [11] to develop AI-enabled solutions to identify infected patients without the need for tedious diagnostics. Khan et al. [12] proposed a DL model called coronet, which is based on pretrained Xception network using CXR for COVID-19 infection. The author uses transfer learning (TL) and performs end-to-end learning. They achieved test accuracy of 89.5% and 95% for 4-class and 3-class classification. In another paper [13], the authors extract deep features from CXR images using the DL ResNet50 model. The extracted features are classified into the appropriate class using the SVM classifier. Their proposed DL model obtained an accuracy of 95.38% in binary classification. Ozturk et al. [14] has proposed a DL model named DarkNet. They used Leaky ReLU activation instead of ReLU. The author used 17 convolutional layers and trained the model from the scratch using 125 CXR images. The model generated an accuracy of 87.02% for the multiclass classification. Hemdan et al. [15] used seven different pretrained models and proposed a model called COVIDX-Net. Among the seven models, the DenseNet121 and VGG19 models achieved the highest accuracy rate of 90%. However, the main drawback is that all models were trained on small data sets. As described in Dash et al. [16] research, they tried to train a VGG16 model by unfreezing all layers. The authors used 1272 X-ray images to train the model. By FT the entire model, a classification accuracy of 97.12% was achieved. Farooq and Hafiz [17] proposed a DL model called COVID-ResNet based on the ResNet architecture for COVID-19 detection. The authors reviewed 68 positive COVID-19 images and achieved an accuracy of 96.23. The main drawback of this study is the small number of images used in the experiment. Song et al. [18] modified the ResNet50 model and proposed a new model called DRE-Net. Their proposed method achieved 86% accuracy for detecting COVID-19. Pandit et al. [19] used the VGG16 and TL model to train the network to automatically detect COVID-19. They used 1428 CXR images and achieved 96% for binary classification and 92.5% for 3-class classification. Asnawi and Chavki et al. [20] used seven different DL models and performed a comparative analysis to find the best model for detecting COVID-19. After extensive experimentation, Inception-ResNetV2 proved to be the best model with a classification accuracy of 92.18%. Hussain et al. [21] used a pretrained model and developed a DL model called COVIDRENet. They used TL to extract features and then used SVM to classify features. The proposed model gives an accuracy of 98.3%. However, the main problem is that this architecture is not end to end. Nayak et al. [22] conducted a comprehensive study of COVID-19 detection using eight different pretrained models. They used 396 CXR images to train the model. After experiments, ResNet-34 achieved the highest accuracy of 98.33%. Monshi et al. [23] used various hyperparameter optimization techniques to scale up the VGG19 and ResNet50 models. Data augmentation is used to improve performance. They used the pretrained EfficientNetB0 model to propose a new model called CovidXrayNet and achieved 95.82% detection accuracy. The research work reported in [24] used various existing pretrained models as feature extractors and added new layers for COVID-19 classification using chest radiographs, and the experimental results showed an accuracy of 93.48%. Most previous studies have used a limited number of images, and the models employed in the experiments have not been adequately empirically studied.

Earlier approaches to classifying and detecting lung diseases using chest radiography, such as COVID-19, primarily relied on using pretrained models as feature extractors or training networks from scratch. However, training models from scratch is both time-consuming and computationally expensive, requiring large amounts of annotated medical data. Fine-tuning the entire model, while simpler than starting from scratch, does not always yield the best performance. This study addresses a critical question: Does fine-tuning (FT) pretrained models enhance performance while eliminating the need for training from scratch? This is particularly important given the challenges associated with training deep learning models for medical imaging tasks. To investigate this, we conducted a comprehensive set of experiments comparing four different training strategies on the widely used VGG16 and VGG19 architectures to determine the optimal approach for classifying CXR. The four strategies explored include (1) training the model from scratch, (2) using the model as an off-the-shelf feature extractor, (3) applying model truncation, and (4) block-wise fine-tuning. The dataset comprises 4055 chest radiographs categorized into COVID-19, healthy, and pneumonia cases. Our work is distinct from previous studies that primarily use pretrained models as feature extractors or fine-tune the entire model at once. To the best of our knowledge, this is the first study to systematically investigate these four strategies to identify the most effective training approach. Experimental results revealed that block-wise fine-tuning consistently outperformed other strategies, achieving incremental performance improvements. Importantly, fine-tuning the entire model was found to be suboptimal, while a moderate level of fine-tuning emerged as the most robust and effective approach. The best fine-tuned VGG16 and VGG19 models achieved classification accuracies of 98.73% and 98.44%, respectively. These findings demonstrate the effectiveness of block-wise fine-tuning for improving both performance and robustness in lung disease detection.

1.1 Major Contributions

- Introduction of block-wise fine-tuning for improved performance.
  This study introduces block-wise fine-tuning as a novel training strategy, demonstrating its ability to incrementally enhance classification performance. Unlike existing methods, this approach optimally adapts pretrained models for lung disease detection, achieving superior results.
- Comprehensive comparison of four training strategies.
  We conducted an extensive evaluation of training from scratch, off-the-shelf feature extraction, model truncation, and block-wise fine-tuning. This systematic comparison highlights the advantages of moderate fine-tuning over traditional strategies in terms of accuracy and robustness.
- Demonstration of moderate fine-tuning as the optimal choice.
  The study establishes that moderate levels of fine-tuning strike the best balance between performance and computational efficiency. This approach outperforms shallow or full model fine-tuning, offering a robust and scalable solution for medical imaging tasks.
- Achieving state-of-the-art classification accuracy.
  By fine-tuning VGG16 and VGG19 using the proposed strategy, we achieved classification accuracies of 98.73% and 98.44%, respectively. These results set a new benchmark for lung disease detection using chest radiographs, demonstrating the efficacy of the proposed methodology.

The layout of this chapter is organized in the following subsections as follows. Section 2 gives the details of the dataset, data preprocessing, and deep transfer learning network. Section 3 discusses the model implementation details, visualization techniques and evaluation metrics. Section 4 discusses the results from different experiments, comparative analysis and a brief discussion. Section 5 describes the conclusions and future work of this chapter.

2 Proposed Methodology

2.1 Dataset

Since previous studies have shown great success using CXR to diagnose infectious diseases of the chest, we also considered CXR images because COVID-19 infects the epithelial cells of the respiratory tract. To perform the experiments, we used CXR images from the popular Kaggle COVID-19 radiology database [25]. This dataset contains chest radiographs from three different categories, namely pneumonia, COVID-19, and normal. This dataset was compiled by different physicians along with collaborators from Pakistan, Bangladesh, and Malaysia. In this study, we collected 1361 images of COVID-19 patients, 1349 normal images, and 1345 images of patients with pneumonia, for a total of 4055 images. Figure 1 shows a sample of CXRs used to perform the experiments in this study. Since the authors of this dataset did not provide information on data splitting, we first shuffled the dataset and then split the images into training and testing sets with 1016 COVID-19 images, 1005 normal images, and 1008 pneumonia images used to train the network, and 345 COVID-19, 344 normal, and 337 pneumonia samples were used for testing.

2.2 Pre-processing and Augmentation Process

The X-ray images in the dataset vary in size, so data preprocessing is one of the main steps in resizing the images to facilitate subsequent network training. All images in the dataset are resized to a shape of 224 × 224 × 3 because the VGG network accepts a fixed output shape of 224 × 224 pixels. In addition, data augmentation techniques are used, which helps to expand the number of images. The augmentation addresses the limited size of the dataset, acts as a regularization, and avoids overfitting issues. In this study, we used two augmentation strategies (horizontal flip and vertical flip). These augmentation techniques flip the images into vertical and horizontal orientations.

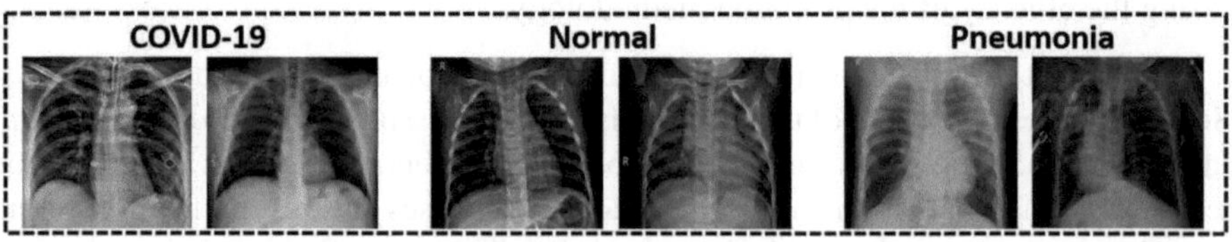

Fig. 1 CXR samples from the dataset

2.3 The Deep Transfer Learning Network

CNN models are a subtype of deep neural networks that have been shown to yield excellent results in a wide range of medical applications. The CNN architecture consists of convolutional layers for extracting features, pooling layers for reducing computational cost and feature maps, and dense layers for classification. However, training a CNN from scratch requires a lot of data and is likely to face the problem of overfitting. In this context, transfer learning is a strategy to eliminate the need of large data required for models trained from scratch [26]. This is a technique that uses a model trained on the ImageNet dataset to solve some different but related problems with a small dataset. This study employs two network architectures: VGG16 and VGG19, which are successful variants of the VGGNet architecture. Both networks accept images of size 224 × 224 as input data. VGGNet [27] model proposed by researchers from Oxford University in 2014. The uniqueness of this model is that it uses a smaller filter size of 3 × 3 instead of 5 × 5, which reduces the parameters in the model. Both models contain 5 different convolutional blocks followed by pooling layers. The convolutional block of VGG16 has 13 convolutional layers, and the convolutional block of VGG19 has 16 convolutional layers. Each model contains 3 dense layers on top for classification. VGG16 won the 2014 ImageNet competition and was evaluated as one of the best architectures for computer vision tasks. The first two blocks of VGG16 and VGG19 each contain two 3 × 3 convolutional layers, where the first block convolutional layer uses 64 filters and the second block convolutional layer uses 128 filters. Each block is accompanied by maximum pooling to handle the reduction in dimensions and computational costs after each block. After that, there are three 3 × 3 convolutional layers in the third block of VGG16 and four 3 × 3 convolutional layers in VGG19, all layers use the same filter size of 256. The fourth and fifth blocks of VGG16 use three 3 × 3 convolutional layers, while VGG19 uses four 3 × 3 convolutional layers with the same filter size of 512. Maximum pooling layer is used after each block to get informative features during training. We chose these models because of its straightforward structure, since our interest is not only in achieving high scores, but also in analyzing different model training scenarios. We removed the fully connected layer from the VGG16 and VGG19 models and added our classifier head, which is simple compared to the original ImageNet head. The new classifier head is connected on top of the VGG16 and VGG19 models, which contain a flatten layer to flatten the output of the last convolutional block, after which a dropout rate of 0.2 is applied to avoid overfitting and provide better regularization, and finally a dense layer containing 3 neurons using a softmax function to obtain the final classification results.

In this study, we analyzed the impact and significance of four different training strategies using the VGGNET architecture to find out which training strategy is best to reduce the potential risk of overfitting and lead to incremental performance improvement for COVID-19 detection. Figures 2 and 3 shows a schematic diagram of the four training strategies implemented to train the VGG16 and VGG19 models for COVID-19 detection. The four different training strategies discussed in this work are: training from scratch, block-wise FT, off-the-shelf features (feature extractor),

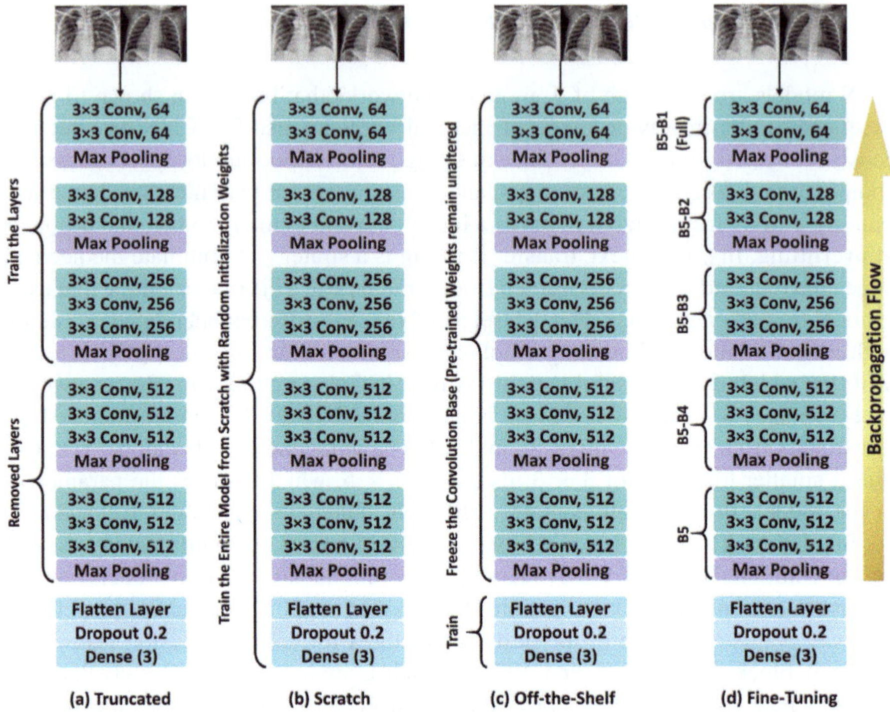

Fig. 2 Schematic diagram of the implementation of different training strategies for the VGG16 model for COVID-19 detection. (**a**) Truncated. (**b**) Scratch. (**c**) Off-the-shelf. (**d**) Fine-tuning

and finally truncating the network structure. It is worth noting that existing studies have not carried out these four different types of training methods to such an extent. We will cover each of these four training strategies in the next four sections.

2.3.1 Truncated Architecture

Due to the large size and parameters present in most deep models, deployment can become a problem in remote areas lacking sufficient computational resources [28]. However, relying only on simple models is not sufficient, especially in medical image analysis, due to the lack of feature extraction capabilities [29]. Unlike other studies, to further generate new findings, this work investigates the impact of the truncation approach on the VGG16 and VGG19 models by eliminating their ImageNet classifiers and truncating the last two blocks, leaving only the input layer and the first three convolutional blocks of the models. This approach provides a fresh perspective to see if the model can still maintain competitive performance and feature generation capabilities with truncated architectures. Figures 2a and 3a illustrate selected blocks and truncated blocks for training VGG16 and VGG19.

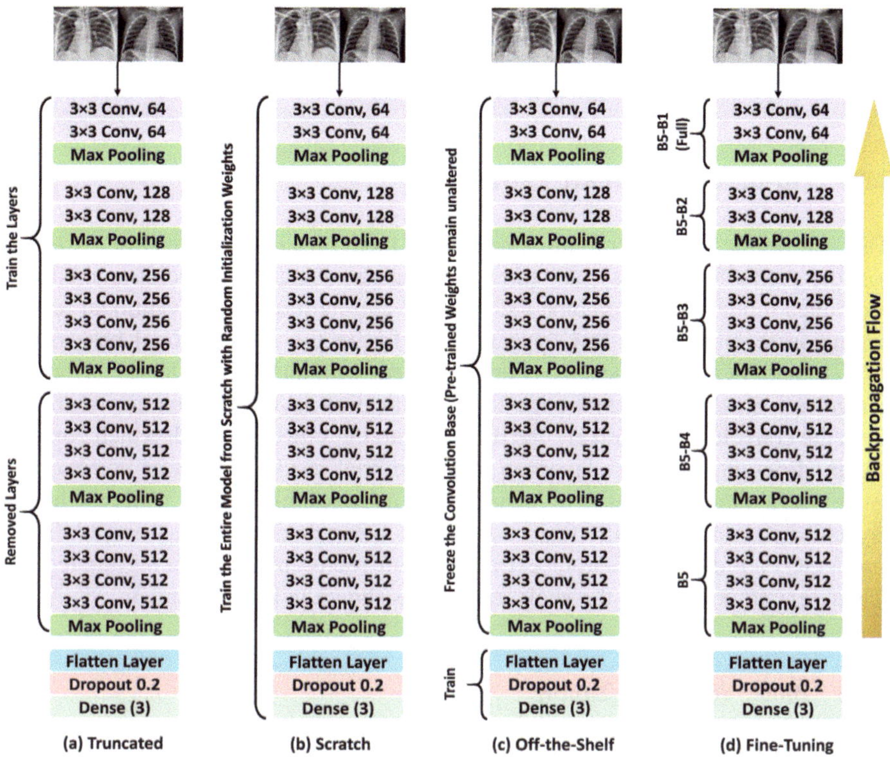

Fig. 3 Schematic diagram of the implementation of different training strategies for the VGG19 model for COVID-19 detection. (**a**) Truncated. (**b**) Scratch. (**c**) Off-the-shelf. (**d**) Fine-tuning

Truncation starts with a shallower network to reduce model complexity, but the core design remains the same. However, in this work, the aforementioned advantages also come with distinct disadvantages. Fewer layers degrade performance due to the smaller number of parameters.

2.3.2 Train from Scratch

Training a network from scratch can be tedious because it requires a lot of data, which can be difficult in medical applications where expert annotations and data are scarce and expensive [30]. This is an important issue because in medical applications, especially in COVID-19, it may not be appropriate to train a model from scratch on limited data. In this study we also aimed to answer this fundamental question in the context of COVID-19 using X-rays, we conducted a comprehensive set of experiments by training the VGG16 and VGG19 model from scratch without importing ImageNet weights. In this approach, both models are trained using randomly initialized weights, without importing ImageNet weights, and then the models are trained from scratch on a new CXR dataset. We denote this strategy as training from scratch. Figures 2b and 3b show the training strategy of both models without ImageNet weights.

2.3.3 Off-the-Shelf (Feature Extractor)

This is a simple form of training a pretrained model using TL as feature extraction (off-the-shelf). It is an easy way to extract features using the convolutional base of pretrained models and overcome the time-consuming flaws of conventional feature extraction techniques. In this approach, we freeze the convolutional base of the VGG16 and VGG19 models in its original form with the weights learned from the ImageNet dataset, and remove the top classification layer. The features extracted from the convolutional base are fed directly into our classifier head, which contains flatten, dropout, and dense layers to make the final result. The lower layers of the model learn natural and general features such as edges, blobs, etc., while the higher layers learn domain-specific features relevant to our dataset. Here, we use VGG16 and VGG19 models as feature extractors, and represent this training strategy as feature extractors and off-the-shelf features, as shown in Figs. 2c and 3c.

2.3.4 Block-Wise Fine-Tuning

During model training, weight initialization is an important step in determining model performance. In the FT strategy, the weights of the pretrained model are transferred to the model we wish to train. Here, we address the following fundamental question in the context of COVID-19 detection: Can using the pretrained model with sufficient FT yield better performance than training a model using truncation, scratch, or feature extractor? This is an important question because it may not be practical to train the model from scratch due to data limitations. To answer this core question, the FT method was further adapted on the VGG16 and VGG19 models. In general, the earlier layers capture general or low-level features, that is, features that are not relevant to the dataset, while the higher layers capture task-specific, high-level features. Therefore, an effective FT strategy is to start with earlier blocks, gradually go deeper into the earlier blocks, and track performance improvements. We call the tuning of the last block "shallow tuning" and we consider the tuning of all blocks as "full training." We would like to point out that the block-wise FT strategy suggested in this work differs from [22], where the pretrained model is used as a feature extractor, and also different from [12, 16, 31], where the entire model is fine-tuned at once. The difference here is that we tend to fine-tune VGG16 and VGG19 block-wise, aiming to find the best block to fine-tune when classifying X-ray images.

To the best of our knowledge, such a block-wise FT strategy has never been tried or discussed before in the X-ray classification method of COVID-19. Figures 2d and 3d illustrate the suggested block-wise FT strategy for the VGG16 and VGG19 models. We perform FT as follows: First, we keep the original structure and remove the original ImageNet classifier, and place our new classifier on top. Second, we divide the VGG16 and VGG19 models into five different blocks (B1–B5). We fine-tune these two models starting with block B5 and freeze all other blocks. To obtain efficient and accurate results and to explore the impact of block-wise (FT), we progressively go deeper down into earlier blocks with a very small learning rate and resume backpropagation to them, and continuously monitor performance.

3 Experiments

The following subsections describe the experimental setup, including model implementation and training details, visualization techniques, and evaluation metrics for performance comparison.

3.1 Model Training and Implementation Details

All experiments are implemented using Google Colab with NVIDIA Tesla K80 GPU and come with Python programming and Keras. A machine configuration using Windows 11 with 16 GB of RAM and 512 GB of storage space is also used. We built a new model using the architectures of VGG16 and VGG19 as input and a new classifier head as output. We added a dropout layer to the classifier head to randomly eliminate neurons in the dense layer with probability 0.2, which also helped reduce overfitting drastically. The four different training strategies discussed in this work are: training from scratch, block-wise FT, off-the-shelf features (feature extractor), and finally truncating the network structure. We trained the model for 20 epochs, but applied an early stopping technique. The early stopping strategy was also employed to train the model with patience set to 8, which is the number of epochs to terminate training if there is no performance improvement. This work also used a ReduceLROnPlateau to reduce the learning rate if there is no improvement in performance. Initial learning rate will decrease by a factor of 0.5 with a minimum learning rate of 1e-6. ModelCheckpoint is also used during training to save models with the highest accuracy. To train all models, we used a batch size of 64 with a learning rate of 1e-3 for off-the-shelf (feature extraction) and truncated strategy, and a low learning rate of 1e-4 is used for FT. We use the Adam optimizer to train all models for faster convergence, which combines the advantages of AdaGrad and RMSProp. It also uses less memory and is computationally more efficient than other optimizers. The categorical cross-entropy is used as a loss function to train all models.

3.2 *Visualization*

To understand which features have been learned and visualize regions of the image, we use the concepts of Grad-CAM [32], Grad-CAM++ [33] and feature maps to investigate how the studied model draws conclusions when distinguishing COVID-19 cases. In other words, when considering the common stigma against the black-box nature of CNNs, it is important to understand what the model is learning. More specifically, Grad-CAM can be used to discover if our model highlights the correct areas of the image to make a particular prediction. To visualize feature maps for models, we iterate through different layers of the model to visualize how the model learns certain features using different filters. As a result, they provide a great deal of insight into the steps a model takes from the input image to the final prediction.

3.3 *Model Evaluation Metrics*

The performance of each model is accomplished using the following evaluation metrics: accuracy, area under the receiver operating characteristic (AUROC), recall, confusion matrix, precision, area under the precision-recall (AUPR), and f1-score.

$$\text{Accuracy} = \frac{\text{True}_{\text{positive}} + \text{True}_{\text{negative}}}{\text{True}_{\text{positive}} + \text{True}_{\text{negative}} + \text{False}_{\text{positive}} + \text{False}_{\text{negative}}} \quad (1)$$

$$\text{Recall} = \frac{\text{True}_{\text{positive}}}{\text{True}_{\text{positive}} + \text{False}_{\text{negative}}} \quad (2)$$

$$\text{Precision} = \frac{\text{True}_{\text{positive}}}{\text{True}_{\text{positive}} + \text{False}_{\text{positive}}} \quad (3)$$

$$F1\text{-score} = 2 \times \frac{\text{Prec} \times \text{Rec}}{\text{Prec} + \text{Rec}} \quad (4)$$

In the above equation, a $\text{True}_{\text{positive}}$ indicates that the model correctly diagnosed an infected patient, while a $\text{True}_{\text{negative}}$ represents a model that correctly diagnosed a normal person. On the other hand, $\text{False}_{\text{positive}}$ indicate that the model incorrectly identified an infectious disease. $\text{False}_{\text{negative}}$ means the model is confused, misclassifying infected as uninfected.

4 Results and Analysis

This section provides experimental results for the VGG16 and VGG19 models using different training strategies. First, we compare the performance of these models using a truncated training strategy. Second, the effect of training the models from scratch is presented. Third, a comparison of VGG16 and VGG19 as an off-the-shelf (feature extractor) is presented. Fourth, the performance comparison of block-wise FT is presented. After that, we visualize the regions activated by the model using Grad-CAM and feature maps. Finally, we discuss the results on how different training strategies affect the performance of the model.

4.1 Performance Analysis of Truncated Model

In this section, we compare VGG16 and VGG19 to explore the impact of truncated training strategy to test the performance of the models. The truncation method provides a fresh perspective to see whether the models can still perform better after significantly reducing the number of layers. Confusion matrices visualize the diagnostics performed by each model in a more straightforward manner. We show the diagnostic results of the truncated VGG16 and VGG19 models using the confusion matrix in Fig. 4. The truncated VGG16 model correctly diagnosed 992 X-ray samples out of 1026 samples in the test set. However, the truncated VGG19 model correctly diagnosed 978 X-ray samples out of 1026 samples. It can be seen that the truncated VGG16 model has a lower misclassification rate than the VGG19 model. Unfortunately, the VGG19 model does not respond very well to the truncation method. Even after truncation, VGG16 maintained substantial diagnostic power because this model received the fewest number of misdiagnosed samples. To summarize the detailed classification results, Table 1 lists the performance metrics of the truncated model. After evaluation, the truncated VGG16 achieves better performance than VGG19 with an accuracy of 96.69%. The lowest performance was

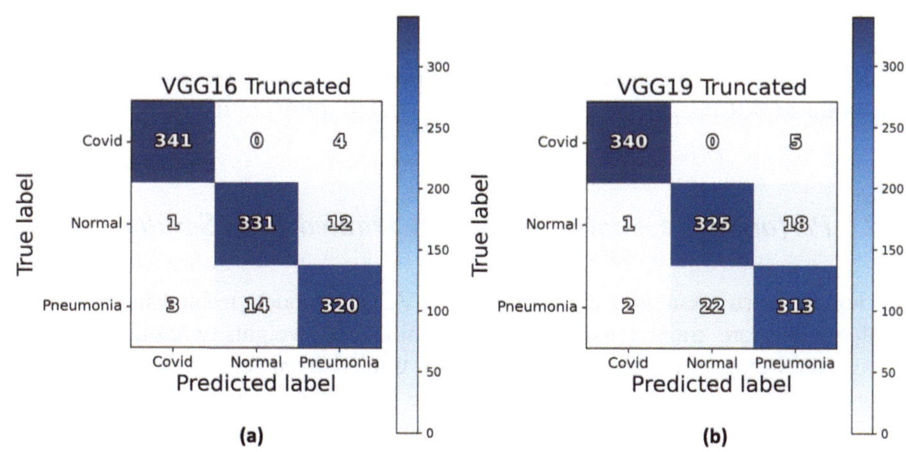

Fig. 4 Confusion matrix of the truncated models (**a**) VGG16, (**b**) VGG19

Table 1 Classification results of truncated models (*TR* truncated)

Model	Accuracy	Precision	Recall	F1-score
VGG16-TR	96.69	96.67	96.67	96.67
VGG19-TR	95.32	95.31	95.30	95.31

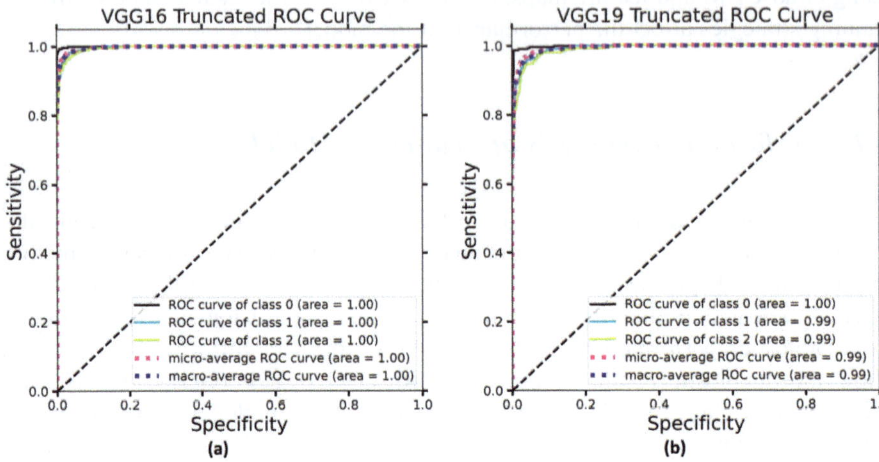

Fig. 5 The AUROC curves of the two models (**a**) VGG16, (**b**) VGG19

again achieved by VGG19-Tr with an accuracy of 95.32%, indicating its difficulty in performing the diagnosis. For a more detailed evaluation, this work has graphically identified the AUROC. The higher the AUROC, the better the performance, but if the AUROC is less than 0.5, it means that the model cannot identify a particular case. Figure 5 shows the AUROC of the truncated model. The AUPR curve is another commonly used metric, as it focuses more on the number of incorrect diagnoses. The AUPR curve of the truncated models in presented in Fig. 6. It is worth mentioning that the truncated training strategy starts a shallower network with fewer layers for feature extraction and replicates its ability to learn features from natural images rather than CXR images, which degrades the overall results of the model.

4.2 Performance Analysis of Model Trained from Scratch

To test the performance of the VGG16 and VGG19 models trained from scratch, both models are trained using randomly initialized weights without importing ImageNet weights, and then the models are trained from scratch on a new CXR dataset. We show the diagnostic results of the VGG16 and VGG19 models trained from scratch using the confusion matrix in Fig. 7. It can be seen that the truncated VGG19 model has a lower misclassification rate than the VGG16 model. To summarize the detailed classification results, Table 2 shows the performance metrics

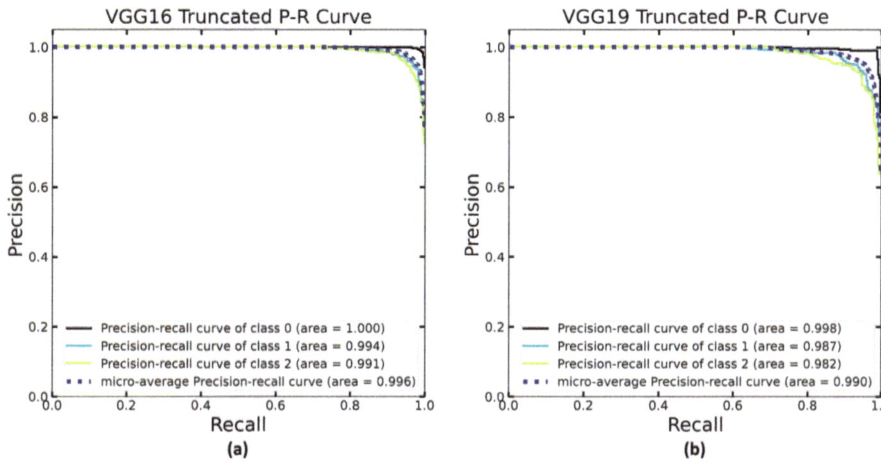

Fig. 6 The AUPR curves of the two models (**a**) VGG16, (**b**) VGG19

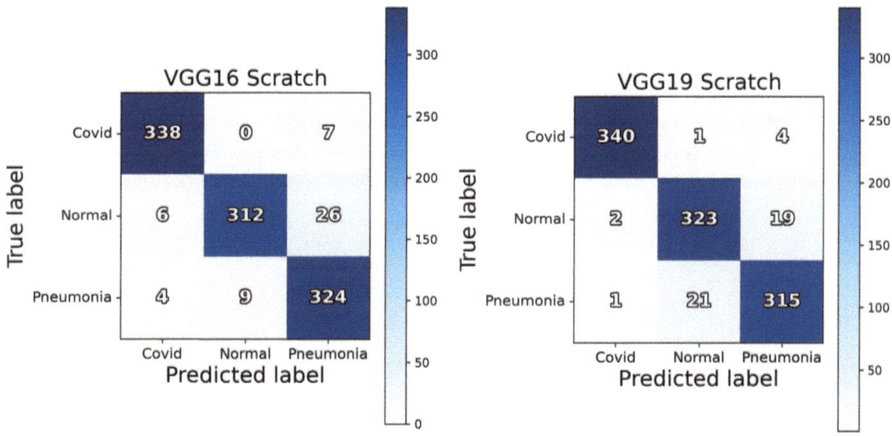

Fig. 7 Confusion matrix of the models trained from scratch

for the model trained from scratch. The main reason for the poor performance of these models trained from scratch is the size of the dataset, which is very small compared to the number of images in the ImageNet dataset. The results seem pretty obvious, where the 4055 CXR images appears too small to train such deep architectures from scratch, so the size of the dataset plays a crucial role in training deep models from scratch. AUROC and AUPR curve analysis was conducted to further evaluate the performance of the model and is shown in Figs. 8 and 9. The main reason for poor performance could be network overfitting caused by a deep architecture trained with a smaller number of images. It is difficult to collect a large dataset, especially in the medical field, so models trained from scratch are often complicated by convergence and overfitting issues, and this training strategy

Table 2 Classification results of models trained from scratch

Model	Accuracy	Precision	Recall	F1-score
VGG16	94.93	95.02	94.93	94.91
VGG19	95.31	95.31	95.30	95.30

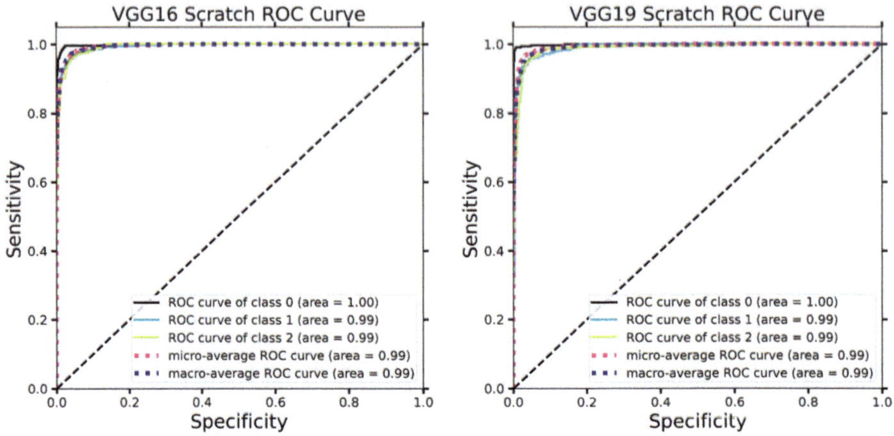

Fig. 8 The AUROC of the two models trained from scratch

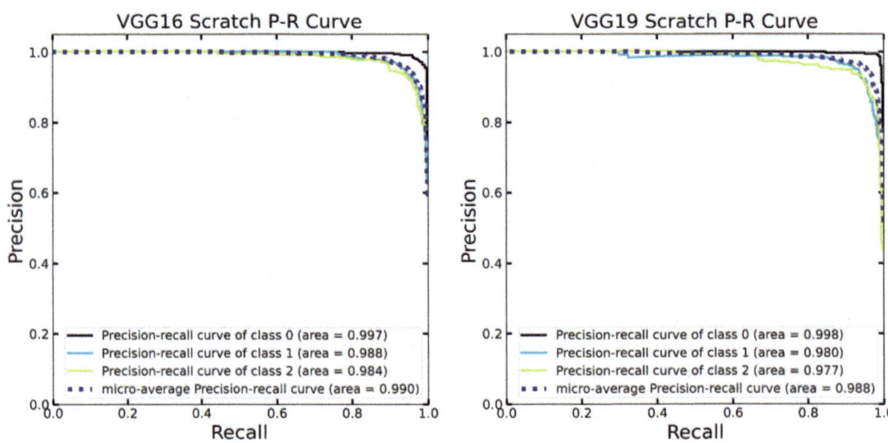

Fig. 9 The AUPR curves of the two models trained from scratch

requires a large dataset, so it is not the best option for a dataset of limited size. A promising alternative to training from scratch is to use two other training strategies: off-the-shelf (feature extractor) and block-wise FT. In the next section, we present the results related to the "off-the-shelf" and FT strategies to achieve higher accuracy.

4.3 Performance Analysis of Off-the-Shelf (Feature Extractor) Model

In this section, we present the results of the VGG16 and VGG19 models used as feature extractors or off-the-shelf features. For these experiments, we freeze the convolutional base of these models pretrained on ImageNet dataset and remove the top classification layer. A new classifier header was added to the top and forward propagation was performed across the models. It can be seen that this training strategy can overcome the drawbacks of traditional feature extraction methods. In addition, the training process is simple compared to models trained from scratch. Figure 10 shows the confusion matrix obtained when training VGG16 and VGG19 as feature extractor. The confusion matrix shows that both models have a lower misclassification rate than other training strategies such as scratch and truncation. Table 3 shows the performance metrics for the models. To further evaluate the performance of the model, AUROC and AUPR curve analysis was performed, as shown in Figs. 11 and 12. Both off-the-shelf models improve the classification accuracy by about 1–2% over the truncated and scratch training strategies. The network trained from scratch performs worse than the off-the-shelf model. This suggests that ImageNet's weights actually perform better than random initialization. Our hypothesis is that ImageNet's weights help the model capture low-level features (e.g., edges, blobs, and colors) and converge to better results compared to randomly initialized weights. The results obtained by the model as a feature extractor are

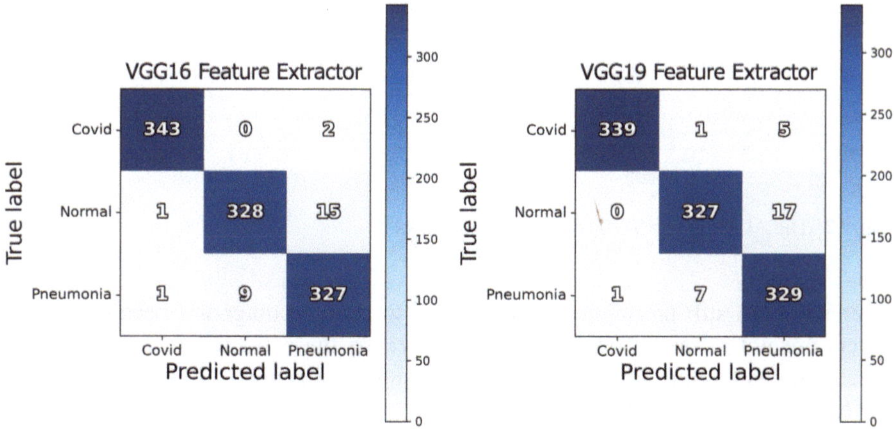

Fig. 10 Confusion matrix of the models as a feature extractor

Table 3 Classification results of models as a feature extractor

Model	Accuracy	Precision	Recall	F1-score
VGG16	97.27	97.27	97.27	97.26
VGG19	96.98	97.02	96.98	96.98

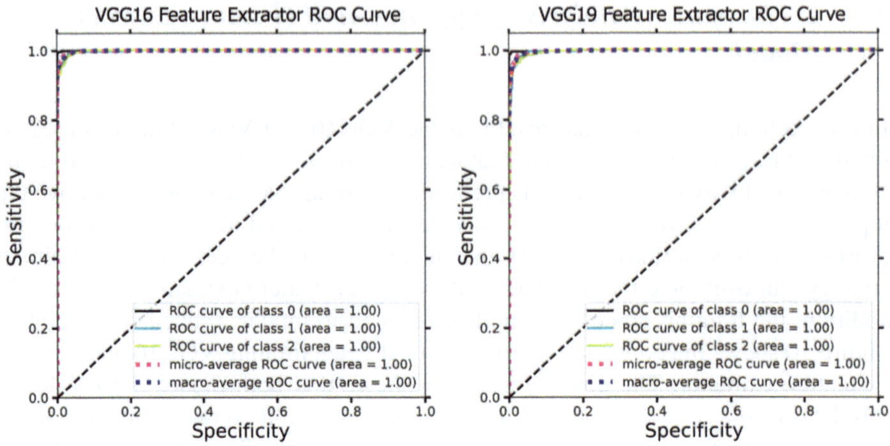

Fig. 11 The AUROC of the VGG16 and VGG19 model

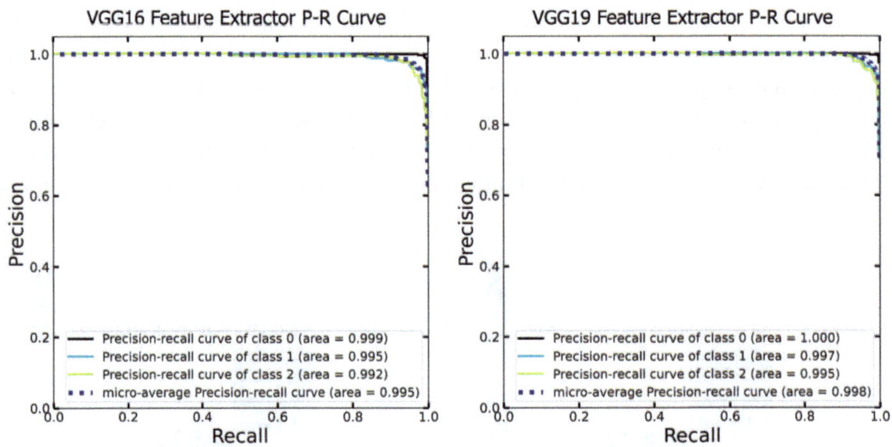

Fig. 12 The AUPR of the VGG16 and VGG19 model

interesting but still unsatisfactory if applied to medical diagnosis because the top layers are not retrained on our X-ray dataset, so the extracted features are low-level features that are useful in computer vision applications. However, CXRs are different from ImageNet images, and if we just use the model by freezing the convolutional base pretrained on ImageNet, it will be difficult for the model to learn domain specific features. In order to learn domain-specific features and get better results, FT is needed. In the next section, we will explore the effect of FT training strategy on VGG16 and VGG19 to achieve higher accuracy.

4.4 Performance Analysis of Block-Wise Fine-Tuning

In this section, we perform extensive experiments to explore the effect of block-wise FT required to achieve optimal performance for classification of CXR images. We test five FT schemes on VGG16 and VGG19 models. Where B5 FT means we unfreeze the last convolution block and classifier head. B5-B1 (full) means that all blocks in the model are fine-tuned and the weights are also updated during full training. The block-wise FT results of VGG16 and VGG19 are shown in Table 4. From the analysis, it can be seen that the performance of the model has improved significantly with the help of proper block-wise FT. It can be inferred from Table 4 that B5 and B5-B4 (shallow FT) achieved the lowest classification accuracy when classifying CXR images compared to other FT strategies. We can see that FT the entire model is not the most suitable option for VGG architectures, as combinations of different block-wise FT are also considered appropriate in certain scenarios. Another important aspect observed in the experiments is that the classification accuracy of VGG16 and VGG19 increases first and then gradually decreases as the FT progresses block by block. The performance improves when the FT is progressively deeper, and this effect can be seen in B5-B3 and B5-B2. The models with B5, B5-B4, and full FT perform worse compared to the B5-B3 and B5-B2 FT schemes. The possible reason is that shallow FT learns low-level features, such as color and edges, which are more beneficial when the source and target tasks are similar, and our dataset is CXR images, which are different from natural images. By adding more blocks to the FT, the performance gradually increases as the image features become more specific. It was also noted that the deep fine-tuned VGG16 and VGG19 models achieved the highest classification accuracy of 98.73% and 98.44%, respectively, and improved accuracy by up to 1%, compared to the models trained from scratch, truncated models. Off-the-shelf models (feature

Table 4 Performance comparison of results obtained with block-wise FT strategy on VGG16 and VGG19

Model	Block	Accuracy	Precision	Recall	F1-score
VGG16	B5	98.44	98.44	98.43	98.43
	B5-B4	98.34	98.35	98.35	98.34
	B5-B3	98.54	98.53	98.53	98.53
	B5-B2	98.73	98.74	98.74	98.73
	B5-B1 (full)	98.54	98.54	98.54	98.53
VGG19	B5	97.27	97.28	97.27	97.27
	B5-B4	98.05	98.06	98.04	98.04
	B5-B3	98.44	98.46	98.45	98.44
	B5-B2	98.44	98.44	98.44	98.44
	B5-B1 (full)	96.98	97.02	96.98	96.97

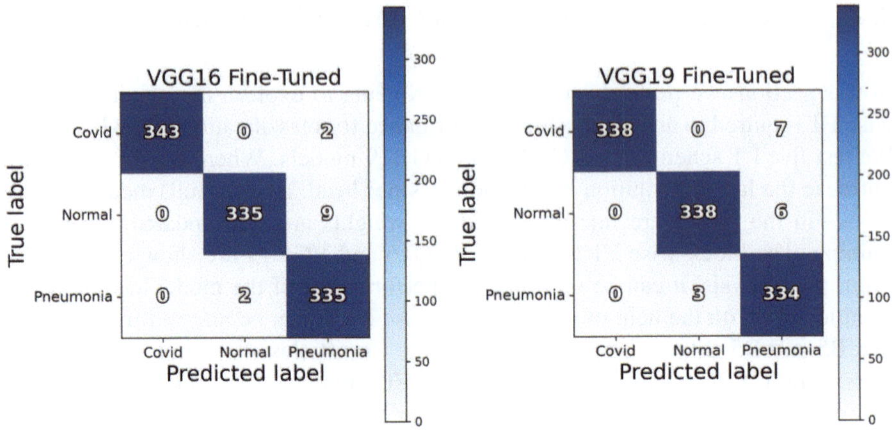

Fig. 13 Confusion matrix of the best fine-tuned models

extractor). These results strongly support the use of a block wise FT over other training strategies. FT the B5-B2 block of VGG16 is the best choice for classifying X-ray images, while FT the B5-B3 and B5-B2 blocks of VGG19 is the best choice for classifying X-ray images. According to the above analytical results, the best classification performance was achieved by FT the B5-B2 block of the VGG16 model and the B5-B3 block of the VGG19. The confusion matrices of the best fine-tuned models are shown in Fig. 13. It is clear from Fig. 13 that the VGG16 model misclassified only two COVID-19 images out of 345 images as pneumonia, and only 9 images out of 344 images were misclassified as pneumonia. We can conclude that out of 1026 tests, our model is correct in 1013 tests. This reflects that this block-wise FT is very robust in discriminating COVID-19 images.

4.5 Grad-CAM and Feature Map Visualization

To better explain and understand which features are learned by the model, this section visualizes Grad-CAM and Grad-CAM++ to investigate how the studied model draws conclusions when distinguishing COVID-19 cases. To achieve this, Fig. 14 shows a comparison of Grad-CAM and Grad-CAM++ interpretations of VGG16 and VGG19 using four different training strategies. In general, the red color emphasizes the most important areas that the model pays the most attention to, and the blue color means that the model pays the least attention. It can be seen from the figure that, compared to other training strategies, the FT strategy in VGG16 and VGG19 concentrates more on lung opacities and depicts the subsequent effects of FT on interpretation abilities. However, among other training strategies, fine-tuned VGG16 and VGG19 allowed better interpretability and more precise localizations, allowing these models to focus more on the infected part of the image. Therefore, the

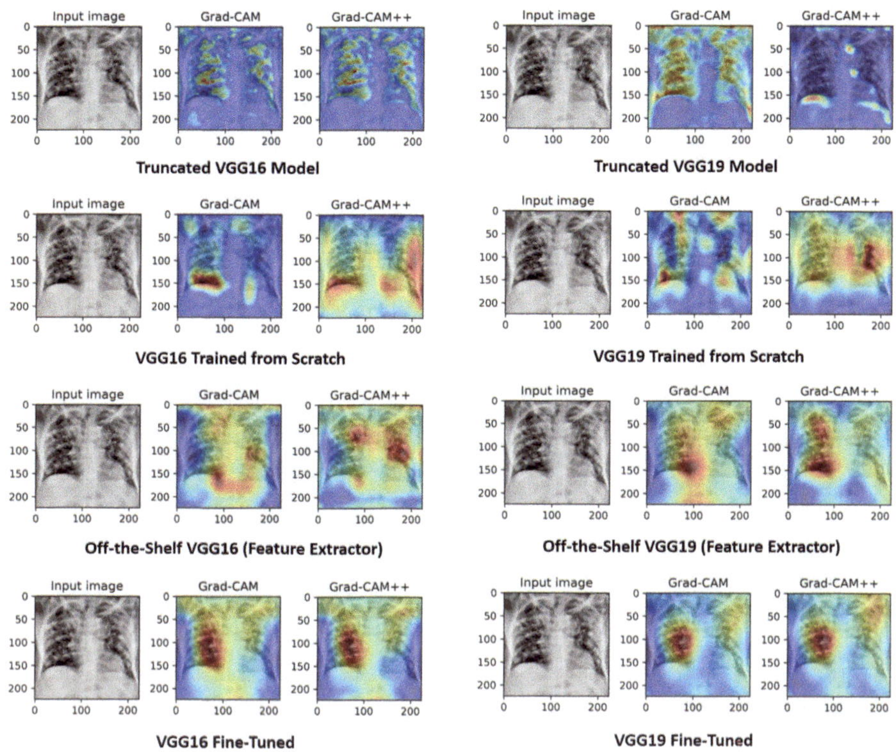

Fig. 14 Comparison of Grad-CAM and Grad-CAM++ using positive COVID-19 X-ray from VGG16 and VGG19 models using different training strategies

block-wise FT applied on both models is consistent with current medical diagnostic techniques. To test the consistency of the visual interpretations obtained with the Grad-CAM and Grad-CAM++ methods, we also used feature map visualization to explore the possibility of transferring knowledge from natural images to the chest radiograph. We just iterated over layers and got feature maps to observe the visual impact of low-level and high-level features from the best-tuned VGG16 model. Figure 15 visualizes the concept of basic feature maps, such as color and edges, while Fig. 16 show the concept of domain-specific features for CXR images. In the early stages of the network, as the first block learn low-level features, over time the model learns high-level features, picking up crazy paving patterns and ground glass opacity. In Fig. 15, we can see that the model starts to learn the basic feature maps from the CXR image. It is clear in the figure that the channels are activated on the color gradient, vertical and horizontal edges of the X-rays. We note that in Fig. 15, the model learns high-level features and tends to focus on more complex lung patterns such as patchy shadows, consolidation, and ground-glass opacity.

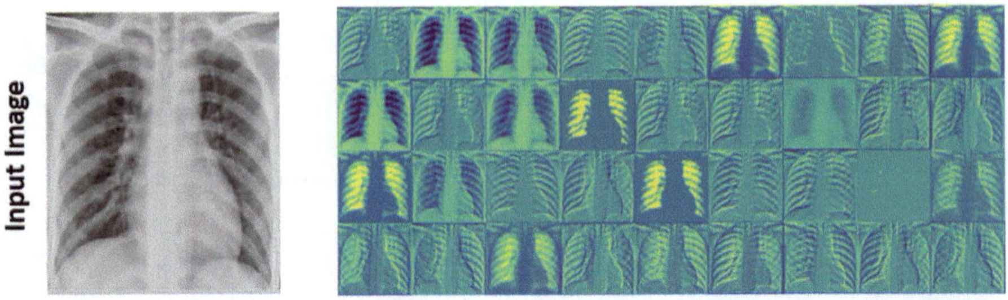

Fig. 15 Feature map visualization of the low-level features learned by the best fine-tuned VGG16 model

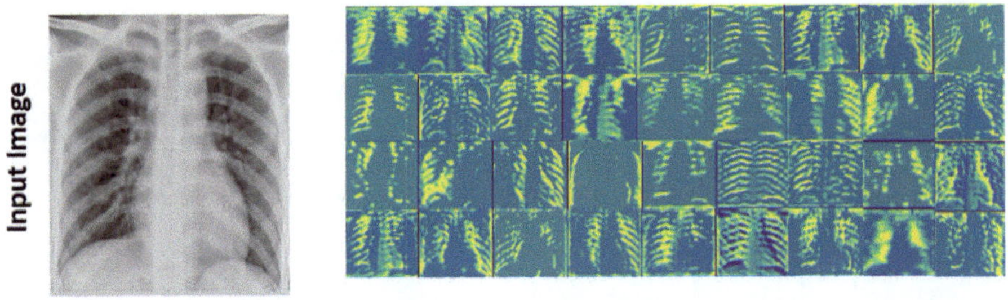

Fig. 16 Feature map visualization of high-level features, such as lung patterns, learned by the best fine-tuned VGG16 model

4.6 Discussion

In the medical field, training a model is a very difficult process due to scarcity of data. DL methods play a leading role as high-performance classifiers in the detection of different chest diseases using radiographs. Accurate prediction of COVID-19 infection using DL methods has attracted significant attention. Given that many new methods have been developed, the aim of this work is to thoroughly investigate four different training strategies on the popular VGG16 and VGG19 architectures to find the best training strategy for classifying COVID-19 using CXR. These four training strategies include, model training from scratch, off-the-shelf (feature extractor), model truncation, and block-wise FT. Different training strategies have not been explored in previous work; instead, most existing work uses pretrained models as feature extractors to extract features. To the best of our knowledge, our work is different from previous works because we experimentally explore the best model training strategy to achieve the best results.

We conducted experiments on CXR dataset containing three different classes: pneumonia, COVID-19, and normal X-ray samples. The experimental results shown in Tables 1, 2, 3, and 4 show that the block-wise FT achieved remarkable performance among all the other training schemes examined in our study. The results show that training the model from scratch is not always the perfect choice. Instead,

Table 5 Classification results of models as a feature extractor

Author	Methods	Accuracy (%)
Dash et al. [16]	VGG16 full training	97.12
Ibrahim et al. [31]	VGG19 + CNN	98.05
Khan et al. [12]	CoroNet	95.00
Pandit et al. [19]	VGG16	92.53
Montalbo et al. [34]	InceptionResNetV2-truncated	97.41
Wang et al. [35]	Modified inception model	89.50
Apostolopoulos et al. [24]	MobileNetV2	94.72
Fayemiwo et al. [36]	VGG16VGG19	93.8592.92
Lee et al. [37]	VGG16	95.90
Proposed study	VGG16 fine-tunedVGG19 fine-tuned	98.7398.44

block-wise FT give the best classification accuracy in the experiment. These findings strongly support the use of a block-wise FT approach over other training schemes. Another important aspect we observe in our experiments is the performance gap, where shallow FT learns generic features, such as color gradients and edges. As the FT goes deeper, the model learns more domain-specific features, resulting in higher performance. Another advantage observes that deep FT outperforms other training schemes and is necessary to achieve accurate image classifiers. Although shallow FT is a FT of the last block that is sufficient for computer vision applications. If we fine-tune the last block, it will be difficult for the model to learn domain-specific features because our CXR dataset is different from natural images. We discovered that a deeper FT is required for medical imaging applications to achieve better performance. For example, we observed a significant performance improvement using deep FT specifically for COVID-19 detection. The difference was also clear when Grad-CAM, Grad-CAM++, and feature maps were compared with other training schemes. As can be seen in Fig. 14, the fine-tuned VGG16 and VGG19 models capture the infected area more accurately and specifically compared to the other training strategies. This may further indicate that deep block-wise FT works best and is a good approach to use deep models for COVID-19 recognition. In addition, we compared the performance results obtained with our best fine-tuned VGG16 and VGG19 models with previous methods for detecting COVID-19, as shown in Table 5. Our chapter distinguishes itself from previous works by not only presenting a comprehensive analysis but also identifying the most effective training strategy for COVID-19 detection. This is the first time we explore what is the best way to train a deep model for COVID-19 detection in this pandemic situation where physicians and medical data are limited. It is clear from the experimental analysis that our block-wise FT provides a significant improvement in performance compared to other recent work in this area. We believe that this strategy is useful for developing a reliable diagnostic model for accurate detection of COVID-19 in this epidemic when the burden of disease is in conflict with available resources.

5 Conclusion and Future Work

Early detection of patients infected with COVID-19 in the initial stages is critical to avoid the spread of the virus. In this article, we try to answer the following key questions in the context of COVID-19 detection. Does FT the pretrained model provide better performance and eliminate the need to train the model from scratch? Given that many new methods have been developed, the importance of this study is to comprehensively explore four different training strategies on the popular VGG16 and VGG19 architectures to find the best training strategy to classify COVID-19 using CXR images. These four training strategies include model training from scratch, off-the-shelf (feature extractor), model truncation, and block-wise FT. To the best of our knowledge, our work is different from previous work because we experimentally explore the best model training strategy to achieve the best results. The study uses 4055 CXR images of COVID-19, pneumonia, and healthy cases. Extensive experiments have shown that our block-wise FT strategy provides a significant improvement in classification performance compared to the other three training strategies. FT the entire model is not an optimal choice and does not yield the best performance. Moderate FT is an optimal choice and is more robust than shallow or deep FT. The block-wise FT strategy focuses more on the infected regions in the Grad-CAM visualization and yields the highest accuracy. The best fine-tuned VGG16 and VGG19 achieve the highest classification accuracy of 98.73% and 98.44% and provide performance comparable to the latest state-of-the-art methods. In future work, we will add more data and study other deep models using different training strategies to produce better and more powerful classifiers.

Declarations Data Availability: The data that support the findings of this study are available from the corresponding author upon reasonable request. Conflicts of Interest: The authors declare no conflict of interest. Ethics Approval: Not applicable.

References

1. World Health Organization, *Getting Your Workplace Ready for COVID-19: How COVID-19 Spreads* (World Health Organization, Geneva, 2020)
2. E. Mahase, *Coronavirus: Covid-19 has Killed More People Than SARS and MERS Combined, Despite Lower Case Fatality Rate* (British Medical Journal Publishing Group, London, 2020)
3. Z. Xu et al., Pathological findings of COVID-19 associated with acute respiratory distress syndrome. Lancet Respir. Med. **8**(4), 420–422 (2020)
4. W. Wang et al., Detection of SARS-CoV-2 in different types of clinical specimens. JAMA **323**(18), 1843–1844 (2020)
5. V.M. Corman et al., Detection of 2019 novel coronavirus (2019-nCoV) by real-time RT-PCR. Eurosurveillance **25**(3), 2000045 (2020)
6. A.K. Giri, D.R. Rana, *Charting the Challenges Behind the Testing of COVID-19 in Developing Countries: Nepal as a Case Study*, vol 2 (Chinese Medical Journals Publishing House Co., Ltd, Beijing, 2020), pp. 53–56

7. W. Yang et al., The role of imaging in 2019 novel coronavirus pneumonia (COVID-19). Eur. Radiol. **30**(9), 4874–4882 (2020)
8. S. Kundu, H. Elhalawani, J.W. Gichoya, C.E. Kahn Jr., How might AI and chest imaging help unravel COVID-19's mysteries? Radiology **2**(3), 53 (2020)
9. A. Bernheim et al., Chest CT findings in coronavirus disease-19 (COVID-19): Relationship to duration of infection. Radiology **295**(3), 200463 (2020)
10. Y. Oh, S. Park, J.C. Ye, Deep learning COVID-19 features on CXR using limited training data sets. IEEE Trans. Med. Imaging **39**(8), 2688–2700 (2020)
11. H. Mohammad-Rahimi, M. Nadimi, A. Ghalyanchi-Langeroudi, M. Taheri, S. Ghafouri-Fard, Application of machine learning in diagnosis of COVID-19 through X-ray and CT images: A scoping review. Front. Cardiovasc. Med. **8**, 638011 (2021)
12. A.I. Khan, J.L. Shah, M.M. Bhat, CoroNet: A deep neural network for detection and diagnosis of COVID-19 from chest X-ray images. Comput. Methods Prog. Biomed. **196**, 105581 (2020)
13. P.K. Sethy, S.K. Behera, Detection of coronavirus disease (covid-19) based on deep features. Int. J. Math. Eng. Manage. Sci. **5**, 643–651 (2020)
14. T. Ozturk, M. Talo, E.A. Yildirim, U.B. Baloglu, O. Yildirim, U.R. Acharya, Automated detection of COVID-19 cases using deep neural networks with X-ray images. Comput. Biol. Med. **121**, 103792 (2020)
15. E.E.-D. Hemdan, M.A. Shouman, M.E. Karar, Covidx-net: A framework of deep learning classifiers to diagnose covid-19 in X-ray images (2020). arXiv preprint arXiv:2003.11055
16. A.K. Dash, P. Mohapatra, A fine-tuned deep convolutional neural network for chest radiography image classification on COVID-19 cases. Multimed. Tools Appl. **81**(1), 1055–1075 (2022)
17. M. Farooq, A. Hafeez, Covid-resnet: A deep learning framework for screening of covid19 from radiographs (2020). arXiv preprint arXiv:2003.14395
18. Y. Song et al., Deep learning enables accurate diagnosis of novel coronavirus (COVID-19) with CT images. IEEE/ACM Trans. Comput. Biol. Bioinform. **18**(6), 2775–2780 (2021)
19. M.K. Pandit, S.A. Banday, R. Naaz, M.A. Chishti, Automatic detection of COVID-19 from chest radiographs using deep learning. Radiography **27**(2), 483–489 (2021)
20. K. El Asnaoui, Y. Chawki, Using X-ray images and deep learning for automated detection of coronavirus disease. J. Biomol. Struct. Dyn. **39**(10), 3615–3626 (2021)
21. S.H. Khan, A. Sohail, M.M. Zafar, A. Khan, Coronavirus disease analysis using chest X-ray images and a novel deep convolutional neural network. Photodiagn. Photodyn. Ther. **35**, 102473 (2021)
22. S.R. Nayak, D.R. Nayak, U. Sinha, V. Arora, R.B. Pachori, Application of deep learning techniques for detection of COVID-19 cases using chest X-ray images: A comprehensive study. Biomed. Signal Process. Control **64**, 102365 (2021)
23. M.M.A. Monshi, J. Poon, V. Chung, F.M. Monshi, CovidXrayNet: Optimizing data augmentation and CNN hyperparameters for improved COVID-19 detection from CXR. Comput. Biol. Med. **133**, 104375 (2021)
24. I.D. Apostolopoulos, T.A. Mpesiana, Covid-19: Automatic detection from X-ray images utilizing transfer learning with convolutional neural networks. Phys. Eng. Sci. Med. **43**(2), 635–640 (2020)
25. M.E. Chowdhury et al., Can AI help in screening viral and COVID-19 pneumonia? IEEE Access **8**, 132665–132676 (2020)
26. H.-C. Shin et al., Deep convolutional neural networks for computer-aided detection: CNN architectures, dataset characteristics and transfer learning. IEEE Trans. Med. Imaging **35**(5), 1285–1298 (2016)
27. K. Simonyan, A. Zisserman, Very deep convolutional networks for large-scale image recognition (2014). arXiv preprint arXiv:1409.1556
28. X.-W. Chen, X. Lin, Big data deep learning: Challenges and perspectives. IEEE Access **2**, 514–525 (2014)
29. T. Hinz, P. Barros, S. Wermter, The effects of regularization on learning facial expressions with convolutional neural networks, in *International Conference on Artificial Neural Networks*, (Springer, Cham, 2016), pp. 80–87

30. D. Erhan, P.-A. Manzagol, Y. Bengio, S. Bengio, P. Vincent, The difficulty of training deep architectures and the effect of unsupervised pre-training, in *Artificial Intelligence and Statistics*, (PMLR, Cambridge, 2009), pp. 153–160
31. D.M. Ibrahim, N.M. Elshennawy, A.M. Sarhan, Deep-chest: Multi-classification deep learning model for diagnosing COVID-19, pneumonia, and lung cancer chest diseases. Comput. Biol. Med. **132**, 104348 (2021)
32. R.R. Selvaraju, M. Cogswell, A. Das, R. Vedantam, D. Parikh, D. Batra, Grad-cam: Visual explanations from deep networks via gradient-based localization, in *Proceedings of the IEEE International Conference on Computer Vision*, (IEEE, New York, 2017), pp. 618–626
33. A. Chattopadhay, A. Sarkar, P. Howlader, V.N. Balasubramanian, Grad-cam++: Generalized gradient-based visual explanations for deep convolutional networks, in *2018 IEEE Winter Conference on Applications of Computer Vision (WACV)*, (IEEE, New York, 2018), pp. 839–847
34. F.J. Montalbo, Truncating fined-tuned vision-based models to lightweight deployable diagnostic tools for SARS-CoV-2 infected chest X-rays and CT-scans. Multimed. Tools Appl. **81**(12), 16411–16439 (2022)
35. S. Wang et al., A deep learning algorithm using CT images to screen for corona virus disease (COVID-19). Eur. Radiol. **31**(8), 6096–6104 (2021)
36. M.A. Fayemiwo et al., Modeling a deep transfer learning framework for the classification of COVID-19 radiology dataset. PeerJ Comput. Sci. **7**, e614 (2021)
37. K.-S. Lee, J.Y. Kim, E.-T. Jeon, W.S. Choi, N.H. Kim, K.Y. Lee, Evaluation of scalability and degree of fine-tuning of deep convolutional neural networks for COVID-19 screening on chest X-ray images using explainable deep-learning algorithm. J. Personal. Med. **10**(4), 213 (2020)

Quantum Neural Network for Robust Image Classification: Applications to Medical and Benchmark Datasets

Hamza Kamel Ahmed, Baraa Tantawi, Malak Magdy, Eman K. Elsayed, and Gehad Ismail Sayed

Abstract In recent years, image classification has undergone significant advancements, notably through the integration of techniques inspired by principles from quantum mechanics. This chapter introduces an image classification model that combines neural network principles with concepts from quantum computing. The process encompasses two main stages: data preprocessing and image classification. During the data preprocessing phase, the original dataset is scaled and normalized. The proposed quantum neural network (QNN) approaches are then applied to the processed dataset. The proposed QNN is based on using quantum circuits instead of traditional convolution filters. A quantum neural network typically consists of three components: an encoder, a quantum layer, and a measurement. The encoder component is formed from a list of gates that are passed. This part has four RY gates, one for each qubit. Then, the ansatz with six trainable parameters and Hadamard non-parameterized circuits is used in the quantum layer. Finally, each qubit is assessed using Pauli-Z. To evaluate the performance of the proposed model, four benchmark datasets are used: two medical datasets (BreastMNIST and PneumoniaMNIST) and two nonmedical datasets (FashionMNIST and MNIST). The experimental results

H. K. Ahmed · B. Tantawi
School of Computer Science, Canadian International College (CIC), Cairo, Egypt

M. Magdy
School of Computer Science, Canadian International College (CIC), Cairo, Egypt

School of Information Technology and Computer Science, Nile University, Giza, Egypt
e-mail: m.magdy2324@nu.edu.com

E. K. Elsayed
Faculty of Science, Al-Azhar University (Girls Branch), Cairo, Egypt

College of Information Technology, Misr University for Science and Technology (MUST), Giza, Egypt
e-mail: eman.karam@must.edu.eg

G. I. Sayed (✉)
Faculty of Informatics and Computer Science, The British University in Egypt (BUE), Cairo, Egypt
e-mail: Gehad.Ismail@bue.edu.eg

N. E. M. Khalifa, M. H. N. Taha (eds.), *Next-Gen Healthcare*,
https://doi.org/10.1007/978-3-032-07267-2_4

revealed that, unlike the state-of-the-art models, the proposed image classification model demonstrated good classification accuracy despite the small input image size. Furthermore, the results showed that the proposed QNN approach can lead to a considerable improvement in the performance of traditional neural networks.

Keywords Image classification · Neural network · Quantum computing · Quantum layer · Machine learning · Medical imaging

Abbreviations

BreakHis	Breast cancer histopathological
CNNs	Convolutional neural networks
FNNs	Feedforward neural networks
MLPs	Multilayer perceptrons
MNIST	Modified National Institute of Standards and Technology
NN	Neural network
QNN	Quantum neural network

1 Introduction

Image classification stands as a pivotal challenge within the realm of computer vision, forming the cornerstone for various applications in visual identification domains. Over recent years, it has garnered significant attention and become a focal point of research endeavors [1]. The quality of a classification model's applications also improves as its performance does, as seen in the cases of people's motion estimates [2], object recognition [3], object tracking [4], segmentation [5], and video classification [6]. Advancing image classification models stands as a pivotal pursuit in propelling the sophistication of computer vision technologies. In recent years, the ubiquitous deployment of machine learning methodologies has experienced a profound surge across various domains, encompassing scholarly research and practical applications such as spam detection, text mining, video recommendation, and notably, image classification. This widespread adoption underscores the burgeoning recognition of machine learning's efficacy in addressing intricate tasks and its transformative potential across diverse sectors reliant on data-driven insights. Within this paradigm, the continual refinement of image classification methodologies not only augments the accuracy and efficiency of computer vision systems but also heralds the advent of innovative applications across industries, including healthcare, automotive, and security, thus underscoring the interdisciplinary impact of advancements in this domain [7]. When it comes to image classification tasks, traditional neural network machine learning algorithms have proven to be incredibly effective [8]. These algorithms, including multilayer perceptrons (MLPs) and feedforward neural networks (FNNs), have received a great deal of attention and are frequently used in computer vision. Complex nonlinear correlations between input characteristics and image classes can be learned particularly well with MLPs. The effectiveness of traditional neural network machine learning methods for image classification tasks has been demonstrated in numerous studies [9, 10].

Convolutional neural networks (CNNs) are a particular type of neural network architecture. They are frequently derived from the network architecture used for image classification and are utilized in a variety of applications, including semantic segmentation, object identification, and object detection. Although convolutional neural networks (CNNs) exhibit remarkable performance in various tasks, they are not devoid of limitations. One significant drawback is their reliance on a substantial volume of training data to achieve optimal performance. Moreover, there is a risk of overfitting, wherein the model becomes overly specialized to the training data and fails to generalize well to unseen data. These limitations underscore the ongoing efforts in research and development aimed at addressing these challenges and enhancing the capabilities of CNNs for more robust and interpretable performance in diverse applications [11]. Additionally, CNNs often use a hierarchical network of convolutional layers to capture local and global information, scanning the image with small receptive fields to detect features. Because the receptive fields are proportionally larger when compared to the input image size, there is a loss of fine-grained information. As a result, the model might be less able to extract precise and discriminative characteristics from the input images. The model's failure to discriminate between minor differences within the images may lead to decreased classification accuracy. Therefore, many researchers have embarked on the quest for pioneering neural network methodologies to address these inherent challenges [10, 12]. Among these forward-looking strategies, the integration of principles inspired by quantum mechanics emerges as a particularly promising avenue. This involves harnessing the foundational principles of quantum mechanics to design novel algorithms and architectures, poised to enhance computational efficiency, resilience, and scalability [10]. By infusing quantum concepts into the framework of neural networks, researchers aspire to chart new frontiers in machine learning, precipitating revolutionary advancements across diverse scientific and technological domains.

Quantum machine learning algorithms have been created as a result of the application of quantum mechanics, a branch of physics, to the field of machine learning. These algorithms are very appealing for a variety of applications since they have significant advantages over traditional machine learning methods [11]. The intrinsic capacity of quantum mechanics to execute computations at accelerated rates and with heightened effectiveness constitutes a fundamental advantage in the domain of machine learning. This advantage arises from the foundational principles governing quantum systems, including superposition and entanglement, which afford them the ability to concurrently process extensive datasets. Such capabilities engender unparalleled computational prowess, offering immense potential for transformative breakthroughs across diverse realms of machine learning research and application [11]. Quantum computers are superior to conventional computers in that they can process vast amounts of data considerably faster and more efficiently. The increased accuracy of quantum machine learning in pattern recognition applications is another benefit. Complex patterns can cause prediction or classification mistakes in traditional machine learning algorithms [10]. However, quantum machine learning techniques have increased these jobs' accuracy, making them more dependable for use in practical applications. In addition to these advantages, quantum mechanics also makes it possible to handle big volumes of data efficiently, which makes quantum machine learning an appropriate option for applications that call for the analysis of enormous amounts of data [12]. The application of quantum mechanics in medical diagnosis holds immense potential for enhancing patient outcomes. Quantum machine learning algorithms offer a novel approach to analyzing medical data, leveraging the inherent computational advantages of quantum systems. Through principles like superposition and entanglement, these algorithms can process complex medical datasets with unprecedented speed and accuracy. By harnessing quantum computational capabilities, healthcare providers can make more informed and timely decisions regarding patient treatment strategies, ultimately leading to improved clinical outcomes. This convergence of quantum mechanics and medical diagnostics represents a paradigm shift in health care, promising significant advancements in diagnostic precision and therapeutic efficacy [13]. Better treatment strategies, quicker and more accurate diagnoses, and ultimately better patient outcomes can all arise from this. One example of how quantum machine learning has the potential to revolutionize numerous industries and significantly enhance our quality of life is the use of quantum mechanics in medical diagnosis.

Recent years have seen the emergence of quantum computing as a promising model that can solve computational issues that traditional computers are unable to handle. However, due to present constraints in quantum technology, quantum-based models, which adopt principles from quantum physics but are replicated on classical systems, have received a lot of interest. These models seek to use benefits like probabilistic reasoning, improved parallelism, and data encoding inspired by nonlinear entanglement without the need for fully functional quantum processors. In this chapter, a new image classification model that combines neural network principles with concepts from quantum computing, called quantum neural networks (QNN), is proposed as a potential way to increase the accuracy of the image classification model and get around some of the drawbacks of traditional neural networks. Preprocessing and classification phases make up the two key components of the proposed image classification model. The original dataset is subjected to image scaling and data normalization during the preprocessing phase. The cleaned-up dataset is then fed into a quantum-network-based neural network (QNN). Three key components make up the proposed QNN: an encoder, a quantum layer, and a measurement. Four RY gates are used in the encoder component's set of gates, one for each qubit. The Hadamard non-parameterized circuits and ansatz with six trainable parameters make up the quantum layer. Pauli-Z is used to measure each qubit in the measurement part. The proposed QNN design is quantum-inspired, which means that it structurally mimics important concepts from quantum computing, namely superposition, entanglement, and quantum measurement, within a neural network framework, even if it is implemented on classical hardware. The encoder converts conventional input data into a quantum-processing-compatible format. The measurement component converts the quantum state into interpretable predictions by extracting observable outputs analogous to quantum measurements, while the quantum layer applies parameterized unitary transformations that capture complex feature interactions and simulate the behavior of quantum circuits. Four benchmark datasets are utilized to evaluate the performance of the proposed model, including two medical imaging datasets—BreastMNIST and PneumoniaMNIST—and two general-purpose datasets—FashionMNIST and MNIST. The following list of points provides a summary of this chapter's major contributions:

(a) A new image classification model based on the principles of quantum computing and neural networks is proposed.
(b) The potential of the proposed QNN approach is highlighted in this study, with a focus on small input image sizes. It indicates that the proposed image classification model may significantly increase classification accuracy while overcoming the drawbacks generally associated with CNNs when working with smaller images.
(c) The performance of the proposed model is tested on four benchmark datasets.
(d) This chapter offers important insights and an understanding of how quantum principles might be leveraged to improve traditional neural network architectures.

The remainder of the chapter is organized as follows. Relevant studies employing quantum computing principles are discussed in the Sect. 2. Section 3 discusses the adopted datasets. A thorough explanation of the proposed image classification model is provided in Sect. 4. The conducted results are discussed in Sect. 5. Section 6 presents a summary of the conducted results as well as its future directions.

2 Literature Review

Quantum machine learning algorithms based on using quantum principles to enable faster processing and enhanced performance on complex tasks compared to classical methods. Some key quantum machine learning algorithms will be further discussed as follows.

Two quantum algorithms for binary classification are presented by the authors in [14]. The first uses a quantum variational classifier, where a variational quantum circuit learns a separating hyperplane through parameter optimization after encoding classical input into a high-dimensional quantum feature space. By utilizing the quantum processor to calculate intricate kernel functions that feed into a classical Support Vector Machine, the second approach applies a quantum kernel estimator. Both algorithms effectively encode and categorize data by taking advantage of the increasingly huge Hilbert space provided by quantum processors. Both techniques were experimentally implemented on two-qubit superconducting quantum processors and showed perfect classification accuracy on maximally separable synthetic datasets. Using TensorFlow quantum, the authors in [15] provide a hybrid architecture that combines classical optimization with quantum convolutional neural networks (QCNNs). Eight data qubits and four ancilla qubits are used in the framework to encode grayscale images into quantum states. Variational quantum convolutions, pooling, and a softmax decision layer are then applied. The accuracy of the QCNN is comparable to that of classical CNNs with a similar number of trainable parameters, according to tests conducted on a 4-class version of MNIST. The results demonstrated the feasibility of using quantum-enhanced deep learning to realistic image identification challenges. Another quantum machine learning model proposed in [16]. In [16], the authors present the quantum multi-class classifier (QMCC), a hybrid variational model that combines classical optimization and quantum circuits. This method uses single-qubit unitary operations to encode classical data into quantum states, and classical backpropagation is used to train parameterized quantum layers. IBM's QX hardware for quantum state preparation was used to implement the concept, and quantum simulators were used for testing. Three benchmark datasets were used to assess QMCC's performance. Strong classification accuracy is demonstrated by the findings, which show that the model performs well in both binary and multi-class classification tasks, with respective scores of 92.10%, 89.50%, and 91.73% for the three adopted datasets.

The authors present two new quantum algorithms for neural networks in [17]. The first is a quantum orthogonal neural network, which effectively performs orthogonal matrix multiplication using a quantum pyramidal circuit; the second is a quantum-assisted neural network, which supports training and inference in classical networks by using quantum inner-product estimation. In addition to reporting comprehensive experiments on medical image classification using genuine quantum hardware and simulators, the authors provide theoretical studies that demonstrate superior scaling for both quantum and traditional training techniques. According to their findings, quantum techniques are as accurate as classical neural networks, suggesting that, pending the development of more sophisticated quantum devices, quantum-enhanced image recognition tasks may be possible. A hybrid quantum-classical convolutional neural network (QCCNN) designed for medical imaging tasks is presented by the authors in [18]. The model experiments with different kernel sizes and encoding techniques, substituting quantum circuit-based convolutional layers for classical ones. The QCCNN uses fewer trainable parameters and performs similarly, and in some cases even better, than the classical CNN baselines when tested on binary (MiraBest) and multi-class (LArTPC) radiological datasets. This implies that in medical image classification, hybrid quantum architectures may provide advantages in robustness and parameter efficiency.

Table 1 Datasets description

	No. of classes	No. of images	Domain
MNIST	10	70,000	Handwritten digits
FashionMNIST	10	70,000	Fashion items
BreastMNIST	2	780	Medical imaging
PneumoniaMNIST	2	5856	Medical imaging

3 Dataset Description

In this chapter, four benchmark datasets [19–21] are utilized. MNIST, Fashion-MNIST, BreastMNIST, and PneumoniaMNIST are these datasets. In machine learning, one of the most used datasets is MNIST (Modified National Institute of Standards and Technology). It includes seventy thousand 28 × 28 pixel grayscale images of handwritten numbers 0–9. There are 10,000 test images and 60,000 training images in the dataset. FashionMNIST is a drop-in alternative to MNIST that is intended to be more difficult. It includes 70,000 28 × 28 pixel grayscale images of ten different types of apparel and accessories (such as T-shirts, trousers, and sneakers). It has 10,000 test images and 60,000 training images, just like MNIST. The Breast Cancer Histopathological Image Classification (BreakHis) dataset is the source of the medical imaging dataset known as BreastMNIST. It includes 780 grayscale images of breast tissue that have been divided into classifications for benign and malignant conditions. To conform to the MNIST standard, the images are scaled to 28 × 28 pixels. It is appropriate for lightweight model testing and is utilized for binary classification jobs in medical imaging. Finally, pneumonia.MNIST is a medical imaging dataset based on the chest X-ray images (pneumonia) dataset. The 5856 grayscale chest X-ray images are divided into two classes: normal and pneumonia. They are reduced to 28 × 28 pixels. It is appropriate for lightweight medical imaging experiments and is utilized for binary classification in disease detection. Table 1 provides a comprehensive summary of the adopted datasets. In addition, Fig. 1 displays samples of these datasets.

4 The Proposed Image Classification Model

The proposed image classification model based on quantum principles consists of two major phases: data preprocessing and image classification. In the preprocessing phase, two primary operations are carried out. Image resizing and image normalization are these steps. In the final phase of classification, the processed images are used to feed the proposed quantum neural network (QNN), which employs quantum mechanics concepts. The block diagram of the proposed model is depicted in Fig. 2. Next, a description of each phase is provided in detail.

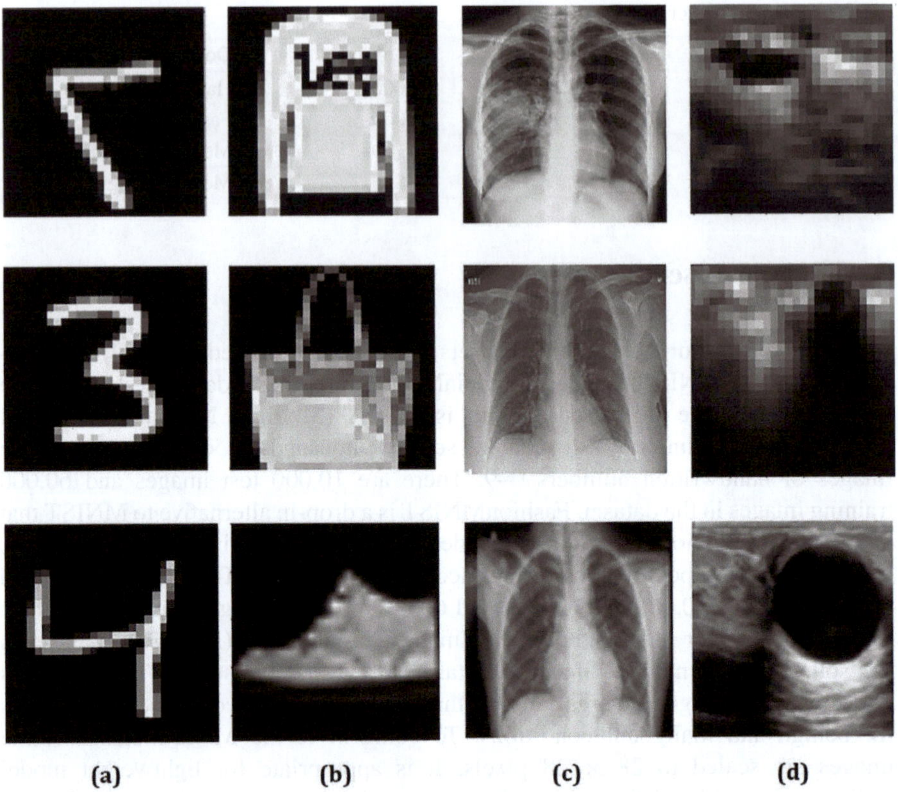

Fig. 1 Samples of the adopted datasets: (**a**) MNIST, (**b**) FashionMNIST, (**c**) PneumoniaMNIST, and (**d**) BreastMNIST

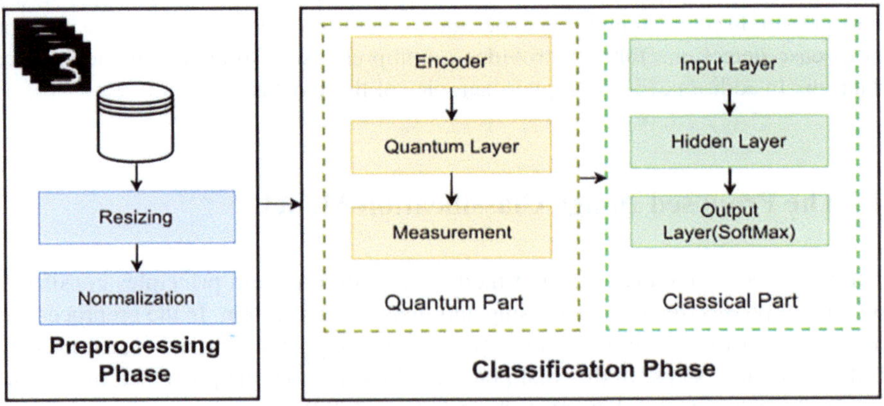

Fig. 2 The block diagram of the proposed image classification model based on QNN

4.1 Preprocessing Phase

During the preprocessing phase, the original images undergo multiple transformations to ensure their quality and consistency. Consequently, it can result in an enhancement of the model's performance. Before applying the QNN method, the images from the original dataset undergo a series of preprocessing steps in this chapter. The original images are first resized to 14×14, with each 7×7 block being processed by a single qubit of the proposed QNN. When developing a neural network model for image processing, the image size is a crucial factor. Due to the limited number of qubits currently available in quantum hardware, exploiting large image sizes in quantum computing is extremely difficult [22]. Quantum computers need exponentially more qubits to process classical data as the amount of input increases. In addition, due to their high computational complexity, current quantum approaches to image processing are not suited for processing large images. It is difficult to process large image sizes with quantum computing due to the limited number of qubits in quantum hardware and the high computational complexity of quantum algorithms. Developing a quantum neural network at the current level of quantum technology necessitates a careful evaluation of the image size. Consequently, this chapter considers input image sizes of 14×14. These images are then normalized. Normalization is regarded as a necessary step for enhancing the convergence of the model during training and enhancing its performance [23, 24]. The processed data is then divided into training sets of 70%, validation sets of 15%, and testing sets of 15%. The training and validation sets are used to train the proposed QNN, while the testing set is used to evaluate the image classification model's overall performance.

4.2 Classification Phase

In this chapter, a quantum neural network (QNN) is proposed. The proposed QNN consists of three main parts: an encoder, a quantum layer, and a measurement. Using the RY gate, the input data is encoded into a quantum state in the encoder section. RY gate is a rotation gate about the Bloch sphere's y-axis. Because it allows for the efficient parameterization of quantum states, it is widely used in quantum machine learning. The angle of the RY gate determines the amplitude of the state, making it a useful tool for encoding input data. The encoded data is then processed in the quantum layer, which combines an ansatz with adjustable parameters and Hadamard circuits without parameters. A series of measurements is performed, one for each qubit in the quantum circuit, to measure each qubit. In this chapter, the output of the model is calculated by measuring each qubit with the Pauli-Z measurement operator. This is accomplished computationally, which is equivalent to measuring the qubit along the z-axis of the Bloch sphere. The classical output of the quantum circuit is either a 0 or a 1, which is the result of each measurement. The overall architecture of

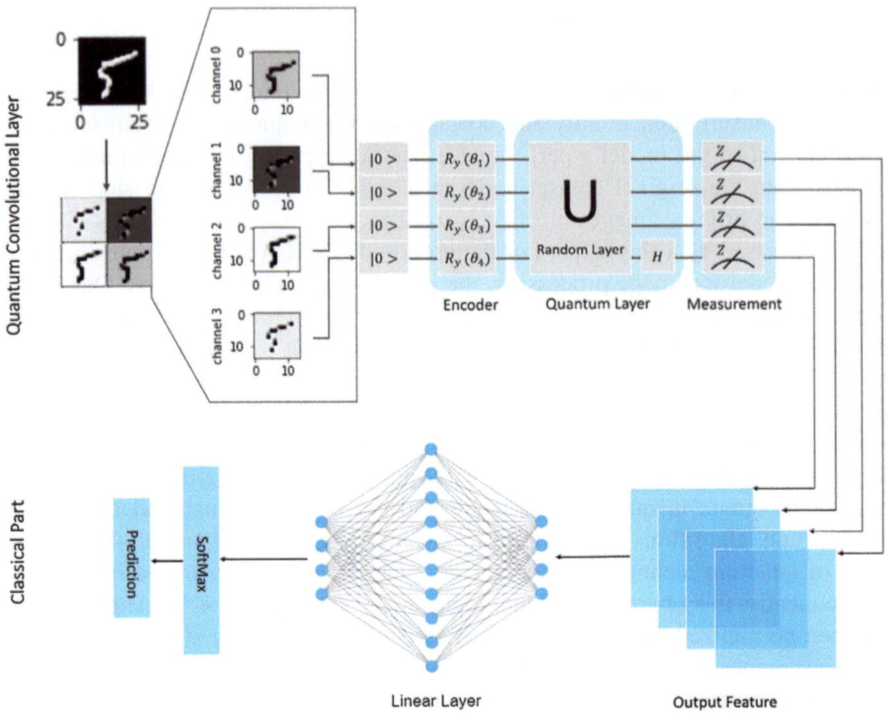

Fig. 3 The Proposed QNN architecture

the proposed QNN method is depicted in Fig. 3. Next, a comprehensive description of each component of QNN is provided.

Encoder Its primary function is to encode the input data into a quantum state that can then be processed by the random layer and measurement components. Creating a quantum circuit that applies the RY gates to each of the input elements in the specified order constitutes the encoding procedure. The circuit's output is a quantum state encoding the input data. This output can then be processed further. A quantum device with four qubits and each with its own wire, is initialized to create the quantum circuit. During the encoding phase, each qubit is subjected to four RY gates. The RY gates play a crucial role in converting the input data into a quantum state that can be further processed by the QNN's random layer and measurement components. The RY gate was chosen due to its ability to perform arbitrary rotations on the state of a qubit, making it suitable for encoding a wide variety of input data.

Quantum Layer The quantum layer is an essential component of the QNN. It includes the ansatz and Hadamard non-parameterized circuits. The ansatz is composed of a series of quantum gates with six adjustable parameters and serves as the core of the quantum layer. These modifiable parameters in the ansatz allow the

QNN to learn and adapt to the particular characteristics of the input data, resulting in an increase in accuracy over time. The non-parameterized Hadamard circuits are also an essential component of the quantum layer. Composed of Hadamard gates that are applied to all qubits [25], it consists of Hadamard gates. These circuits assist in encoding the input data into a quantum state, thereby enabling the QNN to examine a broader range of quantum states and enhancing its classification accuracy. This is accomplished by applying a sequence of quantum gates (unitary operations) generated at random to a given set of quantum wires. In this chapter, the number of operations is set to six, which corresponds to the number of trainable parameters in the ansatz and the range of QNN wires. The integration of the ansatz and Hadamard non-parameterized circuits in the quantum layer, along with the random layer measurement components, produces a flexible and adaptive approach to data, resulting in a complex and dynamic quantum neural network.

Measurement In this step, a measurement operator is applied to each qubit, which collapses the qubits into classical states and determines the model's output. In quantum computing, there are numerous types of measurement operators, including Pauli-X, Pauli-Y, Pauli-Z, and Hadamard operators, each of which collapses the quantum state into a distinct classical state and can be used for a variety of measurement purposes. The choice of measurement operator can significantly impact the QNN's performance. In certain situations, the Pauli-X operator can be used to measure the X-basis of a quantum state, whereas the Pauli-Y operator can be used to measure the Y-basis. Nonetheless, multiple studies have demonstrated the effectiveness of the Pauli-Z measurement operator, particularly for classification tasks [14, 26]. In this chapter, each qubit is measured using the Pauli-Z measurement operator. In the classification task, the output of the measurement phase is used to make predictions.

This study's primary objective is to propose a quantum layer that, when added to a classical neural network (NN), can significantly enhance its performance in image processing applications. This layer is anticipated to leverage the benefits of quantum computing and improve the accuracy of image classification. Unlike the utilized NN machine learning algorithm, in which the original image pixels are treated as features and passed through a linear layer with the softmax activation function, the QNN model adds a quantum layer prior to the linear layer. Figure 4 illustrates how the QNN model's architecture differs from that of the NN model. As can be seen, the NN and QNN models resize the input images to 14×14 pixels. This compact size allows for a clear comparison of the two architectures, highlighting the potential benefits of implementing the proposed QNN. This will be elaborated upon in the results section.

To sum up, for image classification tasks, both QNN and NN employ the same training procedure. Both approaches resize the input images to a fixed size of 14×14 pixels before normalizing the pixel values. The normalized pixel values are used as features in the NN method and are then passed through the linear layer with softmax activation to generate the output class. In contrast, the QNN model has an additional quantum layer preceding the linear layer. The training of the QNN model

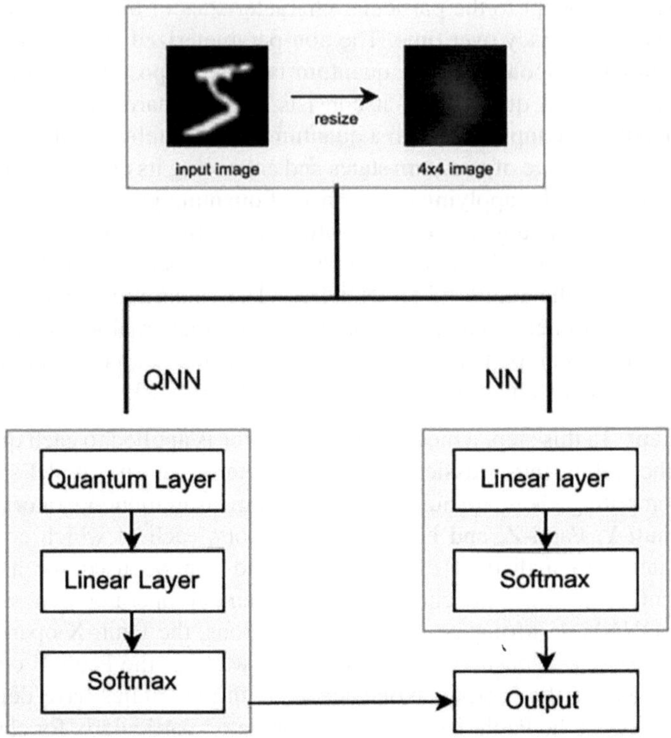

Fig. 4 Architecture of QNN and NN

requires the utilization of a quantum circuit, which was described in the previous section.

Both models are trained using the Adam optimizer algorithm to optimize a loss function. The loss function computes the difference between the expected and observed output of the model. The optimizer algorithm modifies model parameters iteratively to minimize the loss function. In the case of the QNN model, the optimization process involves modifying the quantum circuit parameters. The training processes of both models are repeated for a predetermined number of epochs. This chapter makes use of thirty epochs. The model with the best performance on the validation set is then selected. The trained model is then evaluated on a dataset to determine its performance.

5 Experimental Results and Discussion

In the result section, the outcomes drawn from the image classification algorithm, premised on the introduced quantum neural network (QNN), are meticulously analyzed and evaluated. Four principal empirical investigations have been conducted. The first experiment's objective is to juxtapose the efficacy of the QNN in focus with that of a conventional neural network. The second experiment's purpose is to assess the comprehensive performance of the model in question in relation to accuracy, sensitivity, precision, recall, f-score, and the convergence trajectory. The ultimate experiment is designed to equate the performance of the proffered model with that of other avant-garde models. It is important to underscore that all the investigations implemented were carried out on Google Colab, utilizing PyTorch, Qiskit, and torch quantum libraries. The model was trained for 30 epochs using a batch size of 128 and the Adam optimizer, with an initial learning rate of 5e-3 and a weight decay of 1e-4. All experiments were conducted on a machine equipped with an GPU when available, otherwise defaulting to CPU. The mathematical definition of F1-score, sensitivity, accuracy, and precision is shown in the following equations. Eq. (1) shows the mathematical definition for accuracy, while Eq. (2) shows the mathematical definition for precision, and Eq. (3) shows the mathematical definition for sensitivity or recall measurement. Finally, Eq. (4) shows the mathematical definition for the F1-score measurement.

$$\text{Accuracy} = \frac{\text{TP} + \text{TN}}{\text{TP} + \text{TN} + \text{FN} + \text{FP}} \tag{1}$$

$$\text{Precision} = \frac{\text{TP}}{\text{TP} + \text{FP}} \tag{2}$$

$$\text{Recall (Sensitivity)} = \frac{\text{TP}}{\text{TP} + \text{FN}} \tag{3}$$

$$F1 - \text{Score} = \frac{2\text{TP}}{\text{FN} + \text{FP} + 2\text{TP}} \tag{4}$$

where *FN* indicates the false negative samples, *TP* indicates the true positive samples, *FP* indicates the false positive samples, and *TN* indicates the true negative samples.

Table 2 offers a comparative analysis between the conventional neural network and the QNN, with a focus on quantum circuits, with respect to the mean and standard deviation of the accuracy results. It is noteworthy to mention that the results published in this experiment were deduced from an average of 30 independent trials to evaluate the dependability of the QNN in focus. Moreover, the experiment considered the evaluation of each QNN with an input image size of 14×14, and a neural network with input image sizes of 14×14 and 28×28 within the framework of the proposed image classification model. The size 28×28 was incorporated because it represents the original image size. Evidently, the neural network with an input image size of 28×28 yielded superior results when compared to its 14×14 counterpart. From the aforementioned findings,

Table 2 NN vs. QNN in terms of mean and standard deviation (SD)

	NN (28 × 28)		NN (14 × 14)		QNN (14 × 14)	
	Mean	SD	Mean	SD	Mean	SD
MNIST	91.4	0.01	43.3	0.004	91.6	0.008
PneumoniaMNIST	82.6	0.009	75.4	0.054	83.8	0.005
FashionMNIST	83.4	0.009	54.0	0.007	84.8	0.013
BreastMNIST	79.3	0.04	70.2	0.104	80.5	0.15

it is apparent that an increase in the dimensional size of the input images can substantially influence the effectiveness of a Neural Network. Furthermore, it was noted that the proposed QNN achieved the greatest mean accuracy across all the adopted datasets. Interestingly, the QNN demonstrated the least standard deviation for MNIST, PneumoniaMNIST, and FashionMNIST. It is important to highlight that the QNN, which utilizes an input image size of 14 × 14, exhibited superior results compared to the Neural Network with an input size of 28 × 28. This indicates the significant potential of incorporating quantum computing into traditional Neural Networks, and these results could potentially be augmented by increasing the number of qubits. Considering all the derived results, it is clear that the QNN offers more stability and robustness compared to its conventional counterpart.

To facilitate a more comprehensive examination of the stability inherent in the proposed quantum neural network (QNN) methodology, convergence curves have been constructed for MNIST, FashionMNIST, BreastMNIST, and PneumoniaMNIST, as illustrated in Fig. 5. This figure encapsulates the accuracy outcomes in conjunction with loss value results, obtained from 30 independent runs. In contrast to the conventional convolutional neural network (CNN), the quantum neural network (QNN) shows a substantially faster rate of convergence, as can be seen from the convergence curve. It is clear from this finding that the suggested QNN model can achieve ideal accuracy levels with fewer training cycles. The QNN's fast convergence demonstrates its potential efficiency in learning complicated patterns and achieving high performance early in the training process, which could result in lower computational costs and training time. This behavior suggests that the QNN architecture may outperform classical CNNs, especially in cases where rapid model training and deployment are crucial.

The performance evaluation of the proposed quantum neural network (QNN)-based image classification model, as shown in Fig. 6, highlights its effectiveness across various datasets, including MNIST, PneumoniaMNIST, FashionMNIST, and BreastMNIST. By analyzing accuracy, precision, recall, and F-score, we can assess the model's strengths and identify areas for improvement. On the MNIST dataset, which consists of handwritten digit images, the model achieves outstanding results with an accuracy of 91.6% and nearly equal precision, recall, and F-score values. This balance indicates that the model effectively distinguishes digits while minimizing misclassification, demonstrating strong learning capabilities in general image recognition tasks. Similarly, on FashionMNIST, which contains grayscale

(a)

(b)

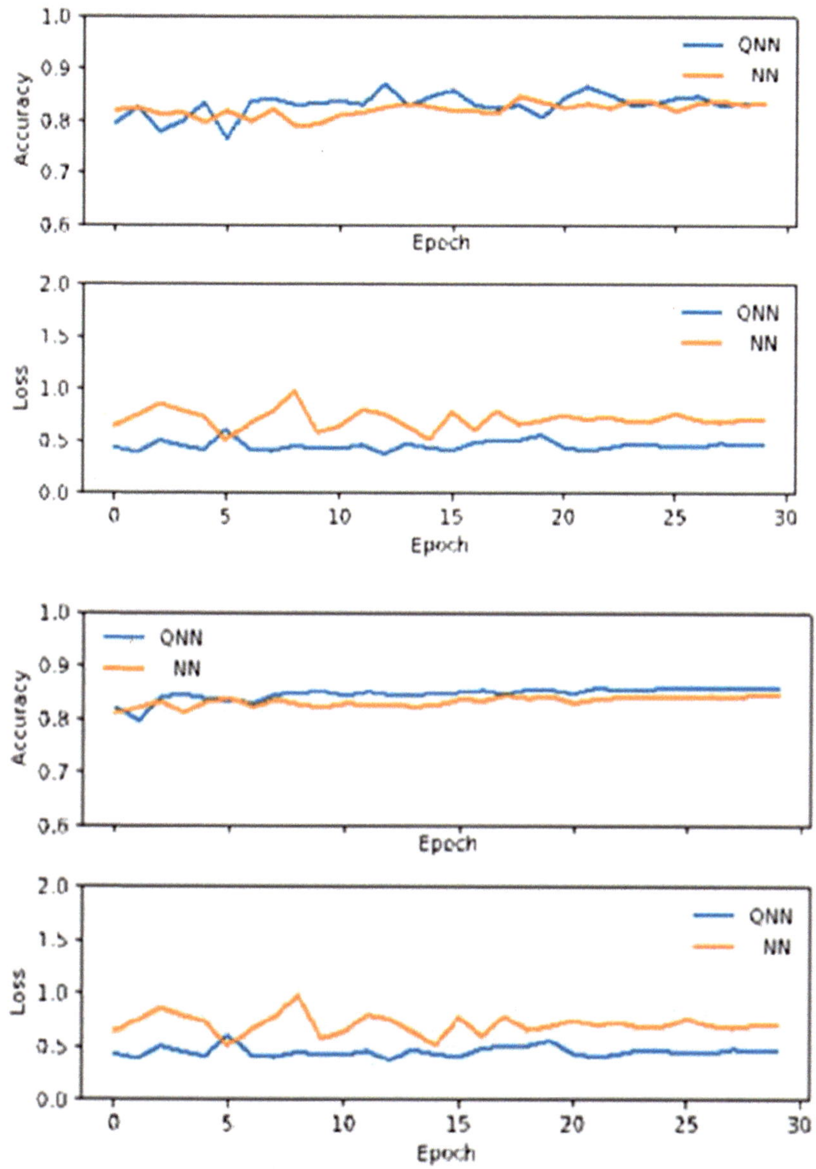

Fig. 5 Convergence curve of the proposed QNN and NN in terms of accuracy and loss for (**a**) PneumoniaMNIST, (**b**) FashionMNIST, (**c**) BreastMNIST, and (**d**) MNIST

(c)

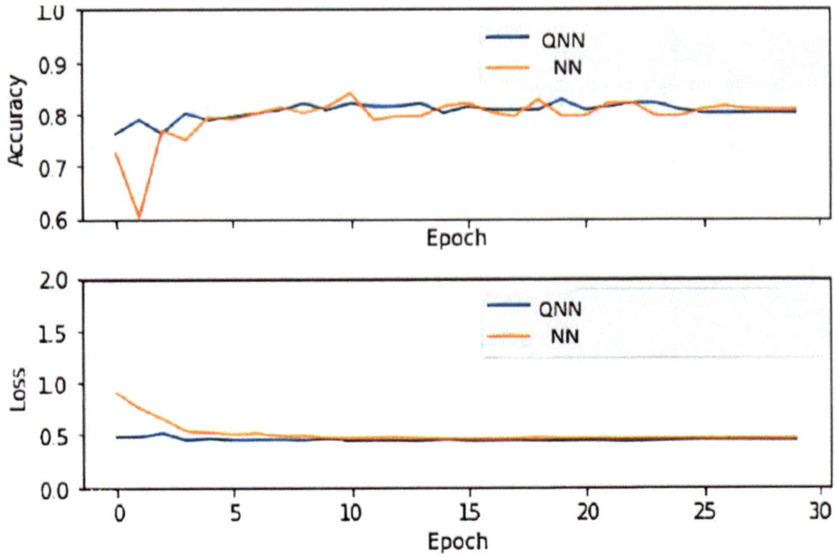

(d)

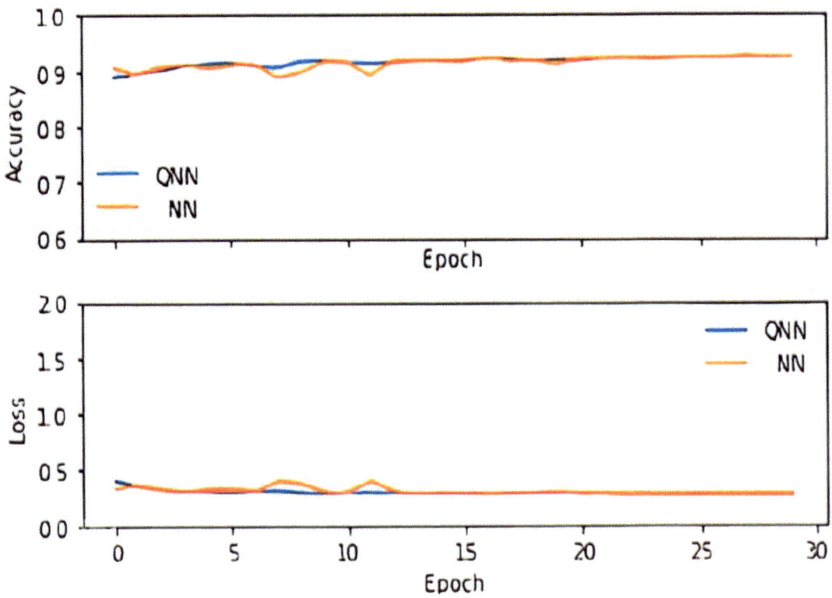

Fig. 5 (continued)

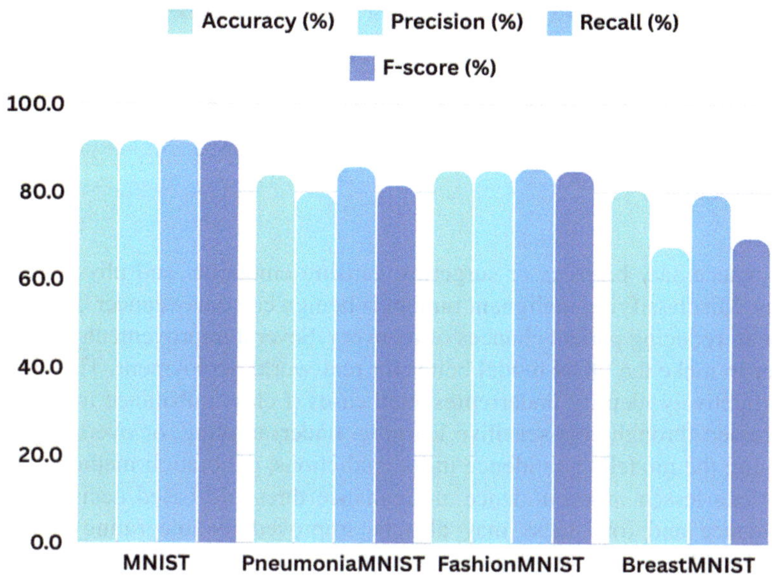

Fig. 6 The performance of QNN for the four adopted datasets in terms of accuracy, precision, recall, and F-score

images of clothing items, the model maintains a high level of performance with an accuracy of 84.8%. The slight advantage in recall (85.3%) suggests that the model prioritizes correctly identifying clothing items over minimizing false positives, which is valuable in classification tasks where sensitivity is important. However, the model's performance declines when applied to medical imaging datasets such as PneumoniaMNIST and BreastMNIST. On PneumoniaMNIST, the model achieves an accuracy of 83.8%, but the lower precision (79.9%) compared to recall (85.7%) suggests a tendency to produce false positives. This imbalance indicates that while the model is effective at detecting pneumonia cases, it may incorrectly classify some healthy cases as pneumonia, which could be problematic in real-world clinical settings. The challenge is even more pronounced in BreastMNIST, where the model records an accuracy of 80.5% but struggles with precision (67.6%) relative to recall (79.5%). This suggests a higher false-positive rate, which could lead to unnecessary follow-up tests or treatments in medical applications where high precision is crucial. Overall, the QNN-based model demonstrates strong performance in general image classification.

The use of medical datasets like BreastMNIST and PneumoniaMNIST presents significant clinical implications when applying machine learning models like the proposed QNN. False positives can lead to unnecessary antibiotic treatments, increased healthcare costs, and psychological distress. False negatives can result in delayed treatment, worsening health conditions, and life-threatening complications, especially for vulnerable populations. In BreastMNIST, false positives can

Table 3 The performance of QNN vs. the state-of-the-art quantum machine learning models

	The proposed QNN	[15]	[16]	[17]	[18]
MNIST	91.6	90.03	77.64	–	–
PneumoniaMNIST	83.8	–	–	87	–
FashionMNIST	84.8	93.63	79.33	–	–
BreastMNIST	80.5	–	–	–	87.5

cause unnecessary biopsies or surgeries, causing emotional and physical harm to patients. Misclassifying malignant tumors is benign can delay cancer diagnosis and treatment, reducing patient chances of recovery. Several improvements are required in order to make the QNN model better for real-world deployment. The model can more effectively identify underrepresented cases if class imbalance in the datasets is addressed through cost-sensitive learning, undersampling, or oversampling. By modifying the model's confidence in its predictions, calibration methods like Platt scaling can lessen overconfidence and enhance threshold-based decision-making. Performance and robustness may also be improved by integrating QNNs with classical models in hybrid or ensemble models.

Table 3 furnishes a comparative study of the performance exhibited by the proposed QNN vs. other cutting-edge quantum machine learning models, all implemented on identical datasets. It can be discerned that the QNN under discussion is highly competitive. The model achieved an accuracy of 86.4% for the ten classes of MNIST and an accuracy of 90.03% for the ten classes of FashionMNIST. However, it is worth mentioning that the quantum models proposed in studies [15, 16] utilize only four classes for both the MNIST and FashionMNIST datasets. Consequently, it is anticipated that the accuracy obtained may witness a decline when the number of classes increases to ten. Furthermore, it is noteworthy to mention that the hybrid quantum-classical convolutional neural networks proposed in the study [18] utilize 8 qubits to achieve the reported accuracy, in contrast to the proposed QNN, which employs merely 4 qubits. A similar observation applies to the quantum-assisted neural networks model proposed in the study [17] wherein the authors employ 8 qubits, as opposed to the QNN under discussion, which utilizes only 4 qubits.

To facilitate a more comprehensive analysis of the performance of the proposed QNN, an additional experiment has been executed. Table 4 compares the performance of the QNN under consideration with two classical convolutional neural network architectures, previously introduced in scholarly literature, on the FashionMNIST dataset. It is essential to note that all comparative architectures employed the same input image size of 14×14. The rationale behind this choice was to ensure a fair comparison, as much as possible. The results generated from this investigation revealed that the proposed QNN is a highly competitive architecture. It achieved optimal results in terms of accuracy, precision, recall, and F1-score. Furthermore, the findings indicated that the QNN model under discussion achieved competitive accuracy despite the constraints imposed by the smaller image size. Additionally, it can be observed that the model proposed in

Table 4 The performance of QNN vs. the state-of-the art classical machine learning models

	The proposed QNN	DARTS [27]	SAM [28]	AlexNet [29]
Accuracy (%)	84.8	81.6	49.1	79.1
Precision (%)	84.8	81.6	49.2	79.2
Recall (%)	85.3	81.5	48.9	79.1
F1 score (%)	84.8	81.4	49.1	79.1

the study [29] employs AlexNet, wherein the input layer must adhere to a specific input size. To navigate this requirement, the images were upsampled to the required input size of 227 × 227 using the zero padding method. Another revelation from the findings is the significant impact of image size on the performance of the model. This observation aligns with the results obtained in Table 2 and underscores the importance of considering image size when designing models for computer vision tasks. The proposed image classification model, which is based on quantum mechanics and neural network principles, shows excellent reliability and resilience based on the obtained results. The study's findings highlight the model's robustness and effectiveness, indicating that it has the potential for larger applications. This method's applicability across many areas can be further validated by expanding its scope to include more complex datasets and real-world use cases.

While the proposed QNN-based image classification model achieves competitive results, it is currently limited to processing downsampled 14 × 14 images and utilizes only 4 qubits for data encoding. While this setting allows for efficient experimentation and demonstration of the proposed QNN architecture, it limits the scalability to higher-resolution images due to the exponential growth of the state space with the number of qubits. Additionally, since the proposed QNN is simulated on classical hardware, the computational cost increases rapidly with more qubits, which constrains the exploration of deeper quantum circuits or larger input dimensions.

6 Conclusion and Future Work

Traditional neural networks usually suffer from small input image sizes because of the limited amount of information that can be analyzed. This chapter presented a quantum neural network (QNN) approach, which effectively employs the concepts of quantum computing to get around this limitation and exhibits encouraging results. The high-dimensional superposition representation of data in a quantum state is made possible by quantum computers. The proposed QNN is utilized for the job of classifying images. In the proposed QNN approach, traditional neural networks are trained for the purpose of image classification using quantum circuits. Using MNIST, PneumoniaMNIST, FashionMNIST, and BreastMNIST as test subjects, the proposed image classification model performed well, with accuracy values of 91.6%, 83.8%, 84.8%, and 80.5%, respectively. The simulation outcomes demonstrated the potential of the proposed model. The results also demonstrated that the proposed QNN approach beat the traditional NN approach and other state-of-the-art models. The results of this study offer a promising framework for additional research in a number of domains. While the proposed QNN-based image classification model achieves competitive results, it is currently limited to processing downsampled 14×14 images and utilizes only 4 qubits for data encoding. Future work will consider expanding the model to handle more qubits, allowing for the processing of larger and more complex image inputs. Furthermore, incorporating quantum-inspired dimensionality reduction or hybrid quantum-classical architectures may assist reduce computational time while improving performance. Furthermore, future research could consider amplitude encoding to represent high-dimensional data effectively with fewer qubits. However, this method has drawbacks such as sensitivity to changes in input, greater processing cost in classical simulation, and complicated state preparation. Furthermore, adopting different quantum circuit architectures (e.g., variational circuits or quantum convolutions) may improve model expressiveness, but also poses challenges such as vanishing gradients, circuit depth constraints, and high simulation complexity. Approximation approaches, circuit optimization, and hybrid quantum-classical methodologies may be required to address these issues.

Acknowledgments We extend our sincere gratitude to Artivay Inc. Company and their Quantum Computing R&D department for their generous sponsorship and invaluable support. Their contribution has been instrumental in the success of our chapter, and we are truly grateful for their partnership.

Statements and Declarations

Statements and Declarations

Author Contributions Design, implementation, methodology, and writing the original draft are performed by H. Kamel, B. Tantawi, and G. Sayed. Data collection and analysis is performed by M. Magdy. Supervision and editing are done by G. Sayed and E. Elsayed. All authors read and approved the final manuscript.

Funding There was no external support for this study.

Data Availability All the adopted datasets are benchmark datasets collected from [19–21].

Disclosure Statement The authors declare that there is no conflict of interest.

Declaration of the Use of AI-Assisted Technologies During the preparation of this work, the authors used Grammarly and ChatGPT to improve the readability and language. After using these tools, the authors reviewed and edited the content as needed and took full responsibility for the content of the publication.

References

1. G. Qu, X. Yu, Z. Wang, Y. Gu, Three quantum neural network architectures for multiclass image classification. ICANCT **13545**, 143–149 (2025). https://doi.org/10.1117/12.3060077
2. A. Toshev, C. Szegedy, Deeppose: Human pose estimation via deep neural networks, in *IEEE/CVF conference on computer vision and pattern recognition*, (IEEE, 2014), pp. 1653–1660. https://doi.org/10.1109/CVPR.2014.214
3. C. Albuquerque, H. Roberto, C. Mauro, Deep learning-based object detection algorithms in medical imaging: Systematic review. Heliyon **11**(1), e41137 (2025)
4. F. Ashiq et al., CNN-based object recognition and tracking system to assist visually impaired people. IEEE Access **10**, 14819–14834 (2022). https://doi.org/10.1109/ACCESS.2022.3148036
5. D. Luo, W. Zeng, J. Chen, W. Tang, Deep learning for automatic image segmentation in stomatology and its clinical application. Front. Med. Technol. (2021). https://doi.org/10.3389/fmedt.2021.767836
6. M. Ramesh, K. Mahesh, Sports video classification framework using enhanced threshold based keyframe selection algorithm and customized CNN on ucf101 and sports1-m dataset. Comput. Intell. Neurosci. **2022**, 1–15 (2022). https://doi.org/10.1155/2022/3218431
7. L. Alzubaidi et al., Review of deep learning: Concepts, CNN architectures, challenges, applications, future directions. J. Big Data **8**, 1–74 (2021). https://doi.org/10.1186/s40537-021-00444-8
8. G. Sayed, M. Soliman, A. Hassanien, Modified optimal foraging algorithm for parameters optimization of support vector machine, in *International conference on advanced machine learning technologies and applications (AMLTA)*, vol. 723, (Springer, 2018), pp. 23–32. https://doi.org/10.1007/978-3-319-74690-6_3
9. L. Chen et al., Review of image classification algorithms based on convolutional neural networks. Remote Sens **13**(22), 1–51 (2021). https://doi.org/10.3390/rs13224712
10. F. Riaz et al., Accurate image multi-class classification neural network model with quantum entanglement approach. Sensors **23**(5), 2753 (2023). https://doi.org/10.3390/s23052753
11. D. Ikemoto et al., Application of neural network-based image analysis to detect sister chromatid cohesion defects. Sci. Rep. **13**(1), 2133 (2023). https://doi.org/10.1038/s41598-023-28742-6
12. O. Kiss, F. Tacchino, S. Vallecorsa, I. Tavernelli, Quantum neural networks force fields generation. Mach. Learn. Sci. Technol. **3**, 1–19 (2022). https://doi.org/10.1088/2632-2153/ac7d3c
13. E. Paquet, F. Soleymani, Quantumleap: Hybrid quantum neural network for financial predictions. Expert Syst. Appl. **195**, 1–7 (2022). https://doi.org/10.1016/j.eswa.2022.116583
14. V. Havlíček et al., Supervised learning with quantum-enhanced feature spaces. Nature **567**(7747), 209–212 (2019). https://doi.org/10.1038/s41586-019-0980-2
15. D. Bokhan et al., Multiclass classification using quantum convolutional neural networks with hybrid quantum-classical learning. Front. Phys. **10**, 1–9 (2022). https://doi.org/10.3389/fphy.2022.1069985
16. A. Chalumuri, R. Kune, B. Manoj, A hybrid classical-quantum approach for multi-class classification. Quantum Inf. Process **20**, 1–19 (2021). https://doi.org/10.1007/s11128-021-03029-9
17. J. Landman et al., Quantum methods for neural networks and application to medical image classification. Quantum **6**, 1–30 (2022). https://doi.org/10.22331/q-2022-12-22-881
18. A. Matic, M. Monnet, J. Lorenz, B. Schachtner, T. Messerer, Quantum-classical convolutional neural networks in radiological image classification, in *QCE24, fifth IEEE international conference on quantum computing and engineering*, (IEEE, 2022), pp. 56–66. https://doi.org/10.1109/QCE53715.2022.00024
19. J. Yang, R. Shi, B. Ni, MedMNIST classification decathlon: A lightweight AutoML benchmark for medical image analysis, in *IEEE international symposium on biomedical imaging*, (IEEE, 2021), pp. 191–195. https://doi.org/10.1109/ISBI48211.2021.9434062

20. H. Xiao, K. Rasul, R. Vollgraf, Fashion-MNIST: a novel image dataset for benchmarking machine learning algorithms (2017). arXiv:1708.07747 [cs.LG]. https://doi.org/10.48550/arXiv.1708.07747
21. L. Deng, The MNIST database of handwritten digit images for machine learning research. IEEE Signal Process. Mag. **29**(6), 141–142 (2012). https://doi.org/10.1109/MSP.2012.2211477
22. C.-F. Chiang, Quantum phase estimation with an arbitrary number of qubits. Int. J. Quant. Inf. **11**(1), 1350008 (2013). https://doi.org/10.1142/S0219749913500081
23. G.I. Sayed, G. Khoriba, M. Haggag, Hybrid quantum salp swarm algorithm for contrast enhancement of natural images. Int. Eng. Syst. **12**(6) (2019). https://doi.org/10.22266/ijies2019.1231.22
24. G.I. Sayed, S. Ibrahim, A. Hassanien, Early detection of red palm weevil in agricultural environment using deep learning. Opt. Mem. Neural Netw. **34**(1), 63–76 (2025). https://doi.org/10.3103/S1060992X24700899
25. W. Liu, W. Li, H. Wang, An improved quantum private set intersection protocol based on Hadamard gates. Int. J. Theor. Phys. **61**, 1–11 (2022). https://doi.org/10.1007/s10773-022-05048-3
26. H. Zhang, L. Ting, L. Fei, Joint mitigation of quantum gate and measurement errors via the Z-mixed-state expression of the Pauli channel. Quantum Inf. Process **23**(6), 213 (2024). https://doi.org/10.1007/s11128-024-04428-4
27. M. Tanveer, M.K. Khan, C. Kyung, Fine tuning DARTS for image classification, in *Proceedings of 16th international conference on pattern recognition*, (IEEE, 2021), pp. 4789–4796. https://doi.org/10.1109/ICPR48806.2021.9412221
28. P. Foret, A. Kleiner, H. Mobahi, B. Neyshabur, Sharpness-aware minimization for efficiently improving generalization (2020). arXiv:2010.01412 [cs.LG]. https://doi.org/10.48550/arXiv.2010.01412
29. M.R. Paul, Classification of garments from fashion-MNIST dataset using AlexNet CNN architecture. EPRA Int. J. Multidiscip. Res. **8**(10), 296–299 (2022)

Explainable Machine Learning Approaches for Cardiovascular Disease Detection: A Comparative Study on the UCI Heart Disease Dataset

Irina Andra Tache and Alina Georgiana Mihăescu

Abstract Cardiovascular disease (CVD) remains the leading cause of mortality and morbidity worldwide, highlighting the necessity for early and accurate risk stratification methods that can improve patient outcomes. This chapter proposes a comparative evaluation of nine supervised machine learning algorithms for the classification of CVD severity. Using the online UCI Heart Disease dataset, each algorithm is evaluated across multiple configurations: a baseline model, three models employing different oversampling techniques, one model with optimized hyperparameters, and finally, the optimized models combined with oversampling.

The presented research findings demonstrate that ensemble-based approaches, particularly CatBoost and XGBoost consistently achieve higher predictive performance than traditional classifiers, especially when combined with oversampling techniques. In addition to performance optimization, this chapter emphasizes explainability to enhance the interpretability of model predictions. SHapley Additive exPlanations are utilized to facilitate clinical integration by improving the transparency of model decision-making. Overall, this study highlights the importance of technical performance and model interpretability in the development of clinically relevant support systems for cardiovascular diagnostics.

Keywords Cardiovascular diseases · Explainable AI · Supervised ensemble learning · Classification

---

I. A. Tache (✉)
Department of Automatic Control and Systems Engineering, National University of Science and Technology Politehnica Bucharest, Bucharest, Romania

Department of Image Fusion and Analysis - Artificial Intelligence, Siemens SRL, Brașov, Romania
e-mail: irina.tache@upb.ro

A. G. Mihăescu
National Institute for Research and Development in Informatics, Bucharest, Romania

Faculty of Automatic Control and Computers, National University of Science and Technology Politehnica Bucharest, Bucharest, Romania
e-mail: alina.mihaescu@ici.ro

N. E. M. Khalifa, M. H. N. Taha (eds.), *Next-Gen Healthcare*,
https://doi.org/10.1007/978-3-032-07267-2_5

Abbreviations

ADASYN	Adaptive synthetic sampling
AUC-ROC	Area under the receiver operating characteristic curve
CatBoost	Categorical boosting
CVD	Cardiovascular disease
EHR	Electronic health record
ENN	Edited nearest neighbors
GDPR	General Data Protection Regulation
KNN	K-nearest neighbor
ML	Machine learning
MLP	Multilayer perceptron
RBF	Radial basis function
RF	Random forest
SHAP	SHapley Additive exPlanations
SMOTE	Synthetic minority oversampling technique
SMOTE-ENN	Synthetic minority oversampling technique with edited nearest neighbors
SVM	Support vector machine
UCI	University of California, Irvine
XAI	Explainable artificial intelligence
XGBoost	Extreme gradient boosting

1 Introduction

Cardiovascular disease (CVD) has become the leading cause of morbidity and mortality worldwide, accounting for over 20 million deaths recorded in 2021 [1].

In the pursuit of improving patient outcomes and reducing adverse clinical events, early and accurate diagnosis of CVD is essential. However, traditional risk assessment models such as the Framingham Risk Score rely heavily on predefined statistical assumptions, therefore lacking patient personalization. The precision of existing methods is not their sole limitation. Current diagnostic workflows are constrained by time, the need for expert interpretation, as well as the lack of feasibility for large-scale preventive screening.

Machine learning (ML) offers an efficient and reliable alternative, identifying complex patterns in clinical datasets, therefore facilitating early detection and assisting clinicians in the diagnosis and treatment of patients, as well as contributing to optimizing patient triage. There are, however, several setbacks when it comes to the adoption of such methods in clinical settings, such as discrepancies between models under real-world class imbalance conditions, the lack of model transparency and interpretability, and challenges in integrating algorithmic observations into clinical reasoning.

The current chapter introduces a comparative study of nine supervised ML algorithms applied to the well-known and frequently used UCI Heart Disease dataset, with the intent of evaluating their diagnostic performance across multiple experimental setups, including baseline, oversampling-enhanced and hyperparameter-tuned configurations. The critical issue of model interpretability is addressed by using the SHAP (SHapley Additive exPlanations) analysis, while the clinical scenarios of clinical data being imbalanced are handled by implementing class-balancing strategies such as SMOTE, SMOTE-ENN and ADASYN.

The fusion of classical performance metrics with model interpretability is aimed at identifying the model configurations that achieve optimal accuracy and offer explanations if the model reached the decision, an essential aspect when it comes to practical clinical adoption.

2 Background and Theoretical Context

2.1 Cardiovascular Disease and Risk Assessment

Cardiovascular diseases include a wide range of pathologies, affecting both the heart and blood vessels, such as coronary artery disease, arrhythmias, and heart failures. Among these, coronary artery disease is the primary contributor to heart attacks and remains an important cause of preventable death globally. In this context, accurate and early detection of cardiovascular disease is essential for reducing clinical complications of patients and improving their quality of life.

Conventional diagnosis approaches such as stress testing, electrocardiography and risk scores are limited by assumptions of linearity, interobserver variability, and lack of ability in capturing complex relationships between risk factors. This might lead to underestimation and misclassification of risk, especially in rare or borderline scenarios [2, 3].

2.2 Machine Learning in Cardiovascular Diagnosis

Machine learning algorithms are data-driven methods, able to detect patterns that may be imperceptible to humans. In the last decades, supervised learning has started to increasingly be utilized on electronic health records (EHR), imaging data, as well as structured clinical datasets to predict cardiovascular outcomes with increasing accuracy. These algorithms rely on the analysis of large datasets to identify patterns and make objective predictions, without the need for human intervention. Unlike traditional approaches that relied on manually hardcoded rule systems, ML systems automatically learn and extract relevant features from data.

This adaptability is particularly useful in cardiac diagnostics, where patient phenotypes are present with overlapping features, resulting in difficult interpretations. The high prevalence of these conditions and the significant impact on population health make the field of cardiology one of the specialties that can most benefit from these models.

ML algorithms can rapidly and accurately analyze large heterogeneous data, from medical history to genetic or lifestyle factors, to develop individual risk prediction models, therefore supporting personalized medicine. Despite these contributions, several concerns remain: lack of transparency, model overfitting, and difficulty in clinical interpretation [4–7].

2.3 *Classification Algorithms*

2.3.1 Logistic Regression

Logistic regression is a probabilistic model, most commonly used to solve classification problems, although it can also be used for regression. It estimates the likelihood of a binary outcome using the logistic (sigmoid) function, transforming a linear combination of predictors into a probability between 0 and 1. This is achieved through the application of the logistic function as shown in Eq. (1):

$$P(y = 1 \mid X) = \frac{1}{1 + e^{-(\beta_0 + \beta_1 X_1 + \cdots + \beta_n X_n)}} \tag{1}$$

Despite its simplicity and computational efficiency, logistic regression assumes that the relationship between features and the target variable is linear, which may not hold in complex clinical datasets. Furthermore, it can suffer from overfitting when applied to high-dimensional data sets. To mitigate this, L1 and L2 regularization techniques can be used [8, 9].

2.3.2 K-Nearest Neighbor

K-nearest neighbor (KNN) is a nonparametric machine learning algorithm for both regression and classification. KNN does not focus on building an internal model but rather stores all instances from the training data into a n-dimensional space, and classifies new instances using a similarity metric. Thus, KNN is based on how similar the vectors are. The algorithm is quite robust to noisy data, but one of its drawbacks is the need for choosing the optimal number of neighbors. Although simple and intuitive, the algorithm suffers from the curse of dimensionality. Its speed decreases as the data volume increases, and its performance can even decrease in the presence of larger data [7–9].

2.3.3 Decision Trees

Decision trees are hierarchical structures used to manage large datasets. It is a rule-based classifier that works by recursively partitioning the feature space into increasingly homogeneous subsets. It usually consists of decision nodes (representing features and splitting criteria), branches (outcomes of the splits), and terminal leaf nodes (predicted classes or values). The splitting process is typically driven by impurity measures such as Gini impurity or entropy.

This algorithm is particularly useful because of its interpretability, and its ability to handle both numerical and categorical data, without any need for prior normalization or transformation. Decision trees are, however, highly susceptible to overfitting, especially when the number of trees grows and begins to introduce noise in the training process. To address this, techniques such as pruning or setting a maximum depth or minimum samples per leaf are implemented. This algorithm serves as the foundation for many models such as random forest and gradient boosting [10].

2.3.4 Random Forest

Random forest (RF) is an ensemble learning algorithm that uses a multitude of decision trees in parallel, on different subsamples of data. Each tree makes its own prediction, and majority voting or averaging determines the final classification. Random forest uses two primary techniques to improve model robustness and reduce variance: bagging and feature randomness. Each tree is trained on a random subset of features considered for splitting at each node. This randomness mitigates overfitting, making the algorithm particularly robust to noise and class imbalance. It manages missing values and maintains high accuracy even with a large number of input features. However, it comes with a relatively high computational cost for large datasets [7, 8, 10].

2.3.5 Support Vector Machine

Support vector machine (SVM) is one of the most widely used supervised learning algorithms, primarily used for binary classifications, though it can be extended to multi-class problems. SVM constructs an optimal hyperplane that maximally separates the data by a margin, so that the decision border can split the n-dimensional space to allow an efficient classification of the new samples. The larger the distance between the hyperplane along with the closest data points from each class, the better the classification performance. However, not all datasets are linearly separable; to address this issue, SVM uses a kernel function to project data into a higher-dimensional space, where a linear separator may exist.

SVM is efficient in high-dimensional spaces and in problems with clear margins of separation. However, its performance is sensitive to parameter tuning, and its computational cost increases with larger datasets [5, 8–10].

2.3.6 Gaussian Naive Bayes

Gaussian naïve Bayes is a widely used machine learning algorithm used to classify data. It is grounded in Bayes' theorem, operating under the simple assumption that all features are statistically independent of each other, given the class label. The Gaussian version of this algorithm is applicable to continuous variables, assuming that their distribution is normal. The model estimates the likelihood of each feature using the Gaussian probability density function. Due to its simple implementation and efficiency, Gaussian naïve Bayes is widely used in the medical field, where interpretability and speed is essential. A major advantage of this algorithm is the fact that it does not need large volumes of data to achieve decent performances. However, the independence assumption is rarely valid in real-world healthcare data, therefore limiting its predictive accuracy in the presence of complex interactions between features [7, 8].

2.3.7 Multilayer Perceptron

A multilayer perceptron is a type of feedforward neural network, a foundational architecture for deep learning networks, designed to learn complex patterns from the input data. They consist of several layers, as follows: an input layer, one or more hidden layers, as well as an output layer. Each neuron computes a weighted sum of its inputs and applies a nonlinear activation function, therefore allowing the model to learn more complex and nonlinear relationships between inputs and outputs.

Training is done by backpropagation, using gradient descent to minimize a loss function, by updating the weights and biases across layers. It offers a large number of adjustable hyperparameters, including the number of hidden layers, learning rate, activation functions, number of epochs, etc. However, its flexibility also leads to increased computational complexity and a greater risk of overfitting, particularly in small or noisy datasets. To address this, techniques such as dropout, early stopping, and L2 regularization are used. In medical applications, MLPs are particularly useful when working with large, structured datasets [8].

2.3.8 XGBoost

XGBoost is an optimized implementation of the gradient boosting algorithm, designed to improve both speed and model performance. It is based on an ensemble learning technique that combines multiple estimators in an iterative manner. It builds and trains a new model, each of these aiming to improve and correct the errors of the previous model. XGBoost extends the principles of previous algorithms by introducing several technical and computational optimizations, including a regularized cost function, which includes an error term and a regularization term that penalizes model complexity, preventing overfitting, parallelization and memory optimization, as well as handling missing values in the dataset, very effective in medical tasks [8, 10].

2.3.9 CatBoost

CatBoost (categorical boosting) is a gradient boosting algorithm designed to improve performance on datasets with categorical features. Unlike other boosting implementations, CatBoost directly handles categorical features without requiring external preprocessing, uses ordered boosting, thus reducing the risk of data leakage and improving generalization. CatBoost is robust to overfitting, requires minimal data preprocessing, and offers high performance, especially on data with many categorical features [11].

2.4 Oversampling Techniques for Class Imbalance

Most clinical datasets suffer from class imbalance, a common challenge in medical data processing that creates major difficulties for ML algorithms which can be biased to favor the majority class. Such imbalances can lead to missed diagnoses through high false negatives rates, or on the contrary, can contribute to high false positive rates, leading to unnecessary additional investigations for the patient. To mitigate this issue, there are implemented three oversampling strategies such as:

Synthetic minority oversampling technique (SMOTE) is one of the most popular oversampling techniques addressing the issue of class imbalance in tasks of supervised learning.

SMOTE operates by identifying the k nearest neighbors for each sample belonging to the minority class and generating synthetic samples along the line segments connecting each minority class sample to its k nearest neighbors from the same class. Given a minority instance x_0, and one of its nearest neighbors x_k, a new synthetic point z is created with linear interpolation, as shown in Eq. (2):

$$z = (1 - \omega)\, x_0 + \omega x_k, \qquad \text{where } \omega \in (0, 1) \tag{2}$$

This interpolation expands the decision region, forcing it to be more general, by spreading the minority class data across its local neighborhood. However, SMOTE has several limitations, including the fact that it may generate data in regions where classes overlap, increasing the risk of ambiguity in classification [12, 13].

Adaptive synthetic sampling (ADASYN) is an extension of SMOTE, developed to address several limitations of this technique. The main advantage of ADASYN is the adaptive generation of synthetic samples depending on the learning difficulty of each instance. Thus, more synthetic samples are created in regions where the minority class samples are more difficult to learn, being surrounded by samples belonging to the majority class.

This adaptive behavior is achieved through a weighting mechanism that quantifies the local learning difficulty for each minority sample x_i. Specifically, the local imbalance degree r_i is calculated as:

$$r_i = \frac{\Delta_i}{K} \quad (3)$$

where Δ_i represents the number of majority class samples among the K-nearest neighbors of x_i. The value $r_i \epsilon$ [0, 1] reflects the complexity of the local region. The higher the value of r_i, the more difficult it is to learn that sample correctly.

Subsequently, a normalized weight is computed to determine the proportion G_i of synthetic samples that should be generated for each sample x_i, based on the overall distribution of difficulty across all minority samples:

$$G_i = \frac{r_i}{\sum_{j=1}^{N_{\min}} r_j} \cdot G \quad (4)$$

where G is the total number of synthetic samples to generate, G_i is the number of synthetic samples to generate for the sample x_i, and $N_{\min}$ is the number of minority samples.

Finally, each synthetic sample z is generated using a linear interpolation between x_i and one of its minority neighbors $x_{i,\,k}$, using a random weight between 0 and 1, as shown in Eq. (5):

$$z = x_i + \delta \cdot \left(x_{i,k} - x_i\right), \qquad \text{where } \delta \in (0, 1) \quad (5)$$

By focusing on difficult areas of the dataset, ADASYN improves the robustness of the models, but it also comes with the additional risk of amplifying noise in the data, especially in the case of regions with high ambiguity [14].

Synthetic minority oversampling technique with edited nearest neighbors (SMOTE-ENN) is a hybrid method, combining the advantages of oversampling via SMOTE with those of informative undersampling via ENN (edited nearest neighbors). After generating synthetic samples using SMOTE, ENN is applied to eliminate those samples that are considered noisy or difficult to classify, by analyzing their nearest neighbors and eliminating instances that differ from the majority of their neighbors. This combination helps to smooth out the decision boundary between classes, eliminating points that present ambiguity or noise, and leads to a clearer separation between classes in the dataset [14, 15].

While several alternative techniques exist to address class imbalance, the proposed approach focuses on oversampling due to its practical advantages in medical datasets. Undersampling may discard informative samples, which is particularly problematic in small datasets. Similarly, class weights require careful hyperparameter tuning, and they still often underperform when the minority class is severely underrepresented. Albattah et al. exemplify that imbalanced datasets are consistently outperformed by balanced ones, highlighting the importance of balancing techniques. Their comparative evaluation, which includes class balancers and distribution-based resampling, shows that synthetic oversampling offers the most scalable and model-agnostic solution. In the current context, oversampling allows the dataset to maintain the original samples while also improving model performance when it comes to the underrepresented cases [16].

2.5 SHAP Analysis for Model Interpretability

Among the most important challenges in the deployment of ML models in clinical settings is their lack of explainability. While these algorithms may achieve state-of-the-art performance metrics values in classification tasks, nontechnical healthcare professionals may be reluctant to use AI predictions in clinical practice, due to their decision processes not being transparent.

To address this, explainable artificial intelligence (XAI) techniques have been developed, making complex models interpretable. One of the most robust and theoretically grounded methods is SHapley Additive exPlanations (SHAP).

SHAP is a multivariate feature importance analysis based on the principles of cooperative game theory, specifically on Shapley values, which assign a value to each player (feature) in a game (model prediction), based on their individual contribution to the outcome.

In the context of a classification model entitled $f(x)$, SHAP aims to express the prediction as an additive combination of feature contributions, as described in Eq. (6):

$$f(x) = \phi_0 + \sum_{i=1}^{M} \phi_i \tag{6}$$

where ϕ_0 is the base value, hence the average model output across all samples, and ϕ_i is the SHAP value representing the contribution of feature i to the deviation from the base value.

Features are rewarded based on their marginal contributions across all possible feature subsets. Therefore, SHAP both ensures transparency and contributes to regulatory compliance (such as GDPR or medical AI guidelines) and ethical AI deployment in healthcare [17, 18].

3 Dataset and Methodology

3.1 UCI Heart Disease Dataset

UCI heart disease is one of the most widely used datasets in scientific literature for predicting and classifying cardiovascular disease using ML techniques. The dataset

Table 1 Description of the dataset features

Feature	Description	Type
Id	Patient ID	Numerical
Age	Patient age	Numerical
Sex	Patient sex ('male', 'female')	Categorical
CP	Type of chest pain ('typical angina', 'asymptomatic', 'non-anginal', 'atypical angina')	Categorical
Trestbps	Resting blood pressure (mmHg)	Numerical
Chol	Serum cholesterol (mg/dl)	Numerical
Fbs	Blood glucose concentration >120 mg/dl (1 = true, 0 = false)	Categorical
Restecg	Resting electrocardiogram results ('lv hypertrophy', 'normal', 'st-t abnormality')	Categorical
Thalach	Maximum heart rate	Numerical
Exang	Exercise induced angina (1 = yes, 0 = no)	Categorical
Oldpeak	ST segment depression	Numerical
Slope	ST slope when exercising ('downsloping', 'flat', 'upsloping')	Categorical
CA	Number of major blood vessels colored with fluoroscopy	Categorical
Thal	Thalassemia test results ('fixed defect', 'normal', 'reversible defect')	Categorical
Num	Cardiovascular disease severity (0–4)	Categorical

is publicly available by accessing the UCI Irvine Machine Learning Repository. The data was originally acquired for medical research purposes, and it is the results of a collaboration between several medical institutions: the Cleveland Clinic Foundation, the Hungarian Institute of Cardiology, University Hospital Zurich and V.A. Medical Center Long Beach.

The dataset contains 920 samples and 16 features, including demographic variables such as age and sex, clinical variables such as blood pressure, cholesterol, as well as results of other clinical tests. The goal is to examine the association between these factors and the severity of heart disease.

The target variable num has values from 0 to 4, representing different levels of the severity of cardiovascular disease. Due to the moderate size of the dataset and the clinical relevance of these features, this dataset represents an ideal case for testing and comparing various ML algorithms across multiple configurations. Table 1 provides a description of the dataset's features, along with their respective types.

Despite its widespread use, the UCI heart disease dataset has several limitations that might affect its generalizability. The first limitation has to do with the nature of the dataset itself and the way the data was acquired. As previously mentioned, it was compiled from four institutions: Cleveland ($n = 304$), Hungary ($n = 293$), VA Long Beach ($n = 200$), and Switzerland ($n = 123$). Figure 1 shows data distribution across these institutions.

While the dataset was constructed using consistent exclusion criteria, subtle differences in clinical environment and data collection practices might introduce variation in the dataset. However, because the study that introduced the dataset provides limited information regarding demographics and instrumentation and

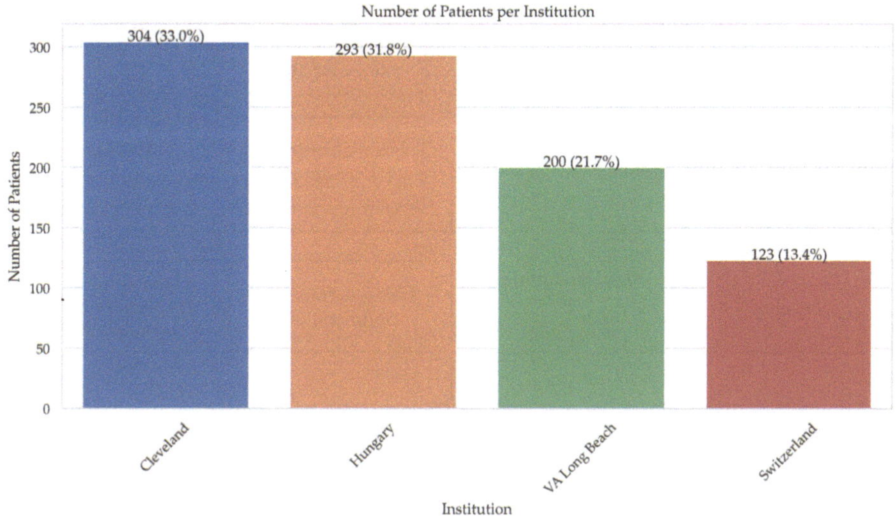

Fig. 1 Data distribution across institutions

diagnostic workflows, it is difficult to assess the extent of such institutional heterogeneity.

Additionally, the dataset lacks information on the race, ethnicity and socioeconomic status of the patients, known factors that contribute to cardiovascular risk assessment and to an important impact on diagnostic accuracy. Since three out of the four institutions are in majority-European countries, it is most likely that the data is highly skewed towards individuals of European descent. Furthermore, there is a temporal gap between the data collection, since it was acquired between 1981 and 1984, and its relatively small sample size further limits applicability in modern populations where disease representation and diagnostic standards have constantly evolved [19].

3.2 Solution Workflow

The proposed solution involves the implementation and comparative evaluation of nine machine learning algorithms for the classification of cardiovascular disease severity using the above-described UCI Heart Disease dataset.

In order to obtain a rigorous and unbiased assessment of model performance and to prevent data leakage, several pipelines were built. Each algorithm was encapsulated within a structured processing pipeline. These pipelines perform numerical data scaling and categorical data encoding and conditionally apply oversampling techniques.

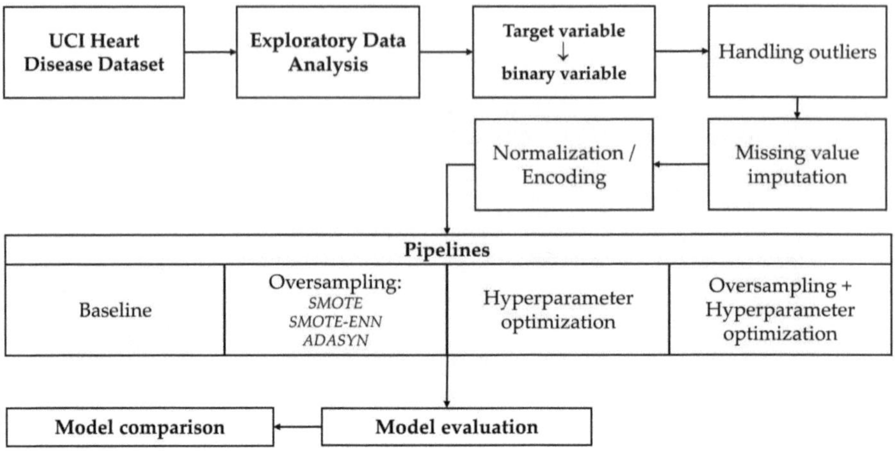

Fig. 2 General workflow diagram

To address the issue of class imbalance, a common challenge in medical datasets, three oversampling methods were evaluated: SMOTE, SMOTE-ENN, and ADASYN. These techniques were applied exclusively to the training data within each pipeline, ensuring that no information from the test set influenced model training or validation. Each model was trained under four distinct configurations, designed to isolate the effects of oversampling and hyperparameter optimization:

- Baseline model: without applying oversampling techniques, with standard hyperparameters.
- Oversampling model: applying the oversampling techniques SMOTE, SMOTE-ENN, and ADASYN.
- Optimized model: using hyperparameter optimization procedures.
- Optimized model and using oversampling techniques: combining both oversampling techniques and hyperparameter optimization.

Model evaluation was performed on previously unseen test sets based on performance metrics such as accuracy, precision, recall, specificity, F1-Score, and AUC-ROC. This approach allows the identification of the best performing model and provides insight into the individual and combined impact of oversampling and parameter optimization on diagnostic performance.

To visually summarize this approach, Fig. 2 presents the general workflow diagram of the proposed solution, illustrating the end-to-end process, including how each algorithm was integrated into a structured configuration to analyze the individual and combined effect of oversampling and hyperparameter optimization on model performance.

3.3 Preprocessing Steps

Data preprocessing is an essential step for any machine learning project, and it directly impacts model performance. The purpose of this process is to ensure data compatibility with the algorithms is to be implemented. Preprocessing involved handling missing values and outliers and normalizing and scaling features.

Target feature conversion to a binary variable. To facilitate the classification task, the target variable num was transformed from a variable with values between 0 and 4 to a binary variable, where 0 indicates the absence of heart disease (corresponding to the original values 0 and 1), and 1 signals the presence of a moderate or severe form of the disease (corresponding to values equal or greater than 2).

The threshold was selected to distinguish between patients with minimal signs of heart disease from those with severe forms of illness, requiring medical attention.

From a clinical perspective, the conversion to a binary target variable aligns with real-world decision making, where detecting whether heart disease is present at all is the primary concern. This approach is more suitable for early disease screening, where the priority is to flag patients potentially at risk and prompt further testing, rather than identifying the severity level.

From a statistical standpoint, the data is highly imbalanced, with most cases falling in the negative category, with a low severity level of heart disease. Maintaining the target variable as a multi-class attribute might lead to unstable estimates and poor generalization, especially for higher severity classes, with fewer samples. Binarizing the variable mitigates this limitation and results in a more robust training and evaluation process.

This binarization strategy has previously been employed by several studies showcasing its impact on model performance. For instance, Kibria et al. compared binary versus multi-class classification using the Cleveland UCI dataset. They have reported a significant performance improvement after converting the target variable to a binary one: while multi-class classification obtained approximately 75% accuracy, binary classification reaches up to 95%, therefore demonstrating the value of this conversion for reliable model performance [20].

To better illustrate the effect of the target variable conversion step, Fig. 3 shows the distribution of data before and after transforming the original multi-class feature into a binary variable. As depicted, the dataset remains imbalanced, negative cases being significantly more prevalent than positive ones.

Data imputation is the process of replacing missing values with appropriate ones, as the presence of incomplete data can introduce significant bias and disrupt algorithm learning [21, 22].

In this study, different imputation strategies were chosen based on the type of variable and the proportion of missingness per feature, guided by the distribution, shown in Fig. 4. For features with more than 30% missing values, Random Forest imputation was used due to its ability to capture non-linear relationships, as well as interactions between variables. This is a non-parametric technique that treats each feature that contains missing values as a target to be predicted from the remaining

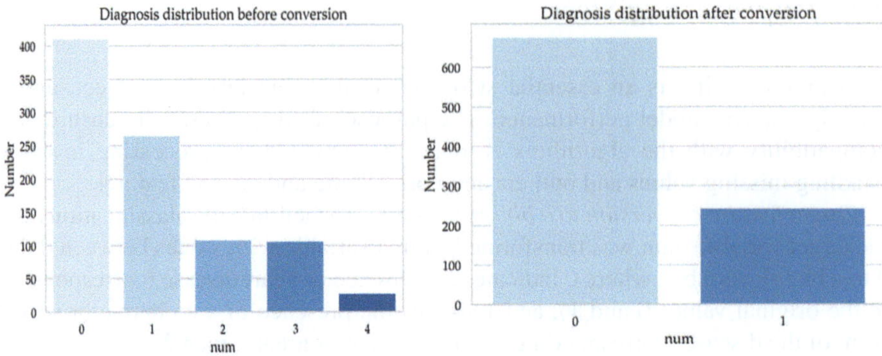

Fig. 3 Data distribution before and after conversion

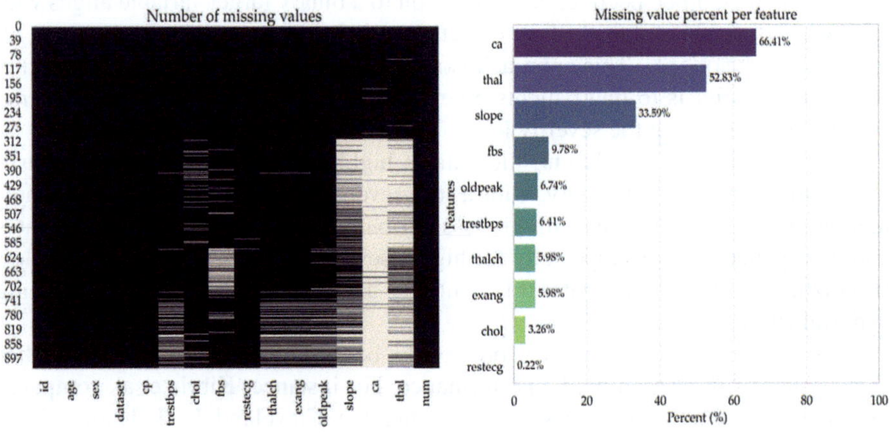

Fig. 4 Distribution of missing values among features

data. It is especially useful in medical data, where the relationships among attributes are complex.

In the case of categorical variables with less than 30% missingness, mode imputation was applied. While this approach is simple, its use is justified by the lack of distortion of class frequencies and the fact that it preserves the most frequent category. Because of its robustness to outliers, for numerical attributes with less than 30% missingness, median imputation was employed. The 30% threshold was chosen based on practical criteria, to be consistent with thresholds commonly used in applied data science.

Outlier Handling Outliers are values that deviate significantly from the rest of the data and can negatively impact the performance of machine learning models, especially those sensitive to scale, such as logistic regression or KNN. Outliers were visually detected by using boxplots for continuous variables. However, it is

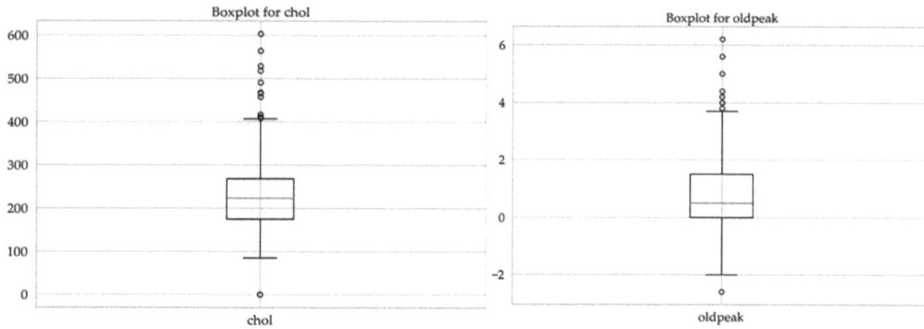

Fig. 5 Outlier detection for cholesterol and ST segment depression

important to note that outliers in medical datasets are not always erroneous or irrelevant but may indicate extreme but clinically plausible situations that could be useful in model prediction. Outliers were identified for the following features:

- Trestbps: Values of 0 mmHg were identified as outliers and were considered erroneous, but values of 175–200 mmHg could be plausible for hypertensive patients. Similarly, a value of 75 mmHg is also possible.
- Chol: Values between 400 and 600 mg/dL, although extreme, may occur in patients with hypercholesterolemia, and should not be discarded. However, values of 0 mg/dL are considered erroneous.
- Thalch: A few values between 60–80 have been observed, which are within acceptable limits for elderly patients or patients with severe cardiovascular problems.
- Oldpeak: A value below −2 has been identified, which is not clinically plausible. Values between 3 and 6 may indicate severe myocardial disease and therefore may appear clinically.

Figure 5 presents two examples of outlier detection using boxplots for assisting the distinction between clinically plausible extremes and data entry errors. Clinically plausible values were retained for their medical significance. However, values of 0 encountered for trestbps or chol were replaced with np.nan and were to be imputed. The value of −2 for oldpeak is most likely a data entry error and was replaced with 0.

Categorical Variable Encoding Machine learning algorithms require numerical representations of data, which is why all categorical variables were transformed using One-Hot Encoding. This process was applied using OneHotEncoder, integrated into a ColumnTransformer, which creates a binary column for each distinct category.

Numerical Features Scaling Numerical features (age, chol, trestbps, thalach, oldpeak) often have different scales and distributions, which can negatively impact the performance of algorithms such as KNN, SVM, or logistic regression. To address this, numerical data standardization was applied. This procedure was performed using the StandardScaler class. As a result, all numerical variables were transformed so that they had a mean of 0 and a standard deviation of 1.

3.4 Model Training Strategies

To ensure reproducibility and methodological rigor, each of the 9 machine learning models was trained under a controlled, standardized pipeline. These pipelines included all necessary preprocessing steps and experimental conditions, such as optional oversampling and hyperparameter optimization.

The models were evaluated using cross-validation technique by splitting the training and testing data using an 80/20 percentage, preserving the original class distribution in both subsets, in order to maintain class balance and to prevent biased evaluation results.

To address the risk of overfitting and to fine-tune model performance, all hyperparameter optimizations were performed using a ten-fold cross-validation. The parameter search was conducted using randomized search, and the scoring metric for cross-validation optimization was AUC-ROC, selected for its robustness to class imbalance.

Each model was evaluated under 8 distinct configurations:

- A baseline model;
- Three models using oversampling: SMOTE, SMOTE-ENN, and ADASYN;
- A model with optimized hyperparameters;
- Three optimized models for which oversampling approach was applied.

All data transformations were applied only to the training set, to avoid data leakage, and for reproducibility and fairness, the same random seed was used across all experiments.

3.5 Evaluation Metrics

For a comprehensive assessment of model performance, several classification metrics were evaluated on the test set. These metrics reflect various aspects of the diagnostic abilities of the models and are particularly relevant in the context of clinical decision-making.

- Accuracy denoting the proportion of correct predictions among all predictions:

$$\text{Accuracy} = \frac{\text{TP} + \text{TN}}{\text{TP} + \text{TN} + \text{FP} + \text{FN}} \tag{7}$$

- Precision is the proportion of true positive predictions among all the positive predictions made by the model:

$$\text{Precision} = \frac{\text{TP}}{\text{FP} + \text{TP}} \tag{8}$$

- Recall (or sensitivity) reflects the proportion of actual positive cases that were correctly identified:

$$\text{Recall} = \frac{\text{TP}}{\text{TP} + \text{FN}} \tag{9}$$

- Specificity denoting the proportion of actual negative cases correctly identified by the model:

$$\text{Specificity} = \frac{\text{TN}}{\text{TN} + \text{FP}} \tag{10}$$

- F1-Score is the harmonic mean of precision and recall, offering a balance between false positive and false negatives:

$$F1 = 2 \cdot \frac{\text{Precision} \cdot \text{Recall}}{\text{Precision} + \text{Recall}} = \frac{2 \cdot \text{TP}}{2 \cdot \text{TP} + \text{FN} + \text{FP}} \tag{11}$$

- AUC-ROC (area under the receiver operating characteristic curve): A threshold independent metric that evaluates the model's ability to distinguish between classes.

4 Results and Comparative Analysis

This chapter presents the experimental findings obtained from a comparison of 9 supervised machine learning models applied to the classification of cardiovascular disease using the UCI heart disease dataset. Each model was evaluated under eight distinct configurations to assess the impact of oversampling and hyperparameter optimization on model performance. The goal was to identify which algorithms and configurations provided the most reliable, robust, accurate and clinically relevant predictions, while maintaining interpretability.

The primary motivation for this analysis stems from the complexity of cardiovascular disease diagnosis, and the fact that overlapping features or subtle patterns make decision frameworks inefficient. In such contexts, predictive models must not only show strong performances but also support clinical workflows through transparency and robustness to data imbalance.

4.1 Models' Performances

Table 2 summarizes the performance metrics obtained across the best performing models and configurations on the test set. As shown, ensemble-based models, and particularly those based on boosting, consistently outperformed linear and non-ensemble baselines. This trend is visible across all metrics but has been highlighted especially in F1-scores and AUC-ROC, reflecting the models' generalization abilities and their ability to manage class imbalance.

CatBoost presented the most robust and highest overall performance across all configurations, especially when combined with ADASYN and hyperparameter tuning. Notably, it achieved the highest AUC-ROC, indicating a superior ability in distinguishing between healthy patients and those with severe cardiovascular disease.

XGBoost followed closely, with high results in both recall and specificity. Its gradient boosting algorithm is resilient across configurations, particularly when applying hyperparameter tuning, where fine adjustments to learning rate and tree depth proved to significantly improve performance.

Random Forest had very strong baseline results, without the need for extensive tuning, indicating that the simple use of multiple decision trees already captured much of the predictive structure necessary for the classification of the dataset. However, this model has been less responsive to oversampling compared to the other models, especially boosting ones.

SVM had great performances in terms of recall, especially when using ADASYN or SMOTE-ENN. This is especially important to note, since for this specific classification task, detecting positive cases is far more important than reducing the rate of false positives. SVM has, however, struggled with recall under imbalance conditions, and has lower precision. Hyperparameter tuning improved the performance slightly, but performance remained sensitive to oversampling techniques.

Multilayer perceptron offered competitive results when hyperparameter tuning was applied. Despite this, performance was more volatile compared to tree-based models, and its sensitivity to feature scaling and parameter initialization made it more difficult to stabilize.

Table 2 The five selected models for best performances

Model	Accuracy	Precision	Recall	Specificity	F1-Score	AUC-ROC
CatBoost + ADASYN	0.886	0.741	0.878	0.889	0.804	0.948
SVM + ADASYN	0.897	0.75	0.918	0.889	0.826	0.936
Optimized XGBoost + ADASYN	0.891	0.764	0.857	0.904	0.808	0.935
Optimized CatBoost + SMOTE	0.87	0.698	0.898	0.859	0.786	0.946
CatBoost + SMOTEENN	0.88	0.714	0.918	0.867	0.804	0.937

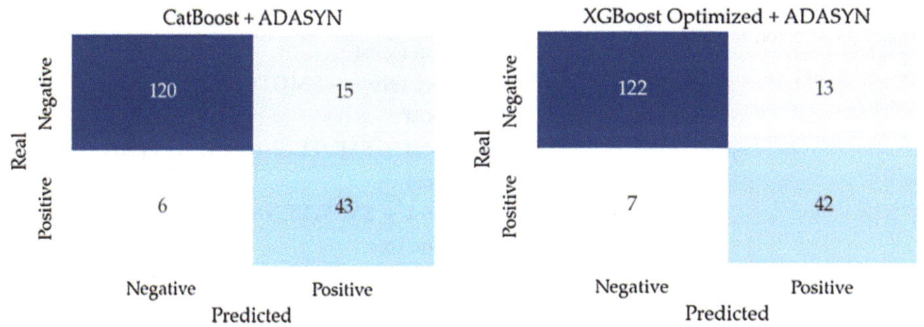

Fig. 6 Confusion matrices for CatBoost + ADASYN and XGBoost Optimized + ADASYN

Logistic regression and Gaussian naïve Bayes demonstrated decent accuracy but were outperformed by nonlinear models in F1-score and AUC-ROC. As expected, naïve Bayes suffered from conditional independence assumptions that do not function well within this dataset. K-nearest neighbors was notably affected by the presence of class imbalance, but its performance improved with oversampling. Figure 6 presents the confusion matrices for two well performing configurations: CatBoost with ADASYN and XGBoost with ADASYN and hyperparameter optimization.

4.2 Impact of Oversampling

Data imbalance is among the most pressing challenges in medical classification tasks, as false negatives may result in missed diagnoses with potentially fatal outcomes. Improving recall without sacrificing overall precision is essential in the development of a clinically adoptable diagnostic tool. To address this, we applied three oversampling techniques across all models: SMOTE, SMOTE-ENN, and ADASYN.

A significant improvement in performance was observed, especially in terms of recall and F1 score. This was expected, given the class imbalance and the fact that the positive class was in the minority. Therefore, SMOTE, SMOTE-ENN and ADASYN had a significant impact on the models that initially had poorer performance in correctly detecting positive cases, that is, those of patients with severe cardiovascular problems.

CatBoost and XGBoost are among the models which showed the best response to oversampling. When combined with ADASYN, both improved their recall (+8–12%) and F1-score (+6–9%) over their respective baseline models. When applying SMOTE-ENN, random forest's recall increases by 10%, with a small decrease in specificity.

Table 3 Oversampling impact on selected models

Model	Recall	F1
Random forest	0.673	0.710
Random forest + SMOTEENN	0.858	0.770
XGBoost	0.755	0.747
XGBoost + SMOTEENN	0.816	0.762
CatBoost	0.816	0.792
CatBoost + SMOTEENN	0.918	0.804
DecisionTree	0.653	0.681
DecisionTree + SMOTEENN	0.775	0.730
LogisticRegression	0.837	0.759
LogisticRegression + ADASYN	0.898	0.765
SVM	0.898	0.822
SVM + ADASYN	0.918	0.826

Oversampling enhanced recall substantially in SVM and MLP, which otherwise underperform in the initial imbalanced scenario. SVM, in particular, had an extreme increase in recall with SMOTE, notable even with a slight decrease in precision.

Simpler models such as KNN, naïve Bayes, and logistic regression had modest gains from oversampling, with small improvements in recall and AUC-ROC. Due to their inherent limitations of capturing complex relationships, they do not benefit as much as ensemble or kernel-based models.

In terms of technique comparison, SMOTE offered general improvements across models, improved recall, but led to drops in precision in sensitive models. SMOTE-ENN, however, delivered the most balanced improvement. It maintained high precision while significantly boosting recall. ADASYN had important increases in F1-score and recall when used with ensemble models, but also SVM and logistic regression.

To quantify the effects of the oversampling techniques, Table 3 presents the recall and F1-score metrics for a selection of models before and after applying oversampling. These values show the improvement in evaluation metrics, particularly for ensemble models like XGBoost and CatBoost.

4.3 Impact of Hyperparameter Optimization

Hyperparameter optimization plays an important role in machine learning performance, especially for those sensitive to parameter selection. Optimal hyperparameters can significantly enhance a model's ability to discriminate between high-risk and low-risk patients.

In this study, hyperparameter tuning was conducted using randomized search with ten-fold cross-validation on the training set. Table 4 presents the hyperparameter search space, along with the corresponding value ranges tested during the tuning phase.

Table 4 Hyperparameters used to tune the models

Algorithm	Hyperparameter	Tested values
Random forest	Number of estimators	100, 200
	Maximum depth	None, 10, 20
	Minimum samples per split	2, 10, 20
	Minimum samples per leaf	1, 2, 5
	Maximum features	Auto, sqrt, log2
	Use bootstrap samples	True, false
Logistic regression	Regularization parameter (C)	0.01, 0.1, 1, 10
	Penalty type	l2, l1
	Solver algorithm	Liblinear, saga
SVM	Kernel coefficient (gamma)	0.1, 1, 10
	Kernel type	Scale, auto
	Degree of polynomial kernel	Linear, poly, rbf
	Number of neighbors	3, 5, 7
KNN	Weight function	3, 5, 7
	Distance metric	Uniform, distance
	Maximum depth	Euclidean, Manhattan
Decision tree	Minimum samples per split	5, 10, 20
	Minimum samples per leaf	2, 10, 20
	Maximum features	1, 2, 5
	Hidden layer sizes	Auto, sqrt
MLP	L2 regularization term (alpha)	(50, 100)
	Activation function	1e-4, 1e-3
	Learning rate	Relu, tanh
	Number of estimators	Constant, invscaling, adaptive
XGBoost	Subsample ratio	100, 200
	Column subsample by tree	3, 5
	Maximum depth	0.01, 0.1, 0.2
	Number of iterations	0.8, 1.0
	L2 leaf regularization	0.8, 1.0
CatBoost	Number of estimators	4, 6
	Maximum depth	0.01, 0.1
	Minimum samples per split	100, 200, 500
	Minimum samples per leaf	1, 3, 5

Hyperparameter optimization had a different impact on each type of machine learning model. While for some models, fine-tuning led to notable performance improvements, for others, these adjustments did not produce significant effects. These variations can be due to several factors: the sensitivity of the model to hyperparameter tuning, the complexity of the parameter space, the robustness of the algorithm to noise, as well as the nature of the dataset.

Among the models with the most significant improvements is XGBoost, for which, in the case of applying ADASYN without optimization, an accuracy of 0.875

Table 5 Model configurations positively impacted by hyperparameter optimization

Model	Accuracy
XGBoost + ADASYN	0.875
XGBoost optimized + ADASYN	0.891
KNN	0.837
KNN optimized	0.859
KNN + ADASYN	0.804
KNN optimized + ADASYN	0.832
XGBoost	0.864
XGBoost optimized	0.875

is obtained. After optimization, the accuracy increases to 0.891. The performance increase is due to the fact that XGBoost is an extremely flexible model, sensitive to hyperparameters such as max_depth, learning_rate, n_estimators and subsample. Optimization allows the control of overfitting, which is otherwise common in models that apply boosting. Similarly, CatBoost showed increased performance across folds and improved handling of class imbalance when tuned, while KNN had a 2–3% improvement in accuracy.

One of the models for which optimization did not have a significant impact on performance is random forest. Accuracy remained constant at 0.853 both before and after optimization, and F1 and AUC-ROC scores stagnated at 0.710 and 0.936, respectively. This behavior can be explained by the fact that the Random Forest algorithm is intrinsically robust to hyperparameter variations, due to the use of multiple decision trees. Thus, performance is often stable, even without optimization. In addition, it is possible that the search space of optimal hyperparameters was too narrow, and it did not include combinations that could generate more significant improvements.

Hyperparameter optimization in the absence of oversampling is an incomplete solution, not fully resolving the issue of class imbalance. Models tuned on imbalanced datasets tend to favor the majority class in the attempt to achieve higher AUC at the cost of clinical usefulness. This reinforces the idea that optimization alone is insufficient in clinical contexts, where recall is a priority. Only when paired with oversampling, did it yield both statistical and clinical improvements.

Table 5 displays configurations for which the performance has improved significantly, especially when combined with oversampling. Notably, models such as XGBoost and KNN had substantial gains in accuracy after optimization. In contrast, Table 6 presents the models that did not have notable improvements in accuracy after tuning. Particularly, random forest showed stable performance across configurations, suggesting its robustness to hyperparameter tuning.

For the five selected models with best performances found in Table 2, the optimal hyperparameter sets were identified and summarized in Table 7. These optimal hyperparameter configurations highlight important tuning adjustments that contribute to improved model performance. For instance, the consistent learning rate of 0.01 across the CatBoost models suggest that this is a step size that balances convergence and speed, while controlling overfitting. The variation observed in tree

Table 6 Model configurations insignificantly impacted by hyperparameter optimization

Model	Accuracy
Random forest	0.853
Random forest optimized	0.853
Random forest + SMOTE	0.864
Random forest optimized + SMOTE	0.875
Random forest + SMOTEENN	0.864
Random forest optimized + SMOTEENN	0.870
Random forest + ADASYN	0.870
Random forest optimized + ADASYN	0.864

Table 7 Hyperparameters for the five selected models with best performance

Model	Hyperparameters
CatBoost with ADASYN	Learning rate = 0.01
	L2 leaf regularization = 5
	Iterations = 500
	Depth = 4
Support vector machine with ADASYN	Kernel = radial basis function (RBF)
	Gamma = 'scale'
	Degree = 7
	Regularization parameter (C) = 1
Optimized XGBoost with ADASYN	Subsample = 0.8
	Number of estimators = 100
	Maximum depth = 5
	Learning rate = 0.1
	Column subsample = 0.8
Optimized CatBoost with SMOTE	Learning rate = 0.01
	L2 leaf regularization = 1
	Iterations = 500
	Depth = 6
CatBoost with SMOTEENN	Learning rate = 0.01
	L2 leaf regularization = 1
	Iterations = 500
	Depth = 6

depth and L2 leaf regularization might indicate that there is a need to adapt model complexity to different oversampling techniques, due to specific data distributions.

Furthermore, an important remark is that the XGBoost model achieved a good performance with a relatively shallow depth and a high learning rate, while the configuration for SVM suggests the need for fine-tuning of the decision boundary to better capture minority class patterns.

Overall, the results highlight the necessity of hyperparameter tuning accompanied by oversampling techniques that enhance the performances of models in imbalanced clinical datasets.

5 Explainability Using SHAP

Recent advancements in machine learning have proved high performance and significant diagnostic abilities. Despite this, their clinical adoption has been slowed by their lack of transparency. In healthcare, predictive accuracy alone is not sufficient. Rather, clinicians need to understand how a model arrived at a specific decision, especially when this output influences diagnoses or treatment plans. To address these issues the study employed the SHAP analysis, an XAI method grounded in game theory, to interpret the best-performing model from our study.

We applied SHAP to the CatBoost model trained with ADASYN oversampling, due to its high predictive performance across all metrics in the study, and SHAP's native support for tree-based models. SHAP was used to produce both global summary plots and individual prediction breakdowns.

The SHAP summary plots rank features by their average absolute SHAP values, indicating the attributes that had the greatest overall impact on the model's decisions. To visually interpret the contributions of each individual feature to the model's output, Fig. 7 presents the SHAP summary plots for the CatBoost + ADASYN configuration.

As the plots show, the type of chest pain, age, ST depression, cholesterol and the maximum pulse are among the most important features for the model. The beeswarm plot indicates the relationship between features and the predicted outcome. For example, asymptomatic chest pain is indicative of a positive diagnosis of the patient, as is male sex and higher blood glucose. In contrast, normal

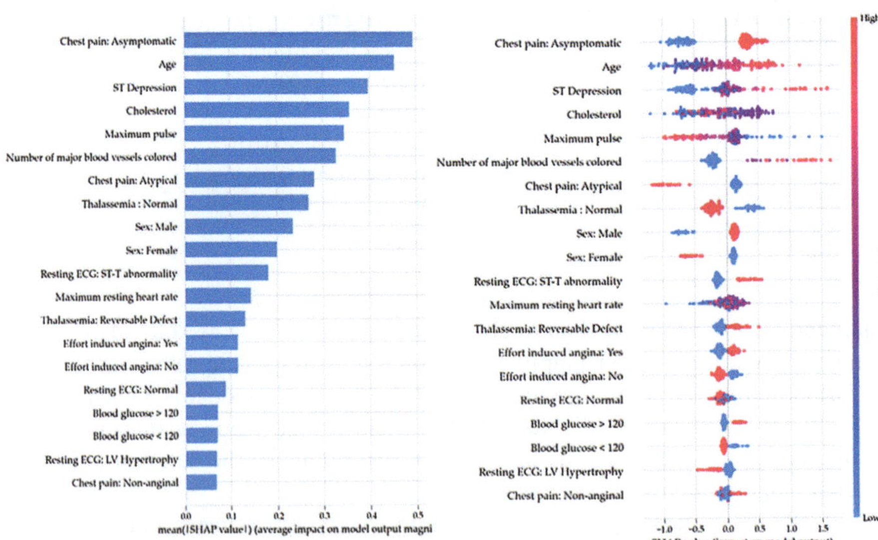

Fig. 7 Summary plots for the interpretability of CatBoost + ADASYN model

thalassemia test results and a lack of angina when exercising, contribute to the negative diagnosis of the patient.

Beyond enhancing model interpretability, SHAP values can directly reveal clinically actionable insights. For example, in a patient instance, a SHAP plot might reveal that ST depression (oldpeak) and asymptomatic chest pain are the most impactful contributors to a positive heart disease prediction. This could potentially prompt the cardiologist to recommend imaging or stress testing to further investigate the case.

Recent studies have demonstrated the real-world value of SHAP in cardiovascular settings. Donmez et al. used SHAP for determining the major contributors to hypertension risk, such as BMI or low physical activity. Even when traditional risk markers such as systolic blood pressure appear normal, this level of explainability allows clinicians to flag cases with hidden risks for further investigation or early intervention [23].

The integration of SHAP in the current workflow offers significant advantages for clinical adoption. It improves trust and transparency, since clinicians can understand the rationale behind the model's predictions, it reveals data quality issues or bias, and it contributes to regulatory alignment.

6 Discussion

The comparative analysis conducted in this chapter provides several key insights into the application of supervised machine learning models for classification of cardiovascular disease. The findings reiterate the idea that algorithm performance alone is not sufficient in clinical contexts. Models must also be interpretable and resilient to data imbalance, frequently encountered in real-world scenarios.

One of the most important takeaways is the superiority of ensemble models, particularly CatBoost and XGBoost in capturing complex and nonlinear relationships within the UCI heart disease dataset. These models outperformed other classifiers such as logistic regression or naïve Bayes across all performance metrics and were especially effective in capturing nonlinear feature interactions.

The introduction of SHAP-based explainability aims to help increase clinical trust on AI models. From a clinical standpoint, the most influential features identified while using SHAP analysis were chest pain type, ST-depression induced by exercise and cholesterol levels, revealing that these selected attributes are consistent with well-established cardiovascular risk factors.

For instance, SHAP plots revealed that asymptomatic chest pain combined with high oldpeak levels had a strong link to heart disease severity, suggesting that these tools could assist clinicians in identifying high-risk patients that traditional scoring systems might overlook.

Another crucial aspect is the use of oversampling techniques, especially ADASYN and SMOTE-ENN. These significantly improved performance by generating synthetic samples for the minority class, addressing class imbalance and enhancing recall without substantially degrading precision.

Hyperparameter optimization was also important in improving model performance, with tree-models and kernel-based models responding particularly well to tuning. Optimization alone, however, is not sufficient to address class imbalance, leading to performance gaps in sensitivity and highlighting again the importance of oversampling.

Despite promising results, while the UCI heart disease is widely used and rather well structured, it is relatively small and may not fully represent the diversity of real-world scenarios, with real-world cardiac patients.

7 Conclusions

This chapter aimed to demonstrate the effectiveness of interpretable machine learning models for cardiovascular disease classification using the multicenter UCI heart disease dataset. A comprehensive comparison of nine algorithms across eight training configurations revealed that CatBoost combined with ADASYN consistently outperformed other models, offering the best balance between predictive accuracy and clinical interpretability. This superior performance is attributed to the complementary strengths of the model along with the oversampling technique.

The CatBoost algorithm handles missing values and categorical features, reducing the need for extensive preprocessing, while ADASYN handles class imbalance by generating synthetic samples for the minority class, improving sensitivity for the underrepresented cases. The use of SHAP analysis provided transparent explanations of model prediction, improving the trustworthiness and clinical acceptance of the system.

From a clinical perspective, this pipeline has the potential to aid cardiologists not only in interpreting the prediction outcomes, but to also identify which features are the most impactful for the classification. These insights support a more personalized approach to patient triage, particularly in resource-limited settings.

Future work will focus on applying the workflow to a real-world clinical dataset collected from a local dataset. This dataset presents a higher-class imbalance and a higher proportion of missing values, posing additional challenges. In this context, the oversampling strategies and hyperparameter tuning are expected to be of even more importance, and lead to an even more accentuated model performance improvement. The models trained on the UCI heart disease dataset could be used in the training stage, while the local dataset may be used for validation and testing, in order to allow for an even more realistic estimation of model performance in contemporary clinical environments.

Another important direction for future work is to investigate the impact of institutional data and to balance the data across sources. In the current study, the models might have overfit patterns from certain subsets, which comprise a larger portion of the dataset. Future studies could implement institution-wise stratified sampling or domain adaptation techniques in order to make sure that models are trained and validated on balanced representations from the institutions. Addressing this variability will help mitigate part of the dataset limitations.

Ultimately, this study aims to highlight the potential of explainable AI to not only improve accuracy of patient diagnosis, but to also improve the trust of clinicians, enhance patient outcomes, and support ethical and transparent deployment of machine learning models in cardiovascular health care.

Acknowledgments The research was supported by the grant from The Executive Agency for Higher Education, Research, Development and Innovation Funding (UEFISCDI) contract no. PN-IV-P7-7.1-PED-2024-1882 entitled HEARTS—Holistic evaluation of coronary collaterals patency in correlation with myocardial viability using artificial intelligence based system.

References

1. M. Di Cesare et al., The heart of the world. Glob. Heart **19**(1), 1288 (2024). https://doi.org/10.5334/gh.1288
2. P. Bovet, N. Banatvala, K.-T. Khaw, K.S. Reddy, Cardiovascular disease, in *Routledge eBooks*, (Routledge, 2023), pp. 45–51. https://doi.org/10.4324/9781003306689-8
3. N. Townsend et al., Epidemiology of cardiovascular disease in Europe. Nat. Rev. Cardiol. **19**(2), 133–143 (2021). https://doi.org/10.1038/s41569-021-00607-3
4. J. Tohka, M. Van Gils, Evaluation of machine learning algorithms for health and wellness applications: A tutorial. Comput. Biol. Med. **132**, 104324 (2021). https://doi.org/10.1016/j.compbiomed.2021.104324
5. J. Komuro, D. Kusumoto, H. Hashimoto, S. Yuasa, Machine learning in cardiology: Clinical application and basic research. J. Cardiol. **82**(2), 128–133 (2023). https://doi.org/10.1016/j.jjcc.2023.04.020
6. G.H. Vardhan, N.S.S. Reddy, K.M. Umamaheswari, Heart disease prediction using machine learning. Int. J. Health Sci. **6**, 7804–7813 (2022). https://doi.org/10.53730/ijhs.v6ns2.6955
7. R. Tr, U.K. Lilhore, P.M.S. Simaiya, A. Kaur, M. Hamdi, Predictive analysis of heart diseases with machine learning approaches. Malays. J. Comput. Sci. **10**, 132–148 (2022). https://doi.org/10.22452/mjcs.sp2022no1.10
8. I.H. Sarker, Machine learning: Algorithms, real-world applications and research directions. SN Comput. Sci. **2**(3), 160 (2021). https://doi.org/10.1007/s42979-021-00592-x
9. G.N. Ahmad, H. Fatima, S. Ullah, A.S. Saidi, N. Imdadullah, Efficient medical diagnosis of human heart diseases using machine learning techniques with and without GridSearchCV. IEEE Access **10**, 80151–80173 (2022). https://doi.org/10.1109/access.2022.3165792
10. C.M. Bhatt, P. Patel, T. Ghetia, P.L. Mazzeo, Effective heart disease prediction using machine learning techniques. Algorithms **16**(2), 88 (2023). https://doi.org/10.3390/a16020088
11. X. Zhang et al., An accurate diagnosis of coronary heart disease by Catboost, with easily accessible data. J. Phys. Conf. Ser. **1955**(1), 012027 (2021). https://doi.org/10.1088/1742-6596/1955/1/012027
12. D. Elreedy, A.F. Atiya, F. Kamalov, A theoretical distribution analysis of synthetic minority oversampling technique (SMOTE) for imbalanced learning. Mach. Learn. **113**(7), 4903–4923 (2023). https://doi.org/10.1007/s10994-022-06296-4
13. N.V. Chawla, K.W. Bowyer, L.O. Hall, W.P. Kegelmeyer, SMOTE: Synthetic minority over-sampling technique. J. Artif. Intell. Res. **16**, 321–357 (2002). https://doi.org/10.1613/jair.953
14. A.M. Halim, M. Dwifebri, F. Nhita, Handling imbalanced data sets using SMOTE and ADASYN to improve classification performance of Ecoli data sets. Build. Inf. Technol. Sci. **5**(1) (2023). https://doi.org/10.47065/bits.v5i1.3647

15. A.X. Wang, V.-T. Le, H.N. Trung, B.P. Nguyen, Addressing imbalance in health data: Synthetic minority oversampling using deep learning. Comput. Biol. Med. **188**, 109830 (2025). https://doi.org/10.1016/j.compbiomed.2025.109830
16. W. Albattah, R.U. Khan, Impact of imbalanced features on large datasets. Front. Big Data **8** (2025). https://doi.org/10.3389/fdata.2025.1455442
17. C. Molnar, *Interpretable machine learning: A guide for making black box models explainable* (Lulu.com, 2025)
18. B. Rozemberczki et al., The Shapley value in machine learning, in *Proceedings of the thirty-first international joint conference on artificial intelligence*, (IJCAI, 2022), pp. 5572–5579. https://doi.org/10.24963/ijcai.2022/778
19. R. Detrano et al., International application of a new probability algorithm for the diagnosis of coronary artery disease. Am. J. Cardiol. **64**(5), 304–310 (1989). https://doi.org/10.1016/0002-9149(89)90524-9
20. H.B. Kibria, A. Matin, The severity prediction of the binary and multi-class cardiovascular disease – A machine learning-based fusion approach. Comput. Biol. Chem. **98**, 107672 (2022). https://doi.org/10.1016/j.compbiolchem.2022.107672
21. B. Bischl et al., Hyperparameter optimization: Foundations, algorithms, best practices, and open challenges. Wiley Interdiscip. Rev. Data Mining Knowl. Discov. **13**(2), e1484 (2023). https://doi.org/10.1002/widm.1484
22. V. Sharma, S. Yadav, M. Gupta, Heart disease prediction using machine learning techniques, in *2020 2nd international conference on advances in computing, communication control and networking (ICACCCN)*, (IEEE, 2020), pp. 177–181. https://doi.org/10.1109/icacccn51052.2020.9362842
23. T.B. Donmez, M. Kutlu, M. Mansour, M.Z. Yildiz, Explainable AI in action: A comparative analysis of hypertension risk factors using SHAP and LIME. Neural Comput. & Applic. **37**(5), 4053–4074 (2024). https://doi.org/10.1007/s00521-024-10724-y

Large Language Models (LLMs) in Medical Error Detection and Correction: A Comprehensive Review

Roshan Chandru, Provia Kadusabe, Asifa Mehmood Qureshi, Shubham Sharma, and Abhishek Kaushik

Abstract The use of Large Language Models (LLMs) in healthcare, specifically for medical error detection and correction, has seen a rise especially in recent years. These errors, if left undetected, can lead to life-threatening consequences; hence, there is a need for advanced solutions. LLMs, with their natural language processing (NLP) ability, can offer valuable opportunities in identifying and correcting medical errors efficiently. This literature review explores various techniques that utilize LLMs for the detection and correction of medical errors. A comprehensive search was conducted across PubMed, IEEE Xplore, and Google Scholar to identify relevant literature. The retrieved research articles were evaluated based on the predefined inclusion and exclusion criteria, and finally, 11 articles were selected. The findings reveal the potential of LLMs in improving healthcare systems by assisting clinicians in their day-to-day work, enhancing clinical decision-making, and automating error detection and correction processes. These models show a promising ability to deliver accurate and timely insights, thereby reducing risks associated with preventable medical errors. Key trends observed include the development and use of fine-tuned medical domain-specific LLMs, integration with electronic health records (EHRs), and applications in real-time clinical settings. Despite their potential, there are still some challenges, such as bias, hallucinations, and ethical concerns. Addressing these issues is crucial to unlock the full potential of LLMs. This review underscores the need for continuous innovation to align LLM capabilities with the dynamic needs of the medical field and procedures.

Keywords Medical error · Large Language Models · detection · correction · EHRs

R. Chandru · P. Kadusabe · A. M. Qureshi · A. Kaushik (✉)
Dundalk Institute of Technology, Dundalk, Co. Louth, Ireland
e-mail: provia.kadusabe@dkit.ie; asifa.mehmood@dkit.ie; abhishek.kaushik@dkit.ie

S. Sharma
Technological University Dublin, Dublin, Ireland
e-mail: shubham.sharma@tudublin.ie

N. E. M. Khalifa, M. H. N. Taha (eds.), *Next-Gen Healthcare*,
https://doi.org/10.1007/978-3-032-07267-2_6

List of Abbreviations

AI	Artificial Intelligence
LLMs	Large Language Models
NLP	Natural Language Processing
EHR	Electronic Health Record
HIT	Healthcare Information Technology
DL	Deep Learning
BERT	Bidirectional Encoder Representations From Transformers
GPT	Generative Pretrained Transformer
QA	Question Answering
CQA	Conversational Question Answering
BioNLP	Biomedical Natural Language Processing
HIPPA	Health Insurance Probability and Accountability Act
GDPR	General Data Protection Regulation
NLI	Natural Language Inference
STS	Semantic Textual Similarity
SQP	Self-Questioning Prompting
ECG	Electrocardiogram
BLURB	Biomedical Language Understanding and Reasoning Benchmark
NER	Named Entity Recognition
RE	Relation Extraction
USMLE	Medical Question-Answering United States Medical Licensing Examination
MMLU	Massive Multitask Language Understanding Medicine
FDA	Food and Drug Administration

1 Introduction

Medical errors are unintentional mistakes in healthcare that happen due to failure to act, taking an incorrect action, or an action that does not achieve its intended goal [1]. These errors can result from performing a planned task incorrectly or deviating from standard care processes. Despite the ongoing efforts to curb them, these errors remain a common problem in healthcare systems around the world.

One of the most prevalent categories of medical errors is medication errors, as shown in Table 1. They arise from factors due to poor handwriting, miscommunication, and lack of standardized protocols for verifying accuracy [2]. Healthcare Information Technology (HIT)-related errors are also prevalent, including issues with the use of Electronic Health Records (EHRs) and ambiguity surrounding medical terms [3, 4]. The occurrence of these errors is often influenced by factors such as resource availability, healthcare system characteristics, and the implementation

Table 1 Common types of medical errors and their definitions

Common medical errors	Definition
Medication errors	Mistakes in prescribing, dispensing, or administering medications
Diagnostic errors	Delays, missed diagnoses, or incorrect diagnoses that lead to improper treatment or no treatment at all
Communication errors	Mistakes that are due to miscommunications among healthcare providers or between providers and patients
Surgical errors	Mistakes made during surgical procedures such as operating on the wrong site or patient
Falls and patient injuries	Physical harm caused to patients due to unsafe conditions or lack of monitoring

of preventive measures including the use of information technology [5], information retrieval [6], natural language processing [7], and Artificial Intelligence (AI) [8].

Medical errors frequently result in fatalities or major injuries; therefore, they represent a serious threat to patient safety. They encompass a wide range of problems, from immediate observable active errors to latent errors that are waiting to happen [9]. The consequences of these errors extend far beyond patient health, placing substantial financial strain on healthcare systems and diminishing overall quality of care. In addition, they have profound emotional and psychological effects on healthcare workers, often leading to distress and feelings of guilt, which can have an impact on their productivity and longevity in the workforce [10]. The financial burden associated with corrective treatments and legal actions further exacerbates the problem, which affects public trust in healthcare systems and leads to increased healthcare avoidance among patients [11].

Estimating the global prevalence of medical errors is challenging due to differences in reporting technique, type of error, and healthcare settings. Additionally, a pervasive blame culture within healthcare institutions may discourage staff from reporting errors [11]. According to a 2016 Johns Hopkins University study, medical errors are responsible for more than 250,000 deaths annually in the United States (U.S), making them the third most common cause of mortality [1]. Another study on diagnostic errors in the U.S.A. estimated that diagnostic error rates range from 2.2% (myocardial infarction) to 62.1% (spinal abscess) across 15 diseases [12].

Despite the ongoing efforts to improve patient safety, substantial challenges remain. Studies continue to highlight critical areas that require attention. For instance, a study conducted in Iran identified that 42.6% of documented medical errors are associated with medication, emphasizing the need to improve healthcare providers' knowledge of pharmacology [13]. Moreover, a recent study indicates that while efforts to address errors have made progress, patient safety has not experienced substantial improvements [14], indicating the need for more effective interventions.

Emerging technology, particularly AI, has shown promise in addressing these challenges. Among these advancements are Large Language Models (LLMs), a

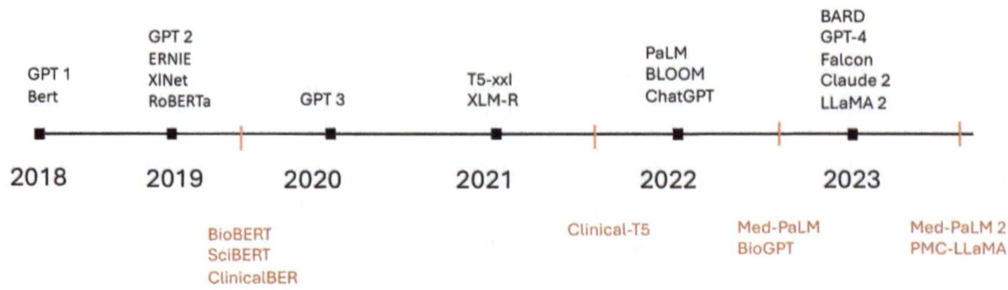

Fig. 1 Chronological display of LLMs releases [15]

subset of AI that is trained on huge amounts of datasets with exceptional capabilities to process, understand, and generate human language [15]. These models have had major successes in other fields, and their application in healthcare holds great potential. Using LLMs in this domain could enhance error detection and correction, ultimately leading to improved patient outcomes. Figure 1 displays the releases of LLMs over time in chronological order.

This review aims to provide a comprehensive overview of how LLMs are being applied to detect and correct a wide range of medical errors across diverse healthcare settings.

The rest of this chapter is organized as follows: Sect. 1.1 presents the motivation for this study, along with the formulated hypothesis, and research questions. Section 1.2 describes the methodology employed to carry out the literature review. Section 2 gives a background on LLMs and also discusses the role of LLMs in medical error detection and correction. Section 3 discusses case studies of LLMs for medical error detection and correction. Section 4 explains the limitations of LLMs in medical error detection and correction. Section 5 discusses the hypothesis and corresponding research questions. Section 6 provides the conclusion and the future work.

1.1 Motivation

Medical error is a global concern and a significant threat to patient safety. It has been estimated to be among the leading causes of death in the US [1], contributing to patient harm, increased healthcare costs, and decline of trust in healthcare institutions [11]. Despite the advancements in healthcare technology and interventions, these errors continue to persist. Traditional error detection methods are often time-consuming, subjective, and lack scalability to handle the growing complexity of healthcare data [16]. The emergence of LLMs presents a transformative opportunity to address these challenges. These models have an ability of processing large amounts of data and generating coherent text. They have been successful in other domains [17, 18], which highlights their potential for medical error detection and correction. This chapter provides an overview of the existing LLM methodologies for medical error detection and correction and identifies key challenges and future directions. Unlike prior work that focuses on specific error types, this review focuses specifically on the role of LLMs across diverse medical errors and clinical contexts. We present a single comprehensive resource for researchers and practitioners, offering informative summaries of existing works to facilitate further advancements in this area.

The formulated hypothesis and corresponding research questions are as follows:

Hypothesis: LLMs improve the detection and correction of medical errors through their advanced capabilities in processing and analyzing data.

RQ1. How effective are LLMs in detecting and correcting medical errors within healthcare systems?

RQ2. What are the primary challenges associated with the use of LLMs for medical error detection and correction, and what approaches can be used to eliminate these challenges?

1.2 Search Methodology

The literature review methodology for assessing LLMs for medical error detection and correction is illustrated in Fig. 2.

We started a focused literature search using major scholarly databases like Google Scholar, IEEE Xplore, and PubMed. These databases were selected due

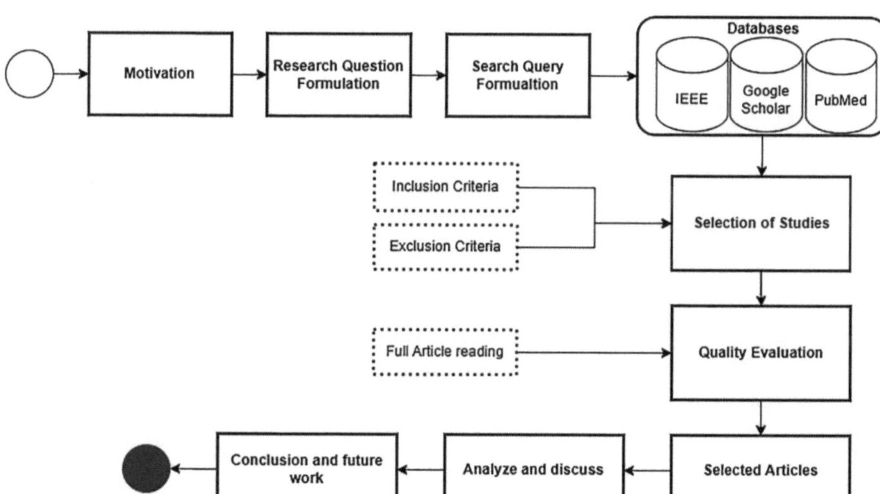

Fig. 2 Methodology workflow for the literature review

to their broad coverage of technological and biomedical research. A search query was formulated to fetch relevant articles. The volume of research in this area was quantified by recording the number of publications retrieved from each database. Our review's breadth was expanded by using PubMed because of its extensive collection of medical literature, IEEE Xplore, because of its focus on engineering and technology research, and Google Scholar, because it covers a larger range of literature. The following query is used to search the aforementioned databases with minimal modifications to optimize the search results:

(("large language model" OR "LLM" OR "BERT" OR "GPT" OR "Transformer") AND ("medical error" OR "diagnostic error" OR "medication error") AND ("detection" OR "correction"))

The search terms were refined based on initial review findings to enhance the specificity and relevance of the results. To capture recent advancements and relevant developments in the use of LLMs for medical error detection and correction, we restricted the search to the period from January 1, 2017, to December 6, 2024.

Our strategy was to analyze and combine the findings from the selected research using a synthesis technique. We established the following inclusion and exclusion criteria to refine our search and include only studies of interest:

1.3 Inclusion Criteria

- Research studies that discuss medical error detection or correction using LLMs.
- Articles published from 2017 to 2024 were included.
- The review includes conferences, journals, books, or proceedings written only in English.

1.4 Exclusion Criteria

- Studies that do not address any of our research questions were not considered.
- Studies unrelated to the use of LLMs for medical error detection or correction were excluded.

The remaining studies were manually refined through full-text reading, resulting in a final selection of 11 articles for review (Fig. 3).

Figure 4 illustrates the yearly submission trends and a cumulative number of reviewed papers that are related to medical error detection and correction using LLMs.

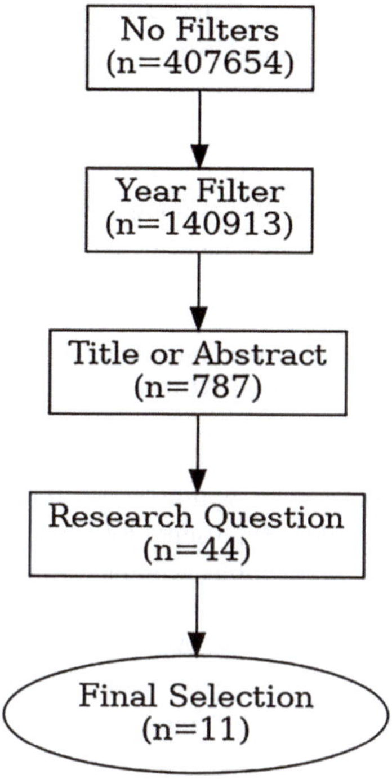

Fig. 3 Flow diagram of included articles

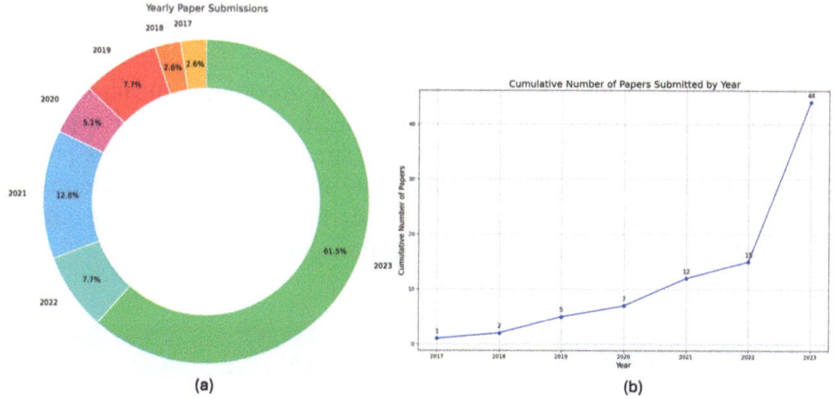

Fig. 4 Distribution of studies: (**a**) Doughnut chart presents the number of papers that are published each year, (**b**) The line chart provides trend of the cumulative number of papers that are submitted each year

2 Large Language Models for Medical Error Detection and Correction

The use of EHRs in healthcare systems generates large volumes of data that can be analyzed to improve patient safety and outcomes. While structured data such as demographics is relatively easy to analyze, unstructured data presents a challenge. Unstructured data including free text notes, admission, and discharge summaries contain vital information but require specialized methods for effective analysis due to its complexity and variability. To address this, Natural Language Processing (NLP) has become a key method for analyzing this type of data.

The use of NLP in medical error detection and correction has evolved over the decades from traditional rule-based approaches to Deep Learning (DL) methods. DL models particularly LLMs have enhanced the ability to analyze context-dependent information within medical texts. Language models like BERT (Bidirectional Encoder Representations From Transformers) have been optimized for medical applications leading to domain-specific models like BioBERT (bidirectional encoder representations from transformers for biomedical text) [19], ClinicalBERT [20], which has further improved NLP's capabilities in handling clinical language [21]. These models can capture semantic relationships within large corpora of clinical documents, which can help in the detection and correction of errors.

2.1 Role of Large Language Models in Enhancing Patient Outcomes

LLM integration in healthcare systems provides an opportunity to enhance patient safety and to provide quality standards. Leveraging their advanced NLP capabilities, LLMs can support clinical decision-making and streamline administrative processes [22]. These models greatly enhance the quality of patient care by offering data-driven insights to patients and physicians [23, 24]. Figure 5 represents the utilization of different LLMs for medical error identification and correction.

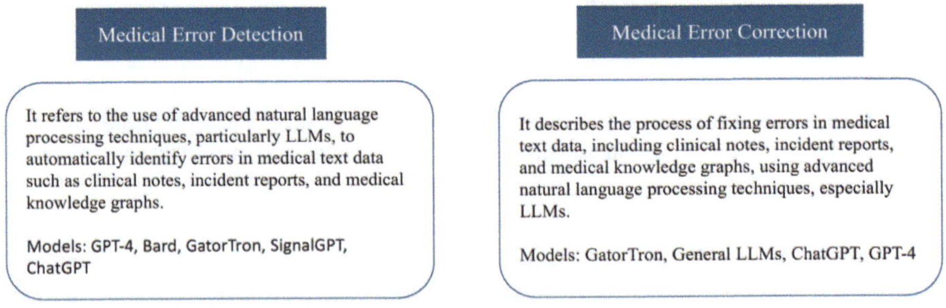

Fig. 5 LLMs used for medical error detection and correction [25, 26]

LLMs show promise in improving medical error detection and correction. Techniques such as the Diagnostic Reasoning Chain of Thought (DR-CoT) illustrate how LLMs may mitigate errors by emulating clinical reasoning used by physicians [27]. Similarly, the Holistically Thought (HoT) approach aids LLMs in performing Medical Conversational Question-Answering (CQA) tasks to provide professional and accurate responses, which can help to minimize errors in patient communications [28].

Moreover, these LLMs can analyze behavioral health data such as cardiac signs and stress level estimation, aiding early detection and prevention of misdiagnoses [29]. This could allow healthcare providers to intervene at earlier stages reducing the likelihood of adverse events.

Additionally, techniques like Biomedical Natural Language Processing (BioNLP) enhanced by LLMs facilitate the extraction of valuable information from the burgeoning biomedical literature. This helps healthcare professionals to keep up with the latest discoveries and minimize errors caused by outdated information or practices [30]. Combining LLMs with bioinformatics methods can further address their limitations, improving their reliability and interpretability of results in clinical applications [31].

The development of specialized models such as ClinicalGPT, specifically designed for clinical settings, showcases the potential of LLMs to surpass conventional models in tasks such as medical knowledge question answering, and diagnostic analysis, underscoring their efficacy in error mitigation [32].

Furthermore, LLMs such as ChatGPT offer the ability to efficiently search databases and provide evidence-based responses that can accelerate the development of practice guidelines and ultimately improve the quality of care provided [23, 33].

Similarly, utilizing LLMs in outpatient treatment support systems shows the potential for personalized treatment recommendations, improving patient adherence and outcomes [17].

LLMs also facilitate administrative efficiency in healthcare by streamlining triage processes, enhancing medical coding accuracy, and improving communication between patients and healthcare providers. These capabilities can lead to operational improvements and better healthcare service delivery [34].

Despite the promising capabilities of LLMs, their implementation requires a cautious and well-regulated approach. Concerns regarding the ability of models to differentiate between accurate and fabricated information pose risks to patient safety. Additionally ensuring adherence to privacy regulations, such as Health Insurance Probability and Accountability Act (HIPPA) and General Data Protection Regulation (GDPR), remains a critical challenge [35]. For LLMs to be successfully incorporated into healthcare systems, it is also essential that their implementation be in line with human values and objectives [23].

The integration of LLMs into healthcare systems holds significant potential for improving safety and quality of care; however, it is crucial to acknowledge and address the associated challenges.

3 Applications of LLMs for Medical Error Detection and Correction

3.1 Case Studies for Medical Error Detection

Medical error detection plays an important role in ensuring patient safety and improving healthcare outcomes. With the vast amount of data generated in medical centers daily, the need for effective and reliable techniques to identify and mitigate errors has never been greater. LLMs could be integrated into hospital EHR systems to monitor and notify healthcare professionals about real-time errors. This could greatly improve safety by enabling the rectification of any identified errors. Transformer-based models are trained to comprehend text, and this capability can be used to understand medical terminology and identify errors by cross-referencing the information from clinical guidelines, and drug interaction databases with medical cases in EHRs to check for inconsistencies [36].

A recent study evaluates the performance of several LLMs (GPT-3.5, GPT-4, and Bard) across various clinical language understanding tasks including Name Entity Recognition (NER), Relation Extraction, Natural Language Inference (NLI), Semantic Textual Similarity (STS), Document Classification, and Question Answering (QA). It introduces a new strategy called Self-Questioning Prompting (SQP), which helps models perform better by generating specific questions and answers to improve their understanding of clinical data. The findings show that GPT-4 consistently outperforms other models in many tasks and also demonstrate that SQP enhances performance compared to traditional prompting methods. However, challenges remain, as the models sometimes struggle with complex medical terminology and misinterpreting negations [37]. The introduction of SQP in this study offers a promising tool for improving model accuracy, which could be applied to detect discrepancies and errors in medical records.

To address issues of medical term complexity, LLMs are being fine-tuned for medical-specific tasks, which has improved their understanding of medical terminology. For instance, ClinicalBERT [20] is one such example, and it was fine-tuned from BERT [38] using MIMIC III dataset [39] that contains medical records of patients admitted to a critical care unit. It was trained to predict 30-day hospital readmissions by analyzing patient notes and calculating a risk score for the likelihood of patient readmission in 30 days. It is designed to handle terminology and context of medical language, which addresses the challenges that general-purpose models face in understanding medical terminology. The model showed improved performance, especially in predictive tasks. Similarly, NYUTron, an advanced clinical language model, was developed by researchers at NYU Langone Health to assist healthcare professionals in making critical, time-sensitive decisions by predicting various clinical and operational events, which can help to mitigate latent errors [40].

Knowledge distillation, a method where a bigger LLM-like GPT-4 is used as a teacher to train a smaller task-specific model known as the student, has also been explored. Such an example is PubMedBert, which was distilled from GPT-3.5. It was examined on biomedical information extraction task, and it achieved a state-of-the-art performance, surpassing its teacher in the task of ADE extraction task without requiring labeled data [41]. This approach can benefit the field with the advantages of bigger LLMs at a fraction of the cost and time.

LLMs work even better when combined with existing procedures compared to using each on their own. Traditionally, the interpretation of medical tests relies solely on medical practitioners, which increases the likelihood of human error. Incorporating an LLM as a supportive tool can assist practitioners in making more accurate assessments, reducing the risk of misinterpretation. For example, a study examines the potential of LLMs in drafting reports for biomedical signals. The study focuses on interpreting electrocardiogram (ECG) signals using SignalGPT, a combination of ChatGPT and a biomedical signal processing system. It aims to develop a signal-to-text (Sig2txt) engine that is capable of processing biomedical signals and generating their textual descriptions. The process involves converting raw ECG signals into text descriptions through a signal-to-text (S2T) engine in the SignalGPT setup. These descriptions are then interpreted using ChatGPT. The results show that SignalGPT outperforms direct applications of ChatGPT interpreting biomedical signals. The system also shows high accuracy in detecting ECG abnormalities with sensitivity rates reaching 100% for conditions like right bundle branch block (RBBB), left bundle branch block (LBBB), and sinus bradycardia (SB). Atrial fibrillation (AF) and first-degree AV block (1dAVb) demonstrated sensitivity rates of 92.31% and 92.86%, respectively [42].

Another study introduces a framework for estimating errors in the outputs of LLMs using a method called pareto optimal learning. This approach generates a POLAR score that quantifies the likelihood of errors in an LLM's response by integrating multiple information sources, such as external knowledge bases. The framework is particularly relevant in high stake fields like medicine, where accurate information is critical. It has been tested on biomedical datasets to extract relationships between chemicals, diseases, and proteins, showcasing its ability to detect errors in domain-specific applications [43].

3.2 *Case Studies for Medical Error Correction*

LLMs are not limited to medical error detection but can also be used for correction. General-purpose models like GPT-4 and domain-specific models are transforming the medical field by automating tasks such as clinical documentation and patient communication, while also assisting in data analysis to enhance diagnosis and treatment efficiency [34].

LLMs integrated into systems to identify errors provide an opportunity to correct the errors before any serious harm. For example, in ClinicalBERT [20], after the model assigns the risk score for a patient's possibility of hospital readmission, the healthcare providers can use the score to determine whether to intervene or not. This can be used to reduce the number of hospital readmissions, ultimately improving the patient's quality of life and saving money [44]. ClinicalBert can also be adapted to other tasks such as mortality risk estimation, and diagnosis prediction which can assist healthcare providers by examining and detecting diagnostic errors and suggesting accurate diagnoses.

Moreover, the practical implementation of integrated LLM systems such as SignalGPT that analyses and interprets biomedical signals like ECGs in clinical environments can assist healthcare professionals by automating the interpretation of ECG signals, thereby supporting informed clinical decision-making [45]. Such systems can reduce clinician workload and enhance diagnostic precision, especially in high-pressure settings like emergency care.

Some errors are caused due to inadequate training among healthcare professionals. LLMs such as GPT-4 have been shown to have the potential to enhance learning by personalizing study materials, generating case studies, supporting curriculum development, and offering interactive teaching tools [46]. This can help avoid errors by continuously training professionals and can be used in medical schools to produce better physicians.

Similarly, the study by Toma et al. addresses the issue of identifying and correcting errors in clinical documentation. The research was conducted as part of the MEDIQA-CORR 2024 shared task, which focused on three distinct objectives: (1) determining whether a clinical text contains an error, (2) identifying the specific erroneous sentence, and (3) generating an accurate correction for the identified error. The authors developed a novel approach using LLMs specifically GPT-4, combined with the DSPy framework, a tool designed to optimize prompt engineering and few-shot learning examples systematically. The methodology showed exceptional performance, achieving the highest scores across all three subtasks. For error detection, the system achieved an accuracy of 86.5%, and for error localization, it achieved an accuracy of 83.6%. In the error correction subtask, the system achieved a composite score of 78.9% using metrics such as ROUGE, BLEURT, and BERTScore [47]. These results underscore the efficacy of combining few-shot learning, chain-of-thought reasoning, and systematic prompt optimization in addressing errors in medical data.

Table 2 shows a summary of the datasets used in some of the case studies reviewed.

3.3 *Advantages of LLMs in Medical Error Detection and Correction*

The following outlines the key advantages of utilizing LLMs for detecting and correcting medical errors:

1. Improved accuracy: The key benefit of utilizing LLMs is that they can analyze huge amounts of medical data and identify errors in clinical documentation,

Table 2 Summary of datasets used in some of the studies reviewed

Study (year)	Dataset name/source	Size (docs/records)	Language	Annotation	Public/private
Huang et al., 2019 [20]	MIMIC-III clinical notes	2M+ notes, 38k+ patients	English	Real-world clinical notes, labeled for hospital readmission	Public (restricted)
Jiang et al., 2023 [40]	NYU Langone Health EHRs	7.25M clinical notes, 387k+ patients	English	Task-specific labeled, real-world EHR	Private
Liu et al., 2023 (preprint) [42]	ECG records from Telehealth Network of Minas Gerais (TNMG) in Brazil	827 ECG tracings	NA	Expert annotated with diagnostic labels for 12-lead ECG recordings	Public
Abacha et al., 2024 [48]	MEDEC benchmark dataset	3800+ notes (train/val/test)	English	Expert annotated for error detection/correction	Public (restricted)
Lee et al., 2020 [19]	PubMed, PMC full text, Wikipedia, BooksCorpus	PubMed: 4.5B words, PMC: 13.5B words, Wikipedia: 2.5B words, BooksCorpus: 0.8B words	English	Self-supervised, no manual annotation	Public
Singhal et al., 2023 [49]	MedQA, MedMCQA, PubMedQA, MMLU	MedQA: 12k+, MedMCQA: 193k+, PubMedQA: 274k+, MMLU: 1212	English	Curated question answer pairs	Public/private
Gu et al., 2021 [50]	BC5-chem, BC5-disease, NCBI-disease, BC2GM, JNLPBA, EBM PICO, ChemProt, DDI, GAD, BIOSSES, HoC, PubMedQA, BioASQ	BC5-chem: 16k, BC5-disease: 13k, NCBI-disease: 6k, BC2GM: 24k, JNLPBA: 60k, EBM PICO: 438k, ChemProt: 46k, DDI: 58k, GAD: 5k, BIOSSES: 100, HoC: 2k, PubMedQA: 1k, BioASQ: 900	English	Mostly manually annotated by experts	Public

prescriptions, and patient records with high precision. This can help minimize human errors caused by fatigue, oversight, or cognitive biases.
2. Clinical decision support: LLMs offer suggestions based on evidence-based guidelines that can help healthcare professionals make better informed decisions.
3. Real-time error detection: LLMs can be integrated into EHR systems to provide real-time alerts for potential errors.
4. Time efficiency: Automating monotonous administrative tasks can reduce documentation errors and reduce administrative burden. This enables healthcare providers to dedicate more attention to patient care.
5. Identifying patterns and anomalies: By rapidly examining enormous volumes of medical data and spotting trends and abnormalities that could point to mistakes, LLMs can increase the accuracy of diagnoses. Additionally, they excel at detecting rare and complex cases by uncovering patterns and irregularities that may be overlooked by humans.
6. Lower costs: The money associated with medical errors and their consequences continues to grow [51]. Leveraging LLMs for error correction can potentially reduce the cost.
7. Improved patient safety: Early detection of errors can prevent adverse events such as medication errors or misdiagnoses, thereby improving overall patient safety.
8. Continuous learning: LLMs have the capacity to continuously learn and adapt to incorporate the latest medical literature and data. This ensures that the detection of medical errors remains aligned with the newest medical knowledge and practices. LLMs can be tailored to comprehend the nuances of medical language and context by integrating domain-specific fine-tuning and expert feedback, which lowers the possibility of missing critical errors [52].

Although LLMs have many benefits, there are still certain issues that must be resolved in order to fully utilize their potential; these issues are discussed in the section that follows.

3.4 Evaluation of LLMs in Medical Error Detection and Correction

Evaluating the performance of LLMs in medical error detection and correction has become increasingly important as these models are introduced into clinical research and workflow settings. Until recently, the field lacked a standardized benchmark tailored to this specific task, limiting meaningful comparisons across models and approaches. MEDEC is the first publically available benchmark specifically designed for medical error detection and correction [48]. It contains 3,848 clinical notes, including 488 real-world examples collected from three U.S. hospital systems. It includes five error categories: diagnosis, management, treatment, pharmacotherapy, and causal organism, and it supports evaluation across three subtasks: error detection, localization, and correction. During the MEDIQA-CORR

Table 3 Comparison of LLM performance across biomedical NLP benchmarks

Benchmark	Task	Models evaluated	Performance comparison
BLURB (Biomedical Language Understanding and Reasoning Benchmark) [50]	NER (Named entity recognition), RE (relation extraction), QA (question answering), similarity, classification	BioLinkBERT-L, PubMedBERT	BioLinkBERT-L: 86.55 > PubMedBERT: 81.10
MedQA (USMLE) (Medical Question Answering United States Medical Licensing Examination) [49, 53, 54]	Multiple-choice medical QA	GPT-4o, Med-PaLM 2, Med-PaLM	GPT-4o: 89% > Med-PaLM 2: 86.5% > Med-PaLM: 67.6%
PubMedQA [53, 55]	Yes/No/Maybe QA from abstracts	BioBERT, Med-PaLM 2, BioGPT-Large	BioGPT-Large: 81% > Med-PaLM 2:75% > BioBERT: 68%
MedMCQA (Medical Multiple-Choice Question Answering) [49, 54]	MCQ from Indian medical exams	GPT-4, Med-PaLM 2	GPT-4: 73.66% > Med-PaLM 2: 72.3%
MMLU (medicine) (massive multitask language understanding medicine) [53, 54, 56]	Medicine, biology, and health MCQs	GPT-4, PaLM, Med-PaLM 2	Med-PaLM 2: 95.2 % > GPT-4: 93.8% > flan PaLM: 63.7%

2024 shared task, state-of-the-art LLMs such as GPT-4, Claude 3.5 Sonnet, and Gemini 2.0 Flash were evaluated in this context. These models demonstrated good performance, with top systems achieving approximately 70% accuracy in error detection and high correction scores across various metrics. However, LLMs still fall short when compared to medical doctors. Beyond MEDEC, LLMs have also been evaluated on broader biomedical and clinical NLP tasks that indirectly reflect their ability to handle medical errors as shown in Table 3.

3.5 Challenges of Deploying LLMs in Clinical Settings

4 Limitations of LLM in Medical Error Detection and Correction

Examples of common limitations of LLMs are illustrated in Fig. 6.

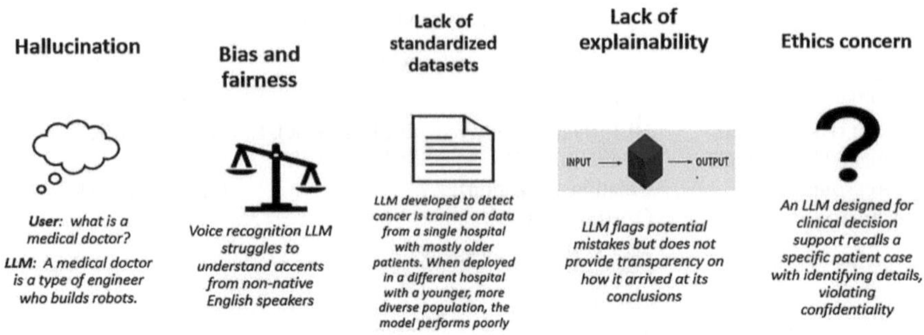

Fig. 6 Common limitations of LLMs for medical error detection and correction with illustrative examples

4.1 Hallucination and Misleading Information

One of the most pressing concerns in using LLMs is their tendency to generate misleading or inaccurate content known as hallucinations. The persuasive and confident tone in which LLMs present their outputs further complicates the matter as healthcare professionals may unintentionally rely on these erroneous suggestions [17].

4.2 Bias and Fairness

LLMs predominantly rely on the data used for training, inherently embedding biases that disproportionately affect underrepresented populations including racial and ethnic minorities, economically disadvantaged groups, and individuals with rare medical conditions. Such biases limit the generalizability of LLMs across diverse populations, languages, and healthcare systems. For example, LLMs trained primarily on data from English-speaking populations, or high-resource healthcare systems may exhibit reduced accuracy when deployed in low-resource settings or among non-English-speaking populations. Furthermore, biases embedded in the training data can exacerbate existing health disparities by systematically underdiagnosing or misdiagnosing certain patient groups, especially those already experiencing healthcare inequities [57].

4.3 Lack of Standardized Datasets

Despite the advancements in technology, evaluation of LLMs within the medical domain remains a challenge mainly due to lack of standardized and comprehensive datasets that are crucial for thorough and reliable assessment [43]. Moreover, the variability in medical documentation formats, terminology, and data quality across different healthcare institutions poses an even bigger challenge for LLMs to achieve consistent performance.

4.4 Lack of Explainability

LLMs operate as "black boxes," which complicates efforts to clearly understand or explain why specific suggestions or error corrections are proposed. This opacity can limit clinician trust and hinder the adoption of AI tools in medical practice, as healthcare decisions require transparent and interpretable reasoning. Enhanced interpretability, potentially achieved through techniques such as attention visualization or model interpretability frameworks such as SHAP [58] or LIME [59], could mitigate this limitation by providing clinicians with clearer insights into the factors influencing AI-generated decisions. Without such transparency, clinicians may remain reluctant to integrate AI recommendations fully into clinical workflows, ultimately restricting the effectiveness and acceptance of these systems [60].

4.5 Ethical Concerns

Ensuring that AI models meet the required ethical standards remains a challenge in healthcare. Safeguarding patient privacy is paramount, as the use of AI necessitates access to sensitive health data and raises concerns regarding unauthorized disclosure and data breaches. Informed consent processes must also be adapted to ensure that patients are aware of AI involvement and its associated limitations. The question of liability in AI-assisted clinical decisions is complex, when AI models influence clinical decisions, determining accountability for errors or adverse outcomes can be ambiguous. Finally, there is also a risk of automation bias, where clinicians may over rely on AI-generated recommendations, potentially overlooking their own clinical judgment or failing to question erroneous outputs [17].

4.6 Deployment Challenges in Clinical Settings

Despite the potential of LLMs to improve medical error detection and correction, their integration into healthcare systems remains difficult. Below, we outline some of the key barriers hindering their clinical deployment.

4.6.1 Integration with Electronic Health Records

Integrating LLMs with existing health IT systems, especially EHRs, poses a major challenge. Hospitals cannot simply introduce a standalone AI tool, and LLMs must communicate with complex, legacy EHR systems to fetch patient data and document outputs. This interoperability is hard to achieve, requiring custom interfaces and significant IT development [61]. Many EHR vendors are beginning to partner with AI companies to embed LLM capabilities directly into their platforms. For example, Epic and Oracle Cerner have announced plans to incorporate GPT-4-driven functions via API integrations [62]. Such closed model approaches (where a proprietary LLM is accessed through an API) offer fast deployment and consistency across sites, but they also raise concerns about data flow and control. In contrast, open model approaches, run locally, offer more control but need costly infrastructure and expertise [62]. Regardless of the model, seamless integration into clinical workflows is crucial to ensure adoption.

4.6.2 Clinician Acceptance and Trust

LLMs can only succeed in clinical settings if clinicians trust and find them useful. At present, many clinicians remain cautious about LLMs. They see the promise of automation but are wary of the pitfalls. A recent survey of practicing clinicians found broad support for using LLMs in supportive roles such as drafting notes or suggesting differential diagnoses but strong reluctance to let an LLM operate autonomously. Concerns include incorrect outputs, lack of empathy, and potential for biased or unsafe recommendations. Building clinician confidence will require demonstrating that LLMs can improve efficiency and quality without compromising safety or the human touch in medicine [63].

4.6.3 Regulatory and Legal Hurdles

The regulatory framework for generative AI in healthcare remains unclear. Current medical device regulations were not crafted with adaptive, self-learning algorithms in mind. In the United States, the Food and Drug Administration (FDA) has approved many AI-based medical devices, but these have typically been "locked" algorithms for specific tasks (like reading an ECG or an X-ray). By contrast, a general-purpose LLM that provides medical advice blurs the line between information tool and medical device. As of 2025, no LLM is formally FDA approved for clinical decision support. Exactly how to regulate LLM-based tools is an open question, traditional approval pathways (involving static hardware/software and clinical trials) may not neatly apply to AI models that continuously learn or update [64]. Legal liability is another major concern. If an LLM recommends a treatment that injures a patient, who is responsible the clinician, the hospital, or the software developer? At present, the law offers little precedent for AI malpractice [61].

4.6.4 Real-World Validation and Evidence

Perhaps the most fundamental challenge is simply proving that LLMs work safely and effectively in real clinical settings. To date, much of the evidence for LLM performance in medicine comes from simulation studies or retrospective datasets. For example, researchers have tested LLMs on medical exam questions, case vignettes, or by seeing if the AI's note summaries align with known diagnoses. While these benchmarks are useful, they do not provide sufficient evidence regarding how LLMs perform in actual clinical settings. There is a pressing need for prospective, real-world validation of LLM tools [61].

5 Discussion

Based on our investigation, LLMs provide significant opportunities for medical error detection and correction. Their advanced capability to process and analyze huge amounts of data, combined with their capacity to generate clear and coherent text, makes them valuable tools in healthcare. The integration of LLMs into healthcare applications can support health practitioners in clinical decision-making, which can help minimize human error, diagnostic errors, and medication errors among others. Moreover, LLMs facilitate task automation, offering fast and efficient solutions to repetitive and time-consuming tasks that are prone to error [18].

Our findings support the hypothesis that LLMs enhance the detection and correction of medical errors due to their advanced data processing capabilities. However, despite their potential, certain limitations must be addressed to fully realize the benefits.

The following sections offer answers to the research questions investigated in this study:

RQ1. **How effective are LLMs in detecting and correcting medical errors within healthcare systems?**

LLMs demonstrate significant potential in detecting and correcting medical errors within healthcare systems. These models leverage their advanced NLP capabilities to analyze clinical documentation, identify inconsistencies, and provide evidence-based recommendations.

For error detection, LLMs are particularly effective in detecting medical errors through the analysis of unstructured data within EHRs. They can identify inconsistencies and anomalies by cross-referencing patient data against established clinical guidelines and protocols. Techniques such as diagnostic reasoning and chain-of-thought prompting enable LLMs to emulate human-like diagnostic processes, improving their accuracy in identifying errors within clinical data [27]. Holistic thought processing can also allow LLMs to consider comprehensive patient data and contextual factors, achieving a more accurate and nuanced understanding of medical cases [28]. Additionally, self-questioning prompting and few-shot learning have been shown to enhance LLM capabilities in detecting errors by improving their reasoning processes and adaptability [47].

In terms of error correction, LLMs provide multiple functionalities that support healthcare providers in addressing identified issues. These models can clarify, rephrase, and complete missing information in clinical documentation to enhance accuracy and consistency. Prompt optimization enhances the responsiveness and precision of LLMs in suggesting appropriate corrections. Knowledge distillation, which transfers knowledge from a larger model to a smaller domain-specific model, enables the smaller model to leverage the accuracy and interpretive capabilities of the larger model while significantly reducing computational costs [41]. Furthermore, LLMs can offer real-time alerts and recommendations that allow healthcare providers to intervene promptly, reducing the potential for errors to escalate into adverse events.

The development of domain-specific models such as ClinicalBERT [20], PubMedBERT [50], and NYUtron [40] has shown promise in enhancing medical error detection and correction. These models are trained on medical literature and clinical data, and possess a deeper understanding of medical terminology and context, enabling them to accurately identify, flag, and rectify errors in clinical documentation. In contrast, general-purpose models like GPT-4 can complement these efforts by aiding in medical education and assisting practitioners in minimizing errors due to insufficient training.

However, despite their potential, LLMs still have several challenges that must be addressed to ensure their full reliability in healthcare systems. Studies reveal that even the most sophisticated LLMs still lack the nuanced understanding and critical thinking skills required to fully match human performance, especially in tasks requiring factual reasoning and comprehension [57]. This suggests that while LLMs can be valuable tools for medical error detection and correction, they cannot fully replace the nuanced reasoning and oversight provided by human experts, underscoring the need for continued development of better detection and correction systems.

***RQ2.* What are the primary challenges associated with the use of LLMs for medical error detection and correction, and what approaches can be used to eliminate these challenges?**

The key challenges associated with the use of LLMs for medical detection and correction are hallucination and misleading information, bias and fairness, lack of standardized datasets, lack of explainability, and ethics concern. The strategies that can be employed to mitigate them include:

1. Implement thorough validation processes by cross-referencing LLM outputs with reliable medical sources. Involve medical professionals in the loop to review and verify the information provided by the LLM [65].
2. Use diverse training datasets that cover different demographics, conditions, and languages. Additionally, apply bias detection tools and continuously monitor model outputs to identify and address any biases that may arise [66].

3. Encourage collaboration among healthcare institutions, researchers, and policy-makers to create and share standardized datasets. This can help improve model training and evaluation consistency across the industry [67].
4. Use interpretable AI techniques such as attention mechanisms, model explainability frameworks (such as SHAP, LIME), and transparency reports [68]. Providing clear explanations alongside model outputs will help build trust among medical professionals.
5. Ensuring compliance with relevant healthcare regulations such as HIPAA, GDPR, and Food and Drug Administration (FDA) guidelines by integrating privacy and security protocols to meet regulations from the start of model development can help align LLMs to ethics and standards.

6 Conclusion and Future Work

This literature review examined the application of LLMs in mitigating the critical issue of medical error detection and correction. The findings highlight that LLMs demonstrate considerable potential in identifying and correcting these errors. This capability is attributed to their advanced NLP abilities, contextual understanding, and capacity to analyze large volumes of data at high speed. By leveraging these strengths, LLMS have the potential to enhance healthcare systems through automation, clinical decision-making support, and provide timely alerts for intervention. Nevertheless, the successful integration of LLMs into clinical practice necessitates addressing several key challenges, including mitigating biases, ensuring model transparency and interpretability, and facilitating access to diverse, high quality, and standardized datasets. Addressing these challenges is crucial to fostering trust and ensuring ethical deployment. Future research should develop standardized benchmarks and evaluation frameworks to assess the reliability and safety of LLM outputs in clinical contexts, create methodologies for bias detection and mitigation specific to medical language and data, design interpretable model architectures or post hoc explanation tools, and curate diverse, high quality, and ethically sourced datasets that better reflect the complexity of clinical environments.

Acknowledgments This research is partially supported by CREATE-DkIT, which is co-funded by the Government of Ireland and the European Union through the ERDF Southern, Eastern and Midland Regional Programme 2021-27 and the Research Ireland under Grant Number 21/FFP-A/9255.

Competing Interests The authors have no conflicts of interest to declare that are relevant to the content of this chapter.

Ethics Approval Not Applicable.

References

1. M.A. Makary, M. Daniel, Medical error–the third leading cause of death in the US. BMJ **353**, i2139 (2016)
2. M. Miladinia, E. Mousavi Nouri, The challenge of medication errors in the emergency department setting. J. Emerg. Pract. Trauma **8**(1), 1–2 (2022)
3. P. Yadhukrishnan, Monitoring and evaluation of medication error in a tertiary care hospital. South Asian Res. J. Pharm. Sci. **2**(2), 16–20 (2020)
4. S. Ekama, A. David, A. Musa, I. Olojo, E. Herbertson, D. Oladele, S. Adaba, M. Chidi, A. Ohihoin, N. Odunukwe et al., Medication errors among healthcare workers in a major HIV treatment centre in Nigeria. J. Adv. Med. Pharmaceut. Sci. **20**(3), 1–9 (2019)
5. A. Kaushik, V. Bhat Ramachandra, G.J. Jones, An interface for agent supported conversational search, in *Proceedings of the 2020 Conference on Human Information Interaction and Retrieval* (2020), pp. 452–456
6. A. Kaushik, G.J. Jones, Exploring current user web search behaviours in analysis tasks to be supported in conversational search. Preprint. arXiv:2104.04501 (2021)
7. G. Kaur, A. Kaushik, S. Sharma, Cooking is creating emotion: a study on hinglish sentiments of Youtube cookery channels using semi-supervised approach. Big Data Cognit. Comput. **3**(3), 37 (2019)
8. M.A. Radwan, *Disclosing Adverse Events in Healthcare: Understanding the Gap Between Knowledge and Practice in Developing Countries* (2022), pp. 82–83
9. T.L. Rodziewicz et al., *Medical Error Reduction and Prevention* (StatPearls, StatPearls Publishing, 2024)
10. J.J. Robertson, B. Long, Suffering in silence: medical error and its impact on health care providers. J. Emerg. Med. **54**(4), 402–409 (2018)
11. T.L. Rodziewicz, J.E. Hipskind, *Medical Error Prevention* (StatPearls Publishing, Treasure Island, 2020)
12. D.E. Newman-Toker, Z. Wang, Y. Zhu, N. Nassery, A.S.S. Tehrani, A.C. Schaffer, C.W. Yu-Moe, G.D. Clemens, M. Fanai, D. Siegal, Rate of diagnostic errors and serious misdiagnosis-related harms for major vascular events, infections, and cancers: toward a national incidence estimate using the "big three". Diagnosis **8**(1), 67–84 (2021)
13. F. Hashemian, M. Farzian, M.H. Bakhshaei, Evaluation of prevalence, distribution and types of drug errors reported in best medical center of Hamadan during 2014–2015 (2019)
14. E. Ahsani-Estahbanati, V. Sergeevich Gordeev, L. Doshmangir, Interventions to reduce the incidence of medical error and its financial burden in health care systems: a systematic review of systematic reviews. Front. Med. **9**, 875426 (2022)
15. H. Naveed, A.U. Khan, S. Qiu, M. Saqib, S. Anwar, M. Usman, N. Barnes, A. Mian, A comprehensive overview of large language models. Preprint. arXiv:2307.06435 (2023)
16. M. Hauskrecht, I. Batal, M. Valko, S. Visweswaran, G.F. Cooper, G. Clermont, Outlier detection for patient monitoring and alerting. J. Biomed. Inf. **46**(1), 47–55 (2013)
17. Z.A. Nazi, W. Peng, Large language models in healthcare and medical domain: a review. Informatics **11**(3) MDPI (2024), 57
18. A.J. Thirunavukarasu, D.S.J. Ting, K. Elangovan, L. Gutierrez, T.F. Tan, D.S.W. Ting, Large language models in medicine. Nat. Med. **29**(8), 1930–1940 (2023)
19. J. Lee, W. Yoon, S. Kim, D. Kim, S. Kim, C.H. So, J. Kang, BioBERT: a pre-trained biomedical language representation model for biomedical text mining. Bioinformatics **36**(4), 1234–1240 (2020)
20. K. Huang, J. Altosaar, R. Ranganath, ClinicalBSRT: modeling clinical notes and predicting hospital readmission. Preprint. arXiv:1904.05342 (2019)

21. A. Abd-Alrazaq, R. AlSaad, D. Alhuwail, A. Ahmed, P.M. Healy, S. Latifi, S. Aziz, R. Damseh, S.A. Alrazak, J. Sheikh et al., Large language models in medical education: opportunities, challenges, and future directions. JMIR Med. Educ. **9**(1), e48291 (2023)
22. B. Meskó, E.J. Topol, The imperative for regulatory oversight of large language models (or generative AI) in healthcare. NPJ Digit. Med. **6**(1), 120 (2023)
23. F. Tustumi, N.A. Andreollo, J.E.d. Aguilar-Nascimento, Future of the language models in healthcare: the role of ChatGPT. ABCD. arquivos brasileiros de cirurgia digestiva (são paulo) **36**, e1727 (2023)
24. J.A. Omiye et al., Large language models propagate race-based medicine. NPJ Digit. Med. **6**(1), 195 (2023). https://doi.org/10.1038/s41746-023-00939-z
25. T. Nguyen, S. Diakiw, M. VerMilyea, A. Dinsmore, M. Perugini, D. Perugini, J. Hall, Efficient automated error detection in medical data using deep-learning and label-clustering. Sci. Rep. **13**(1), 19587 (2023)
26. Z.S. Wong, N. Waters, J. Liu, S. Ushiro, A large dataset of annotated incident reports on medication errors. Sci. Data **11**(1), 260 (2024)
27. C.-K. Wu, W.-L. Chen, H.-H. Chen, Large language models perform diagnostic reasoning. Preprint. arXiv:2307.08922 (2023)
28. Y. Weng, B. Li, F. Xia, M. Zhu, B. Sun, S. He, K. Liu, J. Zhao, Large language models need holistically thought in medical conversational QA. Preprint. arXiv:2305.05410 (2023)
29. X. Liu, D. McDuff, G. Kovacs, I. Galatzer-Levy, J. Sunshine, J. Zhan, M.-Z. Poh, S. Liao, P. Di Achille, S. Patel, Large language models are few-shot health learners. Preprint. arXiv:2305.15525 (2023)
30. Q. Chen, J. Du, Y. Hu, V.K. Keloth, X. Peng, K. Raja, R. Zhang, Z. Lu, H. Xu, Large language models in biomedical natural language processing: benchmarks, baselines, and recommendations. Preprint. arXiv:2305.16326 (2023)
31. S. Lobentanzer, J. Saez-Rodriguez, A platform for the biomedical application of large language models. Preprint. arXiv:2305.06488 (2023)
32. G. Wang, G. Yang, Z. Du, L. Fan, X. Li, ClinicalGPT: large language models finetuned with diverse medical data and comprehensive evaluation. Preprint. arXiv:2306.09968 (2023)
33. OpenAI, Introducing ChatGPT, https://openai.com/blog/chatgpt (2022). Accessed 12 Jun 2024
34. Y. Gao, D.T. Baptista-Hon, K. Zhang, The inevitable transformation of medicine and research by large language models: the possibilities and pitfalls. MedComm–Fut. Med. **2**(2), e49 (2023)
35. A.A. Borkowski, C.E. Jakey, S.M. Mastorides, A.L. Kraus, G. Vidyarthi, N. Viswanadhan, J.L. Lezama, Applications of ChatGPT and large language models in medicine and health care: benefits and pitfalls. Fed. Pract. **40**(6), 170 (2023)
36. H. Naveed, A.U. Khan, S. Qiu, M. Saqib, S. Anwar, M. Usman, N. Akhtar, N. Barnes, A. Mian, A comprehensive overview of large language models. Preprint submitted to Elsevier (2024) [Online]. Available: https://arxiv.org/abs/2307.06435
37. Y. Wang, Y. Zhao, L. Petzold, Are large language models ready for healthcare? A comparative study on clinical language understanding, in *Machine Learning for Healthcare Conference* (PMLR, 2023), pp. 804–823
38. J. Devlin, BERT: pre-training of deep bidirectional transformers for language understanding. Preprint. arXiv:1810.04805 (2018)
39. A.E. Johnson, T.J. Pollard, L. Shen, L.-w.H. Lehman, M. Feng, M. Ghassemi, B. Moody, P. Szolovits, L. Anthony Celi, R.G. Mark, MIMIC-III, a freely accessible critical care database. Sci. Data **3**(1), 1–9 (2016)
40. L.Y. Jiang, X.C. Liu, N.P. Nejatian, M. Nasir-Moin, D. Wang, A. Abidin, K. Eaton, H.A. Riina, I. Laufer, P. Punjabi et al., Health system-scale language models are all-purpose prediction engines. Nature **619**(7969), 357–362 (2023)
41. Y. Gu, S. Zhang, N. Usuyama, Y. Woldesenbet, C. Wong, P. Sanapathi, M. Wei, N. Valluri, E. Strandberg, T. Naumann et al., Distilling large language models for biomedical knowledge extraction: a case study on adverse drug events. Preprint. arXiv:2307.06439 (2023)
42. C. Liu, Y. Ma, K. Kothur, A. Nikpour, O. Kavehei, Biosignal copilot: leveraging the power of LLMS in drafting reports for biomedical signals. medRxiv 2023–06 (2023)

43. T. Zhao, M. Wei, J.S. Preston, H. Poon, LLM calibration and automatic hallucination detection via pareto optimal self-supervision. Preprint. arXiv:2306.16564 (2023)
44. R.B. Zuckerman, S.H. Sheingold, E.J. Orav, J. Ruhter, A.M. Epstein, Readmissions, observation, and the hospital readmissions reduction program. N. Engl. J. Med. **374**(16), 1543–1551 (2016)
45. C. Liu, Y. Ma, K. Kothur, A. Nikpour, O. Kavehei, Biosignal copilot: leveraging the power of LLMS in drafting reports for biomedical signals. medRxiv (2023) [Online]. Available: https://doi.org/10.1101/2023.06.28.23291916
46. A. Abd-alrazaq, R. AlSaad, D. Alhuwail, A. Ahmed, P.M. Healy, S. Latifi, S. Aziz, R. Damseh, S.A. Alrazak, J. Sheikh, Large language models in medical education: opportunities, challenges, and future directions. JMIR Med. Educ. **9**, e48291 (2023) [Online]. Available: https://mededu.jmir.org/2023/1/e48291
47. A. Toma, R. Xie, S. Palayew, P. Lawler, B. Wang, WangLab at MEDIQA-CORR 2024: optimized LLM-based programs for medical error detection and correction, in *Proceedings of the 6th Clinical Natural Language Processing Workshop*, ed. by T. Naumann, A. Ben Abacha, S. Bethard, K. Roberts, and D. Bitterman (Association for Computational Linguistics, Mexico City, 2024), pp. 616–623 [Online]. Available: https://aclanthology.org/2024.clinicalnlp-1.59
48. A.B. Abacha, W.-w. Yim, Y. Fu, Z. Sun, M. Yetisgen, F. Xia, T. Lin, MEDEC: a benchmark for medical error detection and correction in clinical notes. Preprint. arXiv:2412.19260 (2024)
49. K. Singhal, S. Azizi, T. Tu, S.S. Mahdavi, J. Wei, H.W. Chung, N. Scales, A. Tanwani, H. Cole-Lewis, S. Pfohl et al., Large language models encode clinical knowledge. Nature **620**(7972), 172–180 (2023)
50. Y. Gu, R. Tinn, H. Cheng, M. Lucas, N. Usuyama, X. Liu, T. Naumann, J. Gao, H. Poon, Domain-specific language model pretraining for biomedical natural language processing. ACM Trans. Comput. Healthcare **3**(1), 1–23 (2021)
51. K. Dalton, S. Byrne, Role of the pharmacist in reducing health care costs: current insights. Integr. Pharm. Res. Pract. **6**, 37–46 (2017)
52. M. Karabacak, K. Margetis, Embracing large language models for medical applications: opportunities and challenges. Cureus **15**(5) (2023)
53. K. Singhal, T. Tu, J. Gottweis, R. Sayres, E. Wulczyn, M. Amin, L. Hou, K. Clark, S.R. Pfohl, H. Cole-Lewis et al., Toward expert-level medical question answering with large language models. Nat. Med. **31**(3), 943–950 (2025)
54. J. Achiam, S. Adler, S. Agarwal, L. Ahmad, I. Akkaya, F.L. Aleman, D. Almeida, J. Altenschmidt, S. Altman, S. Anadkat et al., Gpt-4 technical report. Preprint. arXiv:2303.08774 (2023)
55. Q. Jin, B. Dhingra, Z. Liu, W.W. Cohen, X. Lu, PubMedQA: a dataset for biomedical research question answering. Preprint. arXiv:1909.06146 (2019)
56. D. Hendrycks, C. Burns, S. Basart, A. Zou, M. Mazeika, D. Song, J. Steinhardt, Measuring massive multitask language understanding. Preprint. arXiv:2009.03300 (2020)
57. A. Albarqawi, Exploring the opportunities and limitations of large language models in biomedical sector (2022)
58. S.M. Lundberg, S.-I. Lee, A unified approach to interpreting model predictions. Adv. Neural Inf. Proces. Syst. **30** (2017)
59. M.T. Ribeiro, S. Singh, C. Guestrin, " why should I trust you?" explaining the predictions of any classifier, in *Proceedings of the 22nd ACM SIGKDD International Conference on Knowledge Discovery and Data Mining* (2016), pp. 1135–1144
60. S. Reddy, J. Fox, M.P. Purohit, Artificial intelligence-enabled healthcare delivery. J. R. Soc. Med. **112**(1), 22–28 (2019)
61. K.-H. Jung, Large language models in medicine: clinical applications, technical challenges, and ethical considerations. Healthcare Inf. Res. **31**(2), 114–124 (2025)
62. F. Dennstädt, J. Hastings, P.M. Putora, M. Schmerder, N. Cihoric, Implementing large language models in healthcare while balancing control, collaboration, costs and security. NPJ Digit. Med. **8**(1), 143 (2025)

63. M. Spotnitz, B. Idnay, E.R. Gordon, R. Shyu, G. Zhang, C. Liu, J.J. Cimino, C. Weng, A survey of clinicians' views of the utility of large language models. Appl. Clin. Inf. **15**(02), 306–312 (2024)
64. G.E. Weissman, T. Mankowitz, G.P. Kanter, Unregulated large language models produce medical device-like output. NPJ Digit. Med. **8**(1), 148 (2025)
65. S. Tonmoy, S. Zaman, V. Jain, A. Rani, V. Rawte, A. Chadha, A. Das, A comprehensive survey of hallucination mitigation techniques in large language models. Preprint. arXiv:2401.01313 (2024)
66. N. Norori, Q. Hu, F.M. Aellen, F.D. Faraci, A. Tzovara, Addressing bias in big data and AI for health care: a call for open science. Patterns **2**(10), 100347 (2021)
67. A. Zhang, X. Lin, Towards secure and privacy-preserving data sharing in e-health systems via consortium blockchain. J. Med. Syst. **42**(8), 140 (2018)
68. P.P. Angelov, E.A. Soares, R. Jiang, N.I. Arnold, P.M. Atkinson, Explainable artificial intelligence: an analytical review. Wiley Interdiscip. Rev.: Data Min. Knowl. Discovery **11**(5), e1424 (2021)

Data Privacy and Security in Large Language Models for Medical Fields

Walid Al-Dhabyani

Abstract Large language models (LLMs) are transforming healthcare through applications such as diagnosis, risk prediction, and treatment planning. While offering improved accuracy and efficiency, their use raises significant privacy and security concerns, including prompt injection, adversarial manipulation, and leakage of sensitive patient data. This chapter reviews key vulnerabilities, attack vectors, and their implications for medical practice. It also includes all medical fields branches and clinical use. We also summarize AI adoption across major medical fields, outlining benefits and challenges. Challenges and mitigation with LLMs in the medical field are illustrated and explained in detail. Some defense approaches with evaluation metrics such as privacy leakage rate, attack success rate, and computational overhead are concluded. Our findings highlight the need for robust, adaptive safeguards to ensure safe and ethical LLM deployment in healthcare. More researches in this direction are still open for academics and industries.

1 Introduction

The use of machine learning (ML) techniques has grown in a number of research fields [1]. A fascinating area of research in the scientific world is the investigation of intelligence and the viability of creating machines with cognitive capacities. Researchers in the field of artificial intelligence (AI) are working hard to improve methods for creating intelligent machines [2]. Large language models (LLMs) are among the most recent developments and are now widely used in both industry and academics. According to [3], these LLMs are remarkably effective and can execute tasks nearly as well as humans. Large text production, text summarization, logical and mathematical reasoning, and code generation are only a few of the challenges that LLMs may handle, in contrast to previous language models (LMs)

W. Al-Dhabyani (✉)
Department of Computer Science, Faculty of Computers and Artificial Intelligence, Cairo University, Giza, Egypt
e-mail: w.aldhabyani@grad.fci-cu.edu.eg

N. E. M. Khalifa, M. H. N. Taha (eds.), *Next-Gen Healthcare*,
https://doi.org/10.1007/978-3-032-07267-2_7

that were restricted to particular tasks like categorization and next-word prediction. Furthermore, without additional training or fine-tuning, LLMs can adapt to various circumstances and/or even complete new jobs with effective rapid engineering [4]. These incredibly effective LLMs are not perfect, though. From a security and privacy standpoint, the vulnerabilities of these LLMs have not been thoroughly investigated on a broad scale [5]. To find these weaknesses, a thorough investigation is essential. Additionally, assessments of LLM concentrated on rationality, correctness, robustness, privacy, and security. We are concentrating on the increasing awareness of the dangers associated with the use of LLM in the medical area. This chapter demonstrates the privacy and security issues with LLMs for healthcare and how they might be resolved to strengthen defenses.

Machine learning (ML) techniques have been increasingly applied across various research domains. Their integration and the advantages they provide have often established them as the primary approach in numerous sectors, including object detection, emotion recognition, speech recognition, and sentiment analysis [6, 7]. ML has also garnered significant interest in the medical community, yielding promising results. Examples of healthcare applications include real-time prioritization [8], personalized medication and care [9], and patient data analytics.

Machine learning (ML) and large language models (LLMs) carry out a variety of tasks in the healthcare industry [10]. These tasks include segmentation and identification, where imaging algorithms identify anatomical structures and identify abnormalities [11]; classification, which groups medical data, such as scans and lab results, into diagnostic groups; and prediction, which forecasts events like hospital readmissions or disease progression [12]. They aid in anomaly discovery by highlighting uncommon or uncommon clinical patterns and risk stratification by assessing the probability of particular illnesses. LLMs provide sophisticated summarization and temporal reasoning, whereas natural language processing (NLP) applications draw structured insights from unstructured information [13]. Additionally, by matching patient profiles with evidence-based treatments, ML and LLMs help guide therapy recommendations. They also support outcome monitoring by continuously analyzing recovery patterns. Drug development gains from expedited candidate selection and literature synthesis, while operational optimization is accomplished through resource forecasting and workflow automation [14]. Additionally, by offering easily available, customized medical information, conversational chatbots driven by LLM improve patient education and engagement.

The chapter focuses on security and privacy of LLMs for healthcare. And it is divided as follows: Sect. 1 introduces machine learning and LLMs, security and privacy, and medical fields. Subsequently, Sect. 2 explores security and privacy of LLMs. Medical fields are illustrated in Sect. 3. Section 4 contains AI application in medical fields. Challenges with LLMs in the medical field and their mitigation strategies are covered in Sects. 5 and 6. Section 7 contains the evaluation and discussion part. Finally, conclusion finalized this chapter in Sect. 8.

2 Privacy and Security of LLMs

As large language models (LLMs) are incorporated into more and more applications, security and privacy threats are becoming serious issues. They are exposed to new types of prompt and input manipulation during interactions with LLMs, which might be used to uncover weaknesses. Finding vulnerabilities and ensuring the responsible and safe deployment of LLMs are the main goals of researching these attacks [15]. Prompt hacking, jailbreaking, and adversarial assaults such as backdoor insertion and data poisoning are some of the main forms of security risks [16]. Regarding privacy, LLMs could unintentionally commit private information to memory and divulge it from their training data [5]. The most common forms of privacy assaults are membership inference attacks (MIA), gradient leaking attacks, and personally identifiable information (PII) leaks that can happen during the inference, fine-tuning, or training stages. The diagram of security and privacy vulnerabilities is illustrated in Fig. 1.

The use of LLMs in healthcare settings raises a number of privacy and security issues that go well beyond conventional data security protocols. The basic conflict between the stringent confidentiality standards of medical information and the data-hungry nature of LLMs is at the heart of these difficulties [17].

2.1 *Security Attacks on LLMs*

Despite its revolutionary potential in a variety of fields, including healthcare, large language models (LLMs) are susceptible to a number of security risks that might compromise their dependability, security, and adherence to privacy laws [18]. These assaults could result in false information, patient injury, or breaches of private health information in high-stakes settings like clinical decision support. Therefore, it is

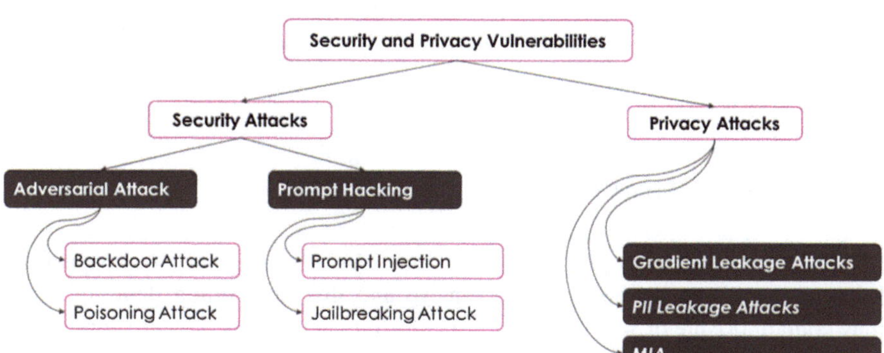

Fig. 1 The diagram of security and privacy vulnerabilities [15]

crucial to comprehend the different kinds of security assaults in order to create effective mitigation plans and guarantee the secure implementation of LLM-based systems. The following are the main types of security attacks:

- **Jailbreaking Attacks (JB)** [19]: The deliberate evasion of security measures, moral limitations, and content filters incorporated into an LLM is known as jailbreaking. Attackers create prompts or instructions that force the model to generate content that is dangerous, restricted, or violates policies. Such attacks have the potential to generate unreliable medical advice in healthcare applications, hence jeopardizing patient safety.
- **Prompt Injection (PI)** [20]: In order to override or change the system's intended behavior, prompt injection entails inserting malicious instructions into user input or external data sources (such as a research document or medical record). This may prompt the LLM to disregard its initial directives or carry out detrimental activities, like disclosing private patient information or making false diagnosis.
- **Adversarial Attacks (AA)** [21]: In order to trick the LLM into generating inaccurate or undesired outputs, adversarial attacks purposefully alter inputs, frequently with minute disruptions that are invisible to the human eye. Token rearrangements, synonym substitutions, or obfuscation strategies that take advantage of model flaws may all be used in text-based systems. Such manipulation could result in faulty treatment recommendations or inaccurate clinical interpretations in the healthcare industry.
- **Backdoor Attacks (BA)** [22]: Backdoor attacks use malicious pretraining checkpoints or compromised datasets to add hidden triggers into the model during training. While operating properly otherwise, the model generates attacker-defined outputs when these triggers are present in the input. In medical settings, where certain trigger phrases or symbols may cause the model to circumvent safety procedures or provide incorrect advice, this can be very risky.
- **Data Poisoning Attacks (DPa)** [23]: When attackers purposefully tamper with training data by adding inaccurate, deceptive, or biased information, this is known as data poisoning. This can lead to systematic errors and deteriorate model performance. Poisoning could provide negative misinformation into clinical support systems, distort treatment outcomes, or bias models against specific groups in healthcare LLMs.

2.2 *Privacy Attacks on LLMs*

LLMs are vulnerable to privacy attacks that take advantage of their capacity to learn and replicate patterns from extensive and diverse training datasets, which may contain private or sensitive data [15]. Such breaches in healthcare applications may lead to patient trust being damaged, regulatory frameworks like HIPAA and GDPR being broken, and protected health information (PHI) being disclosed without authorization [24]. Designing privacy-preserving designs and maintaining regulatory compliance require an understanding of these threats. The following are the main types of privacy attacks:

- **Gradient Leakage Attacks (GLA)** [25]: In order to reconstitute sensitive training data, these attacks take advantage of model gradients that are accessible during training or fine-tuning. Imaging scans, lab findings used in model development, or confidential patient records could all be recovered by an adversary given gradient information.
- **Membership Inference Attacks (MIAs)** [26]: Finding out if a particular data item was included in the model's training set is the goal of MIAs. Such attacks have the ability to disclose sensitive health information in the healthcare industry by revealing if a person took part in a clinical trial.
- **Personally Identifiable Information Leakage (PII-Leak)** [27]: In these attacks, personally identifiable information is extracted from an LLM's outputs either directly or indirectly. Names, addresses, medical record numbers, and information about uncommon conditions that could be used to reidentify patients are examples of this.

3 Medical Fields

Strict regulatory frameworks must be followed, while implementing large language models (LLMs) in the healthcare industry. The main legal foundation for safeguarding patient security and privacy in the USA is the Health Insurance Portability and Accountability Act (HIPAA) [28]. Protected health information (PHI) must be gathered, stored, processed, and shared only under permitted circumstances, with strong security measures in place to prevent unauthorized access. HIPAA compliance necessitates compliance with both the Privacy Rule and the Security Rule.

The phrase "medical fields" refers to a wide range of clinical and surgical specialties, each of which focuses on unique facets of human health. According to organ systems, patient demographics, diagnostic and treatment methods, or whether they entail surgical procedures, these areas are frequently categorized [29]. The main disciplines are then outlined in an organized manner.

3.1 Generalist Care

General Practice/Family Medicine: all-encompassing primary care for people of all ages, with a focus on early detection, prevention, and long-term treatment of common acute and chronic illnesses
Internal Medicine: identification, avoidance, and nonsurgical treatment of complicated adult illnesses, frequently in collaboration with subspecialties based on organs

3.2 Organ- and System-Based Medical Specialties

Cardiology: identification and treatment of cardiac conditions, such as arrhythmias, heart failure, and myocardial infarction
Gastroenterology: illnesses of the pancreas, liver, and digestive system (e.g., hepatitis, inflammatory bowel disease, and peptic ulcer disease)
Pulmonology: respiratory disorders like pneumonia, asthma, and chronic obstructive pulmonary disease
Neurology: illnesses affecting the central and peripheral neurological systems, such as multiple sclerosis, epilepsy, and stroke
Endocrinology: metabolic and hormonal conditions (e.g., thyroid, adrenal, and diabetes mellitus)
Nephrology: chronic kidney disease, nephrolithiasis, electrolyte and acid-base imbalances, dialysis, and transplant medicine are among the kidney diseases
Rheumatology: inflammatory and autoimmune conditions affecting the musculoskeletal system, such as systemic lupus erythematosus and rheumatoid arthritis
Infectious Diseases: infection prevention, antimicrobial stewardship, and the diagnosis and treatment of complicated illnesses
Hematology: blood and hematopoietic system problems, both benign and malignant (e.g., anemia, coagulopathies)
Medical Oncology: systemic cancer treatment, which includes immunotherapy, targeted drugs, and chemotherapy
Geriatrics: care for senior citizens, with a focus on functional status, frailty, and multimorbidity
Pediatrics: healthcare that includes both preventive and therapeutic services for newborns, infants, kids, and teenagers
Psychiatry: prevention, identification, and management of behavioral and mental health issues
Dermatology: conditions affecting the skin, hair, and nails, such as melanoma, psoriasis, and eczema
Ophthalmology: treatment of ocular diseases, such as cataracts and retinal abnormalities, using medicine and surgery
Otolaryngology (ENT): treatment of disorders of the ears, nose, throat, and associated head and neck through medicine and surgery
Urology: disorders of the male reproductive system and urinary tract, such as urologic cancers, benign prostatic hyperplasia, and urolithiasis

3.3 Diagnostic, Interventional, and Laboratory Disciplines

Radiology: diagnosis based on images employing modalities including ultrasound, CT, MRI, and X-rays; incorporates *interventional radiology* for image-guided, less invasive operations

Nuclear Medicine: use of radiopharmaceuticals for both diagnostic and therapeutic purposes (e.g., PET/CT, radionuclide therapy)
Pathology/Laboratory Medicine: molecular diagnostics, tissue and fluid diagnostics (clinical and anatomic pathology), and quality control
Clinical Pharmacology: pharmacovigilance, therapeutics optimization, and the safe and efficient use of pharmaceuticals

3.4 Surgical Specialties

General Surgery: extensive surgical practice that includes certain oncologic, endocrine, and abdominal treatments
Cardiothoracic Surgery: Thoracic organ surgery (e.g., lung excision, valve repair, coronary artery bypass)
Neurosurgery: surgical treatment of conditions affecting the brain, spinal cord, and peripheral nerves
Orthopedic Surgery: musculoskeletal disorders treated surgically (e.g., fracture fixation, arthroplasty)
Plastic and Reconstructive Surgery: cosmetic and reconstructive operations, such as skin grafting and microsurgery
Ophthalmic Surgery: surgical treatment of eye conditions, such as retinal repair and cataract removal
Gynecologic Oncology: surgical management of female reproductive tract cancers
Vascular Surgery: open and endovascular therapy for venous and arterial disorders
Transplant Surgery: solid-organ transplantation and the postoperative treatment that goes along with it
Trauma and Acute Care Surgery: operative and nonoperative time-sensitive care of surgical emergencies and injuries
Otorhinolaryngology—Head and Neck Surgery: surgical treatment of head-neck and ENT disorders
Maxillofacial and Oral Surgery: surgical treatment of dental, oral, and craniofacial structures
Radiation Oncology: cancer treatment using therapeutic radiation, frequently in multimodal regimens combining surgical and medicinal oncology

3.5 Perioperative, Emergency, and Supportive Care

Anesthesiology: critical event management, pain management, and perioperative physiology and anesthesia delivery
Emergency Medicine: prompt diagnosis and care for acute injuries and illnesses in situations that are life-threatening or urgent

Intensive Care/Critical Care Medicine: For severely ill patients, multisystem assistance is frequently provided in conjunction with other disciplines
Physical Medicine and Rehabilitation: recovery from disease or damage in terms of function and quality of life
Palliative Care: control of symptoms and management of treatment goals for severe, life-threatening conditions

3.6 Population and Informatics Disciplines

Public Health and Preventive Medicine: epidemiology, health policy, and health promotion at the population level
Occupational and Environmental Medicine: prevention and control of conditions relating to the workplace and surroundings
Sports Medicine: performance enhancement and nonoperative treatment of sports and activity-related injuries
Clinical Informatics: clinical decision assistance, data standards, and the secure use of digital tools, such as LLMs, into the provision of healthcare

4 AI Applications in Medical Fields

A growing number of medical disciplines are incorporating artificial intelligence (AI), which offers improved workflow efficiency, treatment precision, and diagnostic accuracy. Applications of AI, related advantages, and domain-specific difficulties in seven important medical domains are described in this section. While Table 1 offers a comprehensive breakdown of AI use cases, benefits, and challenges in each domain, Fig. 2 offers a visual summary of these domains and their characteristics.

4.1 Surgery

The Czech dramatist Karel Capek coined the term "robot" a century ago. It referred to a machine with specific mental and physical abilities, or an artificial human. For this reason, I think AI is a component of a robot—more especially, a medical one. As a result, the operating room is currently the scene of another act of this drama [30]. AI-driven technologies are transforming surgical practice by enhancing safety, precision, and intraoperative decision-making [31]:

- **Robotic-Assisted Surgery**: Robotic systems driven by AI make minimally invasive operations more accurate and dexterous.

Table 1 AI applications, benefits, and challenges across key medical fields

Medical field	AI applications	Benefits	Challenges
Surgery	• Robotic-assisted surgery	• Increased precision	• High equipment cost
	• Preoperative planning from scans	• Minimally invasive procedures	• Need for specialized training
	• Intraoperative guidance	• Reduced recovery times	• Risk of system failure during surgery
Emergency medicine	• AI-based triage systems	• Faster treatment decisions	• Data integration across hospital systems
	• Predictive patient deterioration alerts	• Better patient prioritization	• Risk of overreliance on AI decisions
	• Rapid diagnostic support	• Reduced mortality rates	• Privacy concerns in real-time data sharing
Oncology	• AI-driven cancer detection from imaging	• Early cancer detection	• Biased datasets affecting diagnosis
	• Precision oncology (genetic profiling)	• Personalized treatment plans	• Ethical concerns in genetic data use
	• Treatment response prediction	• Better treatment monitoring	• Integration into existing workflows
Cardiology	• Automated ECG interpretation	• Early disease detection	• Need for large, diverse datasets
	• Heart attack risk prediction	• Accurate diagnosis	• Misinterpretation risk in borderline cases
	• Cardiovascular imaging analysis	• Better preventive care	• Regulatory approval delays
Ophthalmology	• Diabetic retinopathy detection	• Early detection of eye diseases	• Variability in skin tone datasets
	• Glaucoma screening	• Reduced specialist workload	• Risk of false positives/negatives
	• Automated retinal image grading	• Increased access in rural areas	• Patient data privacy in telemedicine
Radiology	• Automated image anomaly detection	• Faster report turnaround	• Need for standardization in imaging
	• Workflow prioritization	• Reduced diagnostic errors	• Dependence on high-quality images
	• Error reduction tools	• Increased radiologist efficiency	• Resistance from some practitioners

- **Preoperative Planning**: To create the best surgical plans, machine learning algorithms examine multimodal patient data and imaging.
- **Intraoperative Guidance**: AI feedback in real time helps with anomaly identification, complication risk prediction, and instrument navigation.

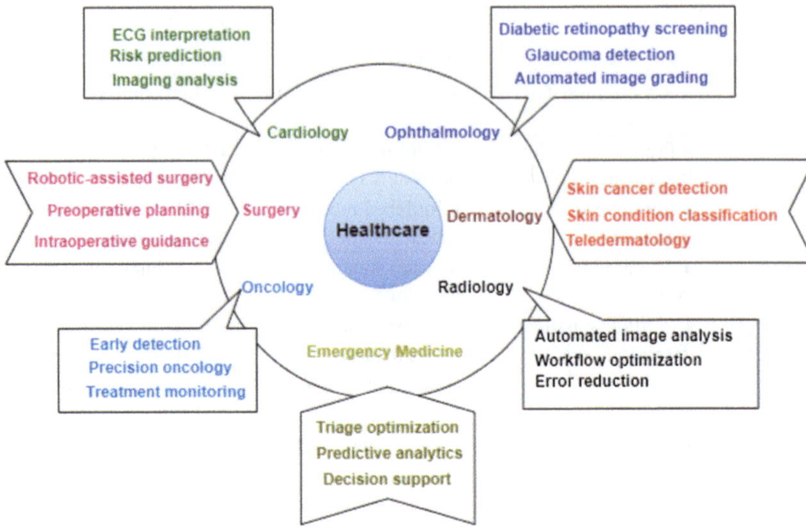

Fig. 2 Overview of selected medical fields and associated AI-related attributes

4.2 Emergency Medicine

During the COVID-19 epidemic, emergency medicine and its services had reached a breaking point. This epidemic has brought to light the shortcomings of a system that requires reexamination and the consideration of innovative solutions. Artificial intelligence (AI) has advanced to the point that it has the potential to drastically change the healthcare industry, with applications in the emergency department showing the most promise [32]. In high-acuity settings, AI supports rapid, evidence-based decision-making under time constraints [33]:

- **Triage Optimization**: AI systems evaluate clinical information and symptoms to rank instances that need immediate attention.
- **Predictive Analytics**: Proactive care is made possible by models that predict patient decline.
- **Decision Support**: AI combines imaging, vitals, and patient history to provide quick diagnostic support.

4.3 Oncology

Oncology's terrain and horizons are being significantly altered by artificial intelligence (AI), which is creating new and significant prospects to enhance cancer patient care. Through an analysis of AI-based devices that have already received formal FDA approval, we demonstrate that the oncology-related field where AI has had the biggest impact on clinical practice is cancer diagnostics [34]. AI in cancer improves early detection, allows for ongoing monitoring, and personalizes treatment [35]:

- **Early Detection**: Earlier than traditional techniques, computer vision algorithms detect cancers in CT scans, mammography, and other imaging modalities.
- **Precision Oncology**: In order to match patients with targeted medicines, genomic and molecular data are evaluated.
- **Treatment Monitoring**: AI models forecast treatment response and monitor tumor growth.

4.4 Cardiology

Cardiology is heavily utilizing artificial intelligence (AI), especially in the areas of risk assessment, treatment planning, diagnostics, and invasive treatments. Even while AI-driven developments have shown promise, there are still significant obstacles preventing their practical application [36]. AI helps in cardiovascular disease management, diagnosis, and prevention [37]:

- **ECG Interpretation**: Algorithms have a high sensitivity and can quickly identify arrhythmias and minor anomalies.
- **Risk Prediction**: Predictive models use lifestyle and history data to assess the risk of myocardial infarction or stroke.
- **Imaging Analysis**: AI improves cardiac MRI, CT angiography, and echocardiography interpretation.

4.5 Ophthalmology

AI improves the early identification and treatment of conditions that endanger vision [38]. Furthermore, researchers can examine the possible applications of LLMs in ocular imaging, focusing on three important areas: creating synthetic data, identifying diseases, and improving images. Moreover, ophthalmologists may make better decisions and treat patients more individually by fusing AI's capabilities with data-driven strategies, innovative biomarkers, and state-of-the-art imaging techniques [39]:

- **Diabetic Retinopathy Screening**: Retinal lesions can be accurately identified by automated image analysis.
- **Glaucoma Detection**: To identify early stages of disease, machine learning evaluates the anatomy of the optic nerve.
- **Automated Image Grading**: AI systems prioritize patient photos for a quicker assessment by specialists.

4.6 Dermatology

Since the COVID-19 pandemic, AI has been increasingly significant in the identification of dermatological disorders. With reports ranging from 81.0% to 99.0%, the majority of the literature on AI in dermatology focuses on the identification of melanoma and nonmelanoma skin cancer. Atopic dermatitis, psoriasis, acne vulgaris, and onychomycosis are among the other conditions that are frequently researched. Even while AI could increase access to dermatological treatment, particularly in underprivileged areas, there are still obstacles in the way of its widespread use [40]. AI systems expedite dermatology diagnosis and streamline therapeutic regimens [41]:

- **Skin Cancer Detection**: Using dermoscopic images, deep learning models detect melanoma and other cancers.
- **Skin Condition Classification**: AI can distinguish between diseases such as infectious rashes, psoriasis, and eczema.
- **Teledermatology**: Access to care is improved by mobile AI applications that allow for remote evaluation of skin lesions.

4.7 Radiology

Applications of AI in radiology are especially useful for tasks involving pattern recognition and classification; for instance, automated feature extraction has improved diagnostic efficiency and accuracy in identifying anomalies across imaging modalities [42]. One of the most developed fields for AI adoption is radiology, which has demonstrated uses in diagnostic imaging:

- **Automated Image Analysis**: AI analyzes CT, MRI, and X-ray data to find vascular anomalies, cancers, and fractures.
- **Workflow Optimization**: Prioritization algorithms identify studies that need to be reviewed right away.
- **Error Reduction**: Both false positives and false negatives are decreased by AI-assisted readings.

5 Challenges with LLMs in the Medical Field

In the digital age, protecting patient privacy has remained a top priority in healthcare information management. Traditional methods have mostly depended on data encryption technologies and rule-based protocols, which usually need a significant amount of IT expertise to execute. Recent developments in large language models (LLMs) have allowed clinical practitioners to use these tools for particular data tasks, while also introducing innovative methods for protecting the privacy of electronic medical records (EMRs) [43].

Researchers and practitioners have created a variety of privacy-preserving methods to meet the inherent privacy difficulties of LLMs in healthcare. These technologies strive to preserve patient anonymity, while maintaining data utility [44]. The integration of LLMs into medical practice presents a wide spectrum of challenges spanning security, privacy, technical, regulatory, and ethical dimensions. These challenges must be addressed to ensure safe, equitable, and legally compliant deployment.

5.1 Security Challenges

LLMs continue to face a number of security threats that could jeopardize their dependability, integrity, and safety, despite their increasing use in clinical and healthcare settings [45]. These weaknesses are especially important in the healthcare industry since breaches or hostile manipulations have the potential to reveal private patient information, jeopardize legal compliance, and ultimately impact patient care. Security challenges can arise from direct system exploitation, malicious user interactions, or adversarial manipulation of inputs and outputs. Prompt injection or hostile inputs that alter model behavior, model inversion, and membership inference approaches that jeopardize confidentiality, and data breaches and cyberattacks that target protected health information (PHI) are the most notable concerns. Each of these attack vectors highlights the need for robust technical safeguards, continuous monitoring, and domain-specific risk mitigation strategies:

- **Data Breaches and Cybersecurity Threats**: Cyberattacks could target LLMs that handle protected health information (PHI). Sensitive data is more likely to be accessed or exfiltrated by unauthorized parties in the absence of strong encryption, access controls, and intrusion detection.
- **Model Inversion and Membership Inference Attacks**: Confidentiality may be jeopardized by adversarial approaches that can reconstruct training data or determine whether a particular patient record was included in the training set.
- **Prompt Injection and Adversarial Inputs**: Carefully constructed inputs need strict input sanitization and monitoring since they can result in harmful recommendations or illegal disclosures from an LLM.

5.2 Privacy Challenges

LLMs provide serious privacy issues in addition to security risks because of their capacity to analyze, retain, and occasionally unintentionally replicate sensitive data [46]. These risks are particularly acute in healthcare, where protected health information (PHI) must be managed under stringent legal and ethical frameworks. Beyond straightforward data leaks, privacy problems also include residual reidentification hazards, legal compliance, and the possible exploitation of recorded interaction logs. Addressing these challenges is essential to maintain patient trust, safeguard confidentiality, and ensure adherence to global privacy regulations. The main categories of privacy challenges include:

- **Compliance with Privacy Regulations**: It is difficult to comply with the regulations of the GDPR in the EU, HIPAA in the USA, and other regional frameworks, particularly when dealing with cross-border data flows.
- **Data Minimization and Deidentification**: Even if deidentification lowers privacy risk, there are still risks of reidentification, especially when using other databases.
- **Data Retention and Secondary Use**: Conversational or inference logs that are kept for an extended period of time may unintentionally be used for reasons other than those for which the original agreement was obtained.

5.3 Other Challenges

Beyond security and privacy, the deployment of large language models (LLMs) in healthcare faces a wide spectrum of additional challenges that are ethical, technical, regulatory, and clinical in nature [47–50]. These challenges are frequently related: Regulatory concerns have a direct effect on workflow integration, while ethical worries about justice may coexist with technological problems of hallucinations. To make sure that LLMs enhance professional judgment and patient trust rather than compromise it, these problems must be resolved. The following lists the main types of challenges.

5.3.1 Ethical Challenges

- **Bias and Fairness**: Biases in training data may be reinforced or amplified by LLM outputs, resulting in recommendations that are unfair to different demographic groups.
- **Transparency and Explainability**: The lack of transparency in LLM decision-making hinders error analysis and reduces clinician trust.
- **Patient Autonomy and Consent**: Concerns over informed consent and shared decision-making may arise because patients may not be aware of the degree of LLM involvement in their care.

5.3.2 Technical Challenges

- **Hallucination of Medical Facts**: LLMs may produce information that is clinically inaccurate but believable, which could be dangerous in therapeutic or diagnostic settings.

- **Contextual Misinterpretation**: Erroneous findings may result from ambiguities in local protocols, medical terminology, or abbreviations.
- **Integration with Clinical Systems**: Adherence to interoperability standards (e.g., HL7, FHIR) is necessary for secure and seamless interoperability with medical equipment and electronic health records (EHRs).

5.3.3 Regulatory and Governance Challenges

- **Certification and Validation**: Standardized frameworks for LLM-specific validation are still in their infancy, yet regulatory agencies like the FDA and EMA need thorough validation for AI-based clinical decision support systems.
- **Liability and Accountability**: Legal culpability is unclear when LLM-generated advice leads to unfavorable results.
- **Auditability and Monitoring**: To identify model drift, new biases, and security flaws, post-deployment monitoring must be ongoing.

5.3.4 Clinical Workflow Challenges

- **Overreliance and Deskilling**: Overreliance on LLM results may impair professionals' ability to diagnose and think critically.
- **Time and Cognitive Load**: If outputs need to be thoroughly verified, poorly integrated systems may make clinicians' workloads heavier rather than lighter.
- **Adaptation to Specialty-Specific Needs**: Development complexity is increased by the need for domain-specific tweaking in high-variance disciplines (such as pathology versus emergency medicine).

A multidisciplinary approach is required to address these issues, including strong cybersecurity safeguards, data processing that protects privacy, regulatory compliance, ethical supervision, and clinical validation. In addition to jeopardizing patient safety and trust, inadequate risk mitigation could impede the long-term use of LLMs in the medical field.

6 Mitigation Strategies for LLM Challenges in Healthcare

To enable the safe, ethical, and effective use of large language models (LLMs) in clinical and public health settings, proactive mitigation strategies must be implemented across technical, regulatory, and organizational domains [51]. The following approaches align with best practices in cybersecurity, health informatics, and medical ethics.

6.1 Security Safeguards

- **Robust Cybersecurity Frameworks**: Use multifactor authentication (MFA), role-based access control (RBAC), and end-to-end encryption for data both in transit and at rest.
- **Adversarial Robustness**: To protect against malicious input manipulation and prompt injection, use prompt sanitization and adversarial training.
- **Regular Penetration Testing**: To find and fix security flaws before they are exploited, do regular penetration testing and vulnerability assessments.

6.2 Privacy Preservation

- **Deidentification and Anonymization**: To reduce the danger of reidentification, use automated PHI redaction and structured deidentification procedures (such as Safe Harbor under HIPAA).
- **Data Minimization**: Do not collect more data than is required for the intended clinical use.
- **Federated and Privacy-Preserving Learning**: To facilitate model training without centralizing sensitive data, use homomorphic encryption, federated learning, or differential privacy.

6.3 Ethical Governance

- **Bias Auditing and Fairness Metrics**: Using verified fairness standards, regularly assess LLM results for demographic bias and, if necessary, implement corrective retraining.
- **Explainable AI (XAI) Tools**: To increase openness and clinician trust, incorporate interpretable model outputs (such as rule-based summaries and attention maps).
- **Informed Consent Protocols**: Patients should be made fully aware of the limits and decision-making boundaries when LLMs are involved in their care.

6.4 Technical Reliability

- **Hallucination Reduction**: Use domain-specific knowledge bases to implement retrieval-augmented generation (RAG), which grounds outputs in validated sources.

- **Contextual Adaptation**: Utilize quick engineering and domain-adapted fine-tuning to incorporate workflows and terminology unique to your specialty.
- **Interoperability Standards**: For smooth interaction with EHRs and imaging systems, follow the DICOM and HL7 FHIR standards.

6.5 Regulatory and Compliance Alignment

- **Model Validation and Certification**: Adhere to existing frameworks for pre-deployment validation, such as FDA SaMD and EMA AI recommendations, which cover usability, safety, and efficacy assessment.
- **Liability Frameworks**: Establish precise accountability frameworks that involve legal, clinical, and IT stakeholders for decisions impacted by LLM outcomes.
- **Audit Logging**: For post-event investigations and compliance audits, keep tamper-proof logs of all inputs, outputs, and system actions.

6.6 Clinical Workflow Integration

- **Human-in-the-Loop (HITL) Review**: All high-risk decisions should be subject to clinical supervision, and LLM findings should be used as advisory rather than independent recommendations.
- **Usability-Centered Design**: Work together with doctors to co-develop LLM interfaces that minimize cognitive load and fit into current workflows.
- **Continuous Education and Training**: Continually educate medical staff on the proper use of LLM, its limits, and how to spot errors.

6.7 Cross-Cutting Measures

- **Continuous Monitoring and Feedback Loops**: Install real-time monitoring tools to identify new biases, accuracy deterioration, and model drift.
- **Ethics and Oversight Committees**: Create interdisciplinary AI governance boards to examine use cases, track results, and authorize updates.
- **Iterative Improvement**: Use a lifetime approach, upgrading protections and models frequently in response to new rules, clinical feedback, and changing risks.

Together, these tactics can help healthcare organizations reduce the most urgent concerns related to the deployment of LLMs, while maximizing their potential to enhance medical research, operational effectiveness, and patient care. An adaptive governance structure that can change with medical practice and AI technology is necessary for effective mitigation, which is not static.

7 Evaluation and Discussion

The evaluation of large language models (LLMs) in the medical field requires a multidimensional approach that extends beyond conventional accuracy metrics to encompass safety, privacy, fairness, and clinical utility [52]. The rapid expansion of LLM research highlights how revolutionary they may be in the medical field. Nonetheless, it will be crucial to address issues including underrepresentation of vital specializations, evaluation unpredictability, and ethical hazards. Standardized frameworks should be given top priority in future initiatives to guarantee the safe, efficient, and just integration of LLM in clinical practice.

7.1 Evaluation Framework

The assessment should include both quantitative and qualitative methods:

- **Clinical Accuracy**: Depending on the type of question-answering or classification task, assessed using task-specific measures including accuracy, recall, F1 score, and perfect match rates.
- **Safety and Reliability**: Evaluated by looking for adherence to accepted clinical criteria, conflicting advice, and hallucinated medical facts.
- **Privacy Compliance**: To identify possible reidentification or inappropriate disclosure, it was tested using simulated input scenarios including deidentified PHI.
- **Bias and Fairness**: In order to identify differences in output quality, performance is analyzed by stratifying it across demographic groupings (such as age, sex, and ethnicity).
- **Usability and Workflow Fit**: Collected by means of standardized physician comments regarding cognitive effort, interpretability, and ease of integration.

7.2 Evaluation Criteria

To assess the effectiveness of the security and privacy of LLMs [15], the evaluation should consider using key metrics as illustrated in Table 2.

7.3 Key Findings

The studies indicate that LLMs demonstrate strong potential in synthesizing medical literature, generating draft clinical documentation, and supporting decision-making in low-risk contexts. However, several limitations were observed:

Table 2 Evaluation criteria for AI privacy and security [15]

Criterion	Description
Privacy leakage rate	Measure of how much private data can be extracted from the model
Attack success rate	Percentage of successful adversarial or prompt injection attacks
False positive rate	Frequency of incorrectly flagged safe inputs or outputs
Model utility	Impact on performance (e.g., accuracy, perplexity) after applying defenses
Adaptability	The system's ability to adapt to novel or unseen threats
Computational overhead	Evaluation of training and inference time increases due to added mechanisms

- *Hallucinations*: In difficult multistep reasoning tasks, clinically significant errors remained even, while retrieval-augmented techniques decreased factual errors.
- *Privacy Risk*: Rarely, models replicated learned training material that looked like PHI, highlighting the necessity of stringent privacy-protection protocols.
- *Domain Variability*: Performance differed significantly by specialty, with lower dependability in high-variance, context-heavy contexts (e.g., emergency care, psychiatry) and higher accuracy in structured, guideline-driven disciplines (e.g., cardiology, oncology).
- *Workflow Integration*: Although they voiced concern about the amount of time needed to validate outputs in critical care settings, they appreciated LLM-generated summaries and guideline lookups.

7.4 Discussion

These findings reinforce the importance of domain-specific adaptation and human-in-the-loop (HITL) oversight for safe LLM deployment in medicine. The observed hallucinations align with documented limitations of generative models in other high-stakes domains, highlighting the necessity of retrieval-augmented generation, constrained decoding, and cross-checking against verified knowledge bases.

From a privacy perspective, even rare reproduction of sensitive patterns presents unacceptable risk under HIPAA and GDPR. Privacy-preserving architectures, such as federated learning with differential privacy, emerge as essential safeguards.

Bias analysis revealed that without targeted mitigation, LLMs can perpetuate existing disparities in healthcare delivery. This necessitates ongoing fairness auditing, inclusive training data, and transparent reporting of subgroup performance.

Clinically, the integration of LLMs must be tailored to the operational tempo and cognitive demands of each specialty. Low-acuity domains (e.g., outpatient documentation) are better suited to early adoption, whereas high-acuity contexts (e.g., trauma surgery, intensive care) require more rigorous validation and fail-safe mechanisms.

7.5 *Implications for LLM Integration*

The breadth and heterogeneity of medical disciplines imply domain-specific requirements for LLM deployment. High-variance, time-critical settings (e.g., emergency and critical care) prioritize reliability, calibration, and uncertainty communication; image-centric fields (e.g., radiology, ophthalmology) require robust multimodal integration; oncology and infectious diseases emphasize guideline concordance and up-to-date evidence synthesis; and population health and clinical informatics stress interoperability, auditability, and governance. Across all domains, alignment with privacy and security safeguards (e.g., HIPAA Privacy and Security Rules) remains foundational [28]. More researches should be applied in the privacy and security of LLMs for medical fields.

8 Conclusion

Large language model integration in healthcare poses a serious barrier to patient privacy and data security, while also offering a previously unheard-of chance to improve medical care. Implementing strong privacy-preserving measures becomes not just a legal need but also a basic obligation to patients and society as healthcare companies embrace these potent technologies more and more. Their use presents serious privacy and security issues, such as rapid insertion, adversarial manipulation, and the disclosure of private patient data, even if they provide increased accuracy and speed. The main weaknesses, attack methods, and their consequences for medical practice are reviewed in this chapter. It also covers clinical use in all branches of medicine. We also provide an overview of the advantages and difficulties of AI adoption in the main medical domains. The difficulties and solutions faced by LLMs in the medical profession are detailed and shown. A few protection strategies are evaluated using parameters like computing overhead, assault success rate, and privacy leakage rate. Our results demonstrate the necessity of strong, flexible safeguards to guarantee the ethical and safe implementation of LLM in healthcare. Both academics and businesses are still welcome to conduct additional study in this area.

Declaration of the Use of AI-Assisted Technologies
The authors declare that large language models were used to assist in language editing, proofreading, and formatting guidance during the preparation of this chapter. All scientific content, interpretation, analysis, and final revisions were thoroughly reviewed and approved by the authors.

References

1. I.H. Sarker, *Machine Learning: Algorithms, Real-world Applications and Research Directions* (Springer, Cham, 2021), pp. 160–172
2. K. Thakur, H.G. Barker, A.-S.K. Pathan, *Artificial Intelligence and Large Language Models: An Introduction to the Technological Future* (Springer, Cham, 2024)
3. Y. Zhuang, Q. Liu, Y. Ning, W. Huang, R. Lv, Z. Huang, G. Zhao, Z. Zhang, Q. Mao, S. Wang, et al., Efficiently measuring the cognitive ability of LLMs: An adaptive testing perspective. Mach. Learn. J. **45**, 123–145 (2024)
4. J. Wei, X. Wang, D. Schuurmans, M. Bosma, F. Xia, E. Chi, Q.V. Le, D. Zhou, et al., Chain-of-thought prompting elicits reasoning in large language models. Adv. Neural Inf. Proces. Syst. **35**, 24824–24837 (2022)
5. B. Yan, K. Li, M. Xu, Y. Dong, Y. Zhang, Z. Ren, X. Cheng, *On Protecting the Data Privacy of Large Language Models (LLMs): A Survey* (Springer, Cham, 2024)
6. M. Wankhade, A.C.S. Rao, C. Kulkarni, *A Survey on Sentiment Analysis Methods, Applications, and Challenges* (Springer, Cham, 2022)
7. R. Magherini, E. Mussi, M. Servi, Y. Volpe, *Emotion Recognition in the Times of COVID-19: Coping with Face Masks* (Springer, Cham, 2022)
8. M. Hardy, H. Harvey, *Artificial Intelligence in Diagnostic Imaging: Impact on the Radiography Profession* (Springer, Cham, 2020)
9. K.B. Johnson, W.-Q. Wei, D. Weeraratne, M.E. Frisse, K. Misulis, K. Rhee, J. Zhao, J.L. Snowdon, *Precision Medicine, AI, and the Future of Personalized Health Care* (Springer, Cham, 2021)
10. R. Magherini, E. Mussi, Y. Volpe, R. Furferi, F. Buonamici, M. Servi, *Machine Learning for Renal Pathologies: An Updated Survey* (Springer, Cham, 2022)
11. S.N. Kumar, A.L. Fred, P.S. Varghese, *An Overview of Segmentation Algorithms for the Analysis of Anomalies on Medical Images* (Springer, Cham, 2019)
12. K. Swanson, E. Wu, A. Zhang, A.A. Alizadeh, J. Zou, *From Patterns to Patients: Advances in Clinical Machine Learning for Cancer Diagnosis, Prognosis, and Treatment* (Springer, Cham, 2023)
13. Y. Zhang, H. Jin, D. Meng, J. Wang, J. Tan, *A Comprehensive Survey on Process-Oriented Automatic Text Summarization with Exploration of LLM-Based Methods* (Springer, Cham, 2024)
14. J.P.S. Saini, A. Thakur, D. Yadav, *AI Driven Innovations in Pharmaceuticals: Optimizing Drug Discovery and Industry Operations* (Springer, Cham, 2025)
15. B.C. Das, M.H. Amini, Y. Wu, *Security and Privacy Challenges of Large Language Models: A Survey* (Springer, Cham, 2025)
16. A.G. Chowdhury, M.M. Islam, V. Kumar, F.H. Shezan, V. Jain, A. Chadha, *Breaking Down the Defenses: A Comparative Survey of Attacks on Large Language Models* (Springer, Cham, 2024)
17. A.B.M.K.I. Riad, M.A. Barek, M.M. Rahman, M.S. Akter, T. Islam, M.A. Rahman, M.R. Mia, H. Shahriar, F. Wu, S.I. Ahamed, Enhancing HIPAA Compliance in AI-driven mHealth Devices Security and Privacy, in *2024 IEEE 48th Annual Computers, Software, and Applications Conference (COMPSAC)* (IEEE, New York, 2024), pp. 2430–2435
18. Z.A. Nazi, W. Peng, *Large Language Models in Healthcare and Medical Domain: A Review* (Springer, Cham, 2024)
19. B. Peng, K. Chen, Q. Niu, Z. Bi, M. Liu, P. Feng, T. Wang, L.K.Q. Yan, Y. Wen, Y. Zhang, et al., *Jailbreaking and Mitigation of Vulnerabilities in Large Language Models* (Springer, Cham, 2024)
20. E. Derner, K. Batistič, J. Zahálka, R. Babuška, *A Security Risk Taxonomy for Prompt-Based Interaction with Large Language Models* (Springer, Cham, 2024)

21. E. Shayegani, M.A.A. Mamun, Y. Fu, P. Zaree, Y. Dong, N. Abu-Ghazaleh, *Survey of Vulnerabilities in Large Language Models Revealed by Adversarial Attacks* (Springer, Cham, 2023)
22. Y. Li, H. Huang, Y. Zhao, X. Ma, J. Sun, *BackdoorLLM: A Comprehensive Benchmark for Backdoor Attacks and Defenses on Large Language Models* (Springer, Cham, 2024)
23. P. Zhao, W. Zhu, P. Jiao, D. Gao, O. Wu, *Data Poisoning in Deep Learning: A Survey* (Springer, Cham, 2025)
24. V.V. Sangaraju, *AI and Data Privacy in Healthcare: Compliance with HIPAA, GDPR, and Emerging Regulations* (Springer, Cham, 2025)
25. J. Dong, J. Chen, X. Xie, J. Lai, H. Chen, *Survey on Adversarial Attack and Defense for Medical Image Analysis: Methods and Challenges* (Springer, Cham, 2024)
26. Z. Li, Y. Wu, Y. Chen, F. Tonin, E. Abad Rocamora, V. Cevher, *Membership Inference Attacks Against Large Vision-Language Models* (Springer, Cham, 2024)
27. X. Zhan, J.C. Carrillo, W. Seymour, J. Such, *Malicious LLM-Based Conversational AI Makes Users Reveal Personal Information* (Springer, Cham, 2025)
28. F. Khan, *Regulating the Revolution: A Legal Roadmap to Optimizing AI in Healthcare* (Springer, Cham, 2023)
29. M. Bath, T. Bashford, J.E. Fitzgerald, *What is 'Global Surgery'? Defining the Multidisciplinary Interface Between Surgery, Anaesthesia and Public Health* (Springer, Cham, 2019)
30. Z. Nawrat, *Introduction to AI-driven Surgical Robots* (Springer, Cham, 2023)
31. N. Abbasi, H.K. Hussain, *Integration of Artificial Intelligence and Smart Technology: AI-Driven Robotics in Surgery: Precision and Efficiency* (Springer, Cham, 2024)
32. G. Chenais, E. Lagarde, C. Gil-Jardiné, *Artificial Intelligence in Emergency Medicine: Viewpoint of Current Applications and Foreseeable Opportunities and Challenges* (Springer, Cham, 2023)
33. A. Kirubarajan, A. Taher, S. Khan, S. Masood, *Artificial Intelligence in Emergency Medicine: A Scoping Review* (Springer, Cham, 2020)
34. C. Luchini, A. Pea, A. Scarpa, *Artificial Intelligence in Oncology: Current Applications and Future Perspectives* (Springer, Cham, 2022)
35. H. Shimizu, K.I. Nakayama, *Artificial Intelligence in Oncology* (Springer, Cham, 2020)
36. G. Biondi-Zoccai, D'Ascenzo, F., S. Giordano, U. Mirzoyev, Ç. Erol, S. Cenciarelli, P. Leone, F. Versaci, *Artificial Intelligence in Cardiology: General Perspectives and Focus on Interventional Cardiology* (Springer, Cham, 2025)
37. F. Lopez-Jimenez, Z. Attia, A.M. Arruda-Olson, R. Carter, P. Chareonthaitawee, H. Jouni, S. Kapa, A. Lerman, C. Luong, J.R. Medina-Inojosa, et al. *Artificial Intelligence in Cardiology: Present and Future* (Springer, Cham, 2020)
38. E. Waisberg, J. Ong, S.A. Kamran, M. Masalkhi, P. Paladugu, N. Zaman, A.G. Lee, A. Tavakkoli, *Generative Artificial Intelligence in Ophthalmology* (Springer, Cham, 2025)
39. H.-N. Costin, M. Fira, L. Goraş, *Artificial Intelligence in Ophthalmology: Advantages and Limits* (Springer, Cham, 2025)
40. S. Biswas, U. Achar, B. Hakim, A. Achar, *Artificial Intelligence in Dermatology: A Systematized Review* (Springer, Cham, 2025)
41. S. Thunga, M. Khan, S.I. Cho, J.I. Na, J. Yoo, *AI in Aesthetic/Cosmetic Dermatology: Current and Future* (Springer, Cham, 2025)
42. R. Obuchowicz, J. Lasek, M. Wodziński, A. Piórkowski, M. Strzelecki, K. Nurzynska, *Artificial Intelligence-Empowered Radiology—Current Status and Critical Review* (Springer, Cham, 2025)
43. M. Gong, Z. Ouyang, D. Ma, E. Cai, C. Liu, D. Shi, B. Zhang, L. Ma, Y. Wei, H. Jiang, et al., *Privacy Protection for Chinese Electronic Medical Records Using Large Language Models: Effectiveness Evaluation and Application of LLM Models in Medical Data Tasks* (Springer, Cham, 2025)
44. Jung, K.-H., *Large Language Models in Medicine: Clinical Applications, Technical Challenges, and Ethical Considerations* (Springer, Cham, 2025)

45. M. Aljohani, J. Hou, S. Kommu, X. Wang, *A Comprehensive Survey on the Trustworthiness of Large Language Models in Healthcare* (Springer, Cham, 2025)
46. C. Nachuma, M.M. Fouda, M.F. Zibran, Security and privacy for LLMs and LMMs across key sectors: a literature survey. In: *International Conference on Information Technology—New Generations* (Springer, Cham, 2025), pp. 25–39
47. M. Al-Garadi, T. Mungle, A. Ahmed, A. Sarker, Z. Miao, M.E. Matheny, *Large Language Models in Healthcare* (Springer, Cham, 2025)
48. S. Maity, M.J. Saikia, *Large Language Models in Healthcare and Medical Applications: A Review* (Springer, Cham, 2025)
49. S. Tripathi, K. Mongeau, D. Alkhulaifat, A. Elahi, T.S. Cook, *Large Language Models in Health Systems: Governance, Challenges, and Solutions* (Springer, Cham, 2025)
50. X. Chen, J. Xiang, S. Lu, Y. Liu, M. He, D. Shi, *Evaluating Large Language Models and Agents in Healthcare: Key Challenges in Clinical Applications* (Springer, Cham, 2025)
51. C. Lin, C.-F. Kuo, *Roles and Potential of Large Language Models in Healthcare: A Comprehensive Review* (Springer, Cham, 2025)
52. S. Shool, S. Adimi, R. Saboori Amleshi, E. Bitaraf, R. Golpira, M. Tara, *A Systematic Review of Large Language Model (LLM) Evaluations in Clinical Medicine* (Springer, Cham, 2025)

Part II
Translational Applications and Disease-Focused Studies Using AI

Advancing Early Alzheimer's Diagnosis with Deep Learning on MRI Data

Aman Yadav, Aman Ahlawat, and Seba Susan

Abstract Alzheimer's disease is a progressive neurodegenerative disorder, and identifying it in its early stages is essential for enabling timely therapeutic intervention. This study investigates the effectiveness of five state-of-the-art deep pretrained convolutional neural networks—VGG19, InceptionV3, ResNet50, InceptionResNetV2, and EfficientNetB0—in classifying Alzheimer's disease using magnetic resonance imaging (MRI) data. Both shallow tuning and deep tuning of the models were explored for effective learning. Furthermore, we fine-tune VGG19 by unfreezing only Blocks 4 and 5, allowing adaptation of high-level features while preserving low-level representations. A cosine annealing learning rate scheduler with warm restarts dynamically adjusts the learning rate to accelerate convergence and mitigate overfitting. The five deep learning models and two machine learning models–SVM and LDA–were trained on brain MRI images from a subset of the ADNI dataset, available online on Kaggle. The dataset comprises three classes representing different stages of Alzheimer's disease and a fourth class representing the control (healthy) group. The three disease-related classes, being minority classes, were merged into a single class, rendering the classification problem binary with a balanced class distribution (diseased versus healthy group). The results indicate that the selectively fine-tuned VGG19 model, trained using a cosine annealing learning rate schedule with warm restarts, achieved superior performance compared to state-of-the-art methods. It attained an accuracy of 97.35%, precision of 0.9751, recall of 0.9706, F1-score of 0.9729, and an AUC of 0.9734, outperforming existing approaches by a significant margin.

Keywords Alzheimer's detection · Pretrained network · Fine-tuning · Deep learning · Learning rate scheduler with warm restarts

---

A. Yadav · A. Ahlawat · S. Susan (✉)
Department of Information Technology, Delhi Technological University, New Delhi, India
e-mail: amanyadav_2k19it014@dtu.ac.in; amanahlawat_2k19it012@dtu.ac.in;
sebasusan@dtu.ac.in

N. E. M. Khalifa, M. H. N. Taha (eds.), *Next-Gen Healthcare*,
https://doi.org/10.1007/978-3-032-07267-2_8

1 Introduction

Alzheimer's disease (AD) is a progressive neurodegenerative brain disorder characterized by a gradual decline in cognitive abilities, including memory, reasoning, and language function [1]. It is the most common cause of dementia in individuals over the age of 85 and is often associated with risk factors such as family history and head trauma [2]. The disease typically follows a variable course, with very mild to mild symptoms often emerging 8–10 years before clinical diagnosis [3].

According to the World Health Organization (WHO), dementia currently affects more than 55 million people worldwide, with nearly ten million new cases reported annually. Alzheimer's disease is the leading contributor to this global burden. In addition to Alzheimer's, several related neurodegenerative disorders—collectively known as Alzheimer's-related dementias (ADRD)—such as vascular dementia, Lewy body dementia, and frontotemporal dementia, exhibit overlapping symptoms and may co-occur with Alzheimer's pathology [4]. This overlap can complicate both diagnosis and treatment, underscoring the need for improved clinical tools and a deeper understanding of disease mechanisms.

Computer-aided brain scans can help diagnose Alzheimer's disease and help in planning effective and timely treatment. Neuroimaging modalities like MRI scans can aid in the automated diagnosis of Alzheimer's disease [5]. Artificial intelligence (AI) tools for processing and analyzing MRI and computed tomography (CT) images have advanced significantly over time, evolving from traditional feature extraction and selection methods, and classical machine learning algorithms, to modern deep neural network approaches. Falahati et al. [6] reviewed several feature selection and machine learning algorithms used to distinguish Alzheimer patients from healthy individuals using structural MRI. The study also highlighted key challenges, including the risk of overfitting arising from limited sample sizes and insufficient patient diversity. In [7], the authors employed minimum redundancy maximum relevance (mRMR) for feature selection and used a random forest classifier on features derived from total variation with L1 norm (TVL1) and gray-level size zone matrix (GLSZM), both of which capture texture irregularities in brain tissue.

Over the past decade, the number of deep learning models proposed for medical image analysis has grown significantly [8]. Most of these models are pretrained on the large-scale ImageNet database and subsequently fine-tuned on smaller, more specialized medical imaging datasets [9]. Deep pretrained convolutional networks are capable of learning the complex and hierarchical feature representations embedded within medical images through the process of transfer learning [10]. This makes them well suited for analyzing Alzheimer's disease MRI scans, where the intricate spatial structure and complexity of brain images present greater challenges than those encountered in conventional medical image analysis tasks. Noor et al. [11] examine the utility of state-of-the-art deep convolutional neural networks (CNN), such as GoogLeNet, AlexNet, ResNet, Inception, and customized CNN architectures, for Alzheimer's diagnosis. The authors highlight the growing use of CNNs for Alzheimer's diagnosis over the past decade and emphasize the need for regular reviews of deep learning model performance in this domain.

In this study, we systematically evaluate five advanced CNN architectures—VGG19, InceptionV3, ResNet50, InceptionResNetV2, and EfficientNetB0—for Alzheimer's disease detection from structural MRI scans. The contributions of this work are summarized as follows:

1. We address the key research gaps by conducting a systematic evaluation of five state-of-the-art convolutional neural network (CNN) architectures—VGG19, InceptionV3, ResNet50, InceptionResNetV2, and EfficientNetB0—for the task of Alzheimer's disease detection using structural MRI scans.
2. We assess the effect of fine-tuning pretrained models on Alzheimer's MRI datasets to determine its influence on classification accuracy and generalizability, building on evidence from prior work that suggests fine-tuning can significantly enhance model performance across various applications.
3. In addition, we employ transfer learning with VGG19, selectively fine-tuning Blocks 4 and 5 while freezing earlier layers to preserve generic features. A cosine annealing learning rate scheduler with warm restarts modulates the learning rate to enhance convergence stability and training efficiency.
4. We also benchmark the performance of the deep learning models against two widely used classical machine learning models—support vector machines (SVM) and linear discriminant analysis (LDA).

The list of abbreviations used in the chapter is given in Table 1.

In the remaining part of the chapter, Sect. 2 discusses some of the existing works, while Sect. 3 describes the methodology followed in the experimentation. Section 4 analyzes the results obtained, while Sect. 5 provides the concluding remarks.

Table 1 List of abbreviations

Abbreviation	Definition
AD	Alzheimer's disease
MRI	Magnetic resonance imaging
CT	Computed tomography
CNN	Convolutional neural network
ReLU	Rectified linear unit
B4	Block 4 (of VGG19)
B5	Block 5 (of VGG19)
LR	Learning rate
AUC	Area under the curve
SVM	Support vector machines
LDA	Linear discriminant analysis

2 Literature Review

A review of the existing literature highlights the significance of deep pretrained networks—particularly some of the more recent architectures—in identifying optimal deep learning models for Alzheimer's disease diagnosis. A recent survey on the application of deep learning for Alzheimer's detection [12] emphasized the role of transfer learning and data augmentation in enhancing brain scan analysis. A notable study by Ghaffari et al. [13] evaluated the performance of several pretrained models, including ResNet, Xception, and InceptionV3, for Alzheimer's detection, with InceptionV3 emerging as the top performer. Another study [14] explored both conventional CNNs and pretrained networks as feature extractors. In [15], researchers trained 2D-CNNs on different MRI slices and applied ensemble learning for Alzheimer's detection. Ebrahimi et al. [16] employed temporal convolutional networks and recurrent neural network to capture the 3D structure within MRI scans. Table 2 provides an overview of key deep learning models for Alzheimer's diagnosis using MRI scans. As observed, the models include both pretrained CNNs, like ResNet and Xception, that leverage transfer learning, and customized CNNs, like DEMNET and ADD-Net, which are trained from scratch. The customized CNNs comprise of convolutional blocks followed by one or more fully connected (dense) layers and a softmax layer for classification. Each convolutional block typically consists of a convolutional layer, a ReLU activation function, and a pooling layer, and may also include batch normalization and dropout.

Beyond MRI-based analysis, alternative biomarkers have also been explored. Al-Shoukry et al. [23] reviewed various biomarkers for Alzheimer's detection, while Gao and Lima [24] advocated for region-of-interest (ROI)-based deep learning approaches to enable effective learning with fewer features. Cheng and Liu [25] implemented a deep learning strategy comprising of an ensemble of deep 3D-CNNs. The 3D-CNNs were trained on local patches of positron emission tomography (PET) brain images to capture generic features. Gharaibeh et al. [26] proposed a deep learning framework utilizing angiogram scans that reflect cerebral blood flow. Their approach employed InceptionV3 and DenseNet201 as feature extractors, followed by feature selection and classification using traditional machine learning algorithms.

3 Methodology

This study aims to evaluate the performance of five deep learning models, namely, VGG19 [27], InceptionV3 [28], ResNet50 [29], InceptionResNetV2 [30], and EfficientNetB0 [31], in detecting Alzheimer's disease from MRI images. While these architectures perform well in general image classification tasks, their effectiveness in neurodegenerative disease detection—and the impact of hyperparameter optimization in medical imaging, particularly for Alzheimer's diagnosis—remains

Table 2 Summary of key deep learning models and approaches for Alzheimer's disease diagnosis using MRI scans

References	Highlights	Model details	Results	Limitations
Ghaffari et al. [13]	Transfer learning using pretrained CNNs	ResNet, Xception, InceptionV3	InceptionV3 performed best (93.33% on the ADNI dataset)	Insufficient training due to the small size of the dataset
Helaly et al. [14]	Training CNNs form scratch versus transfer learning using pretrained CNN VGG19	Simple CNNs, VGG19	CNN architectures trained faster and avoided overfitting, while maintaining comparable effectiveness (within 2%) to VGG19	Trade-off between computational complexity, memory requirement, and accuracy in resource-constrained devices
Pan et al. [15]	Ensemble of CNNs trained on different MRI slices	CNN base model comprising six convolutional blocks and two fully connected layers	Achieved 84% average accuracy in classifying diseased vs. healthy samples	A computationally complex procedure for selecting the five base models with the best generalization ability for each slice orientation
Vanaja et al. [17]	Training CNNs form scratch versus traditional machine learning algorithms	Customized CNN with three convolutional blocks and two fully connected layers	Achieved 87% accuracy on the ADNI dataset, exceeding all other machine learning models	Reduced image quality caused by converting DICOM to JPEG presents a challenge for tailored CNN architectures
Arafa et al. [18]	Training CNNs form scratch versus transfer learning using pretrained CNN VGG16	CNN base model comprising three convolutional blocks and three fully connected layers	Customized CNNs outperformed (99%) the pretrained model VGG16 (97%)	Model performance is highly influenced by the selection of hyperparameters and the configuration of dropout layers with varying dropout rates
Murugan et al. [19]	Novel CNN architecture: DEMentia NETwork (DEMNET) that is trained from scratch	DEMNET base model comprises of two convolutional blocks and three fully connected layers	Achieved 95.23% on the Kaggle dataset	Highly sensitive to class imbalance in the small dataset it is trained on
Fareed et al. [20]	Novel CNN architecture: Alzheimer's disease detection network (ADD-net) that is trained from scratch	ADD-net base model comprises of four convolutional blocks and two fully connected layers	Achieved 98.63% on the Kaggle dataset	Highly sensitive to class imbalance in the small dataset it is trained on

(continued)

Table 2 (continued)

References	Highlights	Model details	Results	Limitations
Abdelaziz et al. [21]	Multiscale deep learning model for multimodal data	CNN base model augmented with attention modules followed by multiscale fusion	Achieved 95.25% accuracy on the ADNI dataset	Lack of inclusion of nonimaging modalities like genetic data
Pradhan et al. [22]	Novel deep CNN architecture that is trained from scratch	CNN base model comprising three convolutional blocks and a fully connected layer	Achieved 98.57% accuracy on the ADNI dataset	Simplistic CNN architecture that works only for the dataset it is trained on

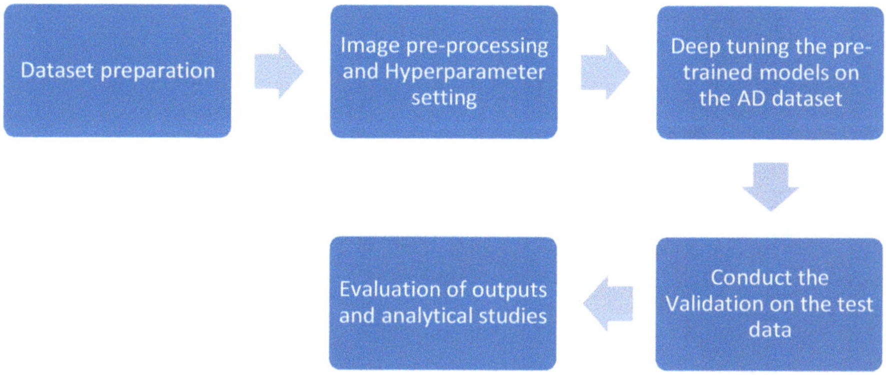

Fig. 1 Process flow for the experimentation

underexplored. In addition, we compare the performance of deep learning models with two traditional machine learning approaches–SVM and LDA—that remain widely used by researchers for Alzheimer's diagnosis based on MRI scans [32, 33].

InceptionResNetV2 was introduced in 2017 and EfficientNetB0 was introduced in 2019, so they can be considered recent models as compared to the more popular VGG19, InceptionV3 and ResNet50 models. The learning rate of EfficientNetB0 was also varied to evaluate its performance.

The process flow diagram in Fig. 1 outlines the end-to-end workflow for Alzheimer's disease (AD) detection. It begins with dataset preparation, where MRI images are sourced, labeled, and partitioned into training and test sets. This is followed by image pre-processing and hyperparameter configuration, including resizing, normalization, and the selection of training parameters such as learning rate, batch size, and number of epochs. Next, deep tuning of pretrained convolutional neural network models (VGG19, InceptionV3, ResNet50, Inception-ResNetV2, and EfficientNetB0) is performed, where network layers are fine-tuned on the training data. The trained models are then subjected to validation using the test set to assess their generalization capabilities. Finally, performance evaluation is conducted using metrics such as accuracy, precision, recall, F1-score, AUC, and confusion matrices to quantify model effectiveness in detecting Alzheimer's disease. After the pre-processing steps, the deep learning models are trained (both shallow- and deep-tuned) on the Alzheimer's disease (AD) dataset comprising of healthy and diseased samples. We implement deep tuning by training the inner layers of the deep models in addition to training the classification layer at the output on the AD dataset, while in shallow tuning, only the output classification layer is trained while all the other layers retain the pretrained ImageNet weights.

Additionally, we implement a transfer learning approach using VGG19, where we apply selective fine-tuning to specific layers of the pretrained model rather than training the entire network from scratch. Specifically, we unfreeze the convolutional layers in Block 4 (B4) and Block 5 (B5), while keeping the earlier layers frozen.

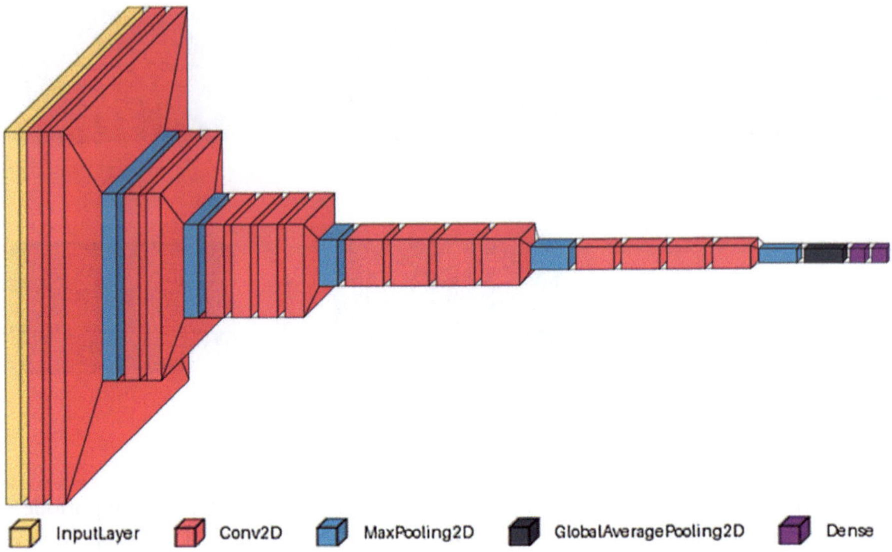

Fig. 2 Architecture of the VGG19 model used for selective fine-tuning, highlighting the custom classification head and trainable layers

This strategy helps retain low-level features learned from large-scale datasets (e.g., ImageNet) while allowing the model to adapt higher-level representations to our target dataset. At the output of each model, a global average pooling layer was added, followed by a dense layer with 128 units and ReLU activation, and a final dense layer with 2 units and softmax activation for binary classification. A cosine annealing learning rate scheduler with warm restarts [34] is employed to dynamically adjust the learning rate during training. This approach reduces training time and mitigates overfitting, especially with limited data. The structure of the VGG19 model with selective fine-tuning and the updated output layers is depicted in Fig. 2.

For all models, we have applied standard image normalization techniques to make the pixel values of the images fall within a standard range. This is done to ensure that the model does not get affected by the brightness and contrast differences in the images.

4 Results and Discussions

All experiments were conducted using Python 3 in a CPU-only environment with 12.7 GB system RAM. Each model took around 55 minutes to train and a few seconds for testing. We used the Kaggle dataset[1] containing 6400 MRI images, each sized 128 × 128, for the classification of Alzheimer's disease. The dataset includes 32 axial (horizontal) MRI slices per subject, capturing comprehensive cross-sectional brain information critical for identifying structural changes associated with Alzheimer's disease. This is a simplified subset of the massive multimodal Alzheimer's disease neuroimaging initiative (ADNI) dataset.[2] The ADNI, launched in 2003, aims to assess the progression of MCI and early Alzheimer's by combining MRI, PET, biomarkers, and clinical evaluations. The Kaggle dataset comprises of four classes corresponding to "Healthy" class [3200 samples], and three grades of Alzheimer's disease–Very Mild [2240], Mild [896], and Moderate [64], which were combined in the current work to form the "Diseased" class [3200 samples]. The class distribution is therefore balanced. This approach has several benefits. It solves the problem of class imbalance, which can cause the model to favor one class over the other. By combining the diseased stages into one group, the number of samples in that class increases, making the model more reliable. It also makes the task easier by turning it into a simple Healthy-vs-Diseased classification, which is more useful for early diagnosis. In addition, it avoids the need for complicated techniques to handle imbalanced data and creates a strong starting point for future research, where models can later be trained to recognize specific stages of the disease when more data is available. Simplifying the task into a binary classification—Healthy vs. Diseased—not only reduces complexity but also aligns with clinical priorities, where the primary goal is early detection of any signs of Alzheimer's. This binary setup supports better model interpretability, as it allows clinicians and researchers to more easily understand and trust the model's predictions. Sample MRI images from the dataset are shown in Fig. 3, highlighting the separation of Healthy and Diseased categories.

This study evaluates several state-of-the-art deep learning models previously used for AD detection, including VGG19, InceptionV3, ResNet50, InceptionResNetV2, and EfficientNetB0 (Table 2). We have not considered customized CNNs due to the relatively higher accuracies achieved by pretrained models due to transfer learning, as reported in Table 2. In prior research on AD detection, these models were commonly employed either as feature extractors [35] (shallow tuning) or fully fine-tuned on smaller AD datasets [13] (deep tuning). In our experiments, we perform both shallow tuning and deep tuning of the pretrained models. In shallow tuning, only the fully connected layers at the output are fine-tuned, while in deep tuning, all layers of the model are trainable. Additionally, we explore selective fine-tuning combined with dynamic learning rate scheduling for training the VGG19 model, which has been widely used in past AD detection studies.

The hyperparameters used in this study were selected through extensive empirical experimentation to identify configurations that yielded stable and high-performing models. The models were trained using the Adam optimizer with a

[1] https://www.kaggle.com/datasets/marcopinamonti/alzheimer-mri-4-classes-dataset.

[2] https://adni.loni.usc.edu/data-samples/adni-data/.

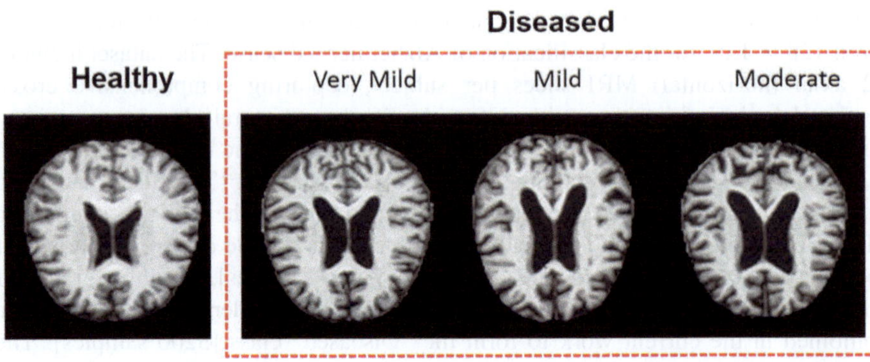

Fig. 3 Examples of MRI images from the Kaggle dataset demonstrating Healthy and different Diseased classes (very mild, mild, moderate)

learning rate of 0.001 and sparse categorical cross-entropy as the loss function. Training was conducted with early stopping, allowing a maximum of 20 epochs and a patience of 3 to prevent overfitting. At the output of each model, a global average pooling layer was added, followed by a dropout layer with a rate of 0.5 (applied only during full fine-tuning), a dense layer with 128 units and ReLU activation, and a final dense layer with 2 units and softmax activation for binary classification. The batch size was set to 32. An 80:20 train-test split was employed, and model evaluation was carried out using five-fold cross-validation to ensure robustness and generalizability. Additionally, we employ a transfer learning approach with VGG19 by selectively fine-tuning Blocks 4 and 5, integrating the same classification head used in other deep learning models—except for the dropout layer, which was removed as regularization is already provided by the cosine annealing learning rate scheduler—resulting in improved performance and reduced overfitting. The training loss and accuracy curves for the five deep learning models—VGG19, InceptionV3, ResNet50, InceptionResNetV2, and EfficientNetB0—are presented in Figs. 4, 5, 6, 7, and 8, respectively. As generally observed from these figures, shallow tuning is computationally efficient and requires less time and data; however, it often results in lower performance, particularly for tasks such as AD detection that diverge significantly from the pretraining distribution. In contrast, deep tuning updates all model weights, enabling the network to better adapt to the new data distribution, which generally leads to higher accuracy—especially when the target dataset is large or substantially different from the original training data.

Table 3 summarizes the test accuracies obtained for the five deep pretrained models on the AD dataset for shallow tuning as well as deep tuning. The confusion matrices corresponding to the five deep learning models are illustrated in Figs. 9, 10, 11, 12, and 13, shown for both shallow tuning and deep tuning (selective fine-tuning in case of VGG19).

Among all evaluated models, VGG19—fine-tuned by unfreezing only the final two convolutional blocks (Blocks 4 and 5) while keeping the earlier layers frozen,

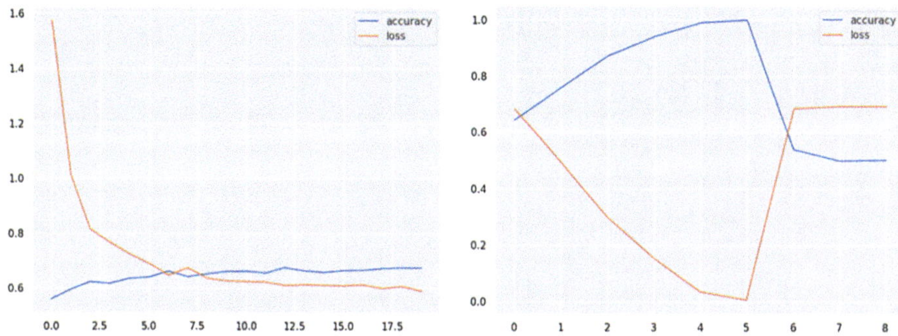

(a) (b)

Fig. 4 Results of (**a**) pretrained (shallow-tuned) and (**b**) selectively fine-tuned VGG19 model (with cosine annealing LR scheduler)

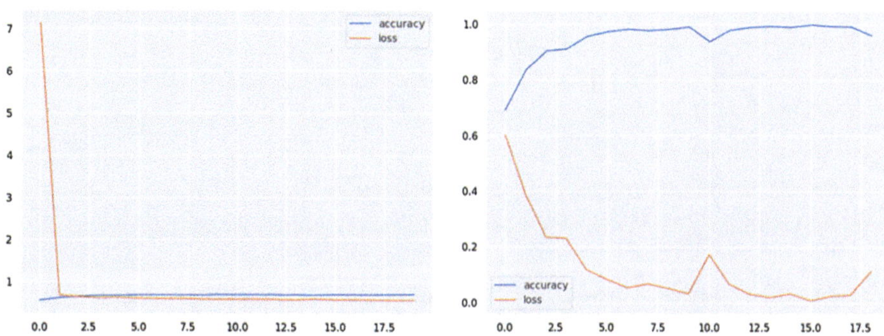

(a) (b)

Fig. 5 Results of (**a**) pretrained (shallow-tuned) and (**b**) fine-tuned (deep-tuned) InceptionV3 model

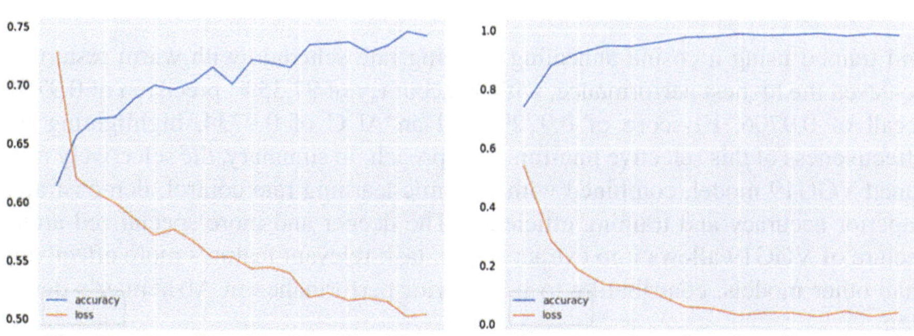

(a) (b)

Fig. 6 Results of (**a**) pretrained (shallow-tuned) and (**b**) fine-tuned (deep-tuned) ResNet50 model

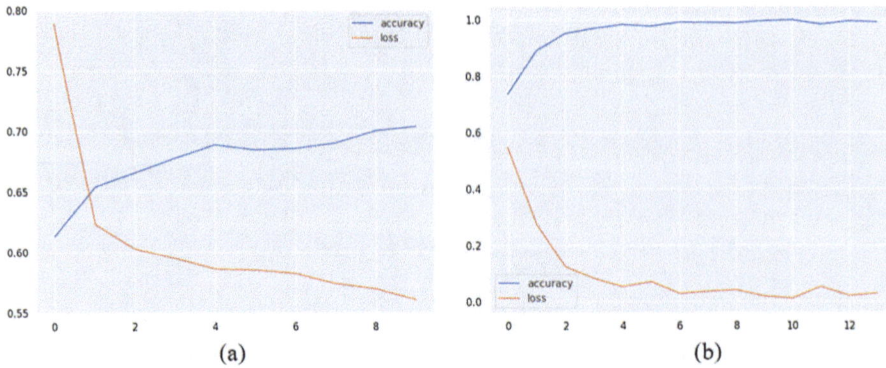

Fig. 7 Results of (**a**) pretrained (shallow-tuned) and (**b**) fine-tuned (deep-tuned) InceptionResNetV2 model

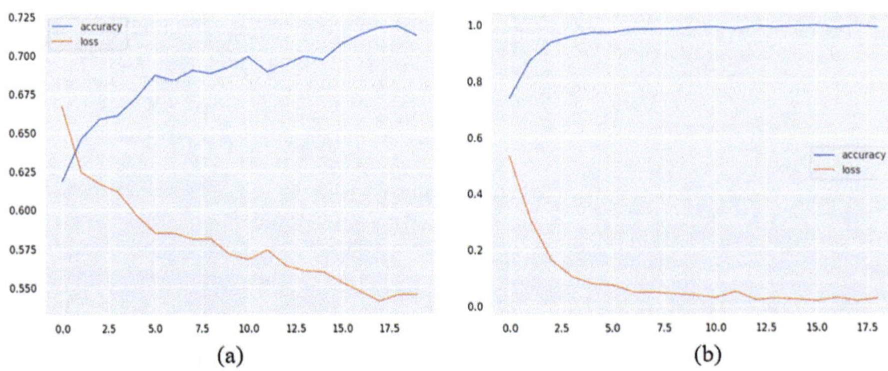

Fig. 8 Results of (**a**) pretrained (shallow-tuned) and (**b**) fine-tuned (deep-tuned) EfficientNetB0 model

and trained using a cosine annealing learning rate schedule with warm restarts—achieved the highest performance, with an accuracy of 97.35%, precision of 0.9751, recall of 0.9706, F1-score of 0.9729, and an AUC of 0.9734, highlighting the effectiveness of this selective fine-tuning approach. In summary, the selectively fine-tuned VGG19 model, combined with dynamic learning rate control, demonstrated superior accuracy and training efficiency. The deeper and more specialized architecture of VGG19 allows it to extract subtle, task-relevant features more effectively than other models, contributing to its superior performance in Alzheimer's detection.

The InceptionResNetV2 model performs second best, though its scores (accuracy = 92.59%, precision = 0.8744, recall = 0.9923, F1-score = 0.9296, and AUC = 0.9267) were notably lower than VGG19, highlighting the advantages of VGG19, with selective fine-tuning and cosine annealing learning rate (LR) scheduler with warm restarts, for the AD detection from MRI signals. Compared

Table 3 Performance comparison of deep learning and classical machine learning models under different training procedures for Alzheimer's detection

Model	Training procedure	Accuracy (%)	Precision	Recall	F1-score	AUC
VGG19	Shallow tuning	71.35	0.6853	0.7589	0.7202	0.7147
VGG19	Selective fine-tuning and LR scheduler	97.35	0.9751	0.9706	0.9729	0.9734
InceptionV3	Shallow tuning	68.55	0.6517	0.7813	0.7107	0.6866
InceptionV3	Deep tuning	83.29	1.000	0.6631	0.7974	0.8315
ResNet50	Shallow tuning	77.02	0.8028	0.7372	0.7686	0.7714
ResNet50	Deep tuning	85.63	0.7793	0.9877	0.8712	0.8584
InceptionResNetV2	Shallow tuning	71.35	0.6908	0.7595	0.7235	0.7141
InceptionResNetV2	Deep tuning	92.59	0.8744	0.9923	0.9296	0.9267
EfficientNetB0	Shallow tuning	74.98	0.7045	0.8425	0.7673	0.7516
EfficientNetB0	Deep tuning	89.04	0.8317	0.9928	0.9051	0.8845
SVM	–	85.56	0.8409	0.8822	0.8610	0.8552
LDA	–	89.87	0.9149	0.8822	0.8983	0.8989

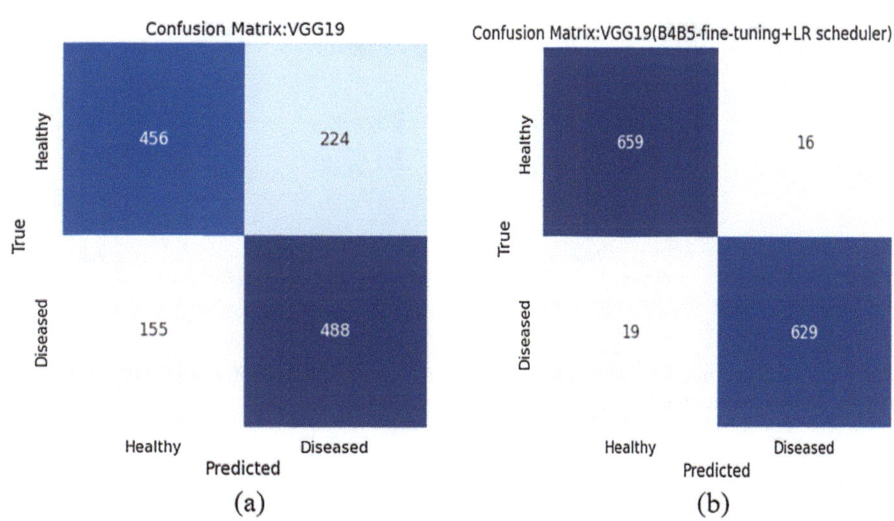

Fig. 9 Confusion matrices illustrating the performance of the VGG19 model using (**a**) shallow tuning and (**b**) fine-tuning

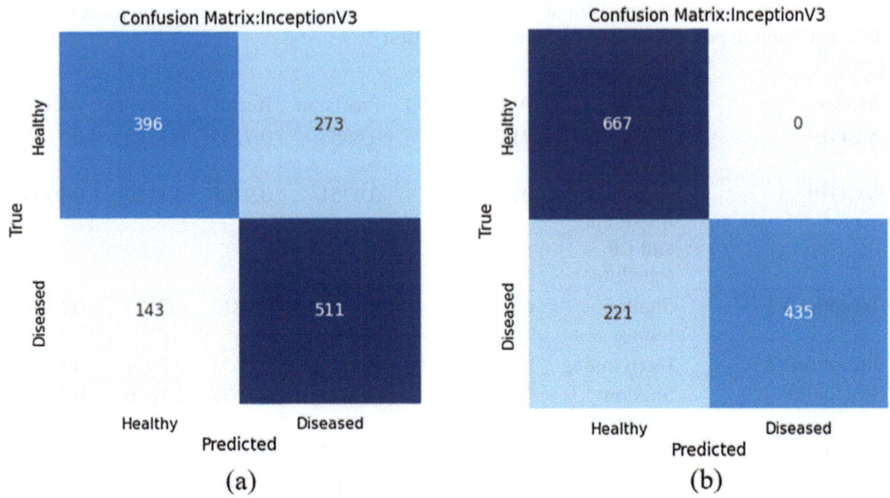

Fig. 10 Confusion matrices illustrating the performance of the InceptionV3 model using (**a**) shallow tuning and (**b**) fine-tuning

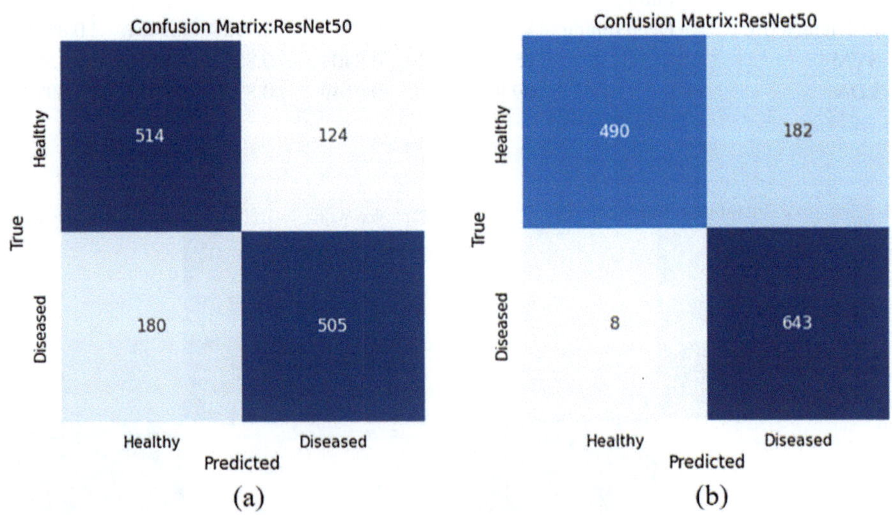

Fig. 11 Confusion matrices illustrating the performance of the ResNet50 model using (**a**) shallow tuning and (**b**) fine-tuning

to VGG19 and InceptionResNetV2, the performance of all other models was substantially lower.

The two machine learning models–SVM and LDA–popularly used in literature for AD detection [32, 33] trained faster while maintaining comparable effectiveness, though the scores were significantly lower than the two best performing deep

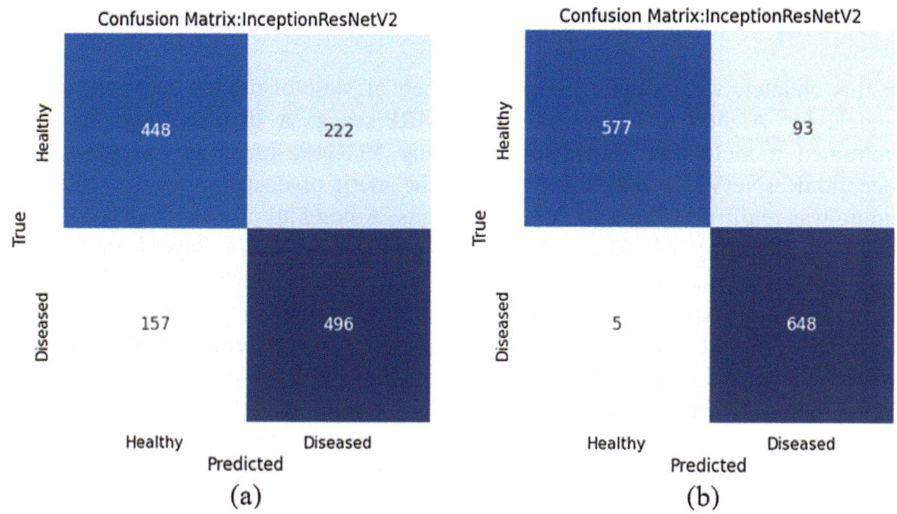

Fig. 12 Confusion matrices illustrating the performance of the InceptionResNetV2 model using (**a**) shallow tuning and (**b**) fine-tuning

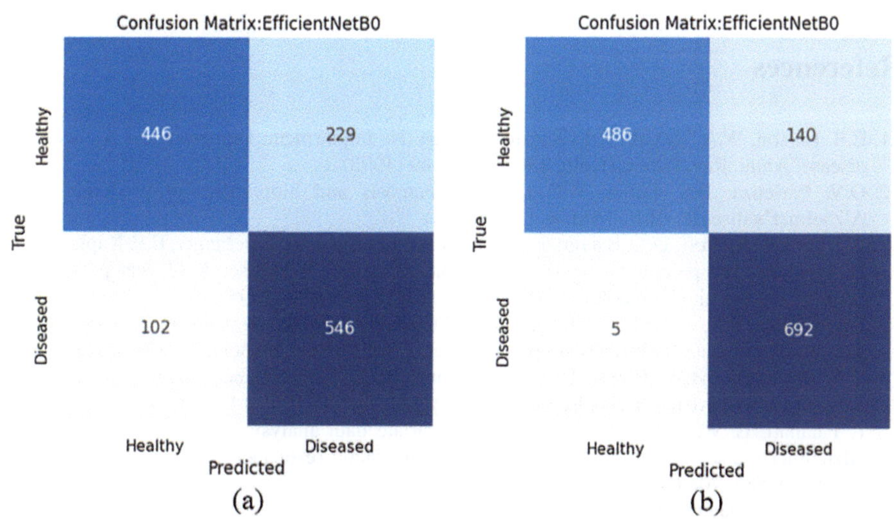

Fig. 13 Confusion matrices illustrating the performance of the EfficientNetB0 model using (**a**) shallow tuning and (**b**) fine-tuning

learning models (VGG19 and InceptionResNetV2). For SVM, the "rbf" kernel was used and the hyperparameters were set by grid search. Out of the two models, LDA achieved higher scores (accuracy = 89.87%, precision = 0.9149, recall = 0.8822, F1-score = 0.8983, and AUC = 0.8989).

5 Conclusion

In this chapter, we evaluate the performance of state-of-the-art deep pretrained models for Alzheimer's detection from MRI scans. A diverse range of deep pretrained models was considered including VGG19, InceptionV3, ResNet50, InceptionResNetV2, and EfficientNetB0. The merit of deep tuning over shallow tuning was reaffirmed through our experiments. Among all models, VGG19—fine-tuned by unfreezing only Blocks 4 and 5 while freezing all earlier layers, and trained with a cosine annealing learning rate schedule with warm restarts—achieved the highest accuracy of 97.35%, precision of 0.9751, recall of 0.9706, F1-score of 0.9729, and an AUC of 0.9734, demonstrating the effectiveness of this targeted training strategy. In future work, we aim to explore the multimodal nature of the ADNI dataset by incorporating additional data sources such as PET scans, clinical assessments, and genetic biomarkers alongside MRI. Investigating multimodal deep learning architectures will allow for more comprehensive modeling of Alzheimer's progression. Furthermore, we plan to focus on the seamless integration of the proposed deep learning models into clinical workflows, with the goal of supporting early diagnosis and decision-making in real-world healthcare settings.

References

1. E.B. Larson, W.A. Kukull, R.L. Katzman, Cognitive impairment: Dementia and Alzheimer's disease. Annu. Rev. Public Health **13**(1), 431–449 (1992)
2. O.V. Forlenza, B.S. Diniz, W.F. Gattaz, Diagnosis and biomarkers of predementia in Alzheimer's disease. BMC Med. **8**, 1–14 (2010)
3. R.T. Linn, P.A. Wolf, D.L. Bachman, J.E. Knoefel, J.L. Cobb, A.J. Belanger, E.F. Kaplan, R.B. D'Agostino, The preclinical phase of probable Alzheimer's disease: A 13-year prospective study of the Framingham cohort. Arch. Neurol. **52**(5), 485–490 (1995)
4. P.A. DeFina, R.S. Moser, M. Glenn, J.D. Lichtenstein, J. Fellus, Alzheimer's disease clinical and research update for health care practitioners. J. Aging Res. **2013**(1), 207178 (2013)
5. C.E. Wierenga, M.W. Bondi, Use of functional magnetic resonance imaging in the early identification of Alzheimer's disease. Neuropsychol. Rev. **17**, 127–143 (2007)
6. F. Falahati, E. Westman, A. Simmons, Multivariate data analysis and machine learning in Alzheimer's disease with a focus on structural magnetic resonance imaging. J Alzheimer's Dis **41**(3), 685–708 (2014)
7. R. HK, H.A. Deepak, M.S. Prapulla Kumar, S. Sharath, G.H. Yogeesh, A robust framework for Alzheimer's disease detection and staging: Incorporating multi-feature integration, MRMR feature selection, and random Forest classification. Multimed. Tools Appl. **84**(22), 24903–24931 (2024)
8. J. Wang, S. Wang, Y. Zhang, Deep learning on medical image analysis. CAAI Trans. Intell. Technol. **10**(1), 1–35 (2025)
9. D. Sethi, K. Arora, S. Susan, Transfer learning by deep tuning of pre-trained networks for pulmonary nodule detection, in *2020 IEEE 15th International Conference on Industrial and Information Systems (ICIIS)*, (IEEE, New York, 2020), pp. 168–173

10. M. Saini, S. Susan, Cervical cancer screening on multi-class imbalanced cervigram dataset using transfer learning, in *2022 15th International Congress on Image and Signal Processing, Biomedical Engineering and Informatics (CISP-BMEI)*, (IEEE, New York, 2022), pp. 1–6
11. M.B. Noor, N.Z. Taj, M.S.K. Zenia, S. Al Mamun, M. Mahmud, Application of deep learning in detecting neurological disorders from magnetic resonance images: a survey on the detection of Alzheimer's disease, Parkinson's disease and schizophrenia. Brain Inf. **7**, 1–21 (2020)
12. A. Ebrahimighahnavieh, S. Luo, R. Chiong, Deep learning to detect Alzheimer's disease from neuroimaging: A systematic literature review. Comput. Methods Prog. Biomed. **187**, 105242 (2020)
13. H. Ghaffari, H. Tavakoli, G.P. Jahromi, Deep transfer learning–based fully automated detection and classification of Alzheimer's disease on brain MRI. Br. J. Radiol. **95**(1136), 20211253 (2022)
14. H.A. Helaly, M. Badawy, A.Y. Haikal, Deep learning approach for early detection of Alzheimer's disease. Cogn. Comput. **14**, 1711–1727 (2021)
15. D. Pan, A. Zeng, L. Jia, Y. Huang, T. Frizzell, X. Song, Early detection of Alzheimer's disease using magnetic resonance imaging: A novel approach combining convolutional neural networks and ensemble learning. Front. Neurosci. **14**, 259 (2020)
16. A. Ebrahimi, S. Luo, R. Chiong, Alzheimer's Disease Neuroimaging Initiative. "Deep sequence modelling for Alzheimer's disease detection using MRI". Comput. Biol. Med. **134**, 104537 (2021)
17. T. Vanaja, K. Shanmugavadivel, M. Subramanian, C.S. Kanimozhiselvi, Advancing Alzheimer's detection: Integrative approaches in MRI analysis with traditional and deep learning models. Neural Comput. & Applic. **37**, 8527–8546 (2025)
18. D.A. Arafa, H.E.-D. Moustafa, H.A. Ali, A.M.T. Ali-Eldin, S.F. Saraya, A deep learning framework for early diagnosis of Alzheimer's disease on MRI images. Multimed. Tools Appl. **83**(2), 3767–3799 (2024)
19. S. Murugan, M.G. Chandran Venkatesan, X.-Z.G. Sumithra, B. Elakkiya, M. Akila, S. Manoharan, DEMNET: A deep learning model for early diagnosis of Alzheimer diseases and dementia from MR images. IEEE Access **9**, 90319–90329 (2021)
20. M.M. Fareed, S.Z. Sadiq, G. Ahmed, S. Mahmood, M. Aslam, S.F. Jillani, A. Moustafa, M. Asad, ADD-net: An effective deep learning model for early detection of Alzheimer disease in MRI scans. IEEE Access **10**, 96930–96951 (2022)
21. M. Abdelaziz, T. Wang, W. Anwaar, A. Elazab, Multi-scale multimodal deep learning framework for Alzheimer's disease diagnosis. Comput. Biol. Med. **184**, 109438 (2025)
22. N. Pradhan, S. Sagar, A.S. Singh, Analysis of MRI image data for Alzheimer disease detection using deep learning techniques. Multimed. Tools Appl. **83**(6), 17729–17752 (2024)
23. S. Al-Shoukry, T.H. Rassem, N.M. Makbol, Alzheimer's diseases detection by using deep learning algorithms: A mini-review. IEEE Access **8**, 77131–77141 (2020)
24. S. Gao, D. Lima, A review of the application of deep learning in the detection of Alzheimer's disease. Int. J. Cogn. Comput. Eng. **3**, 1–8 (2022)
25. D. Cheng, M. Liu, Classification of Alzheimer's disease by cascaded convolutional neural networks using PET images, in *Machine Learning in Medical Imaging: 8th International Workshop, MLMI 2017, Held in Conjunction with MICCAI 2017*, (Springer International Publishing, Cham, 2017), pp. 106–113
26. M. Gharaibeh, M. Almahmoud, M.Z. Ali, A. Al-Badarneh, M. El-Heis, L. Abualigah, M. Altalhi, A. Alaiad, A.H. Gandomi, Early diagnosis of Alzheimer's disease using cerebral catheter angiogram neuroimaging: A novel model based on deep learning approaches. Big Data Cogn. Comput. **6**(1), 2 (2022)
27. K. Simonyan, A. Zisserman, Very deep convolutional networks for large-scale image recognition (2014). arXiv preprint arXiv:1409.1556
28. C. Szegedy, V. Vanhoucke, S. Ioffe, J. Shlens, Z. Wojna, Rethinking the inception architecture for computer vision, in *Proceedings of the IEEE Conference on Computer Vision and Pattern Recognition*, (IEEE, New York, 2016), pp. 2818–2826

29. K. He, X. Zhang, S. Ren, J. Sun, Deep residual learning for image recognition, in *Proceedings of the IEEE Conference on Computer Vision and Pattern Recognition*, (IEEE, New York, 2016), pp. 770–778
30. C. Szegedy, S. Ioffe, V. Vanhoucke, A. Alemi, Inception-v4, inception-resnet and the impact of residual connections on learning, in *Proceedings of the AAAI conference on artificial intelligence*, vol. 31, (AAAI, Philadelphia, 2017)
31. M. Tan, Q. Le, Efficientnet: Rethinking model scaling for convolutional neural networks, in *International Conference on Machine Learning*, (PMLR, Cambridge, 2019), pp. 6105–6114
32. T. Mahmood, A. Rehman, Y. Tanzila Saba, Wang, and Faten S. Alamri., Alzheimer's disease unveiled: Cutting-edge multi-modal neuroimaging and computational methods for enhanced diagnosis. Biomed. Signal Process. Control **97**, 106721 (2024)
33. B. Mabrouk, A.B. Hamida, N. Mabrouki, N. Bouzidi, C. Mhiri, A novel approach to perform linear discriminant analyses for a 4-way Alzheimer's disease diagnosis based on an integration of Pearson's correlation coefficients and empirical cumulative distribution function. Multimed. Tools Appl. **83**(31), 76687–76703 (2024)
34. Z. Liu, Super convergence cosine annealing with warm-up learning rate, in *CAIBDA 2022; 2nd International Conference on Artificial Intelligence, Big Data and Algorithms*, (VDE, Alzenau, 2022), pp. 1–7
35. S. Sharma, K. Guleria, S. Tiwari, S. Kumar, A deep learning based convolutional neural network model with VGG16 feature extractor for the detection of Alzheimer disease using MRI scans. Measure. Sens. **24**, 100506 (2022)

Predictive Models for Early Detection and Prognosis of Dementia Using Artificial Intelligence and Machine Learning

Dipendra Bhattrai, Fareed Ud Din, and Niusha Shafiabady

Abstract Early detection and prognosis of dementia is a critical global health challenge given the rapid aging of populations. Despite the increase in dementia, there is a significant gap in research on early detection and prognosis of dementia, particularly utilizing artificial intelligence (AI) and machine learning (ML) techniques for more accurate and timely diagnosis. This study explores the efficacy of multiple ML algorithms in predicting the onset of dementia using the OASIS dataset, which contains extensive MRI data of individuals aged 60–96 years. Eight state-of-the-art predictive AI/ML algorithms are applied to evaluate dementia classification including support vector machine (SVM), K-nearest neighbors (KNN), decision trees (DT), gradient boosting machine (GBM), random forest (RF), Naïve Bayes (NB), logistics regression (LR), and extra trees (ET). Among the tested models, SVM achieved the overall best performance, with 92% accuracy, 0.92 specificity, and an F1-score of 0.91, highlighting its potential for early dementia classification. Key features such as the mini-mental state examination (MMSE) scores and clinical dementia rating (CDR) are used to train the models. Feature selection was achieved using LASSO and Fisher's exact test. The results indicate that the models achieved high accuracy along with other performance metrics, which highlights the potential of ML techniques in enhancing diagnostic processes and informing early intervention strategies for dementia, potentially improving patient outcomes.

D. Bhattrai · F. U. Din (✉)
School of Science and Technology, University of New England, Armidale, NSW, Australia
e-mail: fuddin@une.edu.au

N. Shafiabady
Department of IT, Peter Faber Business School, Australian Catholic University, North Sydney, NSW, Australia

Faculty of Science and Technology, Charles Darwin University (Sydney Campus), Sydney, NSW, Australia

N. E. M. Khalifa, M. H. N. Taha (eds.), *Next-Gen Healthcare*,
https://doi.org/10.1007/978-3-032-07267-2_9

Keywords Dementia prediction · Alzheimer's disease · machine learning algorithms · MRI data · OASIS dataset · Dementia classification · Feature selection · Early diagnosis · Cognitive decline

Abbreviations

AD	Alzheimer's disease
AI	Artificial intelligence
AUC	Area under the curve
CDR	Clinical dementia rating
DT	Decision tree
GBM	Gradient boosting machine
KNN	K-nearest neighbors
LASSO	Least absolute shrinkage and selection operator
LR	Logistic regression
MCI	Mild cognitive impairment
ML	Machine learning
MMSE	Mini-mental state examination
NB	Naive Bayes
OASIS	Open access series of imaging studies
RF	Random forest
SVM	Support vector machine

1 Introduction

The global population aged 60 and over is projected to be double from 1 billion in 2020 to 2.1 billion by 2050, with two-thirds residing in lower- and middle-income countries [1]. Additionally, individuals aged 80 and above are anticipated to triple in number, reaching 426 million by 2050 [2]. This increase imposes significant social, psychological, and economic strains on the families of those affected. Addressing this, the prevention of dementia has become a critical public health goal. Efforts are underway to develop predictive tests for early intervention, with several prevention trials and prediction models focusing on identifying individuals at risk of developing dementia [3]. Artificial intelligence (AI), particularly machine learning (ML), has shown increasing potential in health informatics, especially in medical imaging, predictive diagnostics, and early disease detection. In particular, image recognition and classification [4] have also significantly improved accuracy and speed in tasks such as object recognition, medical imaging, and quality control. Advances in AI/ML have been harnessed to enhance dementia diagnosis, employing analysis of brain scans and exploration of genetic and risk factor data, extending techniques initially used for other diseases [5] to the realm of dementia prediction and diagnosis

[6]. Dementia symptoms are commonly linked with aging, though some may manifest earlier. Alzheimer's disease alters brain structure and function. Machine learning finds extensive application across industries like health care, finance, transportation, social media, and education. Our research endeavors to create algorithms capable of continuous learning for predictive purposes. Many studies explore machine learning algorithms and their potential for dementia prediction. Yet, no standardized dementia test currently exists [7]. Machine learning methods are a useful tool for determining who has mild cognitive impairment (MCI) or is at risk of dementia. It might be difficult to forecast when a diagnosis will proceed to dementia or when cognitive function will return to normal. To find trends and indicators of cognitive decline, machine learning algorithms can examine a variety of data sources, such as medical histories, demographic data, cognitive tests, and neuroimaging data. Handling diagnoses at the mild cognitive impairment (MCI) stage requires caution, given that research indicates that 10–15% of MCI patients transition to Alzheimer's disease [8].

Various studies have explored machine learning approaches to dementia prediction using diverse datasets and methods, yielding varying levels of performance. For instance, Annette et al. [9] applied ML algorithms on the ADNI and MAS datasets, achieving accuracies of 0.82 and 0.93, respectively. Anastasia et al. [2] investigated dementia diagnosis in patients with Parkinson's disease dementia (PDD) and dementia with Lewy bodies (DLB) using methods such as logistic regression, K-nearest neighbors (K-NNs), support vector machines (SVM), Naive Bayes, and ensemble models. Ahmad Waleed Salehi (2020) employed only the convolutional neural network (CNN) and its variation on the ADNI dataset; however, the comparison with other models is thoroughly addressed. Castellazzi et al. [10] utilized machine learning techniques with MRI features to differentiate between Alzheimer's and vascular dementia, highlighting the importance of imaging data in these models. These studies demonstrate the utility of machine learning across various domains and datasets in improving dementia diagnosis and prognosis.

This research endeavors to utilize multiple ML algorithms on the OASIS dataset [11] to predict the onset of Dementia symptoms at an early stage, thereby aiding physicians in prognosis and diagnostic evaluations. In contrast to prior studies, this research offers a comprehensive examination of supervised machine learning techniques. It has been observed that not many researchers have looked into more than six machine learning algorithms [12], which can provide a comprehensive understanding of AI/ML applicability from varying perspectives. As a result, this study aims to implement eight supervised machine learning techniques including support vector machine (SVM), K-nearest neighbors (KNN), decision tree (DT), gradient boosting machine (GBM), random forest (RF), Naïve Bayes, logistics regression (LR), and extra trees (ET). The efficacy of machine learning in identifying various diseases has been affirmed using a range of methodologies and datasets. AI and ML models, especially those trained on extensive and varied datasets, possess the capability to detect subtle data patterns that may elude human observation [13].

2 Overview of Algorithms

This chapter utilizes a range of statistical and machine learning (ML) methods for feature selection and classification in dementia prediction. Each algorithm offers unique strengths in modelling complex biomedical datasets, and their combined evaluation provides a holistic view of their applicability in clinical decision-making.

Least absolute shrinkage and selection operator (LASSO): LASSO is a regression analysis method that performs both variable selection and regularization to enhance prediction accuracy and interpretability [14]. In dementia research, the challenge often lies in working with datasets containing a large number of potential predictors, such as brain volume measurements, cognitive scores, and demographic factors. Many of these features may be irrelevant or redundant. LASSO addresses this by shrinking the coefficients of less important variables to zero, effectively eliminating them from the model [14]. This not only improves computational efficiency but also reduces the risk of overfitting—a critical issue when working with relatively small clinical datasets. In the present study, LASSO was used to identify the most influential variables for predicting dementia status, helping focus the analysis on clinically meaningful indicators such as MMSE, CDR, and specific neuroimaging features.

Fisher's Exact Test Fisher's exact test is a nonparametric statistical significance test used to determine whether there is a nonrandom association between two categorical variables [6]. It calculates the exact probability of observing a distribution in a contingency table under the null hypothesis. This is particularly useful in small-sample biomedical studies where standard assumptions are invalid. Dementia studies often work with relatively modest sample sizes due to the complexity of data collection and ethical considerations in patient recruitment. Fisher's exact test was employed in this study to evaluate whether particular features (e.g., gender, education level, or cognitive score categories) were significantly associated with dementia status. By removing features that show no meaningful association, we ensured that subsequent modeling efforts concentrated on variables with a statistically demonstrable link to disease presence or progression.

Support Vector Machine (SVM) SVM is a supervised learning method that constructs a hyperplane in a high-dimensional space to separate classes with maximum margin [15]. For nonlinear boundaries, it applies kernel functions such as the radial basis function (RBF). In dementia imaging, SVM excels at identifying subtle MRI-based structural changes. SVM is a powerful supervised learning model that excels in classification tasks involving complex and high-dimensional data [15]. It works by finding the optimal decision boundary that separates classes while maximising the margin between them. In the context of dementia prediction, SVM is particularly well-suited to neuroimaging data, where subtle structural differences in brain scans can be challenging to detect with simpler models. In our analysis, SVM delivered the highest accuracy and specificity, underscoring its robustness in distinguishing early-stage dementia from non-dementia cases.

Decision Tree (DT) A DT is a hierarchical model that recursively splits data based on features that maximise information gain [16]. Its interpretability makes it valuable in healthcare for explaining diagnostic pathways. DT visual structure makes them appealing in clinical contexts, where interpretability is critical. For example, a clinician can follow a sequence of "if-then" rules to understand how a model arrived at a particular classification. In dementia research, DTs can highlight combinations of factors—such as MMSE scores below a threshold combined with reduced intracranial volume—that strongly predict dementia onset. However, single decision trees can be prone to overfitting, which is why they are often used as building blocks in ensemble models like random forests and extra trees as utilized in this study.

Naïve Bayes (NB) NB is a probabilistic classifier based on Bayes' theorem, assuming feature independence. Despite the independence assumption rarely holding in medical datasets, NB is computationally efficient and works well with small training sets [15]. NB is a simple yet effective probabilistic model that applies Bayes' theorem under the assumption that all features are conditionally independent given the outcome. While this assumption is rarely true in real-world medical data, NB can still perform surprisingly well, particularly when the dataset is relatively small and the features are informative. In this study it was useful for preliminary assessment is followed by more computationally intensive modelling.

Logistic Regression (LR) LR is one of the most widely used statistical models for binary classification, and it remains popular in medical research due to its interpretability [17]. LR is a linear model for binary classification that estimates the probability of an outcome via the logistic function. It provides interpretable coefficients, allowing clinicians to quantify the relationship between predictors and disease risk. Although its predictive performance was lower than ensemble methods and SVM, LR's ability to clearly communicate the direction and magnitude of associations makes it invaluable for explaining findings to non-technical audiences, such as clinicians and policy-makers.

Random Forest (RF) RF is an ensemble of decision trees trained on bootstrapped samples, with feature selection at each split to reduce correlation between trees [18]. It improves predictive performance and robustness, making it suitable for heterogeneous clinical data. By averaging across many trees, RF reduces the risk of overfitting while maintaining strong predictive accuracy. It also provides feature importance rankings, which are useful for identifying the most influential variables in dementia classification. In this chapter's analysis, RF was particularly effective at balancing sensitivity and specificity, making it a strong candidate for real-world clinical screening tools.

Gradient Boosting Machine (GBM) GBM builds additive models in a forward stage-wise manner by fitting new models to the residuals of prior models [13]. The method sequentially reduces errors using a differentiable loss function. It is highly effective in handling complex feature interactions common in neuroimaging data. GBM is another ensemble method, but unlike RF, it builds trees sequentially, with each new tree aiming to correct the errors of the previous ones. In our experiments, GBM achieved high precision, suggesting it could help minimise false positives—a valuable trait in diagnostic contexts where misclassification can cause unnecessary stress and resource expenditure.

K-Nearest Neighbors (KNN) KNN is a nonparametric method where classification is based on the majority label among the closest data points in the feature space [19]. While simple, it can perform well for dementia-related pattern recognition when combined with appropriate distance metrics. While KNN is intuitive and nonparametric, it can struggle with high-dimensional data and irrelevant features, which can obscure the "true" neighbourhood relationships. In our study, KNN performed less effectively than other algorithms, indicating that dementia-related data may require more sophisticated models to capture complex patterns.

Extra Trees (ET) ET is similar to RF but selects cut-points at random for each feature split, increasing bias but reducing variance [20]. This randomness can lead to competitive performance with faster computation, particularly in high-dimensional medical datasets. Extra trees are similar to RF but introduce greater randomness in feature selection and split-point choice. ET is particularly advantageous when computational resources are limited or when working with very high-dimensional datasets. In this study, ET performed competitively with RF and GBM, showing that even with added randomness, ensemble tree-based methods can capture the intricate relationships in dementia-related data.

3 Methodology

Dataset: This study utilized the OASIS dataset [11] that includes 150 people aged between 60 and 96 years. The dataset includes people from a larger group who had already taken part in MRI research at Washington University, especially people who had gone for clinical check-ups and MRI scans more than once, and who had at least three MRI images taken each time. All the people included in the dataset were right-handed. Most of these participants were from a long-term group called the WU Alzheimer Disease Research Center. In the first round of tests, 86 people had no signs of dementia, while 98 people had some signs of Alzheimer's disease, ranging from very mild to moderate. Later, some of the people who initially had no signs of dementia were found to have Alzheimer's disease during further evaluations. The term "converts" in this dataset means the people who were later found to have Alzheimer's disease. The dataset utilizes the rating system called clinical dementia rating (CDR) to assess people's condition, where a score of 0 meant no dementia, 0.5 meant very mild symptoms, and 1 meant Alzheimer's disease. If someone's score is 0.5, they are diagnosed with moderate cognitive impairment (MCI) [11].

In this study, 'early stage' refers to individuals with a clinical dementia rating (CDR) of 0.5, which aligns with "very mild dementia" or mild cognitive impairment (MCI). The target variable was defined based on CDR scores as follows:

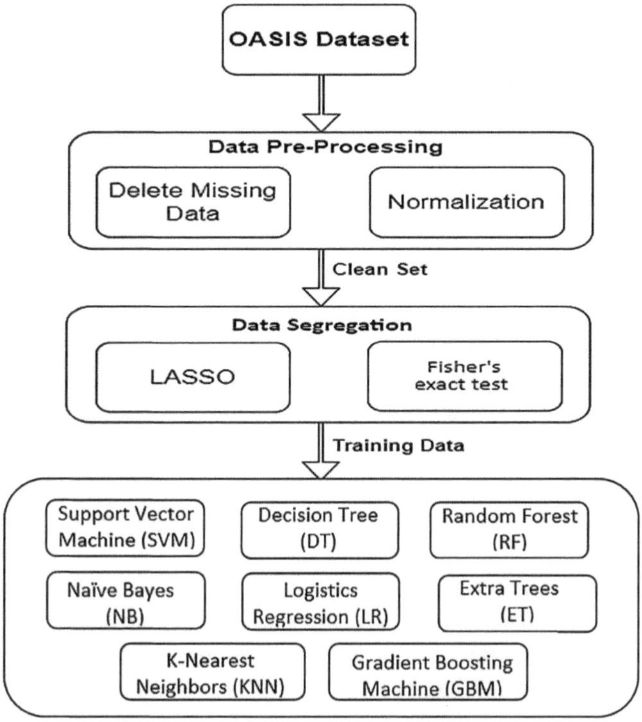

Fig. 1 Data preprocessing pipeline—imputation, outlier removal, normalization, and feature selection

"Non-demented" for CDR $= 0$, "Demented" for CDR ≥ 1, and "Converted" for participants initially with CDR $= 0$ or 0.5 who progressed to a higher CDR score ($\geq$1) in subsequent visits. This classification allows prediction of progression from normal cognition or MCI to diagnosed dementia.

Architecture The proposed model architecture (as depicted in Fig. 1) consists of four major stages: data preparation, data preprocessing, data segregation, and model building. Data preparation involves gathering MRI data and preparing it for subsequent stages. This stage is crucial as it sets the foundation for the entire process. Data preprocessing involves tasks such as data visualization, imputation, transformation, handling missing data, grouping features, outlier removal, normalization, standardization, and feature selection. The output of this stage forms the input for the next stage and significantly impacts the accuracy of the model.

Data segregation involves the division of the dataset into separate subsets for training and testing purposes. This process ensures that the model is trained on one subset of the data and evaluated on another, independent subset. Model building comprises substages such as model training, evaluation, and cross-validation. Various machine learning classifiers are trained, and the model's accuracy is evaluated. Cross-validation techniques are employed to enhance accuracy.

Data Characteristics The dataset comprises an extensive MRI dataset from a longitudinal study involving 150 individuals between the ages of 60 and 96. Utilizing the exact same MRI machine and sequences, 373 imaging sessions were conducted, with participants undergoing at least two sessions spaced a year or more apart. The aim of this study is to evaluate the findings on the use of AI/ML in Dementia early diagnosis and prognosis, with a specific focus on utilizing the mentioned dataset and the impact on the brain among participants categorized as either non-demented or suffering from very mild to mild Alzheimer's disease (AD), as determined by the clinical dementia rating (CDR) [21]. In each session, 4–5 high-contrast MRI scans were taken, enabling in-depth analysis and supporting various computational studies. The utilization of this dataset is demonstrated through the automated measurement of total brain volume [11], highlighting its capability to identify and examine changes due to normal aging and AD.

Missing Data Removal Before analyzing the data properly, it is important to clean it up to deal with missing values or mistakes in the data. One way to do this is by removing the rows that have missing values. In this case, the dataset has been updated by removing the rows that were missing information about SES and MMSE, because these were important for the analysis, and there were 19 rows with missing values for each of these attributes. This helps make sure the dataset is complete and accurate.

Feature Selection This study utilizes two different methods for feature selection: (1) Least absolute shrinkage and selection operator (LASSO) and (2) Fisher's exact test [8]. LASSO is a technique that helps choosing the important variables as well as performing some regularization. Fisher's exact test is utilized in statistics to measure the lack of correlation between features. For this research, Fisher's exact test assessed how the observed count deviated from the expected count, especially in cases where the contingency table cells have small expected counts. Unlike the chi-square test, Fisher's exact test does not rely on any asymptotic assumptions and is particularly useful when dealing with small sample sizes or sparse contingency tables. The formula for Fisher's exact test computes the probability of obtaining a distribution of counts in a 2×2 contingency table, given the marginal totals. After applying Fisher's exact test, the features were ranked based on their significance, as illustrated in Fig. 2.

Features with a p value below 0.05 were considered significant, while others were eliminated. For model training, six features were selected: "Gender," "MMSE," "CDR," "SES," "EDUC," and "eTIV." Six features were eliminated because their p values were greater than 0.05, indicating a lack of significant association with the target variable.

Data Segregation Data preprocessing included removal of 19 rows with missing SES and MMSE values, accounting for approximately 12.7% of the dataset. Missing

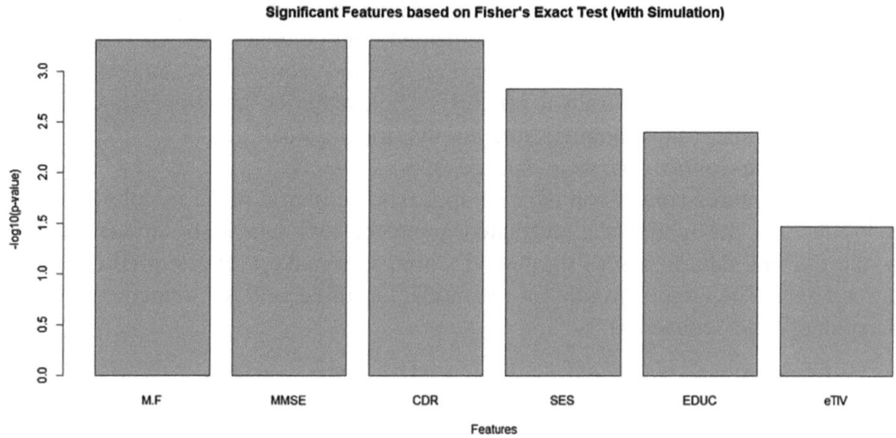

Fig. 2 Feature ranking after applying Fisher's exact test

data were not imputed but removed to maintain data integrity. Standardization and normalization were applied to continuous variables. Outlier detection was conducted using IQR-based thresholds, though no extreme outliers warranted removal beyond the missingness cases. In order to avoid the overfitting problem, the dataset was divided into parts. This helps the model learn well from new data it has not seen before. With the most important selected features the model is tested with the data that is never presented to it before and for that, the model uses fivefold cross-validation. The dataset is divided as per the 30/70 rule into two parts: 70% for training and 30% for testing. A stratified fivefold cross-validation strategy was used to prevent overfitting and maintain class distribution. The dataset was split into 70% training and 30% testing sets. Bootstrapping was not applied. Hyperparameters were tuned using grid search where applicable (e.g., kernel types for SVM, number of trees for RF and GBM), based on maximizing F1-score on validation folds.

Model Building First, we used the data we prepared earlier to build a model. Building a model means teaching a computer program to make guesses (predictions) based on the information it's given. We gave the program some data with both the things we want to predict (i.e., whether someone has dementia or not) and the information we think might help it make predictions (i.e., age or memory test scores). This process is called training the model. The program learned from this training data and made a model. Then, we tested the model using a different set of data we set aside earlier. This data had the same kind of information as the training data but was not used to train the model. This step helps us see how well the model can make predictions on new data it has not seen before. When the model is trained, it learns from the training data. The target variable in our data—what we are trying to predict—has three values: "demented," "non-demented," and "converted." So, the model tries to figure out which of these categories each person in the data belongs to [8].

The model is developed with data containing both the target outcomes (e.g., whether an individual is classified as demented, non-demented, or has transitioned between states) and predictor variables (i.e., age and memory test scores) deemed relevant for prediction to train it properly. The prediction horizon is not defined in absolute time (days/months) due to the longitudinal nature of the OASIS dataset, where follow-ups were spaced approximately 1 year apart. Thus, our prediction captures conversion over an approximate period of 12 months or more. Subsequently, the model was evaluated using the test data with similar features as the training data to assess the model's ability to make accurate predictions on unseen data. The target variable for the model has three values: "demented," "non-demented," and "converted."

4 Results and Discussion

Out of 150 participants, 8 were excluded due to missing data, leading to a final sample of 142 participants (mean age 77.03 ± 7.81 years; 57.63% female) 56 demented, 72 non-demented, and 14 converted participants. The comparison across the demented, non-demented, and converted groups reveals several noteworthy insights as detailed in Table 1. ANOVA tests showed that the individuals in the demented group were slightly younger and less educated. However, the mini-mental state examination score (MMSE) shows a significant difference (p = 7.33E-11), with the Demented group having higher SES levels compared to the non-demented and converted groups. Additionally, there is no significant difference in SES and EDUC scores across the groups, indicating similar cognitive functioning. When considering brain characteristics, while ETIV does not differ significantly between groups, age exhibits a highly significant difference, with the non-demented group having higher volumes.

The chi-square test revealed a significant association between gender and dementia status. Specifically, females were found to be more prevalent in the non-demented and converted groups compared to males. This suggests that gender may play a role in the manifestation or progression of dementia, with females being more likely to be in the non-demented or early-stage dementia categories.

Table 1 Descriptive statistics (mean ± sd) of the numerical variables with ANOVA F tests

Variable	Demented	Non-demented	Converted	p value (ANOVA F test)
Age	76.2 ± 7.35	77.06 ± 8.1	79.76 ± 7.43	0.542575
EDUC	13.83 ± 3.03	15.14 ± 2.74	15.46 ± 2.52	0.1317769
SES	2.77 ± 1.2	2.39 ± 1.05	1.73 ± 0.96	0.3123823
MMSE	24.32 ± 4.66	29.23 ± 0.88	28.68 ± 1.56	7.33E-11
CDR	0.67 ± 0.3	0.01 ± 0.05	0.26 ± 0.25	2.160573E-31
eTIV	1490.7 ± 172.38	1495.5 ± 184.89	1459.27 ± 135.43	0.3281162

Another significant association was observed between education level and dementia status. Higher education levels, such as college graduate, were more prevalent in the non-demented group compared to the demented and converted groups. The details are presented in Table 2, where the finding suggests that higher levels of education may serve as a protective factor against dementia or delay its onset. There was a highly significant association between the clinical dementia rating (CDR) score and dementia status. Participants classified as having no dementia based on CDR score were more prevalent in the non-demented group compared to the demented and converted groups. This highlights the clinical relevance of the CDR score in assessing dementia severity and differentiating between different stages of dementia. In contrast to the other variables, the analysis found no significant difference in mean estimated total intracranial volume (eTIV) across different dementia status categories. This suggests that differences in brain volume, as measured by eTIV, may not be strongly associated with dementia status in this dataset.

The logistic regression model was constructed to explore the relationship between various predictor variables and the likelihood of being classified as demented, as presented in Table 3. The intercept term represents the baseline log-odds of being categorized as demented when all predictor variables are set to zero. The statistically significant intercept ($p < 0.01$) indicates a notable likelihood of being categorized as demented even in the absence of other predictors. Although the coefficient for EDUC did not reach statistical significance at the conventional 0.05 level ($p = 0.6158$), the negative coefficient (−8.30E-02) suggests a potential trend: higher education levels may be linked to a reduced likelihood of being categorized as demented. This finding aligns with previous research indicating a possible protective effect of higher education against dementia. Conversely, the negative coefficient for MMSE (−3.82E-01) was statistically significant ($p < 0.01$), indicating that lower MMSE scores, indicative of cognitive impairment, are strongly associated with a higher likelihood of being categorized as demented. This result corroborates clinical intuition and prior studies highlighting the effectiveness of MMSE in detecting cognitive impairment and dementia.

Similarly, the statistically significant negative coefficient for CDR (4.45E+01, $p < 0.05$) suggests that higher CDR scores, reflecting greater severity of dementia-related symptoms, are linked to a significantly higher likelihood of being categorized as demented. This underscores the importance of clinical assessments such as the CDR in diagnosing and staging dementia. In contrast, the coefficient for eTIV (−0.1.67E-03) was not statistically significant ($p = 0.4556$), indicating that eTIV, a measure of brain volume, does not significantly influence the likelihood of being categorized as demented in this model. Further investigation is warranted to understand the direct relationship between brain atrophy and diagnostic categorization. Additionally, the coefficient for gender (male vs. female) was statistically significant ($p = 0.0386$), suggesting that gender significantly affects the likelihood of being categorized as demented in this model. This result contrasts with some previous studies suggesting a potential gender difference in dementia risk, highlighting the need for further research in this area.

Table 2 Descriptive statistics of key variables with a chi-square test

Variable	Demented	Non-demented	Converted	*p* value (chi-square test)
Gender	Male: 32 (57.14%) Female: 24 (42.86%)	Male: 22 (30.56%) Female: 50 (69.44%)	Male: 4 (28.57%) Female: 10 (71.43%)	3.98E-06
EDUC	Less than high school: 4 High school graduate: 21 Some college: 22 College graduate: 9	Less than high school: 1 High school graduate: 26 Some college: 32 College graduate: 23	Less than high school: 0 High school graduate: 4 Some college: 7 College graduate: 3	0.0001042
MMSE	Severe impairment: 1 Moderate impairment: 9 Mild impairment: 16 No impairment: 30	Severe impairment: 0 Moderate impairment: 0 Mild impairment: 0 No impairment: 72	Severe impairment: 0 Moderate impairment: 0 Mild impairment: 1 No impairment: 13	2.20E-16
CDR	No dementia: 0 Very mild AD: 36 Mild AD: 17 Moderate AD: 3	No dementia: 70 Very mild AD: 2 Mild AD: 0 Moderate AD: 0	No dementia: 1 Very mild AD: 13 Mild AD: 0 Moderate AD: 0	2.20E-16
eTIV	Male mean eTIV: 1557.149 Female mean eTIV: 1389.451	Male mean eTIV: 1670.131 Female mean eTIV: 1413.444	Male mean eTIV: 1593.000 Female mean eTIV: 1386.833	0.259

Table 3 Results from the logistic regression

Description	Estimate	Std. error	*Z* value	Pr (>|*z*|)
(Intercept)	−1.10E+01	1.55E+03	−0.007	0.9943
CDR	4.45E+01	3.10E+03	0.014	0.9886
MMSE	−3.82E-01	1.57E-01	−2.433	0.0150
eTIV	−1.67E-03	2.24E-03	−0.746	0.4556
M.F	1.81E+00	8.76E-01	2.069	0.0386
EDUC	−8.30E-02	1.65E-01	−0.502	0.6158
SES	6.80E-01	3.93E-01	1.731	0.0835

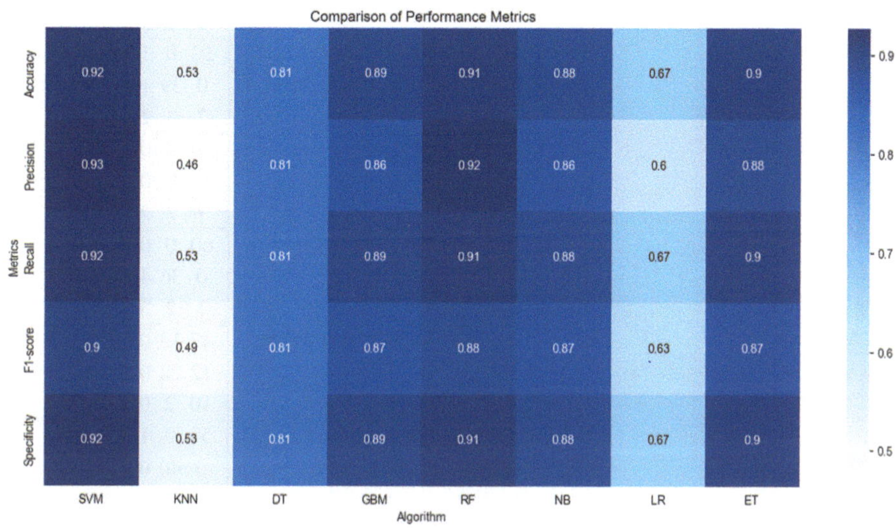

Fig. 3 Comparison of ML algorithmic performance

The heatmap depicted in Fig. 3 illustrates the performance metrics of employed machine learning algorithms including SVM, KNN, DT, GBM, RF, NB, LR, and ET. The metrics analyzed are accuracy, precision, recall, F1-score, and specificity, with each cell indicating the score (ranging from 0 to 1) for a specific metric-algorithm combination. Darker blue shades signify better performance. A closer look at Fig. 2 explains that SVM, GBM, and RF consistently exhibit high scores across all metrics, indicating robust and balanced performance. Notably, GBM has the highest precision (0.92), while SVM leads in accuracy (0.92) and specificity (0.92). ET also shows strong results across metrics, particularly excelling in specificity (0.9) and F1-score (0.87). However, KNN and logistic regression (LR) show lower scores across most metrics, with LR having the lowest precision (0.6) and recall (0.67), indicating struggles with correct positive predictions. Similarly, NB achieves moderate results but falls behind in F1-score (0.63) and specificity (0.67).

While this study focused on traditional performance metrics (accuracy, precision, recall, specificity, F1-score), future work will incorporate area under the receiver operating characteristic (AUROC) and area under the precision-recall

Table 4 Test confusion matrices

Method	Test confusion matrices
SVM	$\begin{bmatrix} 60 & 0 & 0 \\ 0 & 40 & 0 \\ 7 & 2 & 3 \end{bmatrix}$
KNN	$\begin{bmatrix} 42 & 18 & 0 \\ 23 & 17 & 0 \\ 9 & 3 & 0 \end{bmatrix}$
DT	$\begin{bmatrix} 53 & 0 & 7 \\ 3 & 35 & 2 \\ 6 & 3 & 3 \end{bmatrix}$
GBM	$\begin{bmatrix} 59 & 0 & 1 \\ 0 & 39 & 1 \\ 7 & 3 & 2 \end{bmatrix}$
RF	$\begin{bmatrix} 60 & 0 & 0 \\ 0 & 40 & 0 \\ 7 & 3 & 2 \end{bmatrix}$
NB	$\begin{bmatrix} 60 & 0 & 0 \\ 0 & 36 & 4 \\ 7 & 2 & 3 \end{bmatrix}$
Logistic regression	$\begin{bmatrix} 47 & 13 & 0 \\ 12 & 28 & 0 \\ 10 & 2 & 0 \end{bmatrix}$
ET	$\begin{bmatrix} 59 & 0 & 1 \\ 0 & 40 & 0 \\ 7 & 3 & 2 \end{bmatrix}$

curve (AUPRC) to further assess model discrimination, particularly under varying threshold conditions. Given the multi-class nature of the classification task, one-vs-rest AUROC curves will be used to evaluate model performance per class. For all models, the default probability threshold of 0.5 was used to convert predicted probabilities into class labels. Threshold tuning was not applied, which may limit optimal performance in imbalanced cases. Future work will explore threshold optimization using ROC analysis or precision-recall trade-offs.

Precision and recall metrics vary significantly among algorithms, reflecting their ability to correctly identify positive cases, with respect to each algorithm's confusion matrix, as presented in Table 4. Confusion matrices provide an indication of true positives (correctly predicted positive cases), true negatives (correctly predicted negative cases), false positives (incorrectly predicted positive cases), and false negatives (incorrectly predicted negative cases), eventually confirming the robustness of the ML models employed in this study. While high precision indicates fewer false positives, recall measures the model's success in capturing all true positives. F1-scores reflect the balance between precision and recall. Models like SVM and RF perform well due to their balanced predictions. These results suggest that high recall and specificity are critical to minimize false negatives and false

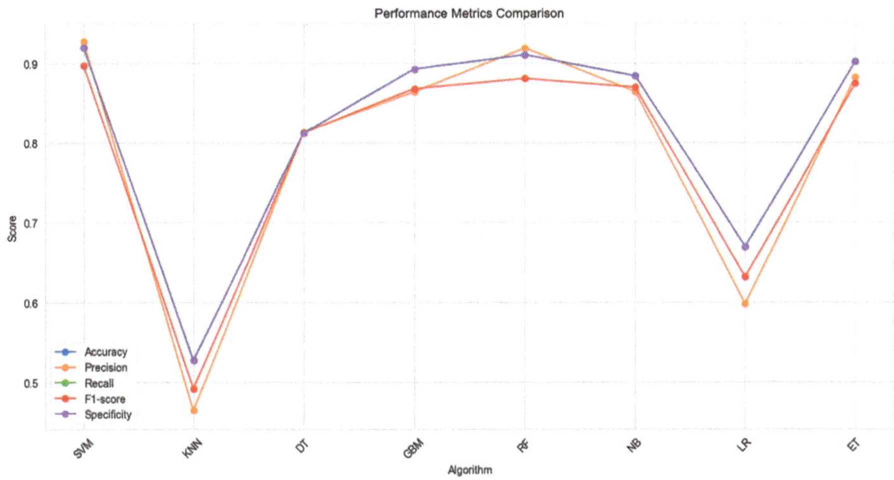

Fig. 4 comparing classification performance of based on metrics, which are macro-averaged across the three classes (demented, non-demented, converted)

positives, suggesting that SVM, RF, and GBM are preferable choices in the context of dementia identification.

Among the algorithms tested, SVM exhibited the most consistent and superior performance across all evaluated metrics, including the highest accuracy (92%), precision (0.90), recall (0.91), and specificity (0.92). This robustness makes SVM the most suitable candidate for clinical application in early-stage dementia detection within our dataset context.

The comparison of the performance metrics, accuracy, precision, recall, F1-score, and specificity, across various machine learning algorithms in the context of dementia diagnosis and prognosis is presented in Fig. 4. SVM, GBM, RF, and ET outperforms other algorithms, particularly in accuracy and specificity, demonstrating robust capabilities for distinguishing between dementia and non-dementia cases. High precision for these algorithms (around 0.9 for SVM and GBM) indicates fewer false positives, which is critical for minimizing misdiagnoses that could lead to unnecessary interventions. High recall and specificity ensure the models effectively capture true dementia cases while correctly identifying non-dementia cases.

KNN and LR show significantly lower scores in most metrics, particularly recall and F1-score. For dementia diagnosis, such models may fail to detect many true positives or maintain a balance between precision and recall. These limitations make them less reliable for applications requiring high sensitivity to capture early signs of dementia. Naive Bayes shows moderate performance but falls behind in F1-score and specificity. This suggests its predictive capability might be affected by dataset features or imbalances, such as skewed class distributions, often observed in medical datasets. In dementia diagnosis and prognosis, accuracy alone is

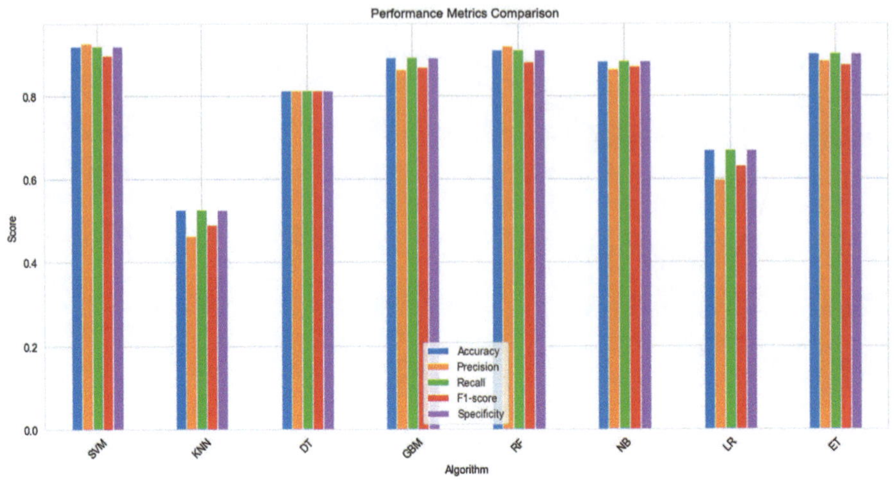

Fig. 5 Computing accuracy, precision, recall, and F1-score for each classification model

insufficient. High recall ensures early detection of dementia cases, which is crucial for timely intervention, while specificity prevents false positives that could cause undue stress to patients. Models like SVM and GBM stand out as they combine high accuracy with balanced precision and recall, making them suitable for clinical applications. The performance of these algorithms reflects their suitability for analyzing complex datasets in dementia studies, such as neuroimaging or cognitive test scores. Algorithms with high specificity and precision, such as RF and GBM, can reduce diagnostic errors, aiding clinicians in accurate decision-making.

Similarly, the comparative visualization in Fig. 5 via a bar graph reinforces the importance of selecting the right algorithm for dementia-related applications, considering both the clinical implications of false predictions and the trade-offs between different performance metrics.

Each key performance metric, including, accuracy, precision, recall, F1-score, and specificity, evaluates a critical dimension of the algorithms' performance in the context of dementia diagnosis and prognosis. Figure 5 clearly spells out that SVM, GBM, RF, and ET consistently achieve high values across all metrics. These algorithms demonstrate their ability to effectively classify dementia cases with a balance of accuracy, precision, and recall. Their high specificity (around 0.9) is particularly noteworthy, indicating a low rate of false positives. Such balanced performance highlights their reliability for medical applications where misdiagnoses can have severe consequences.

Figure 5 also provide a disparity in performance, such as KNN showing significantly lower performance across all metrics. This drop is especially pronounced in precision and recall, suggesting that KNN struggles to differentiate between dementia and non-dementia cases effectively. Similarly, LR underperforms relative to other models, with a noticeable gap in precision and recall. This could indicate limitations in capturing complex, nonlinear relationships in the dataset. Nevertheless, NB achieves moderate scores, maintaining a balance in accuracy and specificity but lagging in precision and recall. This suggests potential challenges with imbalanced or overlapping data distributions, which are common in dementia-related datasets.

For dementia diagnosis, high recall is essential to ensure most true cases are identified, preventing delayed interventions. Meanwhile, high specificity reduces false positives, minimizing unnecessary anxiety and treatment. Algorithms like GBM, RF, and SVM excel in this dual requirement, making them suitable for deployment in clinical or research settings. Similarly, high F1-scores for these models indicate a strong balance between precision and recall, reinforcing their robustness for sensitive applications.

The clear disparity between algorithms underlines the importance of selecting advanced models like GBM or RF for complex medical datasets. Simpler algorithms, such as KNN or LR, may require significant feature engineering or data preprocessing to achieve competitive performance. This visualization emphasizes the critical differences in algorithm performance, particularly in high-stakes contexts like dementia diagnosis, where accurate and reliable predictions are paramount.

One of the primary limitations of this study is the relatively small sample size ($n = 150$, reduced to 142 after preprocessing), which may affect the generalizability of the findings. The limited number of converted cases ($n = 14$) also introduces class imbalance, which can bias model training and evaluation. While stratified cross-validation was used to mitigate this, results should be interpreted with caution. Additionally, the dataset includes only right-handed individuals and is based on a single geographical and institutional cohort, which may not reflect the diversity found in broader clinical populations. Given the limited sample size, especially in the "converted" group, performance metrics may be optimistic due to potential overfitting. Future studies should validate these findings on larger and more diverse datasets to confirm model robustness.

5 Conclusion and Future Work

This study demonstrated the effectiveness of artificial intelligence (AI)/machine learning (ML) algorithms in the early detection and prognosis of dementia. By leveraging the OASIS dataset and employing a variety of models, this study highlights the potential of predictive analytics to identify individuals at risk of dementia. The findings emphasise that AI/ML can offer valuable insights into patient diagnosis, particularly in differentiating between demented, non-demented, and converted cases. Through the analysis of the dataset containing neuroimaging, clinical, and demographic variables, this study determined the main variables to be MMSE scores, CDR scores, and gender, which are linked to support the classification of dementia. Furthermore, this study demonstrated the effectiveness of various machine learning algorithms, including SVM, RF, GBM, DT, and ET, in the early detection and prognosis of dementia. Notably, SVM demonstrated the most balanced and superior performance metrics, reinforcing its utility as a strong candidate for early dementia detection. This study employed a fivefold cross-validation approach with a 70/30 train-test split. The findings demonstrate strong predictive capabilities, particularly with GBM and ET, with notable improvements in specificity and sensitivity. Confusion matrices indicate that GBM and ET are particularly robust, offering significant improvements over other ML models, and highlighting their potential for clinical implementation in dementia care.

The study emphasizes how intricately clinical, neuroimaging, and demographic factors interact to determine dementia classification. Significant correlations between MMSE, CDR, and gender were found by the logistic regression model; higher MMSE scores were associated with a decreased risk of dementia, whereas higher CDR scores were associated with a higher likelihood of dementia. Another important element that surfaced was gender, with females exhibiting a higher probability of being non-demented or converted than males.

While the outcomes are promising, the field of early Dementia prediction still faces significant challenges, for example, a lack of comprehensive longitudinal studies and variability in clinical data hinders the development of universally applicable models. It is also important to investigate a broader range of factors and characteristics that could raise the precision and dependability of dementia prediction algorithms. Future research should focus on enhancing data quality and exploring more sophisticated algorithms to improve prediction accuracy and applicability across diverse populations. Ultimately, the integration of AI/ML techniques in clinical practice has the potential for personalised and timely interventions, improving patient outcomes.

References

1. W.S. Ahmad, B. Preety, B.S. Brij, U. Ankita, G. Gaurav, *A CNN Model: Earlier Diagnosis and Classification* (IEEE, New York, 2020)
2. B. Anastasia, E. Efthymia, S. Ioanna, Z. Panagiotis, A novel machine learning algorithm predicts dementia with Lewy bodies versus Parkinson's disease dementia based on clinical and neuropsychological scores. J. Geriatr. Psychiatry Neurol. **35**, 317–320 (2022)
3. S. Aram, H. Danial, W.P. Kun, S.L. Heui, Early diagnosis of dementia from clinical data by machine learning techniques. Scopus **7**(7), 651 (2017)
4. N. Talha, S. Ahmad, A. Malik, H. Akram, M. Suleman, F. Din, Embedded large scale face recognition in the wild, in *2023 IEEE International Conference on Emerging Trends in Engineering, Sciences and Technology (ICES&T)*, (IEEE, New York, 2023)
5. G. Amrit, U.D. Fareed, Role of data as an interface between primary, secondary and tertiary care: Evidence from literature. Inf. Health **2**(1), 63–72 (2025)
6. Y. Youn, S. Choi, H. Shin, K. Kim, J. Jang, J. Jung, G. Hsiung, S. Kim, Detection of cognitive impairment using a machine-learning algorithm. Neuropsychiatr. Dis. Treat. **14**, 2939–2945 (2018)

7. L. Berg, D. McKeel, J. Miller, Clinicopathologic studies in cognitively healthy aging and Alzheimer disease: Relation of histologic markers to dementia severity, age, sex, and apolipoprotein E genotype. Arch. Neurol. **55**, 326–335 (1998)
8. S. Dhakal, S. Azam, K.M. Hasib, A. Karim, M. Jonkman, F. Al Haque, Dementia prediction using machine learning. Proc. Comput. Sci. **219**, 1297–1308 (2023)
9. S. Annette, C. Emily, S. Arcot, S. Perminder, A.K. Nicole, T. Julian, B. Henry, A comparison of machine learning methods for survival analysis of high-dimensional clinical data for dementia prediction. Sci. Rep. **10**, 20410 (2020)
10. G. Castellazzi, C.M.G.R.M. Cotta, M.D.F. Denaro, A. Ricciardi, P. Vitali, N. Anzalone, S. Bernini, F. Palesi, E. Sinforiani, A. Costa, G. Micieli, E. D'Angelo, G. Magenes, G. Wheeler-Kingshott, A machine learning approach for the differential diagnosis of Alzheimer and vascular dementia fed by MRI selected features. Front. Neuroinform. **14**, 25 (2020)
11. D. Marcus, A. Fotenos, J. Csernansky, J. Morris, R. Buckner, Open access series of imaging studies (OASIS): Longitudinal MRI data in nondemented and demented older adults. J. Cogn. Neurosci. **22**(12), 2677–2684 (2010)
12. A.N. Simonov, T.P. Klyushnik, L. Androsova, N.M. Mikhailova, The use of cluster analysis and logistic regression for assessing the risk of Alzheimer's disease in patients with mild cognitive impairment, amnestic type. Zh. Nevrol. Psikhiatr. Im. S S Korsakova **118**(12), 40–43 (2018)
13. S. Ganesh, T. Chithambaram, N. Krishnan, D. Vincent, J. Kaliappan, K. Srinivasan, Exploring Huntington's disease diagnosis via artificial intelligence models: A comprehensive review. Diagnostics **13**(23), 3592 (2023)
14. P.G. Lim, K.G. Pillay, LASSO and elastic net in the prediction of dementia. Enhanced Knowl. Sci. Technol. **4**(2), 223–232 (2024)
15. N. Shafiabady, N. Hadjinicolaou, F.U. Din, B. Bhandari, R.M. Wu, J. Vakilian, Using artificial intelligence (AI) to predict organizational agility. PLoS One **18**(5), e0283066 (2023)
16. V.G. Costa, C.E. Pedreira, Recent advances in decision trees: An updated survey. Artif. Intell. Rev. **56**(5), 4765–4800 (2023)
17. P. Schober, T.R. Vetter, Logistic regression in medical research. Anesth. Analg. **132**(2), 365–366 (2021)
18. J. Hu, S. Szymczak, A review on longitudinal data analysis with random forest. Brief. Bioinform. **24**(2), bbad002 (2023)
19. S. Zhang, Challenges in KNN classification. IEEE Trans. Knowl. Data Eng. **34**(10), 4663–4675 (2021)
20. A. Sharaff, H. Gupta, Extra-tree classifier with metaheuristics approach for email classification, in *Advances in Computer Communication and Computational Sciences: Proceedings of IC4S 2018*, (Springer, Singapore, 2019), pp. 189–197
21. L. Renjie, W. Xinyi, L. Katherine, G. Saurabh, B. Quan, A. Jane, Applications of artificial intelligence to aid early detection of dementia: A scoping review on current capabilities and future directions. J. Biomed. Inform. **127**, 104030 (2022)

Predicting Drug Response in Diffuse Large B-Cell Lymphoma Patients Using Machine Learning Models

K. Srinika, G. Aramvalartha Nayaki, and Hemalatha Karnan

Abstract Diffuse large B-cell lymphoma (DLBCL) is the most aggressive type of non-Hodgkin's lymphoma (NHL), and it represents approximately 30% of all NHL cases globally. The clinical and molecular diversity of DLBCL renders treatment problematic, as about 30–40% of patients relapse or become resistant to current regimens like R-CHOP (rituximab, cyclophosphamide, doxorubicin, vincristine, and prednisone). The implications are for precision medicine strategies to match treatments with patients' unique genetic, proteomic, and clinical characteristics.

Emerging developments in bioinformatics and genomics have facilitated the generation of large-scale data, including the Genomics of Drug Sensitivity in Cancer (GDSC) database, a useful tool to investigate drug responses. The complex nature and high dimensionality of these data call for sophisticated analysis methods to unveil actionable information. Herein, ML models were utilized to forecast drug reactions in DLBCL patients by utilizing GDSC data to develop precision oncology. Three machine learning models, logistic regression (LR), random forest (RF), and support vector machine (SVM), were trained and tested using some of the major GDSC features, such as Z-score, LN_IC50 (logarithmic half-maximal inhibitory concentration), and AUC (area under the curve).

The outcomes proved that the SVM model, with the radial basis function kernel, had the highest accuracy of 99.88%, performing very well in capturing the intricate, nonlinear relationships of genomic data. Although RF performed well, overfitting was evident. LR, as computationally inexpensive and interpretable as it was, did poorly with the nonlinear patterns in the data, resulting in suboptimal performance.

This study highlights the role of ML in revolutionizing oncology by facilitating targeted treatment regimens in DLBCL. By coupling computational models with clinical care, ML-based approaches have the potential to greatly enhance therapeutic response. Future work needs to address dataset bias and model validation in in vivo settings to increase clinical relevance.

K. Srinika · G. Aramvalartha Nayaki · H. Karnan (✉)
School of Chemical and Biotechnology, SASTRA University, Thanjavur, Tamil Nadu, India
e-mail: 126078016@sastra.ac.in; dpfi0124011938@sastra.ac.in; hemalatha@scbt.sastra.edu

N. E. M. Khalifa, M. H. N. Taha (eds.), *Next-Gen Healthcare*,
https://doi.org/10.1007/978-3-032-07267-2_10

Keywords Diffuse large B-cell lymphoma · Machine learning · Drug response prediction · Logistic regression · Random forest · Support vector machine · Precision medicine

Abbreviations

AUC	Area under the curve
CNN	Convolutional neural network
DL	Deep learning
DLBCL	Diffuse large B-cell lymphoma
EDA	Exploratory data analysis
GDSC	Genomics of drug sensitivity in cancer
LN_IC50	Logarithmic half-maximal inhibitory concentration
LR	Logistic regression
ML	Machine learning
NHL	Non-Hodgkin's lymphoma
RF	Random forest
ROC	Receiver operating characteristic
SVM	Support vector machine

1 Introduction

DLBCL is clinically and molecularly heterogeneous; it represents the most common subtype of non-Hodgkin's lymphoma. Such a case usually grows aggressively as a tumor and has an unfavorable prognosis in cases in which treatment by standard methodologies fails [1, 2]. Globally DLBCL accounts for about 30% of all cases of non-Hodgkin's lymphoma, hence is considered to be among the great contributors to levels of morbidity and mortality associated with cancer [3, 4]. Given the marked improvement in therapeutic regimens with the R-CHOP protocol, still, however, there exists a whole majority of patients who break out or do not even respond appropriately with limited prospects of therapy and dismal survival possibilities [5]. Such findings underscore the strong necessity to develop new ideas that could make treatments specifically personalized to each patient depending on his or her individual genetic and clinical characteristics [6].

DLBCL heterogeneity extends far beyond clinical presentation into being divided into distinct genetic and molecular subtypes that were demonstrated to affect the course of treatment and prognosis in general [7]. For instance, genetic aberrations such as mutations in the BCL2, MYC, and TP53 genes are associated with varying degrees of resistance to chemotherapy and targeted therapies [8]. Advances in high-throughput sequencing and other omics technologies allowed for comprehensive characterization of these molecular subtypes and provided a vast amount of data that can be used for guiding therapeutic strategy [9]. Still, these data volumes and complexities pose significant challenges to actionable insights and clinically applicable translation [10].

Machine learning has been produced during studies in genomics and proteomics and is one of the powerful tools in the analysis of high-dimensional datasets [11]. ML models can predict various outcomes, such as drug response and disease progression, using statistical and computational approaches. Applied to more and more tasks, such as tumor classification, risk stratification, and even prediction of therapeutic response in oncology, ML stands to revolutionize precision medicine [12, 13].

This chapter uses ML models for predicting the response of drugs in patients with DLBCL by utilizing the Genomics of Drug Sensitivity in Cancer dataset [14].

GDSC is one of the richest resources that combine genomics, transcriptomics, and drug response data across a broad range of cancer cell lines. Such a dataset is significant as it offers critical metrics such as Z-score, LN_IC50, and AUC, which point to how drugs are sensitive and potentially effective [15]. Based on these features, one could find the underlying relationships that exist between genetic factors and therapeutic responses, which would be fruitful in understanding the mechanisms responsible for drug resistance and susceptibility [16].

Three ML models specifically logistic regression (LR), random forest (RF), and support vector machine (SVM) have been chosen for this study wherein each model has been taken uniquely based on its individual strengths that could be employed in precise oncology; LR is a simple yet interpretive model, heavily used for performing binary classification tasks [17]. Although this model may not be very efficient if there are nonlinear relationships in the data, LR always gives a base of how the model could perform based on further developments of complexity [18]. RF is an approach to ensemble learning that includes many decision trees to get a better result in the predictability aspect as well as robustness of output [19]. It is especially suitable for high-dimensional data; it gives an idea about which drivers of drug response are more important [20]. SVM is an extremely powerful classification algorithm that is excellent in handling nonlinear relationships and high-dimensional data [21]. SVM can map the input data into higher dimensional spaces by the use of kernel functions, enabling the identification of complex patterns that are not easily discernible in the original feature space [22].

In an effort to deal with drug response prediction difficulties in DLBCL, the study introduces the following major contributions:

- We build and compare three machine learning algorithms LR, RF, and SVM to predict DLBCL drug responses using the GDSC data.
- We explore important genomic and pharmacologic features like Z-score, LN_IC50, and AUC as predictors of significant drug sensitivity and resistance.
- We evaluate the performance of these models using accuracy, precision, recall, F1-score, and AUC, shedding light on their potential for use in clinical practice.
- We also emphasize the drawbacks of current models and suggest directions for enhancing predictive performance, such as overcoming dataset imbalances and adopting deep learning techniques.

- We examine the role of ML-driven strategies in precision oncology, with a focus on their ability to support individualized treatment regimens for patients with DLBCL.

The objective of this study is to evaluate the performance of these ML models in predicting drug responses in DLBCL patients. It compares accuracy, precision, recall, F1-score, and AUC of the different models in order to determine which would be the best for an integration of computational tools with clinical decision-making [23]. Furthermore, the study goes a step further in explaining the biological significance of such crucial characteristics as Z-score, LN_IC50, and AUC; therefore, giving insight into mechanisms of molecular drug sensitivity and resistance [24].

This chapter is structured as follows: The methodology section elucidates the data preprocessing, training procedures, and evaluation metrics of the study. In the results section, it showcases performance metrics of each model in addition to strength and weakness of their applications [25]. Finally, the discussion section discusses these findings against the bigger concept of precision oncology, pointing out areas that require future research and clinical implementation [26]. Finally, the conclusion summarizes the major contributions of this study and gives possible directions for further development of ML-driven approaches in oncology [27].

In short, this research shows that ML models can be used to predict drug responses in DLBCL patients and opens up the avenue to more personalized and effective treatment strategies [28]. With the ability to combine genomic, proteomic, and clinical data, ML will change the landscape of precision medicine, and clinical decisions will be based on clear data, thus helping positively impact patient outcomes [29]. By doing so, the oncology study results will surely testify to the power that ML can bring in these areas while pointing out the necessary steps toward overcoming current hindrances for the sake of harnessing the full benefit of such implementation in clinics [30]. Deep learning (DL) is an emerging technology in precision medicine, particularly for the prediction of drug response to complex diseases such as DLBCL [31]. DLBCL is reported to be the most common subtype of non-Hodgkin's lymphoma, but with substantial genetic and clinical heterogeneity, thus the outcome varies widely in their treatment [32]. It is ineffective in 30–40% cases because of relapse and resistance. Thus, this could be mitigated by incorporating genomics, proteomics, and clinical information in the DL models. It can allow treatment for patients on individualized principles [33]. Unlike conventional machine learning techniques, DL uses multiple layers of artificial neural networks that analyze high-dimensional data sets and identify intricate patterns in such data [34]. Using DL can help clinicians predict drug efficacy much more accurately and, therefore improve therapeutic outcomes [35]. This system predicts drug responses for patients with DLBCL using the newest DL frameworks and genomic datasets like GDSC to revolutionize personalized medicine through optimized treatment regimens and survival.

2 Related Work

Applications of machine learning in the oncology domain have increased gradually as well, particularly in the realm of drug response prediction and patient risk stratification. Table 1 presents a comparison of related works.

2.1 *Neural Networks and Deep Learning*

Neural networks have achieved success in a few instances of cancer outcome prediction. Patel et al. [1] applied feedforward neural networks, achieving accurate predictions at 92% in the cases of DLBCL relapse. However, these techniques are difficult to apply in the real-world field because of the lack of interpretability. Zhang et al. [2] applied deep models for drug response data analysis, achieving high predictive performance but incurring computational inefficiencies due to the size of the dataset.

2.2 *Ensemble Methods*

Ensemble methods such as Random Forest and Gradient Boosting have been shown to be powerful in combining genomics, proteomics, and clinical data. Davis et al. [3] have shown that the ensemble model can be used for stratification of breast cancer by using multi-omics data. However, such models involve many variables, require a lot of preprocessing, and tend to overfit the model if the dataset is not big enough.

2.3 *Linear Models*

Linear models like logistic regression are particularly popular in popular usage because of interpretability and the ease with which further analysis is done.

Table 1 Comparison table of related works

Author and year	Method	Dataset	Accuracy	Limitations
Patel et al. (2022)	Feedforward NN	DLBCL	92%	Poor interpretability
Zhang et al. (2021)	CNN	GDSC	High	High computational cost
Wang et al. (2023)	Deep + multi-omics	Multi-omics	Improved	Dataset bias
This study	LR, RF, SVM	GDSC	Up to 99.88%	In vitro only

However, approaching complex nonlinear datasets, they are significantly inefficient. This chapter attempts to bridge these gaps by testing interpretable and robust models side by side with their performances.

Patel et al. [1] used feedforward neural networks to predict relapse in DLBCL patients. Their model achieved 92% accuracy, and their model showed potential for high-dimensional genomic data analysis. The limitation of its lack of interpretability makes it hard to apply it in clinical decision-making.

Zhang et al. [2] had explored using convolutional neural networks in their analysis of DLBCL patient drug response data based on the concept of deep learning. Their chapter reported high predictive accuracy; it highlighted the ability of deep models to discover latent relations in genomic datasets while identifying challenges in the computational ineligibility of large dataset sizes.

Wang et al. [4] integrated deep learning with multi-omics data, such as genomics, proteomics, and transcriptomics, to predict drug responses. The study showed the power of deep learning in dealing with complex datasets and improved the accuracy of predictions toward the goal of personalized medicine.

Davis et al. [3] investigated the use of recurrent neural networks in predicting drug responses from genomic sequences. The results of this study indicated that RNNs are capable of capturing sequential data well, which made them appropriate for predicting time-dependent drug efficacy. Nonetheless, it was observed that the training complexity was relatively high.

Li et al. [5] applied autoencoders to decrease the dimensionality of drug response data before applying predictive models. This improved the efficiency of deep learning methods from a computational perspective, and in doing so, it highlighted the relationship between feature reduction and predictive modeling.

3 Methodology

The study design is present in Fig. 1. The GDSC dataset was applied for analysis. This consisted of genomic features alongside drug response across multiple cell lines of various cancers, including DLBCL. The main features extracted for further analysis were Z-score, LN_IC50 (half-maximal inhibitory concentration on a logarithmic scale), and AUC (area under the curve of drug response), which are metrics that measure the sensitivity and efficacy of the drug, respectively.

Data preprocessing was done by imputing missing values and outliers to ensure the integrity of the data. Exploratory data analysis was conducted, and it was found that the correlations between the selected features were significant and justified their selection. To predict drug response in DLBCL patients, three machine learning models were adopted: logistic regression (LR), random forest (RF), and support vector machine (SVM). It is selected due to simplicity and interpretability, which really makes it appropriate for clinical applications in which understanding the relationships between features is essential. Z-score, LN_IC50, and AUC were chosen as primary features because they directly measure drug potency, sensitivity,

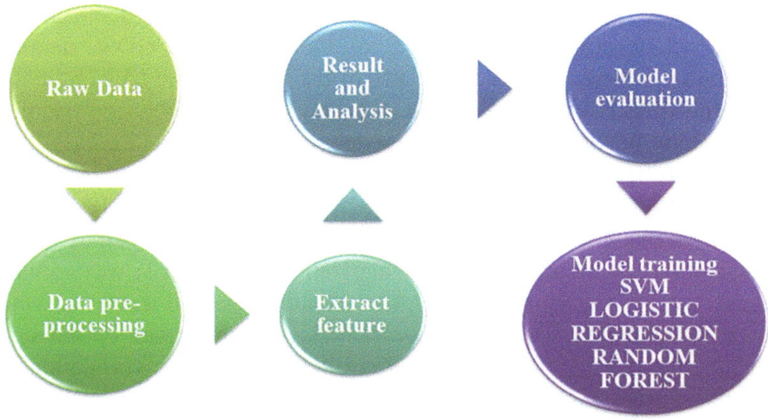

Fig. 1 Study design

and efficacy. For CNN input, the three selected features were normalized to zero mean and unit variance. Although CNNs are typically used for spatial data like images, here the feature vector was treated as a simple 1D input for dense layers, enabling a direct comparison to the other models. Other genomic and transcriptomic features, such as mutation burden and gene expression profiles, were explored but found less predictive due to limited variance within the DLBCL subset. The ensemble model, random forest was used because of robustness and the ability to combine multiple decision trees for an improved accuracy for prediction alongside clarifying the feature importance. A powerful classification algorithm, SVM (support vector machine), was selected as it could cope with complex and nonlinear relationships-the major requirement for genomic datasets that involve intricate patterns. Its performance is largely a matter of kernel choice because the transformation of input data into higher-dimensional spaces is defined by the kernel. Several kernels were tested in this study. The Linear Kernel was used because the data set was separable by lines. This maps the input to the output space without any additional transformations involved. The RBF Kernel was applied since it is sure to map data into a higher dimensional space, handling nonlinear relationships and enhancing the performance of classification. A stratified fivefold cross-validation was used. For LR, regularization strengths ($C = 0.01$–10) were tested. For RF, the number of trees (50–500) and max depth (5–50) were optimized. For SVM, kernel parameters such as gamma and C were adjusted across ranges. A CNN baseline was also tested with a simple architecture: input layer, two dense hidden layers (ReLU), dropout regularization, and softmax output. The polynomial kernel has been used because it would capture feature interaction through polynomial transformations, so there is a chance that if the datasets contain many more complex dependencies between those features, this kind might be able to discover them. Of the kernels applied, the one that worked best for this dataset was RBF. It was able to learn from the data pertaining to nonlinear patterns while having a cost that did not go extremely high; hence it suited well for gaining an in-depth insight into the intricate relationships of the drug response data from the GDSC dataset. This points to the important role that the choice of the kernel in the SVM process plays in optimizing its performance for predictive modelling in precision oncology. To extend the study beyond classical ML models, we implemented a baseline CNN. The architecture includes an input layer that accepts feature vectors representing Z-score, LN_IC50, and AUC values for each sample. This input is reshaped and passed through two dense hidden layers with 64 and 32 neurons respectively, using ReLU activation functions. Dropout regularization (rate = 0.2) was applied after each dense layer to reduce overfitting. The output layer used a softmax activation for binary classification. The CNN was trained using the Adam optimizer with a learning rate of 0.001 for 100 epochs. A stratified five-fold cross-validation strategy ensured robust evaluation of performance.

3.1 Evaluation Metrics

To comprehensively assess model performance, the following metrics were used:

3.1.1 Accuracy

Measures the overall correctness of predictions.

$$\text{Accuracy} = \frac{\text{TN} + \text{TP}}{\text{TP} + \text{TN} + \text{FP} + \text{FN}} \tag{1}$$

3.1.2 Precision

Indicates the proportion of true positives among predicted positives.

$$\text{Precision} = \frac{\text{TP}}{\text{TP} + \text{FP}} \tag{2}$$

3.1.3 Recall (Sensitivity)

Reflects the ability to identify true positives.

$$\text{Recall} = \frac{\text{TP}}{\text{TP} + \text{FN}} \tag{3}$$

3.1.4 F1-Score

Balances precision and recall.

$$\text{F1-score} = 2 * \frac{\text{Precision} * \text{Recall}}{\text{Precision} + \text{Recall}} \tag{4}$$

3.1.5 Area Under the Curve (AUC)

Evaluates the trade-off between sensitivity and specificity across different thresholds. The dataset was stratified into 80% training and 20% testing datasets. Cross-validation using a fivefold method was applied in tuning the hyper-parameters, such as regularization strength for LR, kernel parameters for SVM, and tree depth for RF. The performance was checked by accuracy, precision, recall, F1-score, and area under the curve (AUC). Such an approach made the models' predictions robust and reliable.

4 Results and Analysis

The results of this study highlight the comparative performance of three machine learning models (logistic regression, random forest, and support vector machine) in predicting drug responses using the GDSC dataset. The metrics used for evaluation included accuracy, precision, recall, F1-score, and area under the curve (AUC).

4.1 Exploratory Data Analysis (EDA)

To understand the interaction of features within the GDSC dataset, it has been producing a correlation matrix and displaying it in the form of a heat map. Higher correlations among Z-score, LN_IC50, and AUC are observed that can explain why those features are selected for the models. The heat map is shown in Fig. 2, where darker shades represent greater correlation values.

4.2 Model Performance Metrics

The three machine learning models, namely logistic regression (LR), random forest (RF), and support vector machine (SVM) models, were bench-marked for accuracy, precision, recall, F1-score, and AUC. The confusion matrices for each model are listed to show their performances in classification.

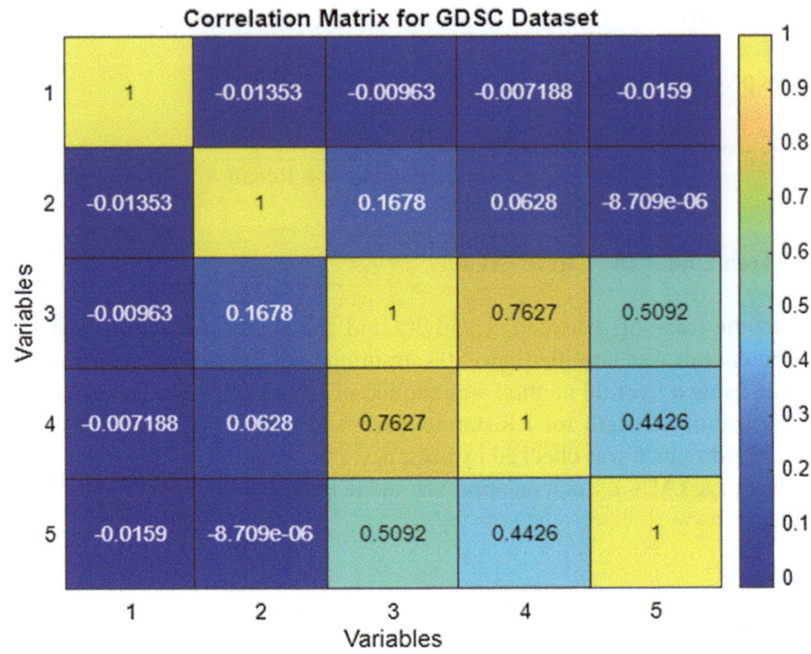

Fig. 2 Correlation matrix

Logistic regression achieved an accuracy of 89.52%, as presented in Fig. 3, indicating moderate predictive power. However, its precision (68.48%) and F1-score (65.53%) were relatively low compared to other models. The confusion matrix revealed that LR struggled to classify complex patterns, primarily due to its inability to handle nonlinear relationships inherent in genomic datasets. This limitation underscores the need for more sophisticated models in this domain.

Random Forest The random forest model, presented in Fig. 4, exhibited high accuracy (99.58%) and provided valuable insights into feature importance, particularly highlighting LN_IC50 as the most influential feature, followed by AUC and Z-score. Despite its impressive accuracy, the RF model showed signs of overfitting, as indicated by its relatively low AUC score of 0.503. This overfitting likely stemmed from the high dimensionality and imbalance of the dataset, which limited the model's generalizability.

Support Vector Machine (SVM) The SVM model, presented in Fig. 5, outperformed both LR and RF, achieving an accuracy of 99.88%, precision of 99.77%, and an AUC of 0.879. The RBF kernel proved to be the most effective, enabling the model to capture complex, nonlinear relationships within the data. The superior performance of SVM underscores its suitability for high-dimensional genomic datasets and its potential for applications in precision oncology.

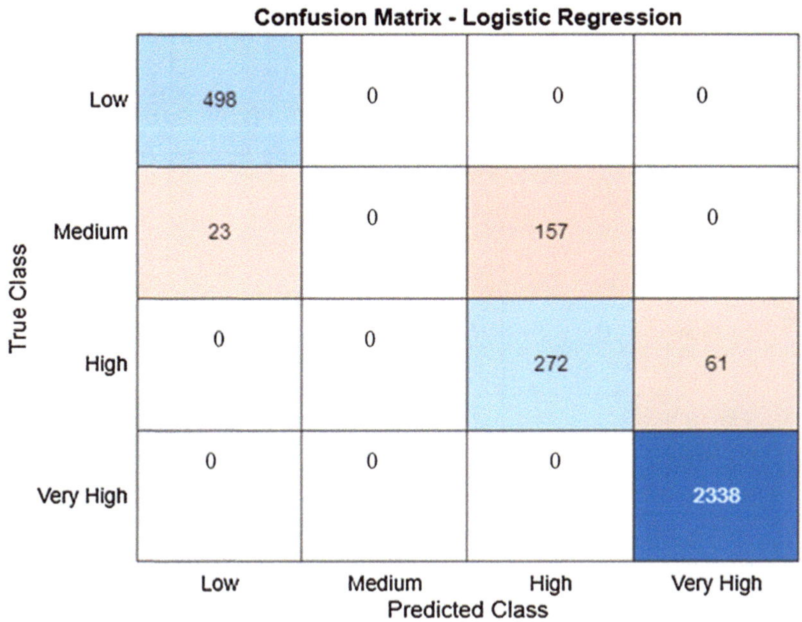

Fig. 3 Confusion matrix for logistic regression

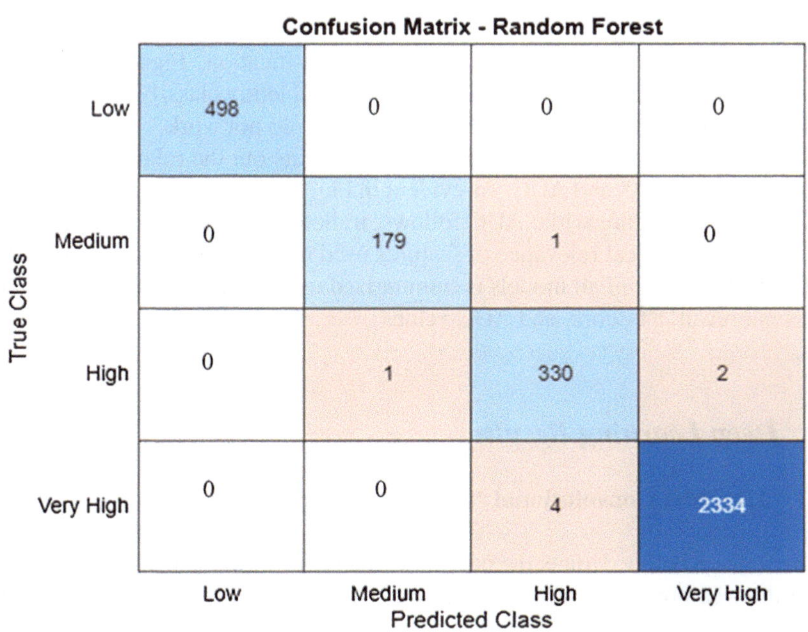

Fig. 4 Confusion matrix for random forest

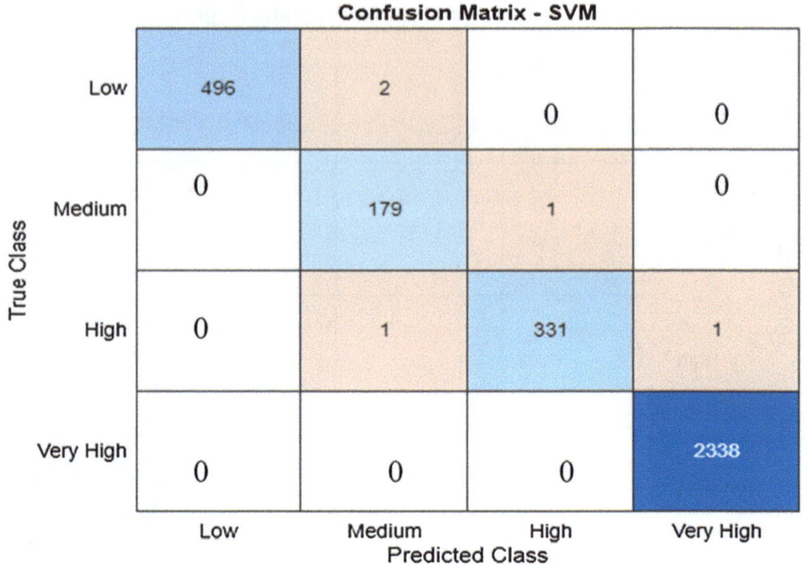

Fig. 5 Confusion matrix for support vector machine

ROC curves in Fig. 6 compare class discriminatory power of models. High AUC values verify SVM to be clearly outperforming; it can exhibit good robustness under nonlinear relationships.

Identify the decision boundary for SVM classification. Figure 7 present the various kernel creates nonlinear boundaries that efficiently classify classes, whereas the linear boundaries of LR and split regions of RF do not work.

The feature importance from random forest points out the relative contributions of Z-score, LN_IC50, and AUC. As evident in Fig. 8, LN_IC50 was identified as the most influential feature while AUC follows, trailed by Z-score. This analysis gives a clue to the biological relevance of features used in prediction of drug responses.

The performance of all models is summarized in Table 2, consolidating accuracy, precision, recall, F1-score, and AUC values.

4.3 Deep Learning Results

4.3.1 1D CNN: Convolutional Neural Network

Figure 9 given below depicts the confusion matrix of CNN, which clearly mentions about the true positives and false negatives. A total number of 325 cases has been predicted correctly as class 0, which classifies low sensitivity drug response from other classes. A highest number of 2266 true positives are identified in class 3 (very high sensitivity). In class 3, there are no cases predicted as class 0, that is, no false

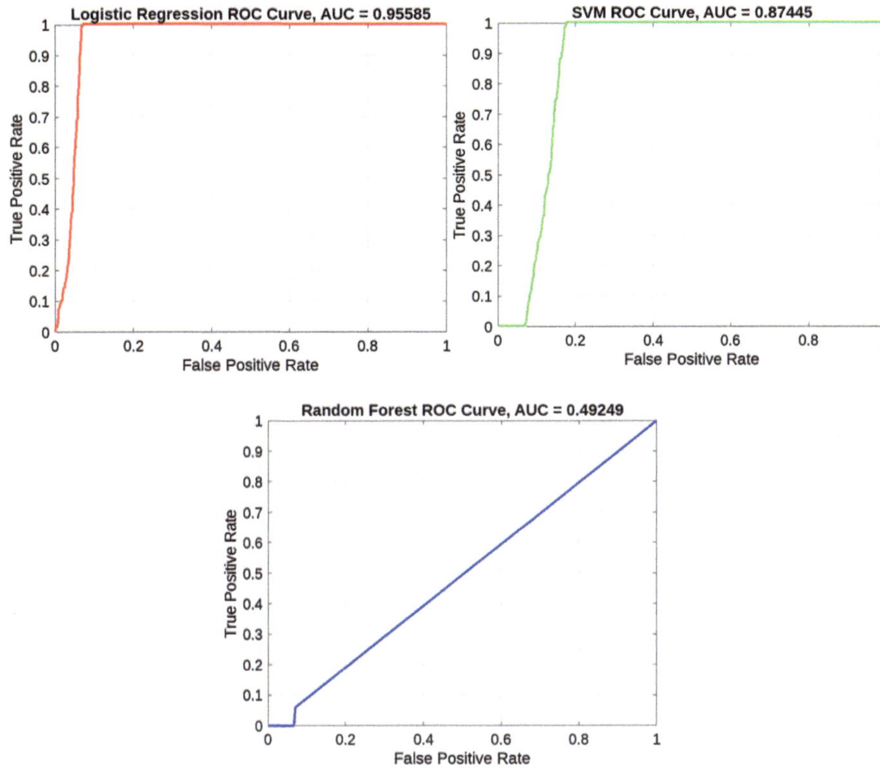

Fig. 6 ROC curves

positives. The number of false positives and true negatives are less when compared to the true positives and false negatives, which clearly tells that the CNN is a good model to use for predicting drug response in DLBCL patients. Similarly, Fig. 10 gives the receiver operating characteristic curve that sketches out the area under the curve (AUC) for each class. The AUC of class 3 is the highest as its true positives, followed by class 0 and class 1. The class 2 has the least AUC function depicting the model's difficulty in distinguishing this class.

5 Discussion

Based on findings from here, there is evidence of the strengths and weaknesses of the three models usedin the estimation of drug response for DLBCL patients. Among the models, SVM shows the highest performance as indicated with 99.88% accuracy, precision of 99.77%, and an AUC of 0.879. Since the genomic datasets have nonlinear relationships, these findings apparently prove that SVM, especially

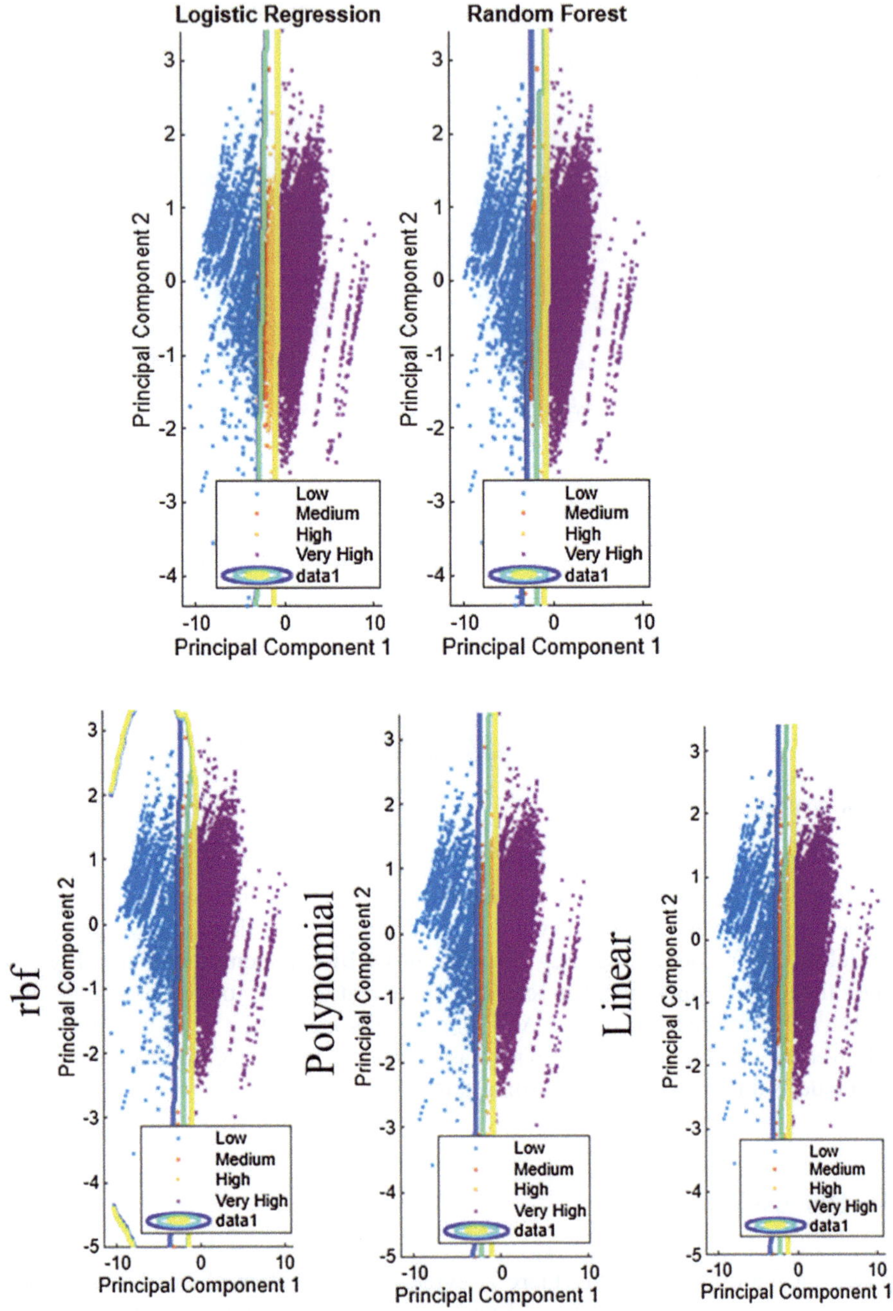

Fig. 7 Decision boundary of SVM in different kernels and for LR and RF

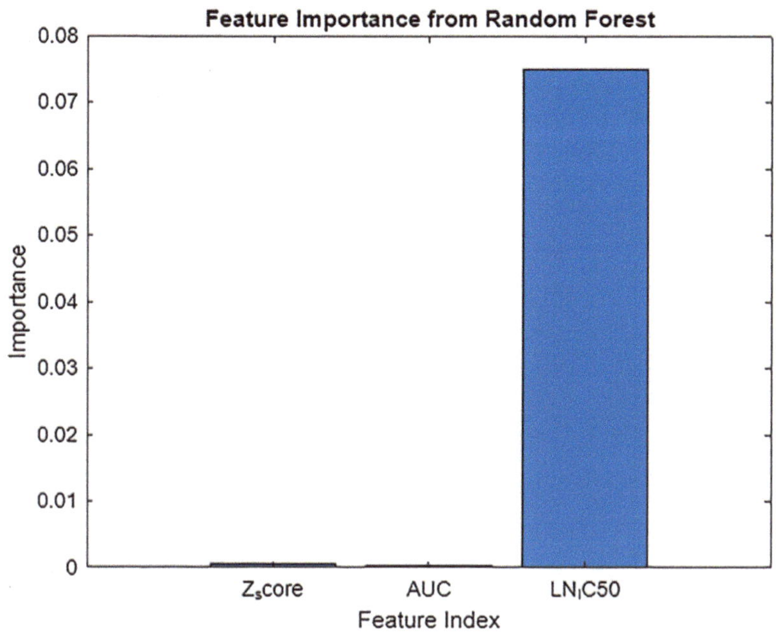

Fig. 8 Feature importance from random forest

Table 2 Model performance metrics

Metric	Logistic regression (%)	Random forest (%)	SVM (%)
Accuracy	89.52	99.58	99.88
Precision	68.48	99.15	99.7
F1-score	65.53	98.83	99.71
AUC	0.959	0.503	0.879

with RBF, is suited to handle it. High-dimensional maps in data by the RBF kernel gave SVM enough capabilities to classify hard patterns against which logistic regression (LR) and random forest (RF) had been lacking. Such strength brings SVM to the forefront as one of the strong candidates for future clinical applications in precision oncology. In addition, random forest achieved an impressive accuracy of 99.58%, a clear display of its power in an ensemble method. However, with an AUC of 0.503 and based on the confusion matrix results, one could argue that the model was overfit due to the very high dimensionality of the data. Despite that, RF provided useful insights into the relative significance of different features born from this study. Most fundamentally, LN_IC50 emerged as the most critical feature, followed by AUC and Z-score. This further explains why these features were chosen and demonstrates the suitability of RF for interpretability and feature selection purposes for this kind of studies. The logistic regression, as interpretable and computationally cheap, yields poor performance metrics, including 89.52%

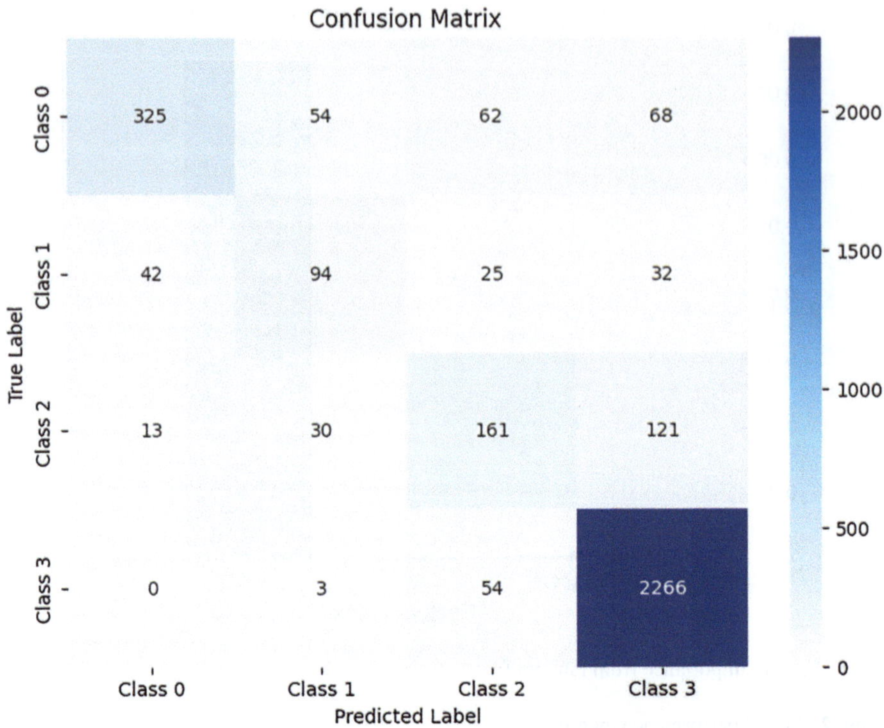

Fig. 9 Confusion matrix of CNN

accuracy and a score of 65.53% of F1-scores. The logistic regression fails to model the complex, non-linear relationships; therefore, its applicability is limited in this framework. However, its simplicity and direct interpretability make it proper for small or separable linear datasets. The CNN model achieved reasonable accuracy but did not outperform the SVM with RBF kernel. Due to the limited feature dimension (three features) and the nonspatial nature of the input, the CNN provided no significant advantage over traditional ML models in this setting. However, it demonstrates the feasibility of extending this framework to more complex multi-omics data, where CNN architectures may be more appropriate for learning intricate patterns.

The chapter indicates that kernel selection is an important step in SVM. Comparing the experimental results of linear, polynomial, sigmoid, and RBF kernels, the authors demonstrated that the RBF kernel is superior to others since it can model effectively the nonlinear interactions between features. This outcome is in line with previous research that showed excellent performance for RBF kernels on genomic as well as clinical datasets. Positive findings notwithstanding, there are limitations to this study. The dataset studied was comprehensive but limited to in vitro cell lines. So, the set of in vivo variability cannot be said to have comprehensively been

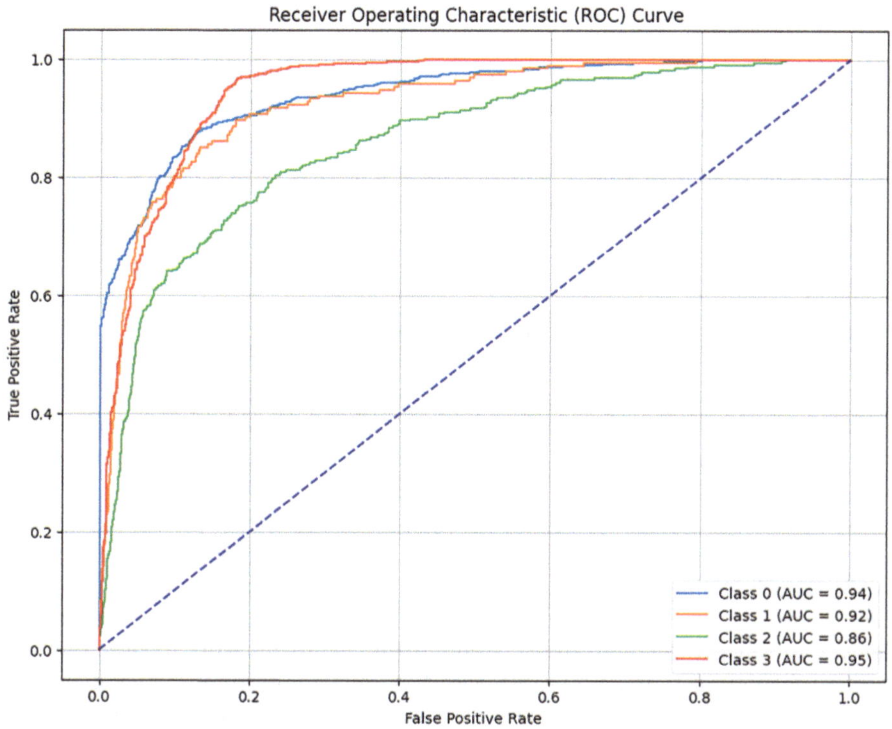

Fig. 10 ROC for CNN

addressed. In addition, the imbalance of classes within the dataset will affect the tendency of the model to favor specific underrepresented drug responses. Thirdly, further improvement over such problems through large and balanced datasets will be crucial for enhancing the validity and applicability of the model after its adaptation for more experiments.

6 Conclusion

This chapter demonstrates that ML models can accurately predict drug response in DLBCL patients using the GDSC dataset. SVM with an RBF kernel emerged as the most effective, outperforming LR and RF in accuracy and robustness. The findings affirm the potential of ML to support personalized medicine by aligning treatment decisions with patient-specific molecular profiles. Future work should validate these models with real-world patient data, incorporate additional omics layers, and adopt explainable frameworks to ensure clinical adoption. It was able to show that machine learning models can predict the responses to medicines in DLBCL patients through the help of GDSC datasets. SVM using the RBF kernel was effective, with highest accuracy at 99.88% and robust performance in all the evaluation metrics. Its ability to handle nonlinear interactions rendered it most appropriate for the complex genomic data set [1]. RF also performed quite well, providing feature importance about guiding biological interpretations that further inform the value of the results [2]. Logistic regression (LR) was easy and interpretable yet failed to exploit the nonlinearities in the data, which led to the poor performance metrics [3]. In short, results like these point toward a strong position of machine learning in driving the next wave of precision oncology toward making treatment strategies patient-centric in nature.

Despite the promising results, this study presents a promising application of machine learning for drug response prediction in DLBCL; however, several limitations must be acknowledged. First, the GDSC dataset is derived entirely from in vitro cell line data, which does not fully replicate the complexity of in vivo tumor microenvironments or patient-specific heterogeneity. Second, despite implementing SMOTE to address class imbalance, there remains a risk that minority classes are underrepresented, which can impact the robustness of predictions for rare drug responses. Another limitation is the risk of overfitting, particularly evident in the random forest model's performance. Although cross-validation helps mitigate this, future studies should incorporate larger, more balanced, and patient-derived datasets to enhance generalizability. Additionally, while this work focused on three primary features Z-score, LN_IC50, and AUC integrating multi-omics data such as gene expression, proteomic, and transcriptomic layers could improve predictive power and biological relevance. Finally, ML models, especially ensemble and deep learning architectures, often function as "black boxes." This lack of interpretability can hinder clinical trust. Future work should integrate Explainable AI (XAI) approaches to make predictions more transparent, aiding clinician understanding and acceptance. While the CNN did not surpass the SVM in this context, future work could explore deeper CNN architectures with larger, multidimensional input data to leverage its full potential.

Future research should focus on expanding datasets to include real-world patient-derived cohorts, developing deep learning techniques to model complex genomic interactions, and validating these models through clinical trials. Additionally, integrating XAI methods will enhance model transparency and clinical usability. Finally, this study highlights the transformative role of machine learning in precision medicine, particularly in DLBCL drug response prediction. By addressing current limitations and pursuing the proposed future directions, ML-driven approaches have the potential to significantly improve patient outcomes and advance the field of personalized oncology.

Acknowledgments The authors declare that large language models were used to assist in language editing, proofreading, and formatting guidance during the preparation of this chapter. All scientific content, interpretation, analysis, and final revisions were thoroughly reviewed and approved by the authors.

References

1. R. Patel et al., Machine learning for predicting patient outcomes in DLBCL. Comput. Oncol. **30**, 412–427 (2022)
2. X. Zhang et al., Genomics and deep learning for drug response prediction in DLBCL. Nat. Biotechnol. **39**, 1013–1021 (2021)
3. K. Davis et al., Personalized treatment approaches in DLBCL. Blood J. **142**, 1062–1074 (2023)
4. X. Wang et al., Integrating genomic and clinical data to predict drug responses. Precis. Med. Cancer Res. **19**, 102–117 (2023)
5. A. Cimino et al., Ensemble methods in precision oncology. J. Oncol. Inf. **25**, 203–221 (2020)
6. L. Qi, *Time Series Analysis in Genomics* (Tsinghua University Press, Beijing, 2019)
7. H. Li, *Statistical Learning for High-Dimensional Data* (Tsinghua University Press, Beijing, 2020)
8. Z. Zhou, *Advances in Machine Learning for Genomic Data* (Springer, Cham, 2021)
9. K. Kim, Support vector machines in precision medicine. Neurocomputing **55**, 307–319 (2020)
10. J. Fan et al., A framework for predicting cancer outcomes. Sci. Oncol. **7**, 1–16 (2021)
11. T. Becker et al., Deep learning for drug sensitivity prediction. J. Comput. Biol. **18**, 215–229 (2021)
12. P. Rao et al., Applications of explainable AI in oncology. Cancer Informat. **15**, 112–128 (2022)
13. D. Singh et al., Precision oncology using multi-omics data. Trends Cancer Res. **25**, 451–468 (2023)
14. R. Gupta et al., Integrating AI in cancer treatment. J. Clin. Oncol. **38**, 2512–2527 (2022)
15. M. Chen et al., Drug response modeling using random forests. IEEE Trans. Biomed. Eng. **68**, 512–524 (2023)
16. S. Lee et al., Kernel optimization in SVM for genomics. Comput. Genom. **35**, 312–328 (2023)
17. F. Carter et al., High-dimensional data analysis in oncology. J. Cancer Inf. **20**, 78–93 (2023)
18. B. Klein et al., Class balancing techniques in cancer datasets. Bioinf. Adv. **15**, 411–426 (2021)
19. G. Yu et al., Enhancing predictive models with SMOTE. Mach. Learn. Appl. **28**, 119–132 (2022)
20. J. Green et al., Validation of ML models in clinical oncology. Ann. Oncol. **33**, 245–260 (2022)
21. N. Brown et al., Evaluating model interpretability in oncology. AI Med. **45**, 512–526 (2022)
22. A. Young et al., Multi-omics data integration for precision medicine. J. Precis. Oncol. **8**, 115–128 (2023)
23. M. Zhang et al., Patient-derived models in drug sensitivity studies. Cancer Res. **78**, 521–532 (2023)
24. E. Johnson et al., AI in predictive oncology. Comput. Oncol. **30**, 132–147 (2023)
25. V. Singh et al., Feature selection techniques in oncology data. J. Data Sci. **12**, 342–356 (2021)
26. H. White et al., Exploring RBF kernels in genomic data analysis. Comp. Med. **17**, 212–227 (2023)
27. K. Sharma et al., Overcoming dataset limitations in ML models. J. Oncol. Data **25**, 319–332 (2022)
28. J. Scott et al., Precision medicine: Challenges and opportunities. Trends Genom. Med. **14**, 78–92 (2023)
29. A. Patel et al., Nonlinear modeling in genomic data. Bioinf. Res. **19**, 62–75 (2022)
30. C. Martinez et al., AI in drug sensitivity prediction. Mach. Learn. Med. **29**, 412–426 (2023)
31. R. Lee et al., Improving ML model robustness in oncology. J. AI Healthc. **23**, 218–232 (2022)
32. M. Xu et al., Leveraging explainable AI in precision oncology. Cancer Informat. **16**, 118–131 (2023)
33. B. Lee et al., Advances in high-dimensional genomic data analysis. AI Bioinf. **24**, 307–321 (2022)
34. F. Kumar et al., Optimizing feature engineering for oncology datasets. J. Bioinf. Adv. **18**, 411–425 (2023)
35. D. Moore et al., Clinical implications of ML in cancer treatment. Ann. Med. Data **19**, 252–226 (2024)

Guideline-Concordant Two-Stage AI for Diabetes Severity Stratification and Pharmacotherapy Recommendation

Hasret Irmak Baran, Nisa Sahinoglu, and Gulay Cicek

Abstract This chapter proposes a guideline-concordant two-stage intelligent system designed to support both the diagnosis and pharmacological management of diabetes. In the first stage, diabetes severity is classified using two distinct datasets—the Pima Indian Diabetes dataset and a local dataset from Iraq—after feature selection and data balancing, applying multiple machine learning and deep learning algorithms with cross-validation. In the second stage, a hybrid drug recommendation module integrates rule-based logic derived from the national diabetes treatment guideline with supervised learning models, incorporating patient-specific variables such as age, body mass index (BMI), glomerular filtration rate (GFR), and comorbidities. The approach achieved high predictive performance in both severity classification and pharmacotherapy recommendation, with random forest and long short-term memory models performing best in their respective categories. By combining clinically interpretable rules with data-driven models and validating on heterogeneous populations, the proposed framework addresses limitations of prior single-task or purely algorithmic approaches and demonstrates potential for real-world clinical decision support. Future work will focus on expanding the dataset, external validation, and deployment in clinical settings to ensure generalizability and safety.

Keywords Diabetes prediction · Machine learning · Deep learning · Drug recommendation · Clinical decision support · Guideline-based treatment · Personalized pharmacotherapy · Precision medicine

H. I. Baran · N. Sahinoglu
Faculty of Engineering and Architecture, Department of Software Engineering, Istanbul Beykent University, Istanbul, Türkiye
e-mail: 2203013009@student.beykent.edu.tr; 2203013022@student.beykent.edu.tr

G. Cicek (✉)
Faculty of Engineering and Architecture, Department of Biomedical Engineering, Istanbul Beykent University, Istanbul, Türkiye
e-mail: gulaycicek@beykent.edu.tr

N. E. M. Khalifa, M. H. N. Taha (eds.), *Next-Gen Healthcare*,
https://doi.org/10.1007/978-3-032-07267-2_11

List of Abbreviations

ADR	Adverse drug reaction
AI	Artificial intelligence
ANN	Artificial neural network
AUC-ROC	Area under the curve-receiver operating characteristic
BMI	Body mass index
Chol	Cholesterol
CNN	Convolutional neural network
Cr	Creatinine
CPU	Central processing unit
CV	Cross-validation
DNN	Deep neural network
DL	Deep learning
DM	Diabetes mellitus
DPP-4	Dipeptidyl peptidase-4
DT	Decision tree
FBG	Fasting blood glucose
FNN	Feedforward neural network
FN	False negative
GFR	Glomerular filtration rate
GLP-1	Glucagon-like peptide-1 receptor
GPU	Graphics processing unit
GRU	Gated recurrent unit
HbA1c	Hemoglobin A1c test
HDL	High-density lipoprotein
KNN	K-nearest neighbors
LSTM	Long short-term memory
LDL	Low-density lipoprotein
LR	Logistic regression
ML	Machine learning
MI	Mutual information
NLP	Natural language processing
OGTT	Oral glucose tolerance test
PID	Pima Indian Diabetes
RBR	Rule-based reasoning
RF	Random forest
RNN	Recurrent neural network
SMOTE	Synthetic minority oversampling technique
SGLT-2	Sodium-glucose co-transporter-2
SVM	Support vector machines
TG	Triglycerides
TP	True positive
Urea	Blood urea nitrogen
VLDL	Very-low-density lipoprotein

1 Introduction

The advancement of artificial intelligence (AI) has enabled the development of applications capable of making highly accurate predictions from large and complex datasets. These applications contribute to improved decision-making accuracy and significantly reduce the time required for clinical evaluations and related processes [1, 2]. This ability of artificial intelligence has been used in many areas such as diagnosis and personalized treatment recommendations in the health field [3–5]. For example, in the field of hematology, applications such as anomaly detection in blood cell images, early diagnosis of hematologic malignancies in leukemia and leukemia-like diseases, and monitoring of treatment response have been developed, and these applications have great potential to be used in different areas as well as having their own development potential [6–8]. In our study, machine learning algorithms were used to predict the treatment responses of acromegaly patients in the fields of endocrinology and metabolism, which we also addressed in our study, and these applications have yielded significant results in terms of improving patients' treatment processes [9]. As another example, in this study, the issue of diabetes was also addressed, and the use of machine learning methods in the diagnosis and treatment management of diabetes can make significant contributions to health services by increasing the accuracy of clinical decision support systems [10, 11]. The potential and results of these applications make it very possible to predict that diseases can be diagnosed more quickly and accurately and that they can be helpful in the treatment process by using artificial intelligence applications.

The focus of this study is diabetes, which has established epidemiological data, diagnostic criteria, and treatment protocols.

1.1 Diabetes Epidemic

Diabetes is a chronic disease that occurs when the body either does not produce enough insulin or cannot utilize the insulin it produces effectively, resulting in elevated blood glucose levels. If left uncontrolled, this can cause serious health problems such as cardiovascular disease, kidney failure, and loss of vision. According to the World Health Organization, around 537 million adults worldwide were living with diabetes in 2021, and this figure is expected to rise to 783 million by 2045 [9]. The financial impact of diabetes is substantial, with global costs for its treatment and management estimated at around $760 billion in 2020 [11].

Diabetes is commonly classified into two primary types: Type 1 and Type 2. Type 1 diabetes typically manifests at a young age and results from the immune system mistakenly attacking the insulin-producing beta cells in the pancreas. Although its exact cause remains unclear, it is believed to result from a combination of genetic predisposition and environmental triggers. People diagnosed with Type 1 diabetes require lifelong insulin treatment [12]. Type 2 diabetes, which is significantly more widespread, is closely associated with factors such as aging, obesity, sedentary lifestyle, and hereditary tendencies. It is characterized by the body's impaired response to insulin (known as insulin resistance) or insufficient insulin production. Most cases of Type 2 diabetes can be managed through lifestyle changes like healthy eating, physical activity, and appropriate medication. Without proper management, it may result in serious complications [13]. Another form, gestational diabetes, emerges during pregnancy and typically disappears after childbirth, though it increases the mother's risk of developing Type 2 diabetes later in life. Careful monitoring during pregnancy is vital to avoid complications for both mother and baby due to elevated blood glucose levels [14].

The primary difference between Type 1 and Type 2 diabetes lies in their underlying causes and typical age of onset. Type 1 generally develops in children or young adults due to an autoimmune reaction, where the immune system mistakenly targets and destroys the insulin-producing cells of the pancreas. On the other hand, Type 2 is largely associated with insulin resistance and tends to affect older individuals, particularly those with excess weight or unhealthy lifestyle habits. While insulin therapy is essential for managing Type 1 diabetes, Type 2 is often controllable through lifestyle modifications, including balanced nutrition, regular physical activity, and medications when necessary. Detecting both types early plays a critical role in preventing long-term health issues and improving quality of life [15].

1.2 Diabetes Epidemic

Accurate diagnostic techniques are crucial for the timely identification and effective management of diabetes. The condition is most commonly identified using tests such as fasting blood glucose (FBG), oral glucose tolerance (OGTT), and hemoglobin A1c (HbA1c).

1.2.1 Fasting Blood Glucose (FBG) Test

One of the simplest and most commonly used methods, the FBG test, measures the glucose level in a blood sample taken after at least 8 hours of fasting. A fasting blood glucose level of 126 mg/dL or higher is considered a significant indicator for a diagnosis of diabetes.

1.2.2 Oral Glucose Tolerance Test (OGTT)

OGTT is a more comprehensive test that is particularly used in individuals with suspected latent diabetes or gestational diabetes. In this test, the individual is given a drink containing a certain amount of glucose, and then blood glucose levels are measured at specific intervals. This test provides more detailed information about how the body uses glucose and helps to assess the risk of diabetes more accurately.

1.2.3 Hemoglobin A1c (HbA1c) Test

The HbA1c test is a measure that reflects the average blood glucose level over the past approximately 3 months. This test is used not only to diagnose diabetes but also to evaluate the response to treatment in individuals with diabetes and to monitor long-term blood glucose control. An HbA1c level of 6.5% or higher is considered a significant indicator for a diagnosis of diabetes [16].

1.3 Diabetes Treatment Process

The treatment process for diabetes requires a personalized and multifaceted approach that, in addition to managing blood sugar levels, may involve addressing cardiovascular diseases, kidney complications, and other metabolic disorders according to individual needs. Today, personalized treatment plans that combine traditional and modern treatment methods are created for patients diagnosed with diabetes [17–19].

Traditional treatment methods, such as dietary modifications and pharmacotherapy, remain the cornerstone of diabetes management. However, advances in modern technologies and innovative therapies are reshaping the landscape of treatment. Procedures like pancreas-kidney transplantation, human islet cell transplantation, and stem cell therapy offer promising alternatives, despite challenges in sustainability and clinical implementation. Nevertheless, personalized drug therapies based on patient-specific factors continue to be the most commonly applied treatments [20–22].

Drug management, one of the cornerstones of the treatment process, is shaped by multifaceted approaches that use different drug classes together. Metformin, which suppresses the liver's glucose production and increases insulin sensitivity, is commonly used as initial therapy [23]. GLP-1 receptor agonists are drugs that can increase insulin secretion and decrease glucagon production; they not only control blood sugar but can also reduce the risk of cardiovascular diseases [24]. SGLT-2 inhibitors prevent glucose from being absorbed by the kidneys, allowing it to be excreted in the urine, which helps lower blood sugar levels and also protects kidney health [25]. Another class, DPP-4 inhibitors, helps regulate blood sugar levels by increasing the effects of incretin hormones, making them a safe alternative for patients who are intolerant to other treatment options [26].

Looking at all these examples, the use of drug combinations in diabetes treatment varies according to the individual needs of patients. During the treatment process, drugs from different classes such as metformin, GLP-1 receptor agonists, SGLT-2 inhibitors, and DPP-4 inhibitors are often used together. However, the interactions between drugs and the overall health status of patients can directly affect the treatment process. For example, the combined use of metformin and SGLT-2 inhibitors can more effectively manage blood sugar but can have effects on kidney function that need to be considered [27–29]. Drug interactions should be carefully monitored and reviewed regularly, especially when several drug combinations are involved.

1.4 Aim of the Study

The main objective in this study is to shorten the diabetes-level assessment and drug recommendation process. The novelty and unique contributions of our study are as follows:

1.5 Aim and Novelty of the Study

The primary aim of this study is to shorten and optimize the diabetes severity assessment and personalized drug recommendation process by leveraging advanced artificial intelligence techniques and clinical guidelines.

The innovations and unique contributions of the study are as follows:

- **Innovative Two-Stage Intelligent System:** A novel two-stage system is proposed that first accurately classifies diabetes severity using machine learning and deep learning models, and then drug classes are recommended through a hybrid decision support system. This integrated approach is designed to enhance both diagnostic accuracy and therapy planning.
- **Personalized Drug Recommendation and Risk Classification:** Unlike traditional drug recommendation systems, potential side effects and drug-interaction risks are evaluated based on individual patient parameters such as age, BMI, kidney function (GFR), and comorbidities. Drugs are classified according to risk levels to ensure safer and more personalized treatment.
- **Integration of Diagnosis and Drug Recommendation Modules:** A unified framework combining diabetes severity classification and drug recommendation is implemented to improve workflow efficiency and provide clinicians with a comprehensive decision support tool. Such integrated systems are rarely reported in the literature.
- **Use of National Clinical Guidelines and Custom Dataset:** The drug recommendation system is built upon a custom dataset derived from national diabetes treatment guidelines, ensuring that clinical relevance and compliance with standard care practices are maintained.

- **Advanced Hybrid Decision Support System:** By combining rule-based logic with supervised classification models, transparent and clinically interpretable recommendations are offered, overcoming the black-box issues common in AI models.
- **Robust Experimental Validation:** Validation has been carried out on two widely used public diabetes datasets for classification and a custom dataset for drug recommendation, with high accuracy achieved, while overfitting issues were addressed through detailed model analyses.

These contributions position this work as a clinically grounded, innovative, and AI-supported practical approach to personalized diabetes management.

The remainder of this chapter is organized as follows: Sect. 2 presents the related literature, Sect. 3 describes the methodology, Sect. 4 presents the results, Sect. 5 offers a discussion within the context of existing research, and Sect. 6 concludes with future research directions.

2 Literature Review

This section summarizes literature studies that examine the applications of machine learning and artificial intelligence-based approaches in various fields such as medical diagnosis, drug recommendation systems, and disease management. Studies have generally used large-scale datasets to comparatively evaluate the performance of various algorithms for problems such as disease prediction, drug-interaction analysis, and adverse drug reaction (ADR) detection. In particular, Tables 1, 2, 3, 4, and 5 systematically present information about the datasets used in each study, sample sizes, methods, results, shortcomings, and suggested areas for improvement. These summaries provide a foundation for understanding the general trends and areas of progress in the literature.

Contribution Beyond Prior Studies

As summarized in Tables 1, 2, 3, 4, and 5, most prior work on diabetes diagnosis and drug recommendation has addressed a single task, used geographically limited datasets, and relied solely on machine learning predictions without incorporating clinical guideline logic. This study introduces a *guideline-concordant two-stage framework* that first stratifies diabetes severity using both international and local datasets and then generates pharmacotherapy recommendations by integrating rule-based logic with data-driven models. This approach enhances both predictive performance and clinical interpretability. The use of two distinct populations allows preliminary testing of generalizability, while explicit drug-drug interaction screening and contraindication handling increase the system's practical applicability in real-world clinical settings.

Table 1 Literature review results

Reference	Publication year	Dataset	Sample size	Methods	Results	Limitations	Future work
[30]	2025	17,773 T2DM patient records (12 years, US VA system)	17,773	Bayesian networks, interpretability via decision trees	Precision = 0.789, Recall = 0.879, F1 = 0.831; personalized medication prescriptions	Single-source dataset (VA); no validation on other populations	Test on different healthcare systems and populations; increase data diversity
[31]	2025	Clinical and laboratory data from various sources	Not specified (large scale)	Random forest, SVM, XGBoost hybrid ensemble	70%+ accuracy; personalized diet and physical activity recommendations	Data imbalance in some datasets; limited feature selection	Use more balanced datasets; expand parameters for lifestyle recommendations
[32]	2024	Biopsy data, medical imaging results, and patient records related to liver diseases	The datasets used in the study are not fully specified, but it is emphasized that multicenter and large-scale data sources were used	Deep learning algorithms for image processing, support vector machines, and regression analysis for prediction models	AI has achieved high accuracy rates in diagnosing liver diseases, contributing to clinical decision support systems for treatment recommendations. It has also shown strong performance in predicting disease progression	The use of AI in liver diseases is limited due to the lack of diversity and standardization of datasets. Additionally, integrating models into clinical use is challenging	Increasing data standardization, developing explainable AI applications, and wider adoption of AI tools in clinical settings are necessary
[33]	2024	Various clinical data of diabetic individuals	Extensive data compiled from different datasets in the literature	Machine learning, big data analytics, natural language processing (NLP)	AI-based systems provide significant advantages in early diagnosis and treatment optimization of diabetes	Limited data diversity, generalizability of AI systems, and clinical integration process not fully tested	Increasing data diversity, testing algorithms on larger populations, and conducting further research on their applicability in clinical practice

[34]	2024	CKD dataset from the US National Kidney Foundation	Approximately 1000 data samples	Ensemble learning techniques, RF, GBM, XGBoost algorithm	Model accuracy exceeded 90%. Ensemble approach achieved higher success compared to individual algorithms	Dataset size is limited; this may affect the model's generalizability. Additionally, manual intervention is required during feature selection	Using larger and more diverse datasets. Automating feature selection. Testing and adapting the model to clinical applications
[35]	2024	19 studies, a total of 304,076 samples; participants aged´ 37–71	109–96,653	GBM, RF, ANN, LR, LightGBM, SVM, AdaBoost, and other ML algorithms	High AUROC (0.85+), sensitivity, specificity, and accuracy; performance varied across algorithms	Lack of external validation; low data quality in some studies; insufficient standardized criteria; limited model generalizability	Using larger and more diverse datasets; increasing external validation; combining different algorithms; applying more homogeneous criteria for AKI definition
[36]	2024	BRFSS dataset; large population with class imbalance	Not specified	RF, SVM, NB, and SMOTE	Data augmentation improved accuracy and other metrics	Class imbalance led to poor performance of some models; limited data diversity	Using larger, balanced datasets; detailed investigation of deep learning techniques
[37]	2024	BRFSS dataset	Not specified	Decision trees, SVMs	Data augmentation and machine learning improved diabetes diagnosis	Lack of data diversity; model interpretability	Larger and more diverse datasets; improving data augmentation techniques; enhancing model interpretability

Table 2 Literature review summary

Reference	Publication year	Dataset	Sample size	Methods	Results	Limitations	Future work
[38]	2024	Various medical datasets for chronic disease management	Not specified; large-scale medical data analyzed	Neural networks, machine learning, risk factor identification, personalized treatment planning	DNNs provide higher accuracy in disease diagnosis and management compared to traditional methods	Data security, model transparency, ethical concerns, and general usability challenges	Integration with wearable devices, alignment with genomic data, model interpretability, and further advancements in ethical frameworks
[39]	2023	Medical datasets including clinical data and survey results of diabetic patients	Large-scale datasets, hundreds of patient samples	Machine learning algorithms such as decision trees, support vector machines, k-nearest neighbors	Machine learning algorithms achieved high accuracy in diabetes diagnosis	Limited dataset diversity and improvements can be made in model generalizability	Using larger and more diverse datasets, reducing false positive rates, and improving model generalizability
[40]	2023	Large dataset containing clinical data of type 2 diabetes patients from various healthcare institutions	Over 50,000 samples	Hybrid meta-heuristic algorithms, genetic algorithms, particle swarm optimization, decision trees, support vector machines (SVMs)	Hybrid meta-heuristic algorithms achieved 5–10% higher accuracy rates compared to traditional methods	Using datasets from a single source may limit the model's generalization capacity. Additionally, more information is needed about the hyperparameter settings of some hybrid algorithms	Using larger and more diverse datasets from various healthcare data sources can improve the model's generalization performance. Additionally, testing algorithms with different hyperparameter combinations can improve results

[41]	2023	Data from clinical studies on diabetes treatment and pharma-cotherapy	Various datasets from literature; sample sizes not specified	Supervised and unsupervised machine learning, subgroup analysis, data processing algorithms	Personalized treatment approaches proposed, especially improvements in drug effects for subgroups	Lack of data diversity and standardization; limited generalizability of some algorithms	Increasing accuracy and predictive power of algorithms with larger and more diverse datasets
[42]	2023	Extensive datasets including medical history and patient records	Large-scale datasets with numerous patient samples	Machine learning algorithms such as decision trees, random forests, support vector machines, artificial neural networks	Machine learning algorithms achieved successful results in disease prediction and drug recommendation	Limited dataset diversity and size, improvements need to be made in model generalizability	Diversifying datasets and using larger datasets. Improving model accuracy through parameter optimization and ensuring the generalizability of algorithms to different patient groups

Table 3 Literature review summary

Reference	Publication year	Dataset	Sample size	Methods	Results	Limitations	Future work
[43]	2023	Clinical datasets of diabetic patients and blood glucose measurements	Data from different studies, totaling over 100,000 samples	Decision trees, artificial neural networks (ANNs), support vector machines (SVMs), regression models	The study stated that ANN and SVM algorithms achieved higher accuracy rates compared to other methods	Datasets used are generally limited and based on a single geographic region, making generalization difficult	The generalizability of models should be improved by using larger and more diverse datasets, and they should be tested on different population groups. Additionally, incorporating biomarkers and genetic data is recommended
[44]	2023	Large-scale datasets containing genetic data, biomedical diseases, and patient health information	Datasets typically consist of millions of samples	Deep learning algorithms (deep neural networks, convolutional neural networks, long short-term memory (LSTM)), feature extraction, genetic algorithms	Deep learning methods achieve high accuracy rates in genomic data analysis and effective results in diagnosing biomedical diseases	Limitations of datasets and the heterogeneous nature of biomedical data limit the model's overall performance. Additionally, interpretability of deep learning models remains a significant challenge	Using larger and more diverse biomedical datasets, improving model interpretability, and developing more robust solutions for health data privacy are needed

[45]	2023	Large datasets containing clinical patient data, drug interactions, biological responses, and genetic data	Datasets contain millions of samples and cover a wide range of patient groups	Machine learning algorithms (decision trees, support vector machines, artificial neural networks), AI-based prediction models, modeling of drug interactions	AI and machine learning methods have achieved high accuracy rates in the early detection of ADRs and drug-induced toxic effects. These methods can improve safety monitoring processes in pharmacovigilance	Diversity and quality of datasets can limit the generalizability of models. Additionally, interpretability of models remains a significant challenge	Using more and more diverse datasets, improving model interpretability, and better modeling of drug interactions are needed. Furthermore, the integration of early detection systems into clinical settings should be ensured
[46]	2022	Extensive dataset on medical emergencies and drug interactions	Tested on various medical emergencies and drug combinations	Stacked artificial neural networks (ANNs)	Model provides accurate and safe drug recommendations for medical emergencies	System should be tested with larger datasets and lacks clinical validation	Model needs to be tested with more medical emergencies and patient profiles. Additionally, the model's accuracy should be further analyzed in clinical settings
[47]	2022	Clinical blood test data	Not specified, but likely limited	Logistic regression, decision trees	High accuracy in anemia detection	Small dataset size may limit model generalizability	Using larger and more diverse datasets; trying more sophisticated methods like deep learning
[48]	2022	PIMA Indian, LMCH Diabetes datasets	768 in PIMA; not specified in LMCH	Spearman correlation for feature selection, polynomial regression for missing value imputation, RF, SVM, 2GDNN for classification	2GDNN achieved 97.34% accuracy, 97.24% sensitivity, 97.26% F1 score	More data analysis in imputation and feature selection; model generalizability not tested	Testing with larger and more diverse datasets; using different hyperparameter optimization techniques

Table 4 Literature review summary

Reference	Publication year	Dataset	Sample size	Methods	Results	Limitations	Future work
[49]	2022	UCI CKD dataset	400 data samples	Feature optimization techniques: PCA, RFE, LASSO; classification algorithms: SVM, random forest, XGBoost	Features optimized with PCA and RFE increased accuracy to 94%	Limited generalization ability due to small dataset. High time cost in the optimization process	Using larger and more diverse datasets. Accelerating feature optimization processes
[50]	2022	Medical data and patient records related to drug treatment protocols and side effects	Large-scale datasets from different patient groups	Decision trees, KNN, ANN, SVM	Machine learning-based recommendation systems accurately match disease-drug relationships and side effects	Limited data diversity and low generalizability of the model to different patient groups	Increasing data diversity and performing parameter optimization. Developing more sensitive models for predicting drug side effects
[51]	2021	Extensive dataset containing chemical and biological interaction data	Thousands of interaction instances from different drug-target interaction data	Knowledge graphs, recommen-dation systems, machine learning algorithms	Unified framework achieved high accuracy in drug-target interaction prediction	Limited data diversity and data quality need improvement	Using larger and more diverse datasets, improving model generalizability. Further applications in clinical trials and drug discovery processes

[52]	2021	Clinical and biological data of diabetes patients	Detailed sample size not specified in the study, but large-scale datasets were studied	Machine learning algorithms, regression models, and classification techniques	Some machine learning algorithms were found to have high accuracy, but results varied across different datasets	Methods used have not been validated with real clinical data and are based on theoretical results only	Accuracy of algorithms should be improved with more datasets tested in real clinical settings. Additionally, more personalized models can be developed by integrating biomarkers and genetic data
[43]	2020	Clinical data of diabetic and healthy individuals	Large dataset consisting of clinical data from various patient groups	Artificial neural network (ANN) classification algorithm	ANN model was found to provide high accuracy rates in diabetes diagnosis	The model's generalizability has not been tested on different patient groups	Improving model accuracy by using larger datasets. Optimizing parameters and applying the model to more diverse patient groups
[53]	2020	UCI Pima Indian Diabetes dataset	768	Hybrid ensemble model (REP Tree, Naïve Bayes, Decorate)	High accuracy, outperformed other methods	Class imbalance; lack of feature selection	Better data preprocessing techniques, algorithm optimization

Table 5 Literature review results

Reference	Publication year	Dataset	Sample size	Methods	Results	Limitations	Future work
[54]	2019	Various datasets containing clinical data and biomarkers of diabetic patients	Over 10,000 samples	Decision trees, support vector machines (SVMs), logistic regression	Support vector machines (SVMs) showed the best performance with high accuracy rates	Limited diversity and geographic constraints of the datasets used make generalization difficult. Additionally, sufficient details were not provided on the hyperparameter settings of some algorithms	Using larger and more diverse datasets from different geographic regions can improve the model's generalizability. Additionally, integrating more biomarkers and genetic data can increase model accuracy
[8]	2018	Over 60,000 blood test samples from a Slovenian hospital	60,000+	RF, gradient boosting, SVM, nonparametric statistical methods	86–88% accuracy in predicting five different diseases; comparable performance to clinical experts	Dataset from a single source; limited generalizability	Testing with more diverse datasets; applying deep learning techniques
[55]	2018	Datasets from studies on genetics, biomarkers, and environmental factors	Specific sample size not specified; biomarker data from various patients used	Genetic testing, biomarker analysis, modeling with lifestyle changes	Precision medicine offers significant potential for early diagnosis and personalized treatment of diabetes	Methods not widely validated with clinical trials and genetic testing may not be suitable for all individuals	Biomarkers and genetic tests should be validated with larger datasets and more clinical studies. Additionally, these approaches should be tested on a wider population

[56]	2017	Datasets containing various medical data and survey results of diabetes patients	Large-scale datasets with thousands of patient samples	Supervised learning (logistic regression, decision trees, support vector machines) and clustering methods	Machine learning techniques achieved successful results in early diagnosis and treatment of diabetes	Limitations in model accuracy and generalizability	Using larger and more diverse datasets, improving model accuracy, and ensuring generalizability with more clinical data
[57]	2015	DBS parameters and medication information of Parkinson's patients	Not specified, but clinical data was used	Machine learning algorithms: parameter optimization and combination analysis	Significant improvements in symptoms observed with optimized DBS and medication treatment	Not tested on a larger patient population; limited information provided about the dataset	Expanding studies to different patient groups, increasing real-time adaptability of algorithms, and performing side effect analyses
[58]	2015	DDI-2013 dataset, commonly used for drug-drug interaction extraction	Collection of biomedical texts containing drug interactions	Supervised machine learning models, text mining, and NLP for classifying and extracting drug names and DDIs	Model successfully identified and classified drug interactions, achieving higher F scores than previous methods	Relies on existing datasets and has difficulty generalizing to unknown biomedical texts	Including larger and more diverse datasets to enable the model to better handle more complex medical terminology and domain-specific contexts
[59]	2011	Labeled text data from biological literature containing protein-protein interactions	Tested on a limited number of interaction data	Support vector machines (SVMs) and feature selection methods	Model successfully extracts protein interactions but has a high false positive rate	Dataset is limited, and further development is needed to reduce false positives	Using larger and more diverse datasets, reducing false positives, and improving the model's generalization ability

3 Method

The system developed in this study provides personalized drug recommendations specifically for diabetes patients, while also performing diabetes prediction. By analyzing demographic and clinical data obtained from patients, the system operates in two main tasks:

Drug Recommendation Module: The drug recommendation system developed in this study is designed using a combination of rule-based approaches and classification algorithms. The system provides drug recommendations that comply with predefined medical rules and clinical guidelines by considering patient information (age, gender, health condition) and disease diagnosis. The rule-based system ranks appropriate treatment options by taking into account drug interactions, contraindications, and patient-specific risk factors. Personalized parameters such as patient age, HbA1c level, GFR level, complication history, obesity status, and hypoglycemia risk are analyzed to shape the treatment recommendation. Based on this information, suitable drug groups are suggested according to the rules specified in the Diabetes Guidelines of the Turkish Endocrinology Society. The active ingredients in the recommended drug groups are compared with the patient's existing medications to assess potential interactions. Drug interactions are classified only into medium and high-risk levels. High-risk drugs are not recommended, while medium-risk options and dose adjustments are provided. The module minimizes drug interactions and potential side effects, offering a customized treatment plan tailored to the individual needs of the patient. This approach provides an effective solution to reduce user errors and accelerate treatment processes, while also featuring a self-improving structure that enhances the accuracy of treatment recommendations over time. Diabetes Prediction Module: The system is designed to predict the diabetes level of patients. This module analyzes features such as blood pressure, body mass index (BMI), and blood glucose levels to generate predictions. The prediction process is supported by machine learning and deep learning models. Both modules provide clinical decision support by evaluating individual patient data and facilitating early disease diagnosis. The data on which this system is based has been meticulously processed to enhance model performance and ensure clinical accuracy.

3.1 Dataset

3.1.1 Data Source

This study employs three different datasets. The first is the Pima Indian Diabetes Dataset available on Kaggle, which contains 768 instances with nine attributes. The independent variables include the number of pregnancies, glucose concentration, blood pressure, skinfold thickness, insulin level, diabetes pedigree function, body mass index (BMI), and age. The dependent variable, "Outcome," indicates diabetes status, with two possible classes: 0 (nondiabetic) and 1 (diabetic). Analysis of the dataset reveals that approximately 65% of the cases are nondiabetic and 35% are diabetic, resulting in a class imbalance that may influence model performance. Therefore, class balancing techniques are necessary during model training.

The second dataset, Diabetes Dataset from the Iraqi population, was compiled from the Medical City Hospital and the Specialized Center for Endocrinology and Diabetes at Al-Kindy Teaching Hospital. Data collection involved systematic review of patient records and extraction of relevant medical and laboratory information. Variables include patient age, gender, blood glucose, creatinine ratio (Cr), BMI, urea, total cholesterol (Chol), LDL, VLDL, HDL, triglycerides (TG), and HbA1C. The target variable represents a three-class classification: diabetic, nondiabetic, and prediabetic. Compared to the binary structure of the Pima dataset, this multiclass design provides a more nuanced diagnostic classification.

The third dataset, referred to as the custom drug-interaction dataset, is publicly accessible on GitHub at this link. This dataset was meticulously curated based on the 2022 guidelines of the Turkish Society of Endocrinology and Metabolism and comprises 109 records detailing drug pairs commonly prescribed in diabetes treatment, their interaction mechanisms, and associated risk levels. Both the dataset and the corresponding code used in this study are available in the repository to promote transparency and support further research in pharmacological risk assessment within diabetes care.

3.1.2 Data Type

All variables in the Pima dataset are numeric. Pregnancy count, glucose, blood pressure, and skinfold thickness are integers; BMI and the diabetes pedigree function are floating-point numbers. Age is also an integer, while the target variable is binary (0/1).

The Diabetes dataset contains both categorical and numerical data. Gender is categorical (F/M), age is integer, and laboratory measurements along with BMI are floating-point values. The target variable is multiclass: class 0 (nondiabetic)—102 cases, class 1 (diabetic)—839 cases, and class 2 (prediabetic)—53 cases. The distribution reveals a significant imbalance, with the diabetic class dominating and the prediabetic class being underrepresented.

The drug-interaction dataset contains both categorical and numeric fields: "Drug1" and "Drug2" identify interacting drug pairs, "Interaction Mechanism" provides a textual explanation of the pharmacological or biochemical interaction, and "Risk Level" is a numeric value ranging from 1 to 2.

3.1.3 Dataset Size

The Pima dataset comprises 768 observations and nine variables, with a total size of approximately 6.144 KB. Its compact size allows for efficient computation, while still providing sufficient data for statistical analysis and machine learning model development.

The Diabetes dataset consists of 994 records and 12 variables, totaling about 48.4 KB. Compared to the Pima dataset, it is 29% larger in terms of sample size and has a broader feature set. Its multiclass structure and larger volume make it particularly valuable for evaluating model performance across different clinical and demographic characteristics.

The drug-interaction dataset contains 105 records and four attributes, occupying approximately 4.8 KB. While small in scale, it offers meaningful insights into drug-interaction risks and can be quickly processed for model training and analysis.

3.2 Data Preprocessing

In many raw medical datasets, inconsistencies, incomplete entries, and errors from different data sources are common. Such issues can undermine the quality of the data and, in turn, reduce the performance of machine learning models. To ensure the reliability of subsequent analyses, a thorough *data preprocessing* stage is essential. This process involves identifying and handling missing values, detecting and managing outliers, addressing class imbalances, normalizing or transforming variables, and, when appropriate, reducing dimensionality [60].

The first step, *data cleaning*, focused on identifying physiologically implausible measurements in both the Pima Indian Diabetes and Diabetes datasets. In several biomedical and anthropometric variables—including glucose, blood pressure, skin thickness, insulin, BMI, urea, creatinine ratio, HbA1c, cholesterol, and lipid profile values—recorded zeros do not represent actual physiological measurements. Clinically, values such as a plasma glucose concentration of 0 mg/dL, a blood pressure of 0 mmHg, a BMI of 0, or a serum urea/creatinine level of 0 are incompatible with life. Such readings indicate either unrecorded measurements or data entry errors. Consequently, all zero values in these variables were reclassified as missing data (*NaN*) and replaced with either the median or mean of the respective feature to preserve dataset integrity and mitigate bias introduced by nonrandom missingness.

Outliers were identified using the Z-score method:

$$Z = \frac{X - \mu}{\sigma} \tag{1}$$

where X denotes the observed value, μ is the mean, and σ is the standard deviation. Observations with $|Z| > 3$ were considered potential outliers. Following this, *Z-score normalization* was applied to standardize the variables:

$$X' = \frac{X - \mu}{\sigma} \tag{2}$$

In some cases, *Min–Max normalization* was used to rescale values to the [0, 1] range:

$$X' = \frac{X - \min(X)}{\max(X) - \min(X)} \tag{3}$$

These normalization methods help improve the performance of models, especially those sensitive to variable scales, such as distance-based and nonlinear algorithms.

Where appropriate, *dimensionality reduction* was applied to produce more compact datasets without losing critical information. For data compiled from multiple sources, *data integration* ensured consistent formatting and semantics.

For model evaluation, the data was divided into training, validation, and testing subsets. When the number of samples was limited, *K-fold cross-validation* was employed, ensuring that each observation contributed to both training and testing, thereby yielding a more robust performance estimate [61].

In the Pima dataset, after handling zero values as described above, the target variable (*Outcome*) was redefined into three categories based on glucose thresholds: "normal," "prediabetes," and "diabetes," encoded as 0, 1, and 2, respectively. In the Diabetes dataset, the target variable (*CLASS*) originally included three labels: "N" (nondiabetic), "Y" (diabetic), and "P" (Predict-Diabetic), which were mapped to 0, 1, and 2. The categorical variable *gender* was encoded numerically (0: Female, 1: Male). Finally, mutual information analysis was performed to identify the most informative features in both datasets, resulting in optimized datasets for classification tasks.

3.3 Feature Extraction

In this study, all variables from each dataset were utilized without applying any feature selection process. For the Pima Indian Diabetes Dataset, the eight available attributes were included in the analysis: *pregnancies, plasma glucose concentration, diastolic blood pressure, triceps skinfold thickness, two-hour serum insulin, body mass index (BMI), diabetes pedigree function*, and *age*. These attributes represent a combination of anthropometric, biochemical, and demographic factors, each of which has established relevance to diabetes risk assessment.

For the Diabetes Dataset, all 12 variables were considered: *gender, age, urea, creatinine ratio (Cr), glycated hemoglobin (HbA1c), total cholesterol (Chol), triglycerides (TG), high-density lipoprotein cholesterol (HDL), low-density lipoprotein cholesterol (LDL), very low-density lipoprotein cholesterol (VLDL), body mass index (BMI)*, and *CLASS*. These variables encompass demographic details, renal function indicators, long-term blood glucose control markers, and a complete lipid profile, offering a comprehensive set of clinical parameters for diabetes classification.

Both datasets were analyzed independently, allowing the evaluation of model performance on different demographic and clinical populations, while making full use of the available data in each case.

3.4 *Feature Selection*

Feature selection is a critical preprocessing step in machine learning and data science applications. This process involves selecting the most meaningful and least collinear features from the raw variables in the dataset that will maximize the model's performance. Its primary goal is to eliminate unnecessary, noisy, or misleading features, thereby improving the model's accuracy, interpretability, and computational efficiency. Feature selection prevents overfitting through dimensionality reduction, enhances the model's generalization ability, and conserves computational resources.

Feature selection algorithms are generally classified into three categories: filter methods (based on statistical tests), wrapper methods (which select features according to model performance), and embedded methods (which integrate feature selection within the algorithm). These algorithms use techniques like correlation analysis, information gain, mutual information, Lasso regression, and random forest feature importance to identify key features and enhance model performance.

3.4.1 Mutual Extraction

Mutual extraction is an information extraction technique aimed at discovering symmetric and complementary relationships between two datasets or entities. This method is commonly used in applications such as natural language processing, knowledge graph construction, and recommendation systems. Mutual extraction makes bidirectional inferences by predicting one entity based on the other.

Mutual Extraction Steps:

- **Data Preparation:** The dataset to be inferred is prepared, and this data is converted into an appropriate format. In this step, necessary preprocessing steps are applied to the input data (e.g., data cleaning or normalization).
- **Initial Seed Set Determination:** The first relationship or entity pair is determined. This seed set serves as the starting point for the extraction process.
- **Feature Extraction:** Features that define the relationships between entities are extracted. These features can be determined through methods such as text mining, contextual information, or semantic analysis.

$$\text{Feature}_i = f(\text{Entity}_i, \text{Context}_i) \tag{4}$$

- **Dual Extraction:** Both directions of the relationships are examined. That is, the second dataset is predicted using the first dataset, and then inferences about the first dataset are made using this prediction.
- **Model Update:** New relationships obtained through the extraction steps are added to the model, and the model is retrained. This step allows the inferences to expand to cover more relationships.
- **Validation and Evaluation:** The accuracy of feature extractions is assessed using a validation set or a labeled dataset. Common evaluation metrics include accuracy and F1 score.
- **Extraction of Results:** The final results ensure that the extracted relationships or entities are accurately represented.
- **Iterative Process:** The mutual extraction process continues iteratively until new relationships are found or a stopping criterion is reached.

To identify the most important features from both datasets, the *mutual information (MI)* technique was employed. For the Pima Indian Diabetes dataset, this approach led to the selection of *five key features*. Similarly, for the Diabetes dataset, comprehensive data preprocessing was performed, including handling missing values by replacing zero values with NaN in numerical columns (Urea, Cr, HbA1c, Chol, TG, HDL, LDL, VLDL, BMI) and subsequently imputing them using *median imputation* with SimpleImputer. Categorical variables were encoded numerically, with gender mapped as F=0, M=1, and class labels transformed from N/Y/P to 0/1/2, respectively. The *mutual information technique* was then applied to rank all features, and the *top 5 highest-scoring features* were selected for model training. Numerical features with varying scales were standardized using *z-score standardization (StandardScaler)*, ensuring a mean of 0 and a standard deviation of 1. Given the class imbalance in the datasets, the *SMOTE (synthetic minority oversampling technique)* method was applied to balance the classes by generating an equal number of samples for each class. This approach helped ensure that the model treated each class equally. Finally, both datasets were evaluated using *k-fold cross-validation*.

3.5 Model Selection

3.5.1 Machine Learning

Machine learning, a subset of artificial intelligence (AI), allows computers to learn from data and improve their performance through experience. Unlike traditional programming, where software follows fixed instructions, machine learning enables systems to analyze data, identify patterns, and make decisions. Over time, this learning process enhances the accuracy and effectiveness of the system's results.

Machine learning holds significant importance, particularly in the field of healthcare. Its ability is to analyze data quickly and accurately facilitate critical applications ranging from early disease diagnosis to personalized treatment plans.

3.5.2 Machine Learning Algorithms

The algorithms listed below are those that can be applied to our dataset effectively in this study:

- **Logistic Regression:** Logistic regression is a model widely used for binary classification problems. It can predict whether individuals are diabetic or not. Advantages: Simple, fast, and interpretable [62]. Formula:

$$p = \frac{1}{1 + e^{-(b_0 + b_1 x_1 + b_2 x_2 + \cdots + b_n x_n)}} \tag{5}$$

  Here, p is the probability of the event, $-(b_0 + b_1x_1 + b_2x_2 + \cdots + b_nx_n)$ represents the model parameters, and $(x_1, x_2, \ldots, x_n)$ are the features.
- **Decision Trees:** Decision trees classify data through a series of yes/no questions. In diabetes diagnosis, they make decisions based on various test results to determine whether an individual is at risk of diabetes. Advantages: Easy to understand and visually represent. Formula: Decision trees do not have a specific formula, but at each decision node, they split data based on a particular feature [63].
- **Support Vector Machines (SVMs):** SVM is an algorithm that attempts to find the best hyperplane (decision boundary) to classify the data. In diabetes diagnosis, it performs optimal classification to separate diabetic and nondiabetic individuals. Advantages: Effective in high-dimensional data and has strong generalization power [64]. Formula:

$$f(x) = w^T x + b \tag{6}$$

  Here, w is the vector defining the decision boundary, x is the input data, and b is the bias term.
- **K-Nearest Neighbors (KNNs):** KNN classifies a new instance based on the class of its nearest neighbors. In diabetes diagnosis, the classification of the individual is determined using the classification information of the nearest k neighbors. Advantages: Simple, nonparametric, and flexible [65]. Formula:

$$y = \frac{1}{k} \sum_{i=1}^{k} y_i \tag{7}$$

  Here, y is the predicted class, k is the number of neighbors, and y_i is the class label of each neighbor.

- **Random Forest:** Random forest is an ensemble technique that merges the predictions of several decision trees to improve accuracy and robustness in tasks such as diabetes diagnosis. By combining the output of multiple trees, it generates more reliable predictions.
  Advantages: It helps minimize overfitting and delivers strong overall performance.
  Formula: The predictions are averaged from the various decision trees [66].

3.5.3 Deep Learning

Deep learning is an advanced machine learning technique inspired by the structure and functioning of the human brain, utilizing layered artificial neural networks. This approach allows for the automatic learning of complex patterns and abstract features from data. Unlike traditional machine learning methods, deep learning models can directly extract hierarchical features from raw input.

The key benefits of deep learning include its ability to handle large, complex datasets with high performance, eliminate the need for manual feature engineering, and succeed in fields like image processing, natural language processing, and speech recognition. By learning directly from data, these models require less human involvement and are highly effective at identifying intricate patterns.

Activation functions play a critical role in deep learning models, enabling the networks to learn complex relationships through nonlinear transformations. Commonly used activation functions include:

- **ReLU (Rectified Linear Unit):** A simple and computationally efficient function that sets negative values to zero, while leaving positive values unchanged.
- **Sigmoid:** Constrains the output between 0 and 1, commonly used in binary classification problems.
- **Tanh (Hyperbolic Tangent):** Similar to sigmoid but constrains the output between -1 and 1.
- **Softmax:** Converts outputs into a probability distribution, often used in multi-class classification problems.

Deep learning has revolutionized artificial intelligence by endowing artificial systems with human-like learning and decision-making capabilities. It has transformative impacts in fields such as image recognition, natural language processing, autonomous systems, and medical diagnosis.

3.6 Model Training and Evaluation

To optimize the performance of the machine learning and deep learning models, a rigorous hyperparameter-tuning process was conducted. For machine learning models, parameters such as the number of estimators, maximum depth, and neighborhood size were fine-tuned. In deep learning models, critical parameters like the number of layers, neurons per layer, activation functions, dropout rates, and regularization techniques were carefully selected. The Adam optimizer and appropriate loss functions were employed during the training phase. Model robustness was evaluated using K-Fold cross-validation, and the SMOTE algorithm was utilized to address class imbalances within the dataset, ensuring the models deliver accurate and generalizable results.

3.6.1 Addressing Overfitting and Underfitting

Overfitting occurs when a model becomes excessively specialized to the training data, compromising its ability to generalize to new, unseen data. To combat this, we implemented techniques such as early stopping, which terminates the training process when the model's performance on a validation set ceases to improve. We also managed model complexity by selecting simpler architectures when appropriate. In contrast, *underfitting* arises when a model is too simplistic to capture the underlying patterns in the data, leading to poor performance on both training and test sets. When this was observed, we increased the model's capacity by adding more parameters or deeper layers.

3.6.2 Evaluation Metrics

The models' effectiveness was comprehensively evaluated using a suite of critical metrics. Initially, a *confusion matrix* was generated to provide a clear visualization of classification outcomes by enumerating true positives, false positives, true negatives, and false negatives. This matrix offers a detailed view of the model's performance, distinguishing between accurate and erroneous predictions:

- **True Positive (TP):** Cases correctly identified as positive
- **False Positive (FP):** Cases incorrectly identified as positive
- **True Negative (TN):** Cases correctly identified as negative
- **False Negative (FN):** Cases incorrectly identified as negative

Beyond the confusion matrix components, other key metrics were calculated to further analyze model performance: *accuracy* (the ratio of correct predictions), *recall* (the proportion of actual positives correctly identified), *precision* (the proportion of positive predictions that were actually correct), and the *F1 score* (the harmonic mean of precision and recall). The formulas for these metrics are as follows:

$$\text{Accuracy} = \frac{\text{TP} + \text{TN}}{\text{TP} + \text{TN} + \text{FP} + \text{FN}} \tag{8}$$

$$\text{Recall} = \frac{\text{TP}}{\text{TP} + \text{FN}} \tag{9}$$

$$\text{Specificity} = \frac{\text{TN}}{\text{TN} + \text{FP}} \tag{10}$$

$$F1 = 2 \cdot \frac{\text{Precision} \cdot \text{Recall}}{\text{Precision} + \text{Recall}} \tag{11}$$

AUC-ROC (Area Under the Curve—Receiver Operating Characteristic) This metric evaluates the model's classification performance and indicates its ability to correctly predict the positive class. Taking a value between 0 and 1, a score closer to 1 signifies better class separation capability. A score of 0.5 represents random classification, while 1 indicates perfect classification. By comparing false positive and true positive rates at different thresholds, the model's overall classification quality is assessed. Typically, a value between 0.7 and 0.8 is considered good, 0.8 to 0.9 is very good, and above 0.9 is excellent.

$$\text{AUC} = \int_0^1 \text{TPR}(FPR)\, d(FPR) \tag{12}$$

These metrics were used to thoroughly analyze the model's accuracy in diagnosing diabetes and ensured balanced performance across both classes.

4 Experimental Results

Under the experimental results section, the performance of classification algorithms in predicting diabetes levels and determining the risk levels of medications addressed in this study will be evaluated.

4.1 Diabetes Prediction

4.1.1 Data Preprocessing

To improve model accuracy, initial preprocessing focused on data cleaning. In the Pima Indian Diabetes dataset, zero values in *glucose*, *BloodPressure*, *SkinThickness*, *insulin*, and *BMI* columns were considered clinically invalid. For example, a glucose level of 0 mg/dL, a blood pressure of 0 mmHg, or a BMI of 0 are incompatible with life; such entries indicate either missing measurements or recording errors. Therefore, these values were treated as missing (*NaN*) and replaced with the column mean. Subsequently, the *glucose* variable was used to classify individuals into "normal," "prediabetes," and "diabetes" groups, and these categories were encoded numerically. Similarly, in the Iraqi Diabetes dataset, zero values in *urea*, *Cr*, *TG*, *HDL*, *LDL*, and *VLDL* were deemed physiologically impossible and treated as

Table 6 First five rows of the dataset after outcome labeling (Pima Indian Diabetes dataset)

Pregnancies	Glucose	BP	SkinTh	Insulin	BMI	DPF	Age	Outcome
6	148.0	72.0	35.00	155.54	33.6	0.627	50	2
1	85.0	66.0	29.00	155.54	26.6	0.351	31	1
8	183.0	64.0	29.15	155.54	23.3	0.672	32	2
1	89.0	66.0	23.00	94.00	28.1	0.167	21	1
0	137.0	40.0	35.00	168.00	43.1	2.288	33	2

Table 7 First five rows after label encoding (Diabetes dataset)

Gender	AGE	Urea	Cr	HbA1c	Chol	TG	HDL	LDL	VLDL	BMI	CLASS
0	50	4.7	46	4.9	4.2	1.0	2.4	1.4	0.5	24.0	0
1	26	4.5	62	4.9	3.7	1.4	1.1	2.1	0.6	23.0	0
0	50	4.7	46	4.9	4.2	1.0	2.4	1.4	0.5	24.0	0
0	50	4.7	46	4.9	4.2	1.0	2.4	1.4	0.5	24.0	0
1	33	7.1	46	4.9	4.9	1.0	0.8	2.0	0.4	21.0	0

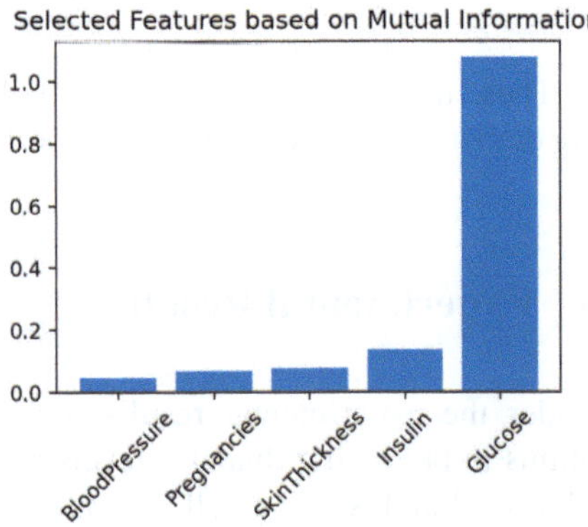

Fig. 1 Mutual information-based selected features (Pima Indian Diabetes dataset)

missing. These entries were replaced with *NaN* and imputed using the median of each column. Categorical variables (*gender* and *CLASS*) were cleaned and label-encoded. As a result, both datasets were prepared in a clean and structured form, ready for analysis (Tables 6 and 7).

In feature selection, mutual information was used to evaluate the dependency between the target variable and each feature. As a result of this process, the five most significant features in the datasets were identified. The selected features stood out as variables with the potential to improve model accuracy and carry more information. Finally, these selected features were combined with the outcome column to create a new dataset, making it more suitable for efficient model performance (Figs. 1 and 2, Tables 8 and 9).

In the newly formed dataset, features and target labels were separated, and the entire dataset was trained and tested using the k-fold cross-validation method. Each fold in the dataset allowed testing the model's overall accuracy with different training and validation splits.

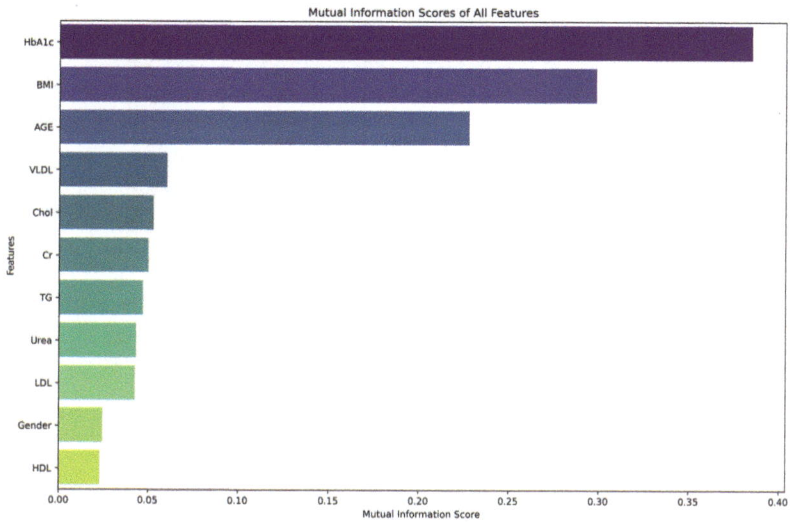

Fig. 2 Mutual information-based selected features (Diabetes dataset)

Table 8 The first five rows of the final dataset created with the selected features and outcome (Pima Indian Diabetes dataset)

SkinTh	BP	Age	Insulin	*Glucose*	Outcome
35.00000	72.0	50	155.548223	148.0	2
29.00000	66.0	31	155.548223	85.0	0
29.15342	64.0	32	155.548223	183.0	2
23.00000	66.0	21	94.000000	89.0	0
35.00000	40.0	33	168.000000	137.0	2

Table 9 First five rows of the new dataset with selected features and CLASS (Diabetes dataset)

HbA1c	BMI	AGE	VLDL	Chol	CLASS
4.9	24.0	50	0.5	4.2	0
4.9	23.0	26	0.6	3.7	0
4.9	24.0	50	0.5	4.2	0
4.9	24.0	50	0.5	4.2	0
4.9	21.0	33	0.4	4.9	0

In the next step, data was scaled to prevent the negative impact of differently scaled features on the model's learning process. Specifically, algorithms such as support vector machines (SVMs) and k-nearest neighbors (KNNs) perform more efficiently with differently scaled data, while uniform scaling enhances model accuracy.

Since imbalanced classes were encountered in the training set, synthetic samples were generated using the SMOTE method, preventing class imbalances from affecting the model's learning process (Figs. 3 and 4). These steps ensured that the model was trained in a more balanced and accurate manner.

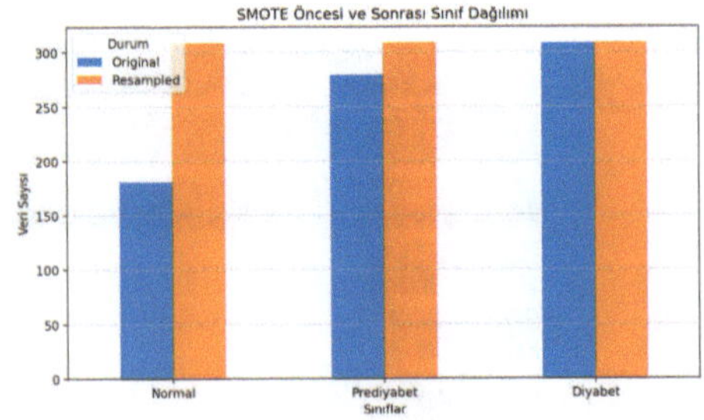

Fig. 3 Class distributions before and after SMOTE (Pima Indian Diabetes dataset)

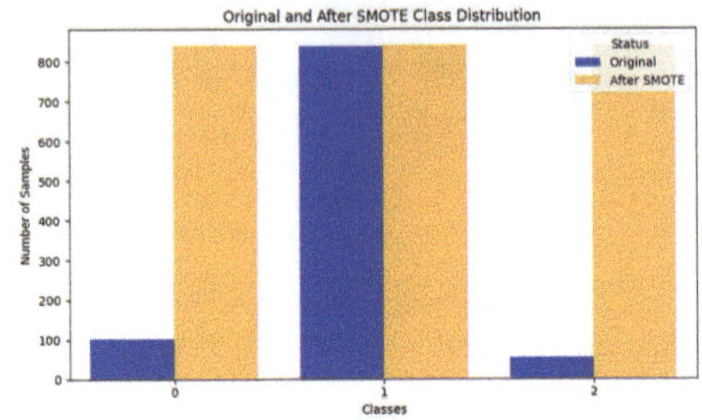

Fig. 4 Class distributions before and after SMOTE ("Diabetes dataset")

4.1.2 Model Performances and Evaluation

During training, five machine learning models—logistic regression, random forest, support vector machines, k-nearest neighbors, and decision trees—and four deep learning models—artificial neural network, deep artificial neural network, convolutional neural network, and long short-term memory—were evaluated. Model performance was assessed using multiple metrics: accuracy (overall correctness), sensitivity/recall (correct detection of positives), specificity (correct detection of negatives), precision (accuracy of positive predictions), F1 score (balance of precision and recall), and AUC-ROC (class separation ability across thresholds). These metrics, particularly valuable for imbalanced datasets, provide a more detailed performance view.

This section presents a comparative analysis of the models based on these metrics, alongside cross-validation and test results, to evaluate generalization and detect overfitting or underfitting. The findings highlight each model's strengths and limitations, supporting the choice of the most appropriate method for the task.

The aggregate results in Tables 10 and 11 were appraised using accuracy, sensitivity, specificity, precision, F1 score, and AUC; the bar charts in Figs. 5 and 6 visualize the relative ordering across models.

Random Forest (RF)

RF delivers the most accurate solution on the *Pima Indian* dataset, reaching *98.70%* accuracy with *AUC* $\approx$ *0.9986*, and—critically—near-perfect balance between

Table 10 Average results (Pima Indian Diabetes dataset)

Model%	Accuracy%	Sensitivity%	Specificity%	Precision%	F1 score%	AUC%
LR	92.961	92.961	93.115	93.199	92.984	0.9769
RF	98.701	98.701	98.705	98.747	98.702	0.9986
SVM	94.696	94.696	94.784	94.849	94.685	0.9789
KNN	89.068	89.068	89.868	89.950	89.159	0.9743
DT	86.687	86.687	88.071	88.187	86.823	0.9604
ANN	97.616	97.616	97.654	97.669	97.620	0.9979
DNN	96.967	96.967	97.015	97.035	96.972	0.9975
CNN	50.317	50.317	47.809	48.223	47.708	0.6987
LSTM	97.185	97.185	97.211	97.276	97.183	0.9988

Table 11 Average results (Diabetes dataset)

Model%	Accuracy%	Sensitivity%	Specificity%	Precision%	F1 score%	AUC%
LR	95.83%	95.83%	97.91%	95.96%	95.82%	98.39%
RF	97.81%	97.81%	98.90%	97.88%	97.80%	99.83%
SVM	96.90%	96.90%	98.45%	97.03%	96.88%	99.09%
KNN	96.50%	96.50%	98.25%	96.67%	96.49%	99.48%
DT	95.23%	95.23%	97.62%	95.31%	95.22%	99.39%
ANN	98.93%	98.93%	99.46%	98.96%	98.92%	99.91%
DNN	98.77%	98.77%	99.38%	98.81%	98.77%	99.91%
CNN	98.01%	98.01%	99.00%	98.06%	98.00%	99.51%
LSTM	97.46%	97.46%	98.73%	97.54%	97.45%	99.51%

sensitivity (*98.70%*) and specificity (*98.71%*). This symmetry indicates that the ensemble is not trading recall for precision, but rather capturing complementary partitions of the feature space. On the *Diabetes* dataset, RF remains highly competitive (*97.81%* accuracy; *AUC = 99.83%*) despite the presence of stronger deep models; the uplift in specificity (*98.90%*) suggests effective handling of the majority class without suppressing minority recall. Taken together, RF emerges as a robust tabular baseline: It scales gracefully across heterogeneous covariates, resists overfitting through bagging, and maintains stable operating points (balanced errors) without heavy hyperparameter sensitivity.

Artificial Neural Network (ANN)

ANN consistently ranks among the top performers on both datasets and becomes the *overall leader* on *Diabetes* with *98.93%* accuracy and *AUC = 99.91%*. Its metrics remain uniformly high—precision (*98.96%*), sensitivity (*98.93%*), specificity (*99.46%*), and F1 (*98.92%*)—indicating that the network is not merely optimizing a single metric but achieving a well-calibrated classifier. On *Pima*,

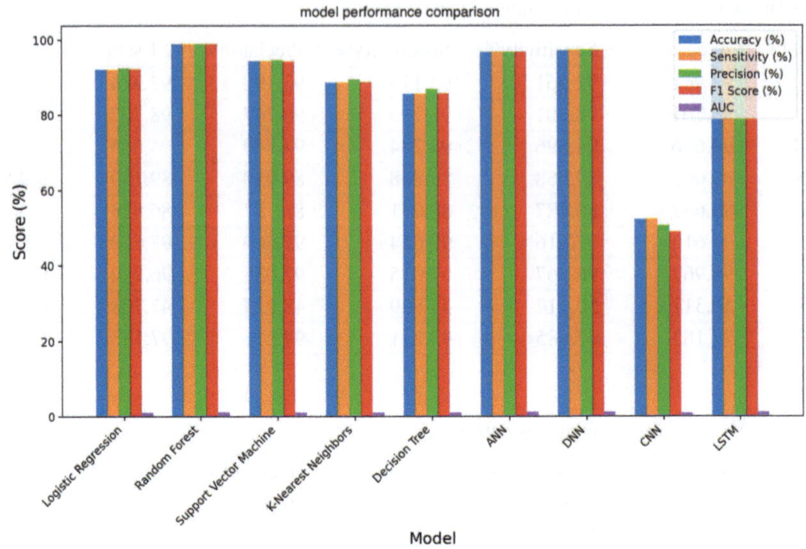

Fig. 5 Detailed performance results of the models (Pima Indian Diabetes dataset)

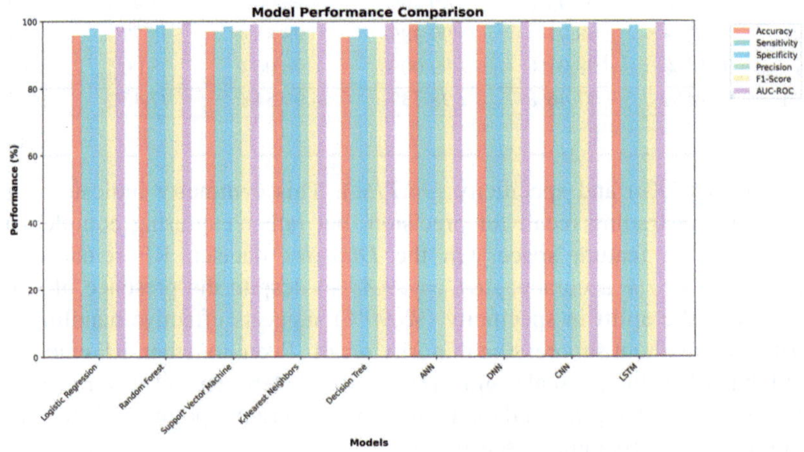

Fig. 6 Detailed performance results of the models (Diabetes dataset)

ANN sustains *97.62%* accuracy (*AUC* $\approx$ *0.9979*), again with tightly clustered sensitivity/specificity, which is consistent with a model that internalizes nonlinear interactions among metabolic and anthropometric variables. In practical terms, ANN's advantage over tree ensembles is modest on Pima but becomes salient on Diabetes, where the richer laboratory panel appears to reward higher-capacity nonlinear mappings.

Long Short-Term Memory (LSTM)

Although the inputs are tabular rather than sequential, LSTM functions as a gated deep classifier and posts *near-ANN performance* on both cohorts: *97.19%* accuracy (*AUC* $\approx$ *0.9988*) on *Pima* and *97.46%* (*AUC* = *99.51%*) on *Diabetes*. The close alignment of sensitivity/specificity across datasets ($\approx$97–99%) indicates stable decision thresholds and limited variance across folds. Relative to ANN, LSTM is fractionally lower in accuracy on Diabetes yet retains *very high AUC*, suggesting strong rank-ordering of risks even when hard thresholds differ. From a deployment perspective, LSTM offers a reliable alternative to feedforward architectures when additional temporal or panel-wise structure is anticipated in future datasets.

For completeness, the remaining models are summarized briefly without extended analysis. *DNN* tracks ANN closely—*98.77%* accuracy (AUC *99.91%*) on Diabetes and *96.97%* (AUC $\approx$*0.9975*) on Pima—yet does not consistently surpass it. *SVM* and *LR* provide strong linear/maximum-margin baselines (Pima: *94.70%* and *92.96%*; Diabetes: *96.90%* and *95.83%*), with solid AUC values that make them attractive when model simplicity and interpretability are prioritized. *KNN* is markedly dataset-sensitive (*89.07%* on Pima vs. *96.50%* on Diabetes), reflecting reliance on local density and scale. *Decision tree* improves from *86.69%* (Pima) to *95.23%* (Diabetes) but remains more variance-prone than RF. *CNN* attains *98.01%* accuracy (AUC *99.51%*) on Diabetes yet collapses to *50.32%* (AUC *0.70*) on Pima, underscoring that convolutional inductive biases are ill-matched to nonspatial tabular inputs.

Overall, a Consistent Picture Emerges RF dominates on Pima's purely tabular structure; ANN leads on the more feature-rich Diabetes dataset; LSTM stays competitive across both, offering deep learning gains with stable operating characteristics. DNN and SVM form strong second-tier options depending on computational budget and interpretability needs, whereas CNN should be reserved for settings where its architectural prior aligns with the data geometry.

Error Analysis

Error analysis is an important evaluation method used to examine the performance of classification models in depth. This analysis reveals the correct and incorrect classifications of the models, showing what types of errors were made. To address the data imbalance during model training, the SMOTE (synthetic minority oversampling technique) method was used. This helped reduce the imbalance between classes. Overfitting and underfitting issues will be discussed in detail in the following paragraphs.

The confusion matrices for different classification models are shown in Figs. 7 and 8. Confusion matrices are a powerful tool for evaluating the performance of models by comparing actual and predicted classification results. Each matrix provides a detailed breakdown of the model's true positives (TP), true negatives (TN), false positives (FP), and false negatives (FN) rates.

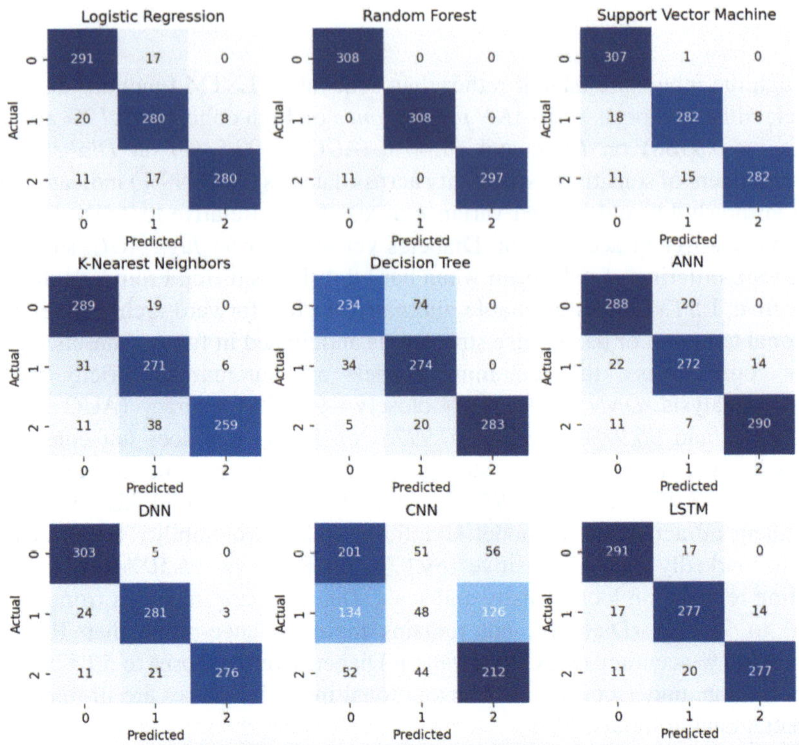

Fig. 7 The confusion matrix of all models (Pima Indian Diabetes dataset)

Comparative Analysis

The comparative analysis reveals distinct performance patterns across both datasets. For the Pima Indian Diabetes dataset, random forest achieved the highest accuracy with minimal errors, followed by support vector machine and deep neural network. The CNN model showed significantly poor performance on this dataset, suggesting its unsuitability for this particular classification problem.

For the Diabetes dataset, neural network-based models (ANN, DNN, LSTM) demonstrated superior performance with perfect or near-perfect classification for classes 0 and 2. Random forest and support vector machine also exhibited excellent results with minimal misclassifications. Notably, the decision tree model showed the highest error rates across both datasets, particularly for class 2 in the Diabetes dataset, indicating consistent overfitting tendencies.

Key Observations

Across both datasets, class 1 appears to be the most challenging to classify, with consistent misclassifications observed in most models. This suggests potential feature overlap with adjacent classes or insufficient class separation in the feature

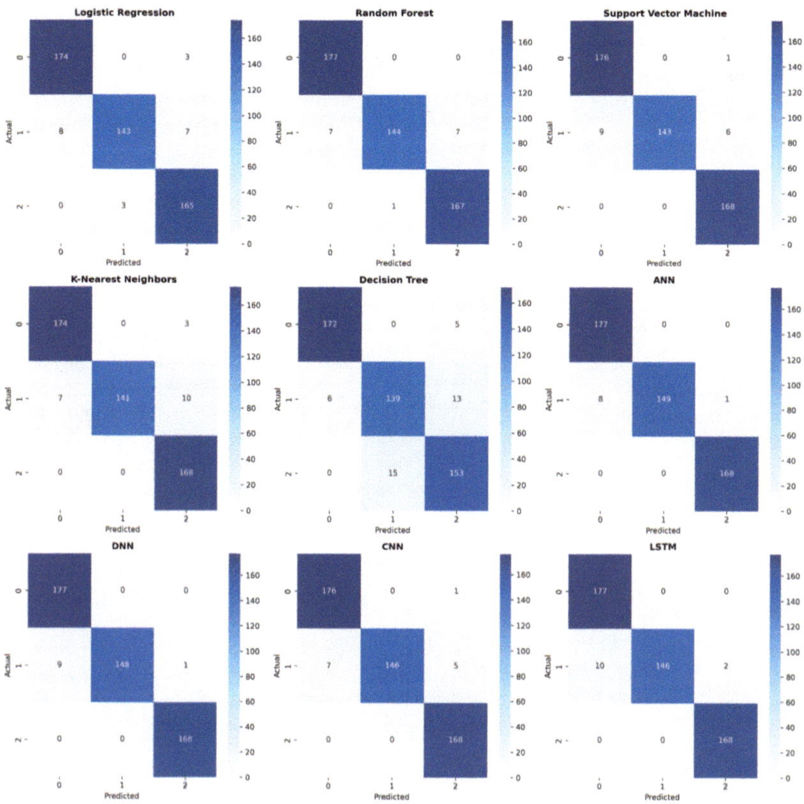

Fig. 8 The confusion matrix of all models (Diabetes dataset)

space. The neural network architectures generally performed better on the Diabetes dataset compared to the Pima Indian dataset, while traditional machine learning algorithms like random forest and SVM maintained consistent performance across both datasets.

As a result, the analysis based on confusion matrices provides a comprehensive comparison of model performance across different datasets, revealing that model selection should be dataset-specific, with neural networks excelling on the Diabetes dataset and ensemble methods like random forest performing exceptionally well on the Pima Indian Diabetes dataset.

4.1.3 Evaluation of Training and Test Performance

Comparing training and test accuracy is crucial for assessing a model's generalization capability. In this process, the ability of the models to successfully transfer the knowledge learned from the training set to the test set is analyzed. Differences

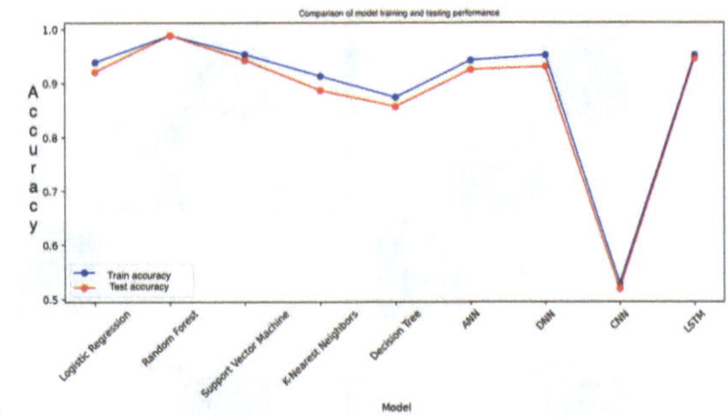

Fig. 9 Comparison of training and test performance (Pima Indian Diabetes dataset)

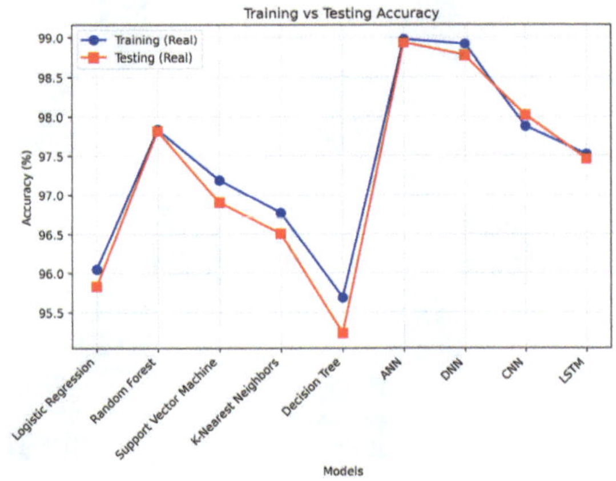

Fig. 10 Comparison of training and test performance (Diabetes dataset)

in training and test performances can indicate overfitting (excessive learning) or underfitting (insufficient learning). The following graphs display the training and test accuracies of various models. The graphs visualize how well the information modeled during training applies to the test data.

Based on the comparison charts, Figs. 9 and 10, for both the Pima Indian Diabetes and Diabetes datasets, the training and test accuracy curves demonstrate remarkably consistent alignment across most machine learning models. The parallel trajectories between training (blue) and testing (red) performance lines indicate that models such as logistic regression, random forest, SVM, and deep learning approaches maintain balanced learning without significant overfitting. Particularly notable is how the accuracy gaps remain minimal throughout different model architectures, suggesting robust generalization capabilities across both datasets. The consistent performance patterns observed in both figures reinforce that the selected models successfully avoid memorizing training data while maintaining strong predictive power on unseen test samples, which is essential for reliable clinical decision support systems in diabetes prediction tasks.

Performance Analysis on Training and Validation Loss in Deep Learning Models

- **Performance Analysis Based on Training and Validation Loss:** (Figs. 11 and 12)

Training and validation losses provide critical insights into model generalization performance. Although both ANN and DNN models exhibit rapid convergence in training loss, the DNN demonstrates pronounced fluctuations in validation loss, indicating severe overfitting and poor generalization. The ANN also showed moderate overfitting, as the validation loss plateaued, while training loss continued decreasing. CNN maintained higher training and validation losses throughout, reflecting underfitting along with minor overfitting due to slight validation loss increase. The LSTM model displayed more parallel trends in training and validation

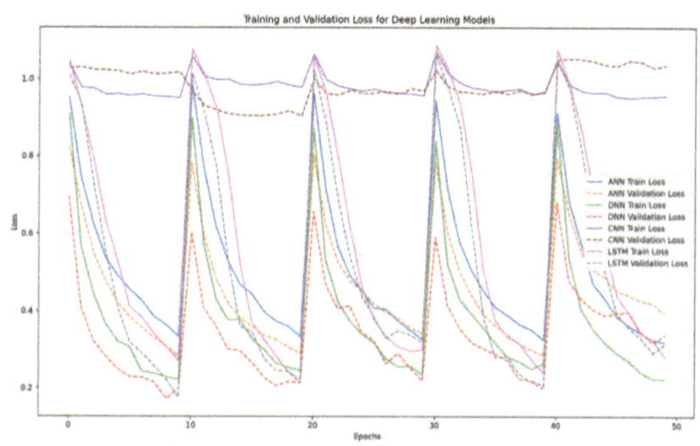

Fig. 11 The graph showing the training and validation losses of deep learning models (Pima Indian Diabetes dataset)

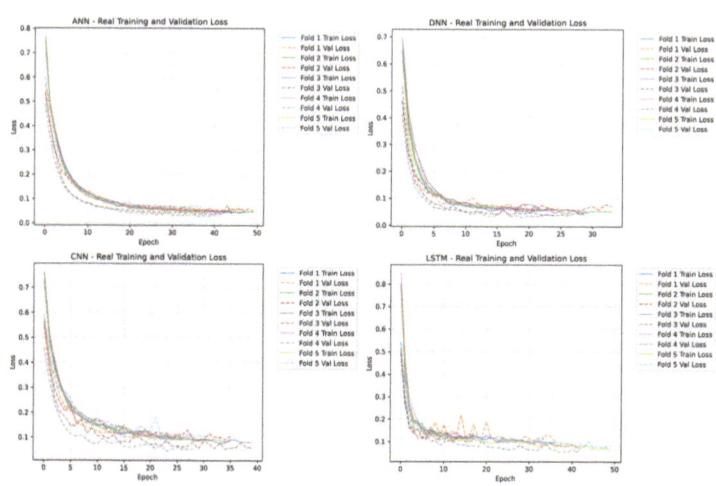

Fig. 12 The graph showing the training and validation losses of deep learning models (Diabetes dataset)

losses, suggesting lower overfitting, though its relatively high loss levels indicate a risk of underfitting.

Models trained on the Diabetes dataset exhibited consistent and stable learning behavior across k-fold cross-validation. Both ANN and DNN achieved very low training losses; however, slight divergence between the training and validation loss curves was observed, indicating the presence of moderate overfitting. CNN and LSTM maintained closer training-validation trajectories across folds, with CNN showing mild underfitting and LSTM demonstrating better generalization, albeit with occasional fluctuations hinting at variance between folds. These results suggest the models' performance improved with the Diabetes dataset, particularly in terms of validation stability and generalization.

4.1.4 Evaluation of Time and Resource Usage

In this section, the training and test durations of the models, as well as their usage of hardware resources, have been analyzed (Figs. 13 and 14). The models were compared based on the metrics of training time (s), test time (s), CPU usage (%), memory usage (%), and GPU usage (MB). The lack of GPU usage has made the comparison CPU-focused:

- **Training and Test Times:** For the Pima Indian dataset, the LR model has the shortest training time (0.0229 s) and test time (0.0006 s), offering a significant advantage for real-time applications. Conversely, the LSTM model shows the highest training (8.3010 s) and testing (1.0857 s) times due to its complex

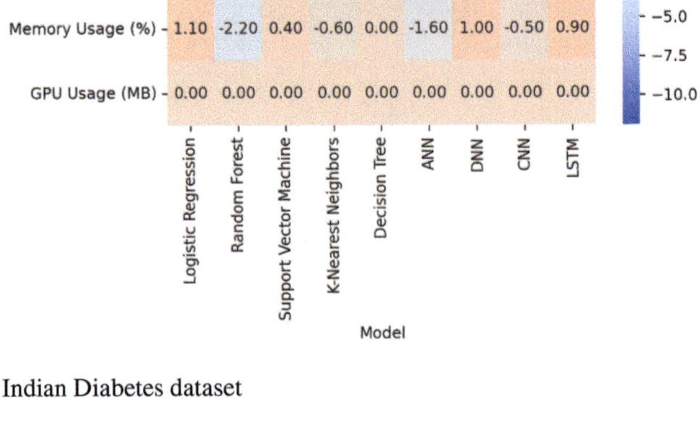

Fig. 13 Pima Indian Diabetes dataset

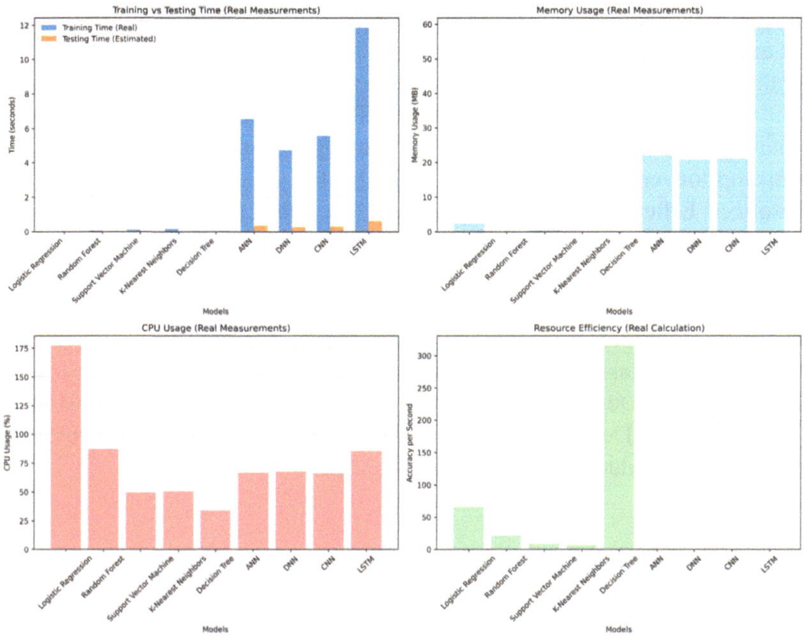

Fig. 14 Diabetes dataset

sequential structure. Deep learning models (ANN, DNN, CNN) generally require longer training and testing durations than traditional models.

Similarly, in the Diabetes dataset, LR again exhibits the fastest processing, with both training and testing times remaining under a second. Deep learning models show a significant increase in time requirements. LSTM, in particular, reaches over 12 seconds of training time, reinforcing its high computational demand. ANN, DNN, and CNN also follow this trend with moderately high training durations.

- **CPU Usage:** In the Pima Indian dataset, the decision tree (DT) model shows the highest CPU usage at %10.4, possibly due to frequent branching operations. Negative CPU values observed in some models (RF, SVM, ANN, DNN, LSTM) may be the result of measurement inaccuracies or system-level factors such as background process interference or idle CPU states.

  On the other hand, for the Diabetes dataset, logistic regression shows the highest CPU usage (over 170%), potentially due to intensive parallelization. Deep learning models like LSTM, CNN, and DNN also show considerable CPU usage (around 70–80%), which can be attributed to the lack of GPU acceleration. KNN and SVM display relatively low CPU usage, possibly benefiting from simpler test-time computations.
- **Memory Usage:** In both datasets, deep learning models exhibit considerably higher memory usage. For Pima Indian, ANN and LSTM report memory

consumption rates of %2.2 and %1.0, respectively, while simpler models like LR and DT consume almost negligible memory.

In the Diabetes dataset, this trend is even more evident. LSTM consumes nearly 60 MB, and other deep models like ANN, DNN, and CNN each use around 20 MB. In contrast, LR and DT remain extremely lightweight in memory consumption, confirming their suitability for low-resource environments.

– **Resource Efficiency:** GPU was not used in either experiment. Therefore, the training and test durations of deep learning models are significantly longer due to CPU-only processing. If GPU support were available, these durations would likely decrease dramatically.

  In terms of efficiency (accuracy per second), the DT model stands out in the Diabetes dataset, achieving the highest performance relative to time and resource usage. Despite its simplicity, it outperforms complex models in speed-efficiency ratio. Deep learning models, while potentially more accurate, show lower efficiency due to high computational costs.

4.1.5 Hyperparameter Settings

The success of machine learning and deep learning models largely depends on correct hyperparameter settings. In this study, detailed hyperparameter tuning has been performed on both traditional machine learning algorithms and deep learning models to optimize the performance of different models. A global seed control (`random_state=42`) was applied across all experiments, including data splitting (K-fold), SMOTE balancing, and model initialization, to ensure reproducibility.

Machine Learning Models

The hyperparameter settings for *logistic regression*, *random forests*, *support vector machines (SVMs)*, *K-nearest neighbors (KNN)*, and *decision trees (DT)* models are as follows:

– **LR:**
  - `max_iter=1500`. Allows sufficient iterations to improve accuracy, while keeping processing time reasonable.
  - `random_state=42` for reproducibility.

– **RF:**
  - `n_estimators=20`, `max_depth=3`, `min_samples_split=3`, `min_samples_leaf=1`, `max_features='sqrt'`.
  - These settings were adjusted from higher complexity defaults to mitigate overfitting observed in initial experiments.
  - `random_state=42` for reproducible bootstrapping and feature selection.

- **SVM:**
  - `kernel='linear'`, `probability=True`.
  - `random_state=42` to ensure reproducibility of shuffling in cross-validation and probability calibration.
- **KNN:**
  - `n_neighbors=15`, `metric='manhattan'`.
  - `random_state=42` applied in upstream data splitting for reproducibility.
- **DT:**
  - `max_depth=15`, `min_samples_split=45`, `min_samples_leaf=45`, `max_features='sqrt'`.
  - `random_state=42` for deterministic tree construction.

Deep Learning Models

The design and hyperparameters of the *artificial neural networks (ANNs)*, *deep neural networks (DNNs)*, *convolutional neural networks (CNNs)*, and *long short-term memory (LSTM)* models are explained below. All models use `seed=42` to control weight initialization and data shuffling:

- **ANN:**
  - Dense(128, `relu`) → Dense(64, `relu`) → Dense(`softmax`).
  - `Dropout=0.3`, L2 regularization $\lambda = 0.001$.
- **DNN:**
  - Layers: 256 → 128 → 64 neurons, all `relu`.
  - `Dropout=0.4`, L2 $\lambda = 0.001$.
- **CNN:**
  - Conv1D(64, kernel=3, `relu`) → MaxPooling1D → `Dropout=0.3`.
  - Dense(128) → Dense(64) → Dense(`softmax`).
- **LSTM:**
  - LSTM(64, `return_sequences=True`) → LSTM(32).
  - Dense(64) → Dense(32) → Dense(`softmax`).

Common Settings:

- Optimizer: Adam; Loss: `categorical_crossentropy`.
- EarlyStopping: monitor=`val_loss`, patience=5, restore_best_weights=True.

Cross-Validation and Use of SMOTE:

- 5-fold K-fold cross-validation (`random_state=42`, `shuffle=True`)
- SMOTE with `random_state=42` to balance classes by generating synthetic minority samples

These settings were optimized to enhance accuracy, precision, and robustness while ensuring reproducibility.

4.2 Drug-Interaction System

The rule-based system recommends specific drug groups for the treatment of diabetes, taking into account the patient's glomerular filtration rate (GFR), age, body mass index (BMI), and any preexisting comorbidities. Following the recommendation of a drug group, each medication is classified as either high or medium risk based on the patient's health parameters and the active ingredients present. For the classification of these drugs, five machine learning algorithms were evaluated: logistic regression, random forest, support vector machines (SVMs), k-nearest neighbors (KNNs), and decision trees. In addition, four deep learning architectures were assessed, including recurrent neural networks (RNNs), long short-term memory networks (LSTMs), feedforward neural networks (FNNs), and gated recurrent units (GRUs).

4.2.1 Model and Performance Evaluation

The effectiveness of each model in predicting drug interactions was rigorously assessed using a comprehensive set of metrics, including accuracy, sensitivity, precision, and the F1 score. These metrics provide a robust framework for comparing the models' performance, particularly their ability to correctly identify drug interactions. Furthermore, both cross-validation and test set results were utilized to evaluate each model's capacity to generalize to unseen data. This dual-approach analysis is crucial for identifying potential issues such as overfitting or underfitting, thereby revealing the unique strengths and weaknesses of each model. The insights gained from this evaluation will be instrumental in selecting the most appropriate and reliable model for accurate drug-interaction prediction, which is essential for ensuring the safety and efficiency of the system.

The performance results provided in Table 12 have been evaluated in terms of accuracy and other metrics. Based on these findings, a detailed performance analysis of the models, error analysis, overfitting analysis, and an assessment of time and resource usage will be conducted in the subsequent sections.

Table 12 Model performance metrics

Model	Accuracy	Precision	Recall	F1 score
RNN	0.775494	0.760001	0.775494	0.762215
Logistic regression	0.747826	0.732137	0.747826	0.736338
LSTM	0.721344	0.695510	0.721344	0.692143
SVM	0.711858	0.685971	0.711858	0.680816
Decision tree	0.702767	0.698342	0.702767	0.692566
FNN	0.694071	0.694088	0.694071	0.641828
Random forest	0.693676	0.693628	0.693676	0.657518
KNN	0.676285	0.657277	0.676285	0.652142
GRU	0.657312	0.462917	0.657312	0.539233

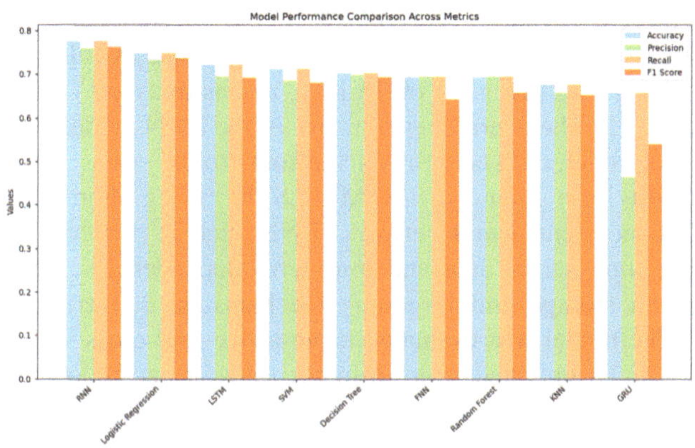

Fig. 15 Detailed performance results of machine and deep learning models

- **Comparison**

  This section presents a comprehensive comparison of the performance metrics for the machine learning and deep learning models utilized in the study. Key indicators such as accuracy, sensitivity, specificity, precision, F1 score, and AUC are systematically analyzed. Initially, a bar chart illustrating the aggregated performance of these models (Fig. 15) is provided. Subsequently, a detailed evaluation based on the average values of each metric across the models will be discussed to highlight their relative strengths and weaknesses.

  The detailed performance results of the top-performing models are presented below:

  - Logistic Regression: The logistic regression model was evaluated using a five-fold cross-validation approach, and performance metrics like accuracy, precision, sensitivity, and F1 score were calculated for each fold. The results show that the model performs consistently in terms of classification. In Fold 1 and Fold 2, the accuracy was %68.18, while Fold 3 saw an increase to %77.27. In Fold 4, the accuracy was again %68.18, and in Fold 5, it rose to %71.43. The average accuracy was 70.65, with precision at %70.58, sensitivity at %70.65, and the F1 score at %69.25. These findings indicate that the logistic regression model maintains stable performance across various data splits and is effective for classification tasks.

- Recurrent Neural Network (RNN): Recurrent neural networks (RNNs) are designed to work with sequential data and have a structure that stores information from previous steps, which influences future predictions. However, traditional RNNs can encounter challenges in learning long-term dependencies.
  When evaluating the accuracy rates obtained across five folds, the highest accuracy of 86.36% was observed in Fold 3. Fold 4 also showed strong performance with an accuracy rate of 81.82%. Accuracy rates of 76.19% in Fold 5, 68.18% in Fold 1, and 63.64% in Fold 2 were recorded.
  The average performance results for the model are as follows: an accuracy rate of 74.64%, a precision of 76.18%, a sensitivity of 74.64%, and an F1 score of 74.89. The overall performance of the RNN model is close to that of the LSTM model, with better results in some folds.
- Long Short-Term Memory (LSTM): LSTM (Long short-term memory) is a type of recurrent neural network (RNN) that is particularly effective for modeling time series data and long-term dependencies. LSTM optimizes information storage and forgetting mechanisms, delivering strong performance. The model was evaluated using a five-fold cross-validation method, and the results obtained from different folds are as follows: The accuracy rate was 68.18% in Fold 1, 77.27% in Fold 2, 77.27% in Fold 3, 77.27% in Fold 4, and 80.95% in Fold 5. The average accuracy was 76.19%, precision was 78.07%, sensitivity was 76.19%, and the F1 score was 73.61%. These results demonstrate that the LSTM model outperforms other models with high accuracy and precision values, showcasing strong performance.

– **Comparative Performance of Other Classifiers** While the LSTM model was the most successful, other models also showed varying levels of efficacy. Feedforward neural networks (FNNs) and recurrent neural networks (RNNs) followed closely behind, achieving average accuracies of 75.24% and 74.64%, respectively. Traditional machine learning models like support vector machines (SVMs) and decision trees provided satisfactory performance, with average accuracies of 75.19% and 73.42%. In contrast, models such as gated recurrent units (GRUs) and K-nearest neighbors (KNNs) lagged significantly, exhibiting average accuracies of just 67.92% and 63.29%, respectively. This wide range of performance underscores the importance of selecting the right model for the specific characteristics of the dataset.

- **Error Analysis**
  Accurate detection of drug interactions is a critical component of effective treatment planning. However, the systems designed for this task are susceptible to various errors, such as false positives, false negatives, missing data, or misclas-

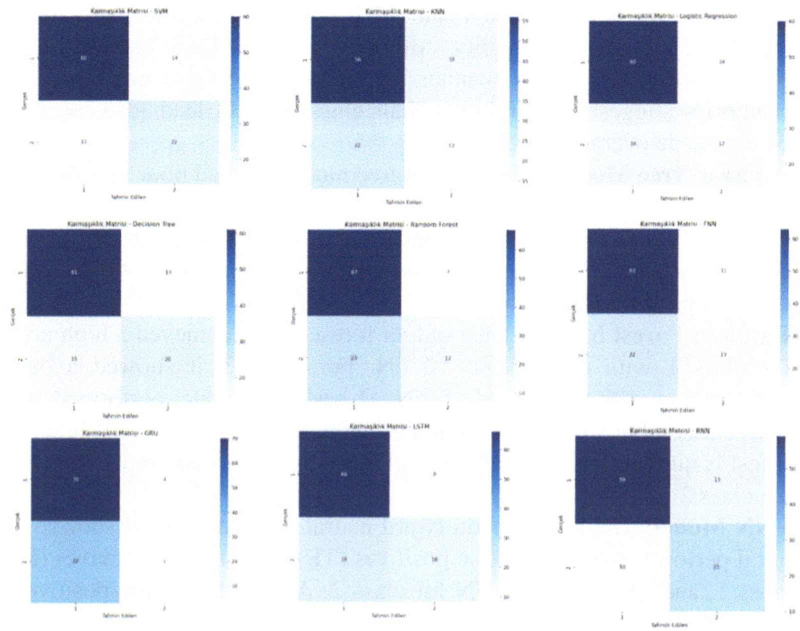

Fig. 16 Confusion matrix

sified interactions. Conducting a thorough error analysis is therefore an essential step to understanding and mitigating these types of mistakes. This section will present the findings of our error analysis on the drug-interaction system. By identifying the model's specific weaknesses, we can pinpoint potential areas for improvement, ultimately enhancing the system's reliability and ensuring its safe and efficient operation.

In Fig. 16, the confusion matrices are discussed in the following paragraphs:

- **SVM Model:** The support vector machine (SVM) model demonstrated a high degree of accuracy, particularly for class 1, achieving 56 true positives (TP) against only one false positive (FP). For class 2, the model performed well with 50 TP, but it exhibited a higher number of false negatives (FN) at 14. This imbalance suggests a need to refine the model to enhance its predictive accuracy specifically for class 2.
- **KNN Model:** The K-nearest neighbors (KNNs) model yielded solid results for class 1, securing 45 TP and 13 FN. However, its performance notably declined for class 2, with only 40 TP and a significantly higher 22 FN. The elevated false negative rate for class 2 indicates that the model struggles with its classification. This area presents a clear opportunity for optimization to improve the model's overall reliability.
- **Logistic Regression Model:** The logistic regression model displayed balanced performance across both classes, correctly identifying 50 TP for each.

It recorded 17 FN for class 1 and 13 FN for class 2, showing a relatively consistent classification ability. Although the model successfully classified both classes in a similar manner, the presence of false negatives in both categories suggests that minor enhancements could lead to a more robust performance overall.

- **Decision Tree Model:** The decision tree model showed poor performance for class 1, with only 13 TP and 20 FP. However, it performed well for class 2 with 61 TP and 15 FN. The model faced significant challenges in correctly classifying class 1. The high FP rate indicates that the model is overfitting and needs improvement for class 1.
- **Random Forest Model:** The random forest model achieved a high accuracy for class 1 with 67 TP and 12 FN. For class 2, it showed a balanced performance with 50 TP and 15 FN. Overall, the model performed well for both classes, but some improvements can be made for class 2. While random forest is quite reliable for class 1, further optimization can reduce the FN rate for class 2.
- **FNN Model:** The FNN (feedforward neural network) model showed a very good performance with 55 true positives (TP) and 14 false negatives (FN) for class 1, and 48 TP and 18 FN for class 2. Although the true positive count is high for both classes, the false negative rate is a bit higher, indicating that the model can still be improved. The model, especially for class 2, could be enhanced by targeting a reduction in the FN rate.
- **GRU Model:** The GRU (gated recurrent unit) model performed well with 51 TP and 16 FN for class 1, and 52 TP and 16 FN for class 2. The true positive counts are quite high for both classes, and the false negative rates are at acceptable levels. However, reducing the FN values in both classes will further improve the model's performance.
- **LSTM Model:** The LSTM (long short-term memory) model achieved good results with 53 TP and 15 FN for class 1, and 49 TP and 19 FN for class 2. However, the 19 FN for class 2 indicates that the model struggled a bit to classify this class correctly. The model requires improvements to reduce the false negatives for class 2.
- **RNN Model:** The RNN (recurrent neural network) model achieved 52 TP and 16 FN for class 1, and 50 TP and 18 FN for class 2. The 18 FN for class 2 indicates that more improvements are needed for this class. The model can deliver better results by reducing false negatives in both classes.

4.3 Evaluation of Training and Test Performances

Comparing training and test performances is crucial for assessing a model's generalization capability. Below is an evaluation of different models based on their training and test accuracies:

- SVM Model: The SVM model achieved high accuracy on the training set and also performed well on the test set. The training and test accuracies are quite close, indicating that the model does not suffer from overfitting or underfitting. The balanced performance suggests strong generalization ability.
- KNN Model: The KNN model also achieved successful results in terms of training and test accuracies. While the training performance was high, the test accuracy was slightly lower for class 2. This indicates that the model faced some challenges in correctly classifying class 2 but generally demonstrated a balanced performance.
- Logistic Regression Model: The logistic regression model maintained a good balance between training and test accuracies. Both performance metrics were at similar levels, showing strong generalization ability. The training loss decreased significantly, while the test loss remained consistently low.
- Decision Tree Model: The decision tree model achieved high accuracy on the training set but performed poorly on class 1 in the test set. The gap between training and test accuracies indicates that the model overfitted the training data. The lower accuracy for class 1 suggests that the model struggles to generalize well for this class.
- Random Forest Model: The random forest model demonstrated a well-balanced performance in terms of training and test accuracies. While the training accuracy remained high, the test accuracy was also consistently high, indicating strong generalization ability.
- FNN Model: The FNN (feedforward neural network) model achieved high accuracy on the training set. However, minor variations in test accuracy were observed. The differences between training and test accuracies suggest that slight improvements could be made to enhance the model's generalization ability.
- GRU Model: The GRU model showed a balanced performance in terms of training and test accuracies. Both metrics were close to each other, indicating that the model has strong generalization capability.
- LSTM Model: The LSTM model generally maintained a balanced performance in training and test accuracies. However, minor deviations in test accuracy suggest that some improvements could be made to enhance its performance on the test set.
- RNN Model: The RNN model achieved good accuracy on the training set but slightly lower accuracy on the test set. The difference between training and test accuracies indicates a risk of overfitting. Improvements can be made to enhance the model's generalization ability.

5 Discussion

Experimental results confirm the efficacy of machine learning and deep learning for diabetes prediction and medication recommendation. Performance varied significantly between the Pima Indian and Diabetes datasets, highlighting the critical role of data characteristics. While the convolutional neural network (CNN) struggled with the Pima Indian dataset (50% accuracy), it excelled on the Diabetes dataset (98.01% accuracy), ranking as the third-best model. This contrast underscores the importance of aligning model architecture with data type, as CNNs are optimized for spatial rather than tabular data. In contrast, random forest, artificial neural networks (ANNs), and long short-term memory (LSTM) models consistently delivered high and stable accuracy across both datasets, establishing them as reliable choices for diverse clinical data. The RNN model showed promising results for drug interaction, but its performance on a limited dataset (109 instances) necessitates validation with larger, clinically verified data to ensure generalization.

5.1 Performance Evaluation

Training the same models on both the Pima Indian and Diabetes datasets revealed significant performance variations, clearly demonstrating the critical impact of dataset characteristics. The random forest and long short-term memory (LSTM) models consistently delivered high and stable performances across both datasets, proving to be the most robust and dependable classifiers.

Other models showed greater performance divergence. For example, the convolutional neural network (CNN) performed poorly on the Pima Indian dataset (approximately 50% accuracy) but excelled on the Diabetes dataset (98.01% accuracy). This contrast highlights the strong dependency of a model's effectiveness on the specific nature and distribution of the data. Similarly, other deep learning models like artificial neural networks (ANNs) and deep neural networks (DNNs) showed signs of overfitting and fluctuation, particularly on the Pima Indian dataset. The stability of the LSTM model, with minimal overfitting, positions it alongside random forest as a top-tier choice for this task.

In the drug-interaction recommendation system, recurrent neural network models, particularly LSTM and RNN variants, showed promising but variable results, reflecting the challenges posed by the dataset's limited size and imbalance. These fluctuations emphasize the necessity for cautious interpretation of performance metrics and underline the importance of extensive validation on larger, more diverse datasets to ensure genuine generalization.

5.2 Cross-Validation and Generalization Ability

Cross-validation analysis provided critical insights into the models' generalization capabilities, with the random forest (RF) model emerging as the most reliable performer. It demonstrated consistent accuracy across all data folds on both datasets, reflecting its inherent ensemble strength in mitigating variance. In contrast, other models like K-nearest neighbors (KNNs), decision tree (DT), and convolutional neural network (CNN) showed significant performance variability, especially on the Pima Indian dataset, indicating susceptibility to overfitting.

For the drug recommendation system, models also exhibited considerable performance fluctuations during cross-validation, a result of the dataset's small size and imbalance. This instability suggests that high accuracy on limited folds likely indicates overfitting rather than true predictive power. These findings emphasize the vital role of cross-validation for both tasks and highlight the urgent need for larger, more representative datasets to ensure trustworthy evaluations.

5.3 Model Selection and Balancing Techniques

Among the models evaluated for diabetes prediction, random forest consistently proved to be a robust and reliable choice, offering an optimal balance of high accuracy and computational efficiency. For deep learning architectures, long short-term memory (LSTM) networks particularly excelled by capturing the complex temporal dependencies often inherent in clinical data, leading to strong and stable predictive outcomes across both the Pima Indian and Diabetes datasets. A key factor in their success was the application of regularization techniques and early stopping during training, which helped them exhibit minimal signs of overfitting.

In the separate application of the drug-interaction recommendation system, recurrent neural network models, particularly LSTM and its variants, showed promising yet highly variable results. This performance instability can be directly attributed to the dataset's limited size and significant imbalance. The fluctuations in performance metrics emphasize the need for a very cautious interpretation of the findings and underscore the critical importance of extensive validation on larger, more diverse datasets to ensure genuine generalization.

Ultimately, this study highlights the critical need to align a model's architecture with the specific characteristics of the data to optimize predictive performance. While random forest and LSTM offer complementary strengths for structured and sequential data, respectively, the instability observed in the drug recommendation system calls for more sophisticated data augmentation, preprocessing, and balanced sampling strategies. These findings align with recent research advocating for hybrid approaches that integrate both machine learning and deep learning techniques to enhance clinical decision-making. In the end, careful model selection, comprehensive cross-validation, and the expansion of datasets remain pivotal for translating these computational advances into reliable, real-world healthcare applications.

5.4 Limitations and Future Work

This study's findings, while promising, are subject to several limitations that must be acknowledged. The custom drug-interaction dataset, comprising only 109 records, represents a relatively small and homogeneous sample size, which constrains the generalizability of the drug recommendation model. Expanding this dataset to include a broader spectrum of drug interactions, particularly those involving comorbidities or polypharmacy scenarios across diverse patient populations, would enhance the robustness and clinical relevance of the system. Moreover, while the current diagnostic models demonstrated strong performance in diabetes classification, their scope is limited to this specific condition. Future research should aim to extend the diagnostic framework to encompass multiple chronic diseases, enabling a more comprehensive clinical decision support system. By integrating multi-disease diagnostic capabilities with an enriched pharmacological interaction database, the ultimate goal is to develop an AI-driven assistant that effectively supports clinicians throughout both diagnosis and treatment phases, thereby optimizing personalized patient care and improving clinical outcomes.

6 Conclusion

This study introduced a two-stage intelligent framework designed to assist in diabetes diagnosis and treatment planning through the application of machine learning and classification algorithms. The system initially predicts a patient's diabetes level based on selected clinical features and subsequently recommends drug classes by evaluating relevant physiological parameters and comorbidities. Individual medications within the recommended drug group are further classified by risk levels, enhancing the personalization of the recommendation process.

The experimental findings indicated that the random forest and long short-term memory (LSTM) models achieved high accuracy in predicting diabetes levels. However, caution is warranted in interpreting these results due to limitations related to dataset size and the absence of real-world clinical validation.

The primary limitations identified in this study include:

- The diabetes classification models were trained on publicly available datasets that lack sufficient size and diversity, potentially impacting the generalizability of the models.
- The drug recommendation system has not been validated using actual patient data in clinical environments, which limits its current reliability and applicability.

Despite these limitations, the proposed framework demonstrates significant potential as a clinical decision support system, particularly in promoting early diagnosis and personalized treatment strategies. Future research could expand this framework to address other chronic diseases, and the drug-interaction database could be enhanced to incorporate polypharmacy scenarios involving medications for comorbid conditions.

Acknowledgments The authors used language editing support tools, including large language models, to assist with grammar correction and clarity improvements during manuscript preparation. All scientific content and interpretations were developed and critically reviewed by the authors.

Competing Interests The authors have no competing interests to declare that are relevant to the content of this chapter.

Ethics Approval This chapter is based on publicly available secondary data and does not involve any direct experimentation on human participants or animals. Hence, ethical approval was not required.

References

1. R. Cioffi, M. Travaglioni, G. Piscitelli, A. Petrillo, F. De Felice, Artificial intelligence and machine learning applications in smart production: progress, trends, and directions. Sustainability **12**(2), 492 (2020)
2. Y. Chen, U. Liebau, S.M. Guruprasad, I. Trofimenko, C. Minke, Advancing life cycle assessment of sustainable green hydrogen production using domain-specific fine-tuning by large language models augmentation. Mach. Learn. Knowl. Extr. **6**(4), 2494–2514 (2024)
3. A. Alhazmi, Y. Alhazmi, A. Makrami, A. Masmali, N. Salawi, K. Masmali, S. Patil, Application of artificial intelligence and machine learning for prediction of oral cancer risk. J. Oral Pathol. Med. **50**(5), 444–450 (2021)
4. M. Liu, X. Shen, W. Pan, Deep reinforcement learning for personalized treatment recommendation. Stat. Med. **41**(20), 4034–4056 (2022)
5. L. Pedersen, M. Mazur-Milecka, J. Ruminski, S. Wagner, A review on machine learning deployment patterns and key features in the prediction of preeclampsia. Mach. Learn. Knowl. Extr. **6**(4), 2515–2569 (2024)
6. L. Alzubaidi, M.A. Fadhel, O. Al-Shamma, J. Zhang, Y. Duan, Deep learning models for classification of red blood cells in microscopy images to aid in sickle cell anemia diagnosis. Electronics **9**(3), 427 (2020)
7. W. Rösler, M. Roiss, C. Widmer, Advancements in machine learning (ML): Transforming the future of blood cancer detection and outcome prediction. Healthbook TIMES Oncol. Hematol. **20**(2), 20–25 (2024)
8. G. Gunčar, M. Kukar, M. Notar, M. Brvar, P. Černelč, M. Notar, M. Notar, An application of machine learning to haematological diagnosis. Sci. Rep. **8**(1), 411 (2018)
9. N. Hong, H. Park, Y. Rhee, Machine learning applications in endocrinology and metabolism research: an overview. Endocrinol. Metab. **35**(1), 71–84 (2020)
10. B.F. Wee, S. Sivakumar, K.H. Lim, W.K. Wong, F.H. Juwono, Diabetes detection based on machine learning and deep learning approaches. Multimed. Tools Appl. **83**(8), 24153–24185 (2024)
11. F.J. Barrera, E.D.L. Brown, A. Rojo, J. Obeso, H. Plata, E.P. Lincango, N. Terry, R. Rodríguez-Gutiérrez, J.E. Hall, S. Shekhar, Application of machine learning and artificial intelligence in the diagnosis and classification of polycystic ovarian syndrome: a systematic review. Front. Endocrinol. **14**, 1106625 (2023)
12. A.W. Purcell, S. Sechi, T.P. DiLorenzo, The evolving landscape of autoantigen discovery and characterization in type 1 diabetes. Diabetes **68**(5), 879–886 (2019)
13. R. Ruze, T. Liu, X. Zou, J. Song, Y. Chen, R. Xu, X. Yin, Q. Xu, Obesity and type 2 diabetes mellitus: connections in epidemiology, pathogenesis, and treatments. Front. Endocrinol. **14**, 1161521 (2023)
14. M.V. Diaz-Santana, K.M. O'Brien, Y.-M.M. Park, D.P. Sandler, C.R. Weinberg, Persistence of risk for type 2 diabetes after gestational diabetes mellitus. Diabetes Care **45**(4), 864–870 (2022)
15. S. Pleus, A. Tytko, R. Landgraf, L. Heinemann, C. Werner, D. Müller-Wieland, A.-G. Ziegler, U.A. Müller, G. Freckmann, H. Kleinwechter, et al., Definition, classification, diagnosis and

differential diagnosis of diabetes mellitus: Update 2023. Exp. Clin. Endocrinol. Diabetes **132**(03), 112–124 (2024)

16. D.B. Sacks, M. Arnold, G.L. Bakris, D.E. Bruns, A.R. Horvath, Å. Lernmark, B.E. Metzger, D.M. Nathan, M.S. Kirkman, Guidelines and recommendations for laboratory analysis in the diagnosis and management of diabetes mellitus. Clin. Chem. **69**(8), 808–868 (2023)
17. D.M. Williams, H. Jones, J.W. Stephens, Personalized type 2 diabetes management: an update on recent advances and recommendations, in *Diabetes, Metabolic Syndrome and Obesity: Targets and Therapy* (2022), pp. 281–295
18. A.T. Arias-Marroquín, F.M.D. Razo-Olvera, Z.M. Castañeda-Bernal, E. Cruz-Juárez, M.F. Camacho-Ramírez, D. Elías-López, M.A. Lara-Sánchez, L. Chalita-Ramos, V. Rebollar-Fernández, C.A. Aguilar-Salinas, Personalized versus non-personalized nutritional recommendations/interventions for type 2 diabetes mellitus remission: a narrative review. Diabetes Therapy **15**(4), 749–761 (2024)
19. J.M. Dennis, Precision medicine in type 2 diabetes: using individualized prediction models to optimize selection of treatment. Diabetes **69**(10), 2075–2085 (2020)
20. J. Su, L. Yang, Z. Sun, X. Zhan, Personalized drug therapy: innovative concept guided with proteoformics. Mol. Cell. Proteomics **23**(3), (e105512) (2024)
21. S. Pernice, A. Maglione, D. Tortarolo, R. Sirovich, M. Clerico, S. Rolla, M. Beccuti, F. Cordero, A new computational workflow to guide personalized drug therapy. J. Biomed. Inform. **148**, 104546 (2023)
22. D.A. Drexler, B. Gergics, M. Puskás, T.P. Haidegger, L.A. Kovács, Personalized therapy using drug delivery devices. IFAC-PapersOnLine **58**(24), 550–555 (2024)
23. C.R. Sirtori, S. Castiglione, C. Pavanello, Metformin: from diabetes to cancer to prolongation of life. Pharmacol. Res., **208**, 107367 (2024)
24. H. Yao, A. Zhang, D. Li, Y. Wu, C.-Z. Wang, J.-Y. Wan, C.-S. Yuan, Comparative effectiveness of glp-1 receptor agonists on glycaemic control, body weight, and lipid profile for type 2 diabetes: systematic review and network meta-analysis. BMJ **384** (2024)
25. R. Pishdad, P.G. Auwaerter, R.R. Kalyani, Diabetes, SGLT-2 inhibitors, and urinary tract infection: a review. Curr. Diab. Rep. **24**(5), 108–117 (2024)
26. D. Mohajan, H.K. Mohajan, Dipeptidyl peptidase-4 (DPP-4) inhibitors: New oral medications for the treatment of type 2 diabetes. Innovation Sci. Technol. **3**(3), 31–35 (2024)
27. D.H. van Raalte, P. Bjornstad, D.Z. Cherney, I.H. de Boer, P. Fioretto, D. Gordin, F. Persson, S.E. Rosas, P. Rossing, J.A. Schaub, et al., Combination therapy for kidney disease in people with diabetes mellitus. Nat. Rev. Nephrol. **20**(7), 433–446 (2024)
28. E. Obeagu, E.E. Ayogu, C.N. Anyanwu, G.U. Obeagu, Drug-drug interactions in the management of coexisting sickle cell anemia and diabetes. Elite J. Health Sci. **2**(2), 1–9 (2024)
29. L.-Y. Lian, G. Targher, C.D. Byrne, W.-Y. Liu, M.-H. Zheng, Resmetirom for mash patients with diabetes: challenges and opportunities in the real world. Metab. Clin. Exp. **156** (2024)
30. M. Zargoush, S. Ghazalbash, M.M. Hosseini, F. Alemi, D. Perri, Machine learning driven diabetes care using predictive-prescriptive analytics for personalized medication prescription. Sci. Rep. **15**(1), 26811 (2025)
31. M. Sajid, K.R. Malik, A.H. Khan, S. Iqbal, A.A. Alaulamie, Q.M. Ilyas, Next-generation diabetes diagnosis and personalized diet-activity management: a hybrid ensemble paradigm. PloS One **20**(1), e0307718 (2025)
32. L. Žigutytė, T. Sorz-Nechay, J. Clusmann, J.N. Kather, Use of artificial intelligence for liver diseases: a survey from the EASL Congress 2024, in *JHEP Reports* (2024), pp. 101209
33. A. Keshtkar, N. Ayareh, F. Atighi, R. Hamidi, P. Yazdanpanahi, A. Karimi, A. Naseri, F. Hosseini, M.H. Dabbaghmanesh, Artificial intelligence in diabetes management: Revolutionizing the diagnosis of diabetes mellitus; a literature review. Shiraz E-Medical J. **25**, e146903 (2024)
34. D. Chhabra, M. Juneja, G. Chutani, An efficient ensemble-based machine learning approach for predicting chronic kidney disease. Curr. Med. Imaging **20**(1), e080523216634 (2024)
35. Y. Lin, T. Shi, G. Kong, Acute kidney injury prognosis prediction using machine learning methods: a systematic review. Kidney Medicine, **7**, 100936 (2024)

36. M.M. Chowdhury, R.S. Ayon, M.S. Hossain, An investigation of machine learning algorithms and data augmentation techniques for diabetes diagnosis using class imbalanced BRFSS dataset. Healthcare Anal. **5**, 100297 (2024)
37. I. Nissar, W.A. Mir, T.A. Shaikh, T. Areen, M. Kashif, S. Khiani, A. Hussain, An intelligent healthcare system for automated diabetes diagnosis and prediction using machine learning. Procedia Comput. Sci. **235**, 2476–2485 (2024)
38. S. Arefin, Chronic disease management through an AI-powered application. J. Serv. Sci. Manag. **17**(4), 305–320 (2024)
39. F.A. Khaleel, A.M. Al-Bakry, Diagnosis of diabetes using machine learning algorithms. Mater. Today Proc. **80**, 3200–3203 (2023)
40. F. Navazi, Y. Yuan, N. Archer, An examination of the hybrid meta-heuristic machine learning algorithms for early diagnosis of type ii diabetes using big data feature selection. Healthcare Anal. **4**, 100227 (2023)
41. X. Zou, Y. Liu, L. Ji, Machine learning in precision pharmacotherapy of type 2 diabetes—a promising future or a glimpse of hope? Digital Health **9**, 20552076231203879 (2023)
42. S.K. Nayak, M. Garanayak, S.K. Swain, S.K. Panda, D. Godavarthi, An intelligent disease prediction and drug recommendation prototype by using multiple approaches of machine learning algorithms. IEEE Access **11**, 99304–99318 (2023)
43. Y. Liu, et al., Artificial intelligence–based neural network for the diagnosis of diabetes: model development. JMIR Med. Inform. **8**(5), e18682 (2020)
44. I. Zafar, S. Anwar, W. Yousaf, F.U. Nisa, T. Kausar, Q.ul Ain, A. Unar, M.A. Kamal, S. Rashid, K.A. Khan, et al., Reviewing methods of deep learning for intelligent healthcare systems in genomics and biomedicine. Biomed. Signal Process. Control **86**, 105263 (2023)
45. S. Yang, S. Kar, Application of artificial intelligence and machine learning in early detection of adverse drug reactions (ADRs) and drug-induced toxicity. Artificial Intelligence Chemistry, **1**, 100011 (2023)
46. U. Bhimavarapu, N. Chintalapudi, G. Battineni, A fair and safe usage drug recommendation system in medical emergencies by a stacked ANN. Algorithms **15**(6), 186 (2022)
47. V. Geetha, C.K. Gomathy, K. Keerthi, N. Pavithra, Diagnostic approach to anemia in adults using machine learning. J. Pharm. Negat. Results, **13**, 3713–3717 (2022)
48. C.C. Olisah, L. Smith, M. Smith, Diabetes mellitus prediction and diagnosis from a data preprocessing and machine learning perspective. Comput. Methods Prog. Biomed. **220**, 106773 (2022)
49. M.M. Hossain, R.A. Swarna, R. Mostafiz, P. Shaha, L.Y. Pinky, M.M. Rahman, W. Rahman, M.S. Hossain, M.E. Hossain, M.S. Iqbal, Analysis of the performance of feature optimization techniques for the diagnosis of machine learning-based chronic kidney disease. Mach. Learn. Appl. **9**, 100330 (2022)
50. K. Tiwari, D.K. Singh, Machine learning-based recommendation system for disease-drug material and adverse drug reaction: comparative review. Mater. Today Proc. **51**, 304–313 (2022)
51. Q. Ye, C.-Y. Hsieh, Z. Yang, Y. Kang, J. Chen, D. Cao, S. He, T. Hou, A unified drug–target interaction prediction framework based on knowledge graph and recommendation system. Nature Commun. **12**(1), 6775 (2021)
52. D. Gupta, A. Choudhury, U. Gupta, P. Singh, M. Prasad, Computational approach to clinical diagnosis of diabetes disease: a comparative study. Multimed. Tools Appl., **80**, 1–26 (2021)
53. A. Sarwar, M. Ali, J. Manhas, V. Sharma, Diagnosis of diabetes type-ii using hybrid machine learning based ensemble model. Int. J. Inf. Technol. **12**, 419–428 (2020)
54. S. Larabi-Marie-Sainte, L. Aburahmah, R. Almohaini, T. Saba, Current techniques for diabetes prediction: review and case study. Appl. Sci. **9**(21), 4604 (2019)
55. F. Xie, J.C.N. Chan, R.C.W. Ma, Precision medicine in diabetes prevention, classification and management. J. Diabetes Investig. **9**(5), 998–1015 (2018)
56. I. Kavakiotis, O. Tsave, A. Salifoglou, N. Maglaveras, I. Vlahavas, I. Chouvarda, Machine learning and data mining methods in diabetes research. Comput. Struct. Biotechnol. J. **15**, 104–116 (2017)

57. R.R. Shamir, T. Dolber, A.M. Noecker, B.L. Walter, C.C. McIntyre, Machine learning approach to optimizing combined stimulation and medication therapies for Parkinson's disease. Brain Stimul. **8**(6), 1025–1032 (2015)
58. A.B. Abacha, M.F.M. Chowdhury, A. Karanasiou, Y. Mrabet, A. Lavelli, P. Zweigenbaum, Text mining for pharmacovigilance: Using machine learning for drug name recognition and drug–drug interaction extraction and classification. J. Biomed. Inform. **58**, 122–132 (2015)
59. Y. Chen, B. Manderick, F. Liu, *Extract Protein-Protein Interactions from the Literature Using Support Vector Machines with Feature Selection* (INTECH Open Access Publisher, New York, 2011)
60. O. Sami, Y. Elsheikh, F. Almasalha, The role of data pre-processing techniques in improving machine learning accuracy for predicting coronary heart disease. Int. J. Adv. Comput. Sci. Appl. **12**(6), 812–820 (2021)
61. X. Zheng, M. Wang, J. Ordieres-Meré, Comparison of data preprocessing approaches for applying deep learning to human activity recognition in the context of Industry 4.0. Sensors **18**(7), 2146 (2018)
62. R. Couronné, P. Probst, A.-L. Boulesteix, Random forest versus logistic regression: a large-scale benchmark experiment. BMC Bioinf. **19**, 1–14 (2018)
63. H.H. Patel, P. Prajapati, Study and analysis of decision tree based classification algorithms. Int. J. Comput. Sci. Eng. **6**(10), 74–78 (2018)
64. M.A. Chandra, S.S. Bedi, Survey on SVM and their application in image classification. Int. J. Inf. Technol. **13**(5), 1–11 (2021)
65. S. Zhang, Challenges in KNN classification. IEEE Trans. Knowl. Data Eng. **34**(10), 4663–4675 (2022)
66. H. Ahmed, A.K. Nandi, *Decision Trees and Random Forests* (2019), pp. 199–224

MOBPITL: Enhancing Diabetic Retinopathy Detection Via PiT-MobileNetV2 Fusion and Lamb Optimization

Youssef Khalaf, Randa Hamada, and Samar Elbedwehy

Abstract Diabetic retinopathy (DR) is a significant eye condition that can lead to vision loss and blindness in diabetic patients, emphasizing the importance of early detection and intervention. DR affects the blood vessels in the retina, often without initial symptoms, making regular comprehensive eye exams crucial for those with diabetes. This study addresses the challenge of DR detection by exploring various state-of-the-art deep learning models, including DeiT, MobileNet-V2 V2, and combinations of PiT architectures with MobileNet-V2. After evaluating these approaches, we focused on optimizing the PiT-Base-224 with MobileNet-V2 model, utilizing both Adam and Lamb optimizers to enhance its performance. By integrating the strengths of transformer-based architectures with pretrained CNNs, we developed a highly accurate and efficient diagnostic system. The results demonstrate the potential of this optimized model to enhance DR detection, achieving high accuracy and paving the way for accessible and reliable diagnostic tools in diabetic care with 99.43, 99.6, and 99.4 for accuracy, precision, and recall, respectively. This study highlights the effectiveness of our hybrid model and optimization strategy in accurately diagnosing diabetic retinopathy, emphasizing the importance of early detection and intervention in preventing vision loss.

Keywords Diabetic retinopathy · Early detection · Medical diagnostics · Deep learning

Y. Khalaf · R. Hamada
Faculty of Artificial Intelligence, Kafrelsheikh University, Kafrelsheikh, Egypt
e-mail: youssef_768a@ai.kfs.edu.eg; randa_664a@ai.kfs.edu.eg

S. Elbedwehy (✉)
Faculty of Artificial Intelligence, Kafrelsheikh University, Kafrelsheikh, Egypt

University of Science and Technology, Zewail City of Science and Technology, Giza, Egypt
e-mail: samarelbedwehy@ai.kfs.edu.eg

N. E. M. Khalifa, M. H. N. Taha (eds.), *Next-Gen Healthcare*,
https://doi.org/10.1007/978-3-032-07267-2_12

1 Introduction

Diabetic retinopathy (also known as diabetic eye disease) is a medical condition in which damage occurs to the retina due to diabetes. It is a leading cause of blindness in developed countries and one of the leading causes of sight loss in the world, even though there are many new therapies and improved treatments for helping people live with diabetes. Diabetic retinopathy affects up to 80% of those who have had both type 1 and type 2 diabetes for 20 years or more. In at least 90% of new cases, progression to more aggressive forms of sight-threatening retinopathy and maculopathy could be reduced with proper treatment and monitoring of the eyes. The longer a person has diabetes, the higher his or her chances of developing diabetic retinopathy. Each year in the United States, diabetic retinopathy accounts for 12% of all new cases of blindness. It is also the leading cause of blindness in people aged 20–64 [1].

Also, a cross-sectional study conducted over 3 years at a major ophthalmology referral center in Assiut City, Upper Egypt, reported a diabetic retinopathy (DR) prevalence of 18.2% among 2178 adult diabetic patients. DR was significantly associated with factors such as poor glycemic control, longer diabetes duration, hypertension, smoking, older age, dyslipidemia, female sex, and insulin use. These findings underscore the need for efficient, early DR detection strategies to mitigate associated complications [2].

Once vision is lost due to diabetic retinopathy, it cannot be restored. Traditionally, the diagnosis of DR relies on manual examination of retinal fundus photographs by ophthalmologists, which is time-consuming and subject to human error.

In recent years, deep learning has emerged as a transformative technology in the field of medical imaging, offering powerful tools for the automated detection and classification of diseases such as diabetic retinopathy (DR) [3–6]. DR, which involves damage to the retinal blood vessels due to prolonged high blood sugar levels, often progresses silently and can lead to irreversible vision loss if not detected early. Traditional screening methods require expert ophthalmologists to manually examine retinal fundus images, a process that is time-consuming, resource-intensive, and prone to interobserver variability. Deep learning models, particularly convolutional neural networks (CNNs) and transformer-based architectures, have shown exceptional capabilities in learning complex visual patterns directly from large datasets, enabling them to identify early signs of DR such as microaneurysms, hemorrhages, and exudates with high accuracy. These models can analyze retinal images at scale and provide consistent, objective results, making them valuable tools in both clinical and screening environments. As such, deep learning is playing a crucial role in advancing the early detection and monitoring of diabetic retinopathy, contributing to improved outcomes and reduced vision loss among diabetic patients.

The main contributions of this study are as follows:

- Innovative classification technique: This chapter presents a new method for classifying diabetic retinopathy that performs strongly across multiple datasets, underscoring the significance of interpretability and explainability in clinical applications.

- Advanced integration of neural networks: this study integrates features from MobileNet-V2 and PiTtransformer to create a comprehensive and informative feature representation. This fusion leverages the strengths of both architectures, resulting in superior performance compared to individual models.
- Improved model performance: By integrating MobileNet-V2 with PiT, the chapter attained enhanced discriminative ability, effectively capturing a wider spectrum of visual features and outperforming the individual models.
- Optimized training process: This study introduced a custom optimization technique based on lamb that dynamically adjusts the step size according to the gradient norm, leading to more efficient convergence in training the merged MobileNet-V2 and PiTmodels.

The remainder of the chapter is structured as follows: the next Sect. 2 presents a literature review. Section 3 discusses the underlying motivation for the study. In Sect. 4, the methodology employed in this research is detailed, followed by Sect. 5, which outlines the findings. Finally, Sect. 6 wraps up the chapter and suggests directions for future work.

2 Literature Review

The classification of diabetic retinopathy (DR) is a crucial research area that significantly impacts clinical diagnosis, treatment strategies, and patient management. As our understanding of retinal disorders and the effect of diabetes evolves, there has been an increasing amount of literature focused on various methodologies for accurately classifying DR. This literature review aims to provide a comprehensive overview of the current research landscape, exploring the diverse approaches used to categorize the stages of diabetic retinopathy, from traditional techniques to recent advancements in machine learning and deep learning. By distilling key insights and trends, this review highlights the progress made in improving diagnostic accuracy and facilitating more effective therapeutic interventions, while also identifying potential directions for future research and technological innovation in this vital field.

Khalifa et al. [7] investigated deep transfer learning models for the early detection of diabetic retinopathy (DR) to improve recovery and reduce vision loss. Using the APTOS 2019 dataset, they evaluated models such as AlexNet, ResNet18, SqueezeNet, GoogleNet, VGG16, and VGG19, with AlexNet achieving the highest test accuracy of 97.9%. Adrimana et al. [8] developed a hybrid system for detecting and classifying diabetic retinopathy (DR) by combining local binary patterns (LBP) for texture feature extraction with deep learning models like ResNet, DenseNet, and DetNet. The system achieved accuracies of 96.35% (ResNet), 84.05% (DenseNet), and 93.99% (DetNet). The authors recommended future improvements focusing on advanced LBP variants, such as circular-LBP, and hyperparameter optimization to enhance performance. Mushtaq et al. [9] focused on the application of deep learning models for classifying diabetic retinopathy (DR) severity levels. They proposed a DenseNet-169 model, which was trained using a combination of datasets: Diabetic Retinopathy Detection 2015 and APTOS 2019 Blindness Detection. The model achieved a training accuracy of 95.3% and a validation accuracy of 90.34% upon evaluation. Additionally, a regression model was applied to the dataset, achieving a validation accuracy of 78.9%. The proposed DenseNet-169 model outperformed the regression model, demonstrating its superior capability in classifying DR severity levels.

Minarno et al. [10] proposed a deep learning method utilizing the EfficientNet-B7 model for the automatic identification of diabetic retinopathy (DR). The research applied three preprocessing techniques to the APTOS 2019 Blindness Detection dataset, with the Usuyama technique achieving the highest accuracy of 89% in training data and 84% in test data. In comparison, the Harikrishnan technique reached 82% accuracy, and the Ben Grahamtechnique achieved 81% accuracy in test data. The study also incorporated an augmentation process to reduce overfitting due to the limited size of the dataset. Overall, these preprocessing and augmentation techniques significantly enhanced the performance of the EfficientNet-B7 model in classifying DR. Obayya et al. [11] introduced the XAITO-DRGC model for detecting diabetic retinopathy (DR) using OphthoAI IoMT headsets for remote monitoring. Their approach involves preprocessing steps such as median filtering and contrast enhancement, followed by U-Net-based image segmentation and SqueezeNet-based feature extraction. For classification, they utilized the Archimedes optimization algorithm (AOA) and a bidirectional gated recurrent convolutional unit (BGRCU). The model achieved an accuracy of 98.24%, significantly surpassing the CNN512-dropout model at 84.10% accuracy on the DDR dataset. Future research will explore fusion-based deep learning models to further improve detection capabilities.

Mohanty et al. [12] proposed two deep learning approaches for diabetic retinopathy (DR) detection: a hybrid network combining VGG16 with an XGBoost Classifier and the DenseNet 121 network. These models were evaluated using retinal images from the APTOS 2019 Blindness Detection Kaggle dataset achieving an accuracy of 79.50% and 97.30%, respectively. Akgül et al. [13] conducted a study utilizing the VGG16 model for detecting diabetic retinopathy (DR) from retinal images. They enhanced the original VGG16 architecture by creating two variants: one version incorporated a dropout layer solely in the classification layers, while the other applied dropout across all model blocks. When they evaluated on APTOS 2019 Blindness Detection Kaggle dataset They enhanced the performance from the original VGG16 model with an accuracy of 75.48% to 81.74% with the newly proposed model that featured a dense first layer and progressively decreasing convolutional layers.

Akyel et al. [14] developed a hybrid approach to diagnosing diabetic retinopathy (DR) by combining blood vessel segmentation with machine learning-based ensemble models. They used the LinkNet-RCB7 model to segment blood vessels in fundus images, improving image quality for diagnosis. Their classification model, utilizing gray-level co-occurrence matrix (GLCM) features, achieved a Dice coefficient of 85.95% for segmentation and 97.46% accuracy for binary classification. Additionally, they classified DR into five stages with an accuracy of 96.10% using the APTOS 2019 dataset. This method enhances classification accuracy while reducing computational load, making it viable for resource-constrained settings. Moustari et al. [15] developed a two-stage deep learning system for classifying the severity of diabetic retinopathy (DR) using an attention-guided convolutional neural network (AG-CNN). The system features two branches: one for global attention on the entire image and another that focuses on specific regions to enhance local features. Their baseline model, DenseNet-121, achieved an accuracy of 97.46% and an AUC of 0.995. By adding the local branch, accuracy improved to 98.48% and AUC to 0.998. They also employed gradient-weighted class activation mapping (Grad-CAM) for preprocessing, enhancing image quality and classification accuracy by highlighting relevant features.Jain et al. [16] proposed an innovative approach that integrates quantum computing with machine learning to enhance the detection of diabetic retinopathy (DR). Their methodology employs a hybrid quantum transfer learning technique, utilizing various pretrained deep neural networks (DNNs), including ResNet-18, ResNet34, ResNet50, ResNet101, ResNet152, and Inception V3 for initial feature extraction. The final classification is performed using a Variational Quantum Classifier (VQC), and the model was evaluated on the APTOS 2019 Blindness Detection dataset, achieving an impressive accuracy of 97% with the ResNet-18 architecture. Ikram et al. [17] proposed the ResViT FusionNet model, a hybrid approach combining ResNet-50 CNNs and vision transformers to automate the grading of diabetic retinopathy (DR) from retinal images. This fusion leverages CNNs for capturing local features and ViTs for modeling global image context, achieving a high overall accuracy of 93.01%. The model also incorporates explainable AI techniques like LIME and Grad-CAM to provide visual interpretations of its predictions, enhancing clinical trust. Despite its strong performance in identifying healthy and moderate DR cases, the model shows lower recall and F1-scores for severe DR, indicating difficulties in precisely distinguishing advanced disease stages.

Folorunsho et al. [18] proposed an explainable ensemble deep learning model for predicting diabetic retinopathy using the APTOS 2019 eye dataset. This model combines multiple state-of-the-art neural networks—such as EfficientNet, DenseNet, and ResNeXt—into an ensemble to leverage their complementary strengths, resulting in improved accuracy and robustness in classifying the various stages of diabetic retinopathy. The approach includes extensive image preprocessing and data augmentation to handle the class imbalance and variability present in the dataset. Additionally, the model integrates explainability techniques like Grad-CAM to generate visual explanations, highlighting the key regions in retinal images that influenced its predictions, thereby enhancing clinical interpretability and trust. The ensemble achieves an accuracy between 79% and 81%, outperforming individual models, but it also faces limitations including high computational complexity and sensitivity to data quality. Related works in APTOS dataset are presented in Table 1.

Table 1 Related work in APTOS classification

References	Year	Methodology	Dataset	Evaluation
Khalifa et al. [7]	2019	Investigated deep transfer learning models (AlexNet, ResNet18, SqueezeNet, GoogleNet, VGG16, and VGG19)	APTOS 2019	AlexNet achieved the highest test accuracy: 97.9%
Adrimana et al. [8]	2020	Hybrid system: local binary patterns (LBP) with ResNet, DenseNet, and DetNet	APTOS 2019	Accuracy: 96.35% (ResNet); 93.99% (DetNet); 84.05% (DenseNet)
Mushtaq et al. [9]	2021	DenseNet-169 trained on combined datasets with regression model comparison	DR Detection 2015, APTOS 2019	Validation accuracy: 90.34% (DenseNet-169); 78.9% (regression)
Minarno et al. [10]	2022	EfficientNet-B7 with preprocessing techniques (Usuyama, Harikrishnan, ben Graham) and augmentation	APTOS 2019	Test accuracy: 84% (Usuyama preprocessing)
Obayya et al. [11]	2022	XAITO-DRGC model with median filtering, U-net segmentation, SqueezeNet feature extraction, and BGRCU classification	DDR	Accuracy: 98.24% (XAITO-DRGC); 84.10% (CNN512-dropout)
Mohanty et al. [12]	2023	Two approaches: VGG16 with XGBoost classifier and DenseNet-121	APTOS 2019	Accuracy: 97.30% (DenseNet-121); 79.50% (VGG16)
Akgül et al. [13]	2023	Enhanced VGG16 with dropout layers in classification and model blocks	APTOS 2019	Accuracy: 81.74%
Moustari et al. [14]	2024	Attention-guided CNN (AG-CNN) with DenseNet-121 baseline and grad-CAM for preprocessing	APTOS 2019	Accuracy: 98.48%; AUC: 0.998 with local branch

(continued)

Table 1 (continued)

References	Year	Methodology	Dataset	Evaluation
Akyel et al. [15]	2024	Hybrid approach: LinkNet-RCB7 for blood vessel segmentation and GLCM-based ensemble models	APTOS 2019	DR stage accuracy: 96.10%; binary classification accuracy: 97.46%
Jain et al. [16]	2024	Hybrid quantum transfer learning using pretrained DNNs (e.g., ResNet-18) and variational quantum classifier (VQC)	APTOS 2019	Accuracy: 97%
Ikram et al. [17]	2025	ResViT FusionNet which merges ResNet50 and ViT	APTOS 2019	Accuracy: 93.01%
Folorunsho et al. [18]	2025	CNN, long short-term memory (LSTM) networks, simple recurrent neural networks (SRNN), and XGBoost in an ensemble model (EM)	APTOS 2019	Accuracy: 95.63%

3 Motivation

The pressing need to enhance patient care and diagnostic accuracy in diabetic eye health is a key motivator for research into diabetic retinopathy (DR) detection. DR poses a significant global health challenge, potentially leading to severe vision impairment if not detected and treated in a timely manner. Accurate and prompt identification of DR is crucial for formulating effective treatment plans and improving patient management.

Several factors highlight the importance of advancing DR detection techniques:

- Clinical significance: Diagnosing diabetic retinopathy accurately can be complex due to the diverse ways it manifests and progresses. Improving detection methods enables healthcare providers to gain a deeper understanding of the condition and customize treatment approaches based on individual patient characteristics.
- Importance of early detection: Identifying DR at an early stage is vital for implementing timely interventions that can halt or slow the disease's progression, ultimately enhancing patient outcomes. Advanced classification systems can recognize early signs of retinal changes associated with DR, allowing for more focused and proactive treatment strategies.

- Utilization of cutting-edge technologies: Recent developments in machine learning, deep learning, and image analysis have opened new avenues for creating advanced models for DR detection. Leveraging these technologies has the potential to significantly improve diagnostic precision and efficiency, fundamentally changing how healthcare professionals manage diabetic eye health.

4 Proposed Methodology

In this work, we propose a hybrid architecture that integrates the pooling-based vision transformer (PiT) with the lightweight MobileNet-V2 model to address the unique challenges of diabetic retinopathy (DR) detection, particularly in resource-constrained and real-time diagnostic settings. DR detection from fundus images requires both fine-grained local feature extraction (e.g., microaneurysms, exudates) and the ability to capture broader contextual information across the retina (e.g., spatial distribution of lesions).

MobileNet-V2 [19] is a family of lightweight convolutional neural networks specifically designed for efficient performance on mobile and embedded devices. It achieves computational efficiency primarily through the use of depthwise separable convolutions, which significantly reduce the number of parameters and multiply-accumulate operations compared to standard convolutions. Notable advantages of MobileNet-V2 include its low latency, minimal memory footprint, and fast inference time—making it an excellent choice for real-time applications and deployment on resource-constrained devices. Furthermore, MobileNet-V2 is scalable in terms of width, depth, and resolution, allowing for customizable trade-offs between accuracy and computational cost. However, its lightweight design may lead to reduced representational power, especially when handling complex datasets or high-resolution images. Additionally, since MobileNet-V2 primarily focuses on local feature extraction, it may struggle to model long-range dependencies and global context—capabilities that transformer-based models are better equipped to handle.

PiT (pooling-based vision transformer) [20] is a vision transformer architecture that integrates pooling layers within transformer blocks to enhance computational efficiency and spatial generalization. Unlike traditional vision transformers such as ViT, which suffer from high computational complexity due to the global self-attention mechanism applied across all image patches, PiT introduces pooling to progressively reduce spatial dimensions, making the model more scalable. This architectural innovation allows PiT to effectively capture both local and global features while maintaining a relatively low computational footprint. Its strength lies in modeling long-range dependencies and contextual relationships across the image—attributes particularly valuable for tasks such as object detection, semantic segmentation, and DR detection. However, transformers generally require large datasets for effective training and tend to converge more slowly than convolutional networks, especially when trained from scratch on smaller datasets.

To integrate the lightweight local feature extraction capability of MobileNet-V2 with the global context modeling strength of PiT, we remove the classification head from MobileNet-V2 and retain its convolutional backbone as a feature extractor. The output feature map from the final convolutional layer is reshaped into a sequence of flattened patches. These patches are then passed through a linear projection layer to reduce dimensionality and are augmented with positional encodings to preserve spatial information. The resulting sequence forms the input to the PiT transformer block, enabling the model to capture both local features and long-range dependencies in a unified architecture.

Training of the proposed model is optimized using the layer-wise adaptive moments (LAMB) optimizer [21], which is particularly effective for training deep networks with large batch sizes. LAMB extends the widely used Adam optimizer by incorporating layer-wise adaptive learning rate scaling as in Eq. (1), enabling each layer to adjust its update magnitude based on its weight norm as in Eq. (2). This results in more stable training and faster convergence, particularly for large-scale models such as transformers. So, the key innovation of LAMB lies in its "trust ratio," a layer-wise adaptive scaling factor that distinguishes it from optimizers like Adam and SGD.

$$\text{trsut ratio} = \frac{\|\theta_t\|}{\|r_t\|} \tag{1}$$

While the final parameter update is

$$\theta_{t+1} = \theta_t - n_t.\text{trust ratio}.r_t \tag{2}$$

where $\|\theta_t\|$ the norm of the parameter for the layer is, $\|r_t\|$ is the norm of the Adam-like update for the layer and n_t is the learning rate.

For the images in the preprocessing phase, we applied the CLAHE filter [22] that was utilized for contrast enhancement by segmenting every image into small regions, equalizing the histograms locally in those regions, and thus adjusting the contrast with noise control. Besides, black background pixels of intensity values close to zero were excluded to ensure that the model focused on significant retinal features.

The overall process of our proposed method is illustrated in Fig. 1 and follows a structured pipeline. Data preprocessing involves preparing the dataset through normalization, augmentation then applies CLAHE filter [14], and splitting into training and validation subsets. In the feature extraction and model fusion stage, features are independently extracted from PiT and MobileNet-V2 models, and then concatenated to create a unified representation that leverages the strengths of both architectures. Model optimization is carried out using the LAMB optimizer, which ensures efficient and stable training, particularly in large-batch scenarios. Finally, in the performance evaluation phase, the effectiveness of the proposed method is assessed using a range of evaluation metrics to determine its accuracy, robustness, and generalization performance.

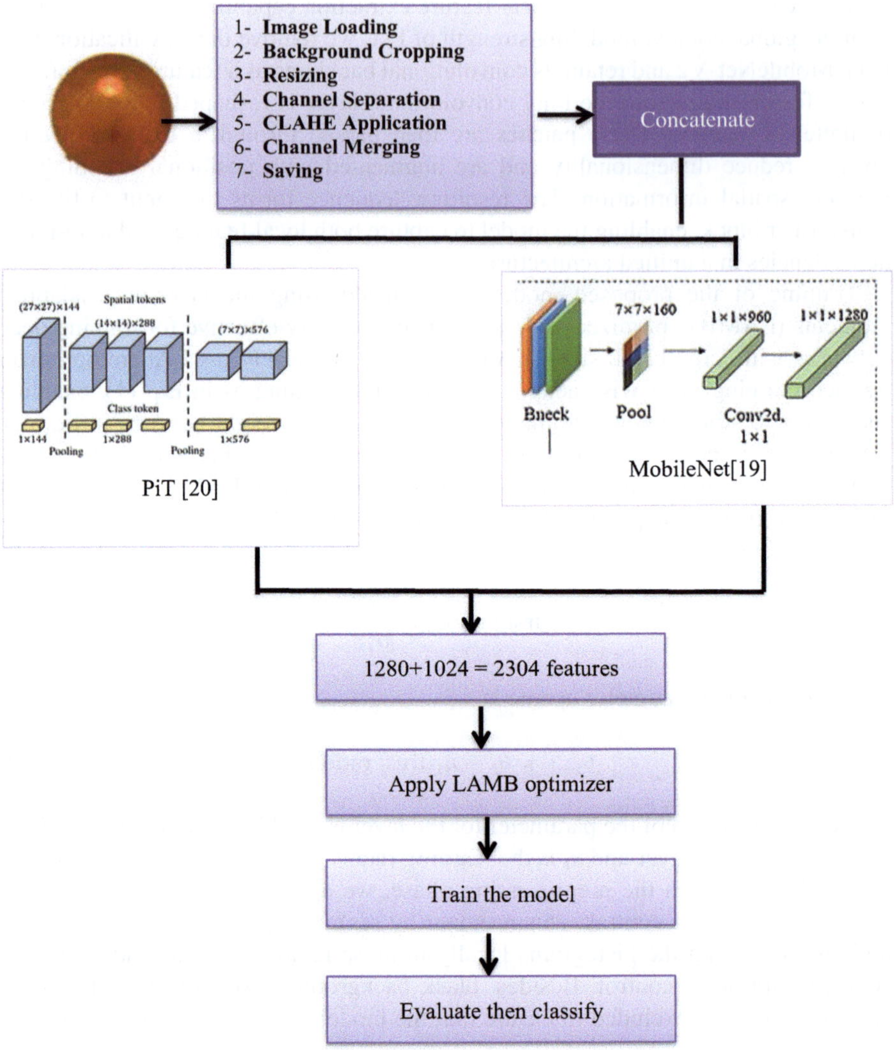

Fig. 1 The pipeline steps of our proposed model

4.1 Datasets

The APTOS 2019 dataset from https://www.kaggle.com/datasets/mariaherrerot/aptos2019, which was a part of the Blindness Detection competition, comprises 3662 retinal fundus images, labeled into five categories according to the International Clinical Diabetic Retinopathy scale: No DR, mild, moderate, severe, and proliferative DR as in Table 2.

Table 2 The APTOS 2019 dataset's class distribution

Class name	Number of samples
No DR	1805 samples
Mild DR	370 samples
Moderate DR	999 samples
Severe DR	193 samples
Proliferative DR	295 samples

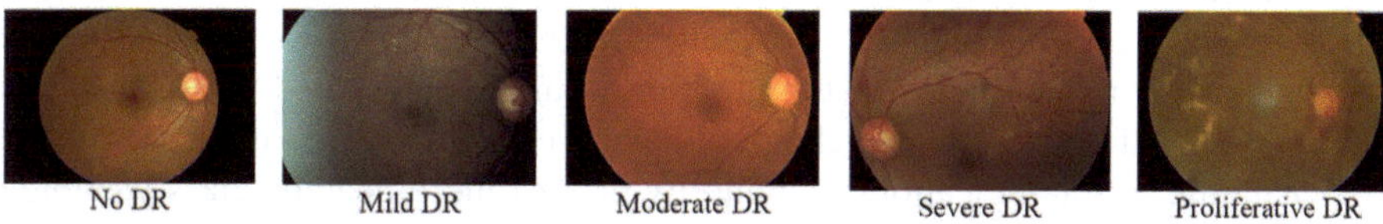

Fig. 2 Samples of the dataset

While no DR means no visibility abnormalities in the retina. Also, there are no signs of diabetic retinopathy such as microaneurysms, hemorrhages, or exudates. The retina appears healthy and unaffected by diabetes-related damage. But, mild DR is characterized by the presence of microaneurysms, which are small bulges in the retinal blood vessels. These are usually the earliest visible signs of DR. At this point, vision is typically unaffected, but the disease has begun. With moderate DR, there are an increased number of microaneurysms and retinal hemorrhages, along with possible hard exudates (lipid deposits). The damage is more widespread, and blood vessels may begin to leak fluid into the retina, potentially affecting vision. But with severe DR, there is extensive retinal damage with numerous hemorrhages and microaneurysms in all four quadrants of the retina, along with venous beading and intraretinal microvascular abnormalities (IRMA). This stage is a critical point before the retina begins to develop new abnormal blood vessels. The risk of progression to proliferative DR is high. While proliferative DR is the most advanced stage, where the retina begins to grow new, fragile blood vessels (neovascularization) as a response to poor oxygen supply. These vessels are prone to leaking and bleeding into the vitreous, potentially leading to retinal detachment, scar tissue, and vision loss. Immediate medical intervention is typically required as in Fig. 2.

To ensure consistent image quality and effective learning, all fundus images were subjected to a standardized preprocessing pipeline:

1. Image loading: Raw images were loaded from the original dataset.
2. Background cropping: The black background was removed by applying a grayscale threshold to isolate the circular fundus region.
3. Resizing: Images were resized to a uniform size of 224 × 224 pixels to match the input requirements of MobileNet-V2 and PiT.
4. Channel separation: Images were split into blue, green, and red (BGR) channels to perform localized enhancements.
5. CLAHE application: Contrast limited adaptive histogram equalization (CLAHE) was applied to each channel individually to enhance local contrast.

6. Channel merging: The enhanced B, G, and R channels were merged back into a single RGB image.
7. Saving: The preprocessed image was saved to a new directory for training and evaluation.

To address the significant class imbalance present in the APTOS 2019 dataset, we employed a class-weighted loss function during training. Specifically, we used a weighted categorical cross-entropy loss, where the weight assigned to each class was inversely proportional to its frequency in the training data. This approach ensures that the model pays greater attention to underrepresented classes such as severe and proliferative DR, which are clinically critical but sparse in the dataset. By penalizing misclassifications of minority classes more heavily, class-weighted loss helps balance the learning process and improves the model's sensitivity to rare disease stages without requiring oversampling or data augmentation techniques.

5 Experiments and Results

This research utilized the APTOS 2019 Blindness Detection dataset, which comprises 3662 curated and annotated retinal fundus images categorized into five classes: No DR, mild, moderate, severe, and proliferate DR, as detailed in Table 2. The dataset was divided into training and validation sets after undergoing preprocessing steps such as resizing and normalization. To tackle class imbalance, class weights were calculated based on the distribution of classes, allowing for effective learning from underrepresented categories. The optimal hyperparameter settings for the best-performing model (PiT_base Transformer combined with Mobile Net using the Lamb optimizer) are as follows: LEARNING_RATE = 1e-4 TRAIN_BATCH_SIZE = 32 VALID_BATCH_SIZE = 32 TRAIN_SPLIT = 0.8 NUM_WORKERS = 2 USE_AMP = True EPOCHS = 20, CrossEntropyLoss for the loss function and Lamb as the optimizer. The models were trained using PyTorch on Kaggle with a GPU (P100).

The evaluation of the models involves an analysis based on parameters such as accuracy in training, sensitivity (or recall), precision (or positive predictive value—PPV). To calculate precision and recall, we utilize true positive (TP), false positive (FP), true negative (TN), and false negative (FN) samples. Recall, also known as sensitivity, this is determined by dividing the number of true positives by the sum of true positives and false negatives. In medical diagnosis, the high recall is imperative for accurately identifying individuals with the disease, as overlooking the positive category can result in serious consequences like misdiagnosis and treatment delays. Precision (PPV) becomes crucial when assessing the proportion of predicted positive examples that are genuinely positive. Precision is calculated by dividing the number of true positives by the sum of true positives and false positives.

In the realm of medical imaging, achieving high precision is highly desirable. The F1-score for all models is derived from the sensitivity and precision values. The provided formulas are applied to calculate accuracy, precision, sensitivity, and the F1-score [23].

$$\text{Percision}_i = \frac{\text{TP}_i}{\text{TP}_i + \text{FP}_i} \tag{3}$$

$$\text{Recall}_i = \frac{\text{TP}_i}{\text{TP}_i + \text{FN}_i} \tag{4}$$

$$F\text{-score}_i = \frac{2 * \text{Percision}_i * \text{Recall}_i}{\text{Percision}_i + \text{Recall}_i} \tag{5}$$

where i name of the class for the dataset, *TP* true positive, *FN* false negative, *TN* true negative. Figures 3 and 4 illustrate the training and validation loss and accuracy, respectively, while Fig. 5 presents the precision, recall, and F1-score for the model.

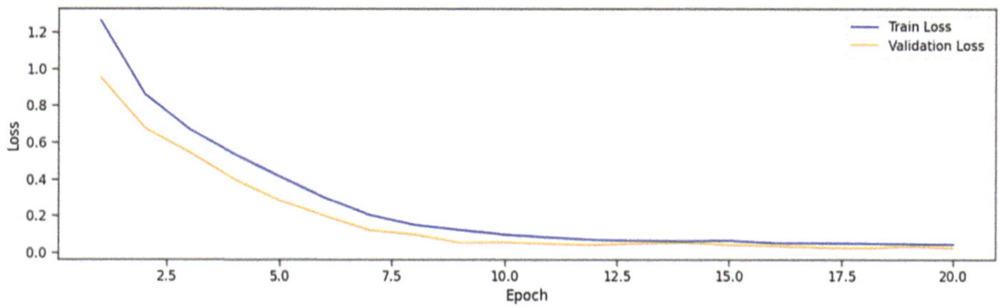

Fig. 3 Training and validation loss per epoch

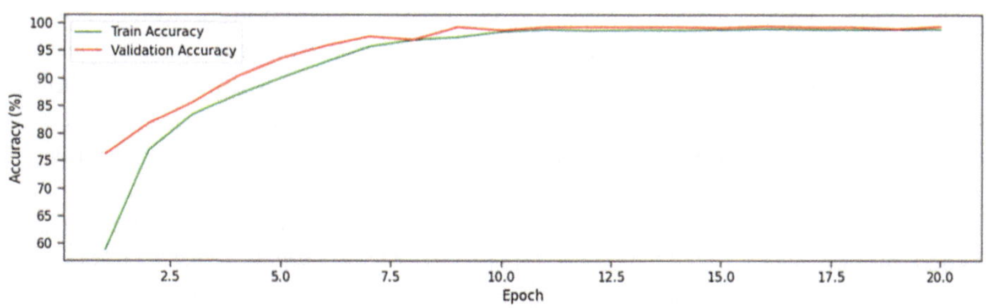

Fig. 4 Training and validation accuracy per epoch for our proposed model

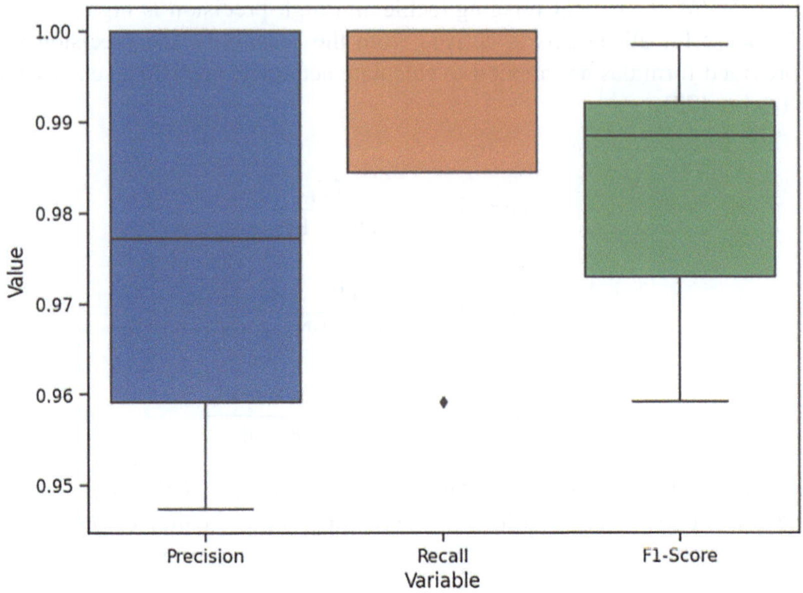

Fig. 5 Precision, recall, and F1-score per class

5.1 Performance Evaluation Methods

The evaluation of transformer-based models for retinopathy detection highlighted the effectiveness of different architectures and optimization techniques. Our approach, PiT_Base_224 with MobileNet-V2, achieved strong performance, reaching 99.43% accuracy with the Lamb optimizer. As in Table 3, the results presented in the table demonstrate the effectiveness of combining different models and optimizers for diabetic retinopathy diagnosis. Overall, the Lamb optimizer consistently outperformed Adam across most model configurations. For the standalone models, PiT-Base-224 achieved a slight improvement in accuracy when switching from Adam (99.15%) to Lamb (99.29%), while MobileNet-V2 showed a similar trend, increasing from 99.29% to 99.43%. In terms of average precision and recall, MobileNet-V2 with Lamb (99% and 98.2%, respectively) performed better than with Adam. The DeiT model maintained the same accuracy with both optimizers but showed higher recall (99.2%) with Lamb compared to Adam. When models were fused, such as DeiT with MobileNet-V2 and PiT-Base-224 with MobileNet-V2, further improvements were observed. Notably, PiT-Base-224 fused with MobileNet-V2 and optimized by Lamb achieved the highest results across all metrics: 99.43% accuracy, 99.6% average precision, and 98.4% average recall. Conversely, some fused models like DeiT with PiT-Base-224 showed less-significant gains. Overall, these findings highlight that model fusion combined with the Lamb optimizer yields superior performance, emphasizing the advantage

Table 3 Comparison between the individual models using the Adam and Lamb optimizer

Model	Optimizer	Accuracy (%)	Avg. precision (%)	Avg. recall (%)
PiT-Base-224	Adam	99.15	98	98.8
	Lamb	99.29	98	98.8
MobileNet-V2	Adam	99.29	98.4	97.4
	Lamb	99.43	99	98.2
DeiT	Adam	99.29	97.6	98.8
	Lamb	99.29	98.2	99.2
DeiT with MobileNet-V2	Adam	99.29	98.6	99.2
	Lamb	99.01	97.8	99
PiT-Base-224 with MobileNet-V2	Adam	99.29	99	98.2
	Lamb	99.43	99.6	98.4
DeiT with PiT-Base-224	Adam	99.01	98.6	97.6
	Lamb	99.01	98.6	98.2

of integrating lightweight architectures with powerful optimization techniques for medical imaging tasks.

Although both MobileNet-V2 with the Lamb optimizer and the fused PiT-Base-224 with MobileNet-V2 model using Lamb achieve the same overall accuracy of 99.43%, there are notable differences in their performance and architecture. The fused model shows a significant improvement in average precision, reaching 99.6% compared to 99% for MobileNet-V2 alone, and a slight improvement in average recall (98.4% vs. 98.2%). This indicates that the fusion of PiT-Base-224 with MobileNet-V2 enhances the model's ability to correctly classify diabetic retinopathy cases with fewer false positives and negatives. Architecturally, MobileNet-V2 is a lightweight convolutional model designed for efficiency, while the fused model combines the strengths of PiT, a compact vision transformer, with MobileNet-V2 to enrich feature extraction. As a result, the fused model is slightly more complex but offers greater robustness and reliability, making it more suitable for sensitive medical applications where precision is critical.

The training and validation loss curves in Fig. 6 show that all models, optimized with the Lamb optimizer, converge well with minimal overfitting. Among them, the PiT-Base-224 combined with DeiT and PiT-Base-224 combined with MobileNet-V2 models (Fig. 6d, f) perform the best, achieving the lowest and most stable losses. Their smooth, early-converging curves and minimal gap between training and validation loss indicate strong learning and generalization, highlighting the advantage of combining models for richer feature representation.

The training results show that the models PiT-Base-224 combined with DeiT Fig. 7d and PiT-Base-224 combined with MobileNet-V2 Fig. 7f perform the best. They achieve the lowest training and validation losses and the highest, most stable accuracies with minimal overfitting. This indicates that combining models captures

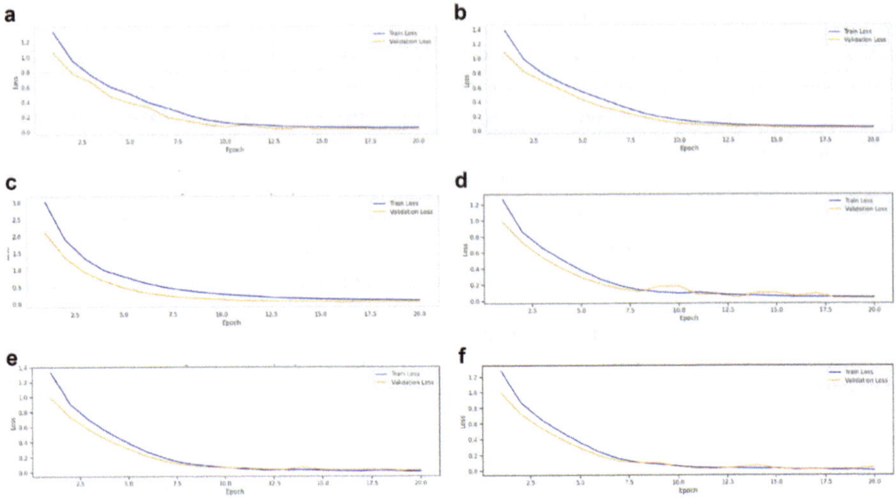

Fig. 6 Training and validation loss curves for each model. (**a**) PiT-Base-224 using Lamb optimizer. (**b**) DeiT using lamb optimizer. (**c**) MobileNet-V2 with Lamb optimizer. (**d**) PiT-Base-224 with DeiT using Lamb optimizer. (**e**) DeiT with MobileNet-V2 using Lamb optimizer. (**f**) PiT-Base-224 with MobileNet-V2using Lamb optimizer

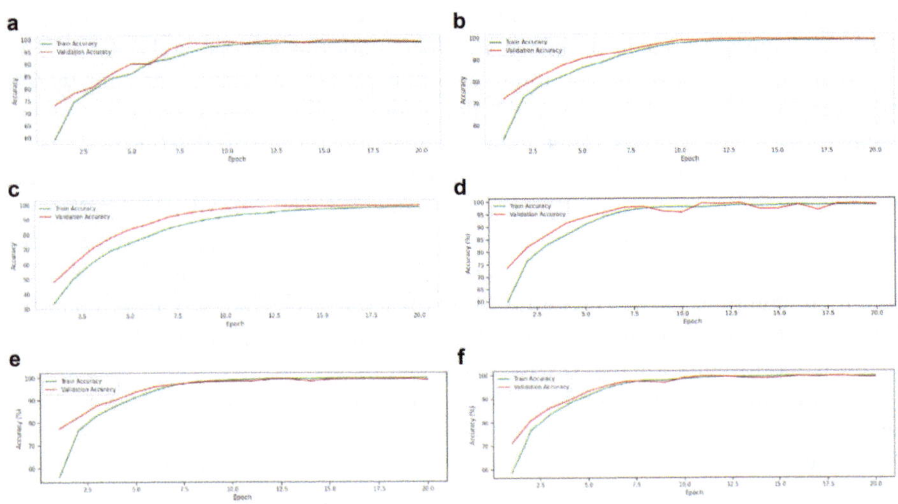

Fig. 7 Accuracy curves for each model. (**a**) PiT-Base-224 using Lamb optimizer. (**b**) DeiT using Lamb optimizer. (**c**) MobileNet-V2 with Lamb optimizer. (**d**) PiT-Base-224 with DeiT using Lamb optimizer. (**e**) DeiT with MobileNet-V2 using Lamb optimizer. (**f**) PiT-Base-224 with MobileNet-V2 V2 using Lamb optimizer

richer features and, with the Lamb optimizer, leads to better convergence and generalization compared to using single models.

In medical diagnosis, precision and recall are crucial for evaluating model performance, as misclassifications can have serious consequences. Our PiT-Base-224 with MobileNet-V2 model, optimized with Lamb, achieves high precision and recall, minimizing false positives and false negatives. The confusion matrix provides a detailed breakdown of predictions, helping assess the model's reliability in medical applications, as in Fig. 8.

In Table 4, we evaluate several deep learning models using two optimizers—Adam and Lamb—based on key performance metrics. The analysis considers not only accuracy, precision, and recall, but also training time and number of parameters, offering a complete view of each model's efficiency and effectiveness. The goal is to identify the best-performing configuration in terms of both predictive power and computational cost.

Based on the comparison of accuracy, precision, recall, training time, and model size, two models clearly stand out. MobileNet-V2 with the Lamb optimizer offers the best balance of performance and efficiency, achieving the highest accuracy (99.43%) with a very small model size (22 million parameters) and the fastest training time among high-performing models (355.67 s). However, the most powerful and well-rounded model overall is the combination of PiT-Base-224 with MobileNet-V2 using the Lamb optimizer. This model not only matches the highest accuracy (99.43%) but also achieves the highest average precision (99.6%) and strong recall (98.4%), making it especially effective in tasks where minimizing false positives is crucial. While it requires more training time (1679.10 s) and a larger model size (74.9 million parameters), it still remains significantly more efficient than heavier alternatives like DeiT + PiT-Base-224. Therefore, PiT + MobileNet with Lamb stands out as the best overall model when both performance and reliability are priorities.

6 Conclusion

This study explored the effectiveness of advanced deep learning models—specifically MobileNet-V2, DeiT, and PiT-based transformer architectures—for the detection of diabetic retinopathy using the APTOS 2019 blindness detection dataset. By integrating the lightweight efficiency of MobileNet-V2 with the global feature representation strengths of vision transformers, we developed a hybrid model that achieved impressive diagnostic accuracy. Among the evaluated approaches, the combination of PiT-Base-224 and MobileNet-V2, optimized with the LAMB optimizer, delivered the best performance, achieving an accuracy of 99.43%, along with high precision and recall. These results highlight the potential of such hybrid architectures in building effective early screening tools for diabetic retinopathy. However, the model is not without limitations. The use of an imbalanced dataset may impact its ability to generalize across varied clinical settings, and the increased complexity resulting from merging distinct architectures could pose challenges for real-time deployment in low-resource environments.

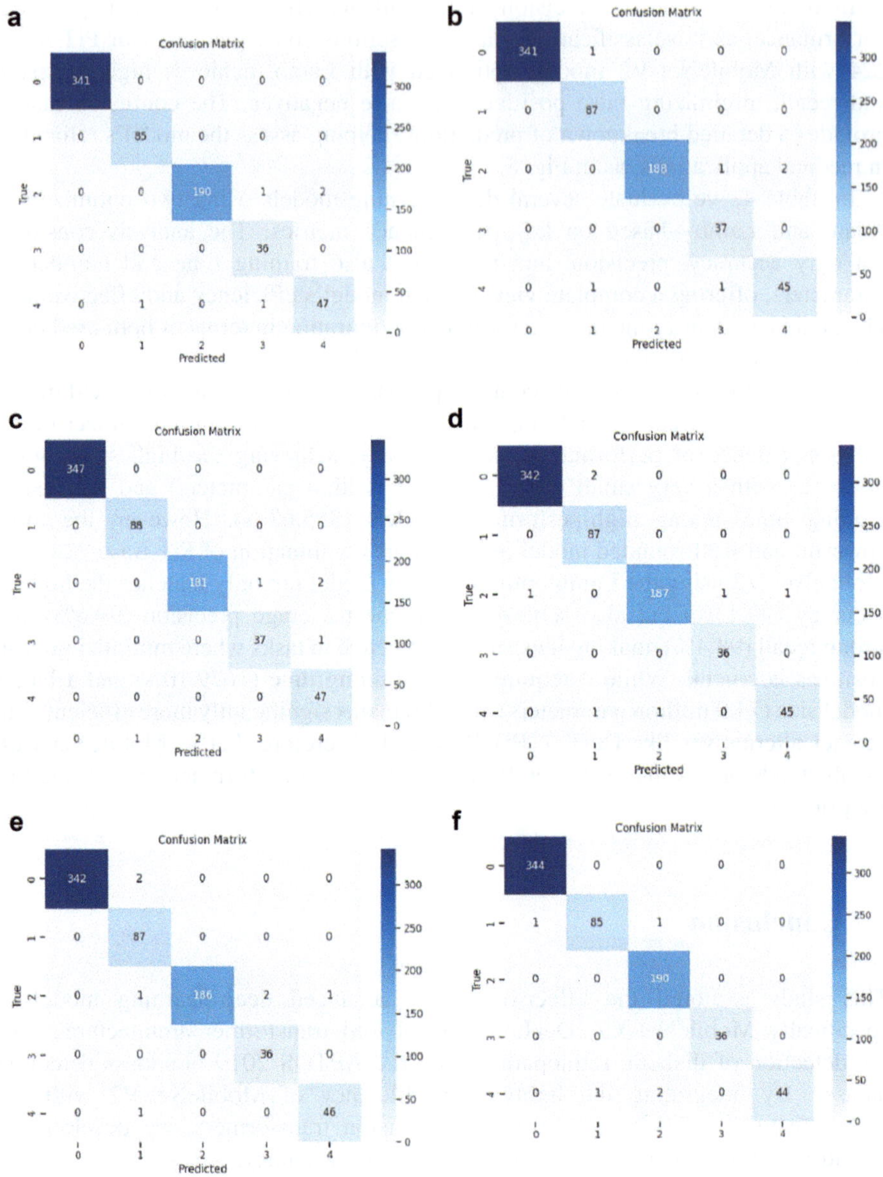

Fig. 8 Confusion matrices for different models using Adam and Lamb optimizers. (**a**) PiT-Base-224 using Lamb optimizer. (**b**) DeiT using Lamb optimizer. (**c**) MobileNet-V2 with Lamb optimizer. (**d**) PiT-Base-224 with DeiT using Lamb optimizer. (**e**) DeiT with MobileNet-V2 using Lamb optimizer. (**f**) PiT-Base-224 with MobileNet-V2 V2 using Lamb optimizer

Table 4 Model performance vs. training time and parameters (Adam vs. Lamb)

Model	Optimizer	Training time (s)	# parameters
PiT-Base-224	Adam	1382.09	72,744,965
	Lamb	1379.67	
MobileNet-V2	Adam	253.97	22,302,77
	Lamb	355.67	
DeiT	Adam	1406.8	85,802,501
	Lamb	1483	
DeiT with MobileNet-V2	Adam	1615.98	88,032,773
	Lamb	1806.83	
PiT-Base-224 with MobileNet-V2	Adam	1463.6	74,975,237
	Lamb	1679.10	
DeiT with PiT-Base-224	Adam	2693.51	158,547,461
	Lamb	2812.4	

Future work will involve evaluating the model on more balanced and diverse datasets, improving computational efficiency, and exploring newer transformer models to further enhance its reliability and applicability.

Data Availability The data used in this chapter are available at https://www.kaggle.com/datasets/mariaherrerot/aptos2019.
Code availability: https://github.com/youssef-khalf/APTOS-Detection

References

1. R. Kommaraju, M.S. Anbarasi, *Detection of Diabetic Retinopathy (DR) Severity from Fundus Photographs Using Swin Transformer* (IEEE, New York, 2023), pp. 1–6. https://doi.org/10.1109/icraie59459.2023.10468500
2. H.S. Yousef, M.E. Ahmed, E.A.G.A.E. Wafa, M.A.K. Salih, Epidemiology and risk factors of diabetic retinopathy in upper Egypt: A 3-year prospective study. J. Egypt. Ophthalmol. Soc. **117**(2), 178–183 (2024). https://doi.org/10.4103/ejos.ejos_6_24
3. J. Wu, R. Hu, Z. Xiao, J. Chen, J. Liu, Vision transformer-based recognition of diabetic retinopathy grade. Med. Phys. **48**(12), 7850–7863 (2021). https://doi.org/10.1002/mp.15312
4. M.Z. Atwany, A.H. Sahyoun, M. Yaqub, Deep learning techniques for diabetic retinopathy classification: A survey. IEEE Access **10**, 28642–28655 (2022). https://doi.org/10.1109/access.2022.3157632
5. N.J. Mohan, R. Murugan, T. Goel, P. Roy, *ViT-DR: Vision Transformers in Diabetic Retinopathy Grading Using Fundus Images* (IEEE, New York, 2022), pp. 167–172. https://doi.org/10.1109/r10-htc54060.2022.9930027
6. B. Menaouer, Z. Dermane, N.E.H. Kebir, N. Matta, Diabetic retinopathy classification using hybrid deep learning approach. SN Comput. Sci. **3**(5), 1–15 (2022). https://doi.org/10.1007/s42979-022-01240-8
7. N. Khalifa, M. Loey, M. Taha, H. Mohamed, Deep transfer learning models for medical diabetic retinopathy detection. Acta Inform. Med. **27**(5), 327 (2019). https://doi.org/10.5455/aim.2019.27.327-332

8. R. Adriman, K. Muchtar, N. Maulina, Performance evaluation of binary classification of diabetic retinopathy through deep learning techniques using texture feature. Proc. Comput. Sci. **179**, 88–94 (2021). https://doi.org/10.1016/j.procs.2020.12.012
9. G. Mushtaq, F. Siddiqui, Detection of diabetic retinopathy using deep learning methodology. IOP Conf. Seri. Mater. Sci. Eng. **1070**(1), 012049 (2021). https://doi.org/10.1088/1757-899x/1070/1/012049
10. A.E. Minarno, M.H.C. Mandiri, Y. Azhar, F. Bimantoro, H.A. Nugroho, Z. Ibrahim, Classification of diabetic retinopathy disease using convolutional neural network. JOIV Int. J. Inf. Visual. **6**(1), 12 (2022). https://doi.org/10.30630/joiv.6.1.857
11. M. Obayya et al., Explainable artificial intelligence enabled TeleOphthalmology for diabetic retinopathy grading and classification. Appl. Sci. **12**(17), 8749 (2022). https://doi.org/10.3390/app12178749
12. C. Mohanty et al., Using deep learning architectures for detection and classification of diabetic retinopathy. Sensors **23**(12), 5726 (2023). https://doi.org/10.3390/s23125726
13. İ. Akgül, Ö.Ç. Yavuz, U. Yavuz, Deep learning based models for detection of diabetic retinopathy. Tehnički Glasnik **17**(4), 581–587 (2023). https://doi.org/10.31803/tg-20220905123827
14. A.M. Moustari, Y. Brik, B. Attallah, R. Bouaouina, Two-stage deep learning classification for diabetic retinopathy using gradient weighted class activation mapping. Automatika **65**(3), 1284–1299 (2024). https://doi.org/10.1080/00051144.2024.2363692
15. C. Akyel, B. Ciylan, Blood vessel segmentation and classification of diabetic retinopathy with machine learning-based ensemble model. J. Adv. Res. Nat. Appl. Sci. **10**(3), 560–570 (2024). https://doi.org/10.28979/jarnas.1482123
16. V. Gupta, Y. Dash, S.C. Sarangi, A. Abraham, Quantum transfer learning for enhanced diabetic retinopathy detection using ResNet architecture, in *Lecture Notes in Networks and Systems*, (Springer, Cham, 2025), pp. 562–571. https://doi.org/10.1007/978-3-031-81080-0_53
17. A. Ikram, A. Imran, ResViT FusionNet model: An explainable AI-driven approach for automated grading of diabetic retinopathy in retinal images. Comput. Biol. Med. **186**, 109656 (2025). https://doi.org/10.1016/j.compbiomed.2025.109656
18. O. Folorunsho, S.E. Akinsanya, O.A. Fagbuagun, S.A. Mogaji, S.K. Raji, Explainable ensemble deep learning model for predicting diabetic retinopathy based on APTOS 2019 eye pack dataset. LAUTECH J. Eng. Technol. **19**(1), 1–14 (2025). https://doi.org/10.36108/laujet/5202.91.0110
19. M. Sandler, A. Howard, M. Zhu, A. Zhmoginov, L.-C. Chen, MobileNetV2: Inverted residuals and linear bottlenecks. arXiv.org (2018), https://arxiv.org/abs/1801.04381
20. B. Heo, S. Yun, D. Han, S. Chun, J. Choe, S.J. Oh, Rethinking spatial dimensions of vision transformers, in *2021 IEEE/CVF International Conference on Computer Vision (ICCV)*, (IEEE, New York, 2021), pp. 11916–11925. https://doi.org/10.1109/iccv48922.2021.01172
21. Y. You, et al., Large batch optimization for deep learning: Training BERT in 76 minutes. OpenReview, https://openreview.net/forum?id=hKsZjzF4H5Z
22. E.A. Tjoa, I.P.Y.N. Suparta, R. Magdalena, N.K. Cp, The use of CLAHE for improving an accuracy of CNN architecture for detecting pneumonia. SHS Web Conf. **139**, 03026 (2022). https://doi.org/10.1051/shsconf/202213903026
23. V. Tuyet, N. Hien, P. Quoc, N. Son, N. Binh, Adaptive content-based medical image retrieval based on local features extraction in Shearlet domain. EAI Endors. Trans. Context-Aware Syst. Appl. **6**(17), 159351 (2019). https://doi.org/10.4108/eai.18-3-2019.159351

A Comprehensive Approach to Skin Lesion Classification Using Machine and Deep Learning

Sultan Tazefidan and Gulay Cicek

Abstract Early diagnosis of skin lesions is crucial due to lack of definitive treatment options, as timely and accurate classification is essential for identifying malignant lesions. This study focuses on classifying malignant and rare skin lesions using the 10,132 images from the ISIC2019 dataset, which comprises eight classes: melanoma, melanocytic nevus, basal cell carcinoma, actinic keratoses and intraepithelial carcinoma, benign keratosis-like lesions, dermatofibroma, vascular lesion, and squamous cell carcinoma. The dataset was augmented to increase its sample size. Classification was performed using both machine learning techniques (KNN, SVM, DT, RF, ANN) and deep learning models (VGG19, Inception-V3, U-Net, CNN, RNN). To address dataset imbalance, a hybrid algorithm integrating SMOTE was developed, and transfer learning was applied to the convolutional layers of VGG16 and ResNet50. The dense and flatten layers were customized according to the dataset. Feature extraction was used to enhance classification performance. Model performance was evaluated using accuracy, recall, specificity, precision, F1 score, and AUC-ROC metrics. The hybrid algorithm achieved 86.48% accuracy on the PCA test set and 88.05% on the LDA test set. This study offers an approach for classifying eight rarely studied skin lesion types. Future research could benefit from data augmentation and strategies to address class imbalance.

Keywords Skin lesion classification · Deep learning · Machine learning · Transfer learning · Hybrid algorithm

---

S. Tazefidan
Software Engineering Department, Faculty of Engineering and Architecture, Istanbul Beykent University, Istanbul, Türkiye
e-mail: 2203013086@student.beykent.edu.tr

G. Cicek (✉)
Biomedical Engineering Department, Faculty of Engineering and Architecture, Istanbul Beykent University, Istanbul, Türkiye
e-mail: gulaycicek@beykent.edu.tr

N. E. M. Khalifa, M. H. N. Taha (eds.), *Next-Gen Healthcare*,
https://doi.org/10.1007/978-3-032-07267-2_13

List of Abbreviations

AI	Artificial intelligence
AKIEC	Actinic keratoses and intraepithelial carcinoma
ANN	Artificial neural network
Adam	Adaptive moment estimation
AdamW	Adam with weight decay regularization
AUC-ROC	Area under the receiver operating characteristic curve
BCC	Basal cell carcinoma
BKL	Benign keratosis-like lesions
CAD	Computer-aided diagnosis
CNN	Convolutional neural network
DF	Dermatofibroma
DL	Deep learning
DT	Decision tree
FNN	Feedforward neural network
GAN	Generative adversarial network
Grid Search	Grid search optimization
KNN	K-nearest neighbors
LDA	Linear discriminant analysis
LSTM	Long short-term memory
MEL	Melanoma
ML	Machine learning
MLP	Multilayer perceptron
NV	Melanocytic nevi
Optuna	Optimization software framework
PCA	Principal component analysis
PSO	Particle swarm optimization
RandomizedSearchCV	Randomized search cross-validation
RF	Random forest
RMSprop	Root mean square propagation
RNN	Recurrent neural network
SCC	Squamous cell carcinoma
SGD	Stochastic gradient descent
SMOTE	Synthetic minority oversampling technique
SVM	Support vector machine
VASC	Vascular lesions
ViT	Visual transformer

1 Introduction

Skin cancer is a malignancy that arises from the uncontrolled proliferation and growth of cells [1]. It is among the most common types of cancer worldwide, and its primary causes include direct exposure to the sun, excessive use of tanning beds and similar devices, as well as various environmental factors [2]. According to research conducted by the World Health Organization, one in every three diagnosed cancers is skin cancer. Although everyone is at risk of developing skin cancer, individuals with fair skin, multiple large moles, and those subjected to prolonged sun exposure are at an elevated risk [3]. Among the contributing factors to cancer, it has been proposed that the diminishing protective capacity of the atmosphere allows greater amounts of UV radiation to reach the Earth's surface, leading to lesions caused by direct sun exposure [4]. Figure 1 illustrates how common types of skin cancer affect different layers of the skin. The image was sourced from iStock and is used with the appropriate license.

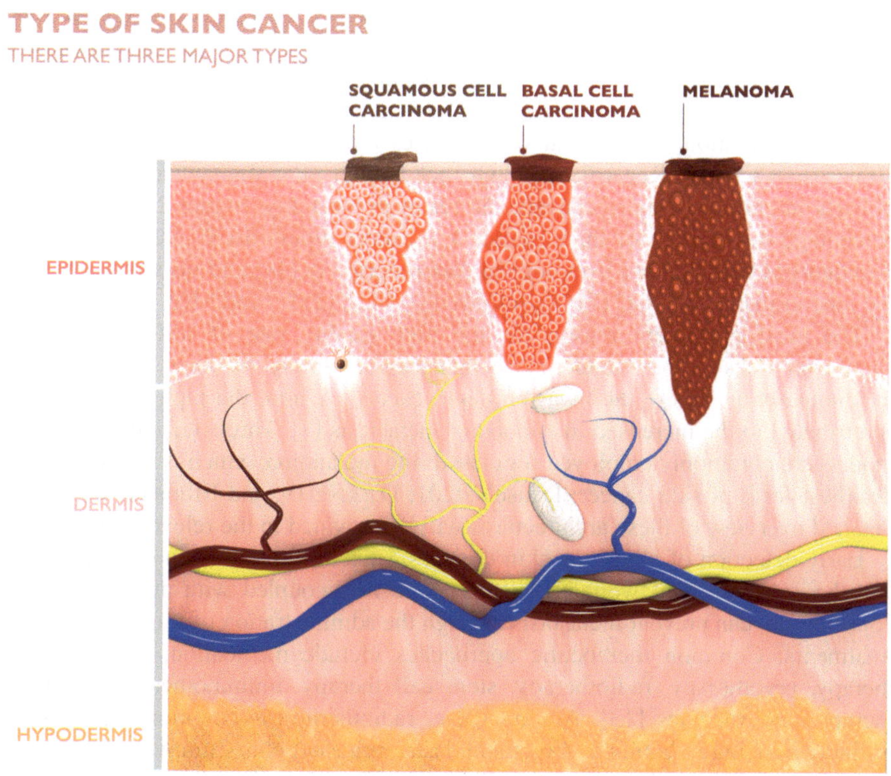

Fig. 1 3D representation of the skin structure (epidermis, dermis, hypodermis) and the typical locations of skin cancer types (squamous cell carcinoma, basal cell carcinoma, melanoma). Source: iStock, licensed for use

Analysis of data on the incidence of skin cancer in our country reveals a 237% increase over the past 30 years [5]. Active cancer registration, initially implemented in only two provinces in 2002, was extended to cover all 81 provinces both in our country and globally by 2013 [6].

According to research conducted by the American Cancer Society, approximately 96,480 cases of melanoma skin cancer were expected to be diagnosed in 2019, with 7,230 of these patients projected to succumb to the disease [7]. Researchers at the University Hospital of Nice in France, using data collected from the World Health Organization's International Agency for Research on Cancer, evaluated the mortality rates associated with skin cancer. The study concluded that in 2020, accounted for 57,000 deaths, while nonmelanoma skin cancers were responsible for 63,700 deaths [8].

Given the data, early diagnosis plays a crucial role in the fight against skin cancer. While there is no definitive cure for this disease, if left untreated, it can be fatal. Early detection of Stage 1 and 2 lesions is associated with a 98% success rate over a five-year period [9]. Research indicates that survival rates are considerably higher when accurate diagnoses are made and appropriate treatments are administered [7]. Among the high-risk malignant cancers, melanoma (MEL) and squamous cell carcinoma (SCC) are recognized as major risk factors. Additionally, basal cell carcinoma (BCC) and actinic keratoses and intraepithelial carcinoma (AKIEC), although generally considered benign, are prevalent conditions. Analysis of case distribution reveals that 6% of cases are SCC, 4% are melanoma, and 80% are BCC [10]. Regardless of whether benign or malignant, in the absence of early intervention, these cancers can result in mortality. Figure 2 illustrates the percentage distribution of three major skin cancer types—BCC, SCC, and MEL. The figure is based on epidemiological data reported in [11] and visually highlights the predominance of BCC (71%), followed by SCC (25%) and MEL (4%).

The most prominent reason for the high fatality rate of lesions that pose significant risks is their tendency to metastasize rapidly to other tissues [7]. In melanoma cases where the invasion depth exceeds 2 mm, the high mortality rate is attributed to the increased likelihood of metastasis [7]. Three deep learning (DL) models are commonly employed for classifying melanoma, which is considered the deadliest form of skin cancer: DenseNet201, DarkNet19, and EfficientNet [12]. A detailed overview of these architectures will be provided in the relevant section.

Early detection of abnormal skin changes, such as alterations in color or shape and the appearance of wounds, blisters, or rashes, coupled with prompt medical consultation, can prevent metastasis through the administration of stage-appropriate treatments. Common therapeutic approaches include medication, surgery, laser therapy, cryotherapy, radiotherapy, stem cell therapy, immunotherapy, hormone therapy, and vaccines [13]. Among these, radiotherapy is commonly employed, utilizing ionizing radiation to target and destroy cancer cells. Curative radiotherapy aims to control or reduce cancer cell proliferation, focusing either on a specific region or the entire body [14]. If a late diagnosis leads to cancer metastasizing to healthy tissues cells, more aggressive treatments, such as chemotherapy, become necessary. Chemotherapy can be categorized into primary induction chemotherapy

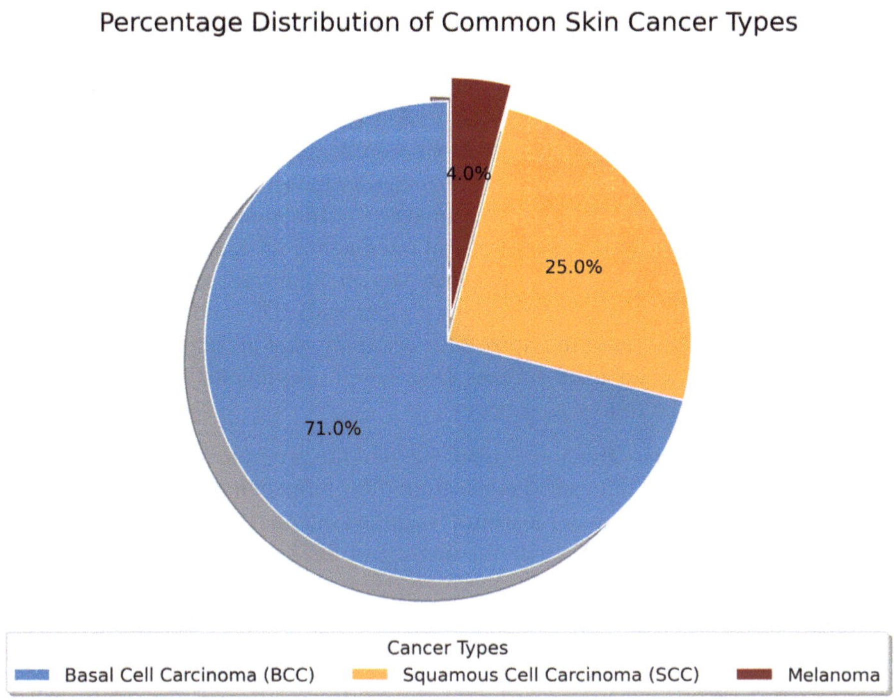

Fig. 2 Percentage distribution of common skin cancer types (BCC, SCC, and MEL), illustrated by the authors for illustrative purposes

and neoadjuvant chemotherapy. Primary induction is used as the initial treatment when other options are no longer viable, while neoadjuvant chemotherapy is employed for localized cancers where surgery alone is insufficient [15].

Even for experts, diagnosing skin lesions can be challenging due to factors such as irregular shapes, unclear boundaries, low contrast, and interference from skin hair, fatty tissue, or air bubbles [10]. Traditional methods have an accuracy rate of only 75–84% [7]. Consequently, automated and reliable computer-aided diagnosis (CAD) systems have been developed to support dermatologists in making more accurate diagnostic decisions [16]. CAD systems operate in three stages: feature extraction, selection, and classification [17]. Additionally, dermoscopy, which magnifies lesion images and eliminates surface artifacts, enhances diagnostic accuracy [18]. Traditional methods often face challenges due to varying contrast values and other complications, which has led to the widespread adoption of GPU-based advancements in image analysis [19]. Image classification challenges include ambiguous images, diverse textures, noise from image features, computational complexity, and high time costs associated with processing [20]. Among all DL models, convolutional neural networks (CNNs) are the most prominent [20]. Studies show that CNNs outperform traditional methods [20]. Moreover, the analysis of CT scans and other diagnostic tests has been enhanced through the use of AI-powered systems [21]. Accurate classification of skin lesions, particularly malignant ones, is crucial, as misdiagnosis can lead to fatal consequences.

The ability of DL models to train on thousands of benign and malignant images has further boosted their adoption [22]. DL-based image classification can be applied directly to raw image pixels without preprocessing; however, this approach neglects the spectral information of the image, which may be valuable for the classification process [23]. To enhance image classification performance, spectra should be taken into account [23]. Artificial intelligence (AI), and particularly deep learning and machine learning, has recently shown significant success in the early detection and classification of skin lesions. In this study, DL- and machine learning (ML)-based models are used to improve the accuracy of skin cancer diagnosis.

This study aims to enhance success rates based on previous research, with its originality lying in the following aspects:

- In this study, the classification extends beyond the prominently featured classes to include additional relevant classes, aiming for more comprehensive results.
- In feature extraction, transfer learning is applied only to the convolutional layers of VGG16 and ResNet50, while the dense and flatten layers are customized to suit the dataset.
- In this architecture, data augmentation is performed using the synthetic minority oversampling technique (SMOTE) to address the small and imbalanced classes within the dataset, with the sampling strategy parameter adjusted according to the specific characteristics of the dataset.
- In this study, Optuna is utilized for hyperparameter optimization, while the AdamW algorithm is chosen to optimize the model.

In Sect. 2, a literature review is presented, comparing the findings of this study with similar research. Section 3 provides detailed information about the dataset utilized and the deep learning model methodology. Section 4 presents the experimental results. In Sect. 5, the findings are discussed, and Sect. 6 highlights the key conclusions.

2 Literature Review

This section presents a tabular review of academic studies focused on the classification of skin lesions as benign or malignant. The tables below (Tables 1, 2, and 3) summarize the key findings derived from these studies. Each table outlines the datasets used, methodologies applied, results obtained, identified limitations, and potential future directions. Alongside the tables, general findings and discussions highlighting the main aspects of the reviewed studies are provided under the subheadings Common Findings and Literature Review—Discussion.

Table 1 Literature review results—part I

Reference	Dataset	Sample numbers	Methods	Results	Deficiencies	Future contributions	Publication year
[24]	ISIC2017	2000 samples (training set: 70%; validation set: 15%; test set: 15%)	EfficientNet, VGG, inception, DenseNet, DarkNet, etc.	Accuracy: 84.00%; specificity:-; recall: 74.96%	A key limitation is the reliance on a single dataset, which may restrict the model's generalizability	Exploring larger, diverse datasets, applying transfer learning, and experimenting with new architectures are planned to improve performance	2025
[25]	ISIC	3.297 samples (training set: 70%, test set: 30%)	DenseNet201, Xception, InceptionV3, ConvNeXt-Large, etc.	Accuracy: 88.49%; specificity: 87.37%; recall: 89.58%	DenseNet201's lower performance suggests a risk of overfitting and limited generalizability	Future work aims to improve performance by working with different datasets	2025
[7]	ISIC 2019 and ISIC 2020	Total 10048 samples (training set: 70%, validation set: 20%, test set: 10%)	CNN	Accuracy: 96.90%; specificity:-; recall: 89%	No reliable method has been developed to reduce hair artifacts and lower their contrast	Images can be classified by extracting features using methods such as GLCM	2024
[26]	HAM 10000	2100 samples (with 300 images evenly distributed across each class)	CNN	CNN accuracy: 82.34%; specificity:-; recall:-	Not all data was used, nor was performance compared with other architectures	Performance may improve by filtering images to reduce noise and artifacts	2024

(conitnued)

Table 1 (continued)

Reference	Dataset	Sample numbers	Methods	Results	Deficiencies	Future contributions	Publication year
[12]	ISIC	3256 samples (benign: 1792, malignant lesion: 1464)	DenseNet201, EfficientNet, DarkNet19	Accuracy: 87%; specificity: 84%; recall: 89%	There is an insufficiency of both quantitative and qualitative data	The effectiveness of classifying different types of lesions can be evaluated across various skin types	2024
[27]	ISIC 2018	10015 samples (MEL: 1113, BKL: 1099, BCC: 514, AK: 327, dermatofibrom: 115, MN: 6705, VL: 142)	CNN, DenseNet201	Accuracy: 99.51%; specificity:-; recall: 98%	Data preprocessing and segmentation have not been performed	A web-based tool will be developed for user interaction, analysis, and result visualization	2024
[28]	ISIC 2019 and Asian Dermoscopy	166326 samples (MEL:28584, MN:87462, BCC:24258, BKL:26022)	CNN, PSO	Accuracy: 99.33%; specificity: 98.87%; recall: 94.65%	The computation time is longer than the minimum acceptable threshold	Local datasets can test system generalizability and robustness	2023
[29]	ISIC	3.297 samples (training set: 60%, test set: 30%, validation set: 10%)	CNN	Accuracy: 84.8%; specificity:-; recall: 80.5%	The diversity and size of the datasets are limited	Data augmentation will be performed to improve the accuracy rate	2023
[30]	Seda Sakaci Cosmetology Center	11500 samples (training set: 70%, validation set: 10%, test set: 20%)	CNN, LTSM	CNN accuracy: 83.75%, LTSM accuracy: 68.90%	More methods should be tested to improve performance	Real-world assessment using human skin images	2023
[31]	Kaggle-2021	3297 samples (benign: 1497, malignant lesion: 1800)	VGGNet	Accuracy: 83%; specificity: -; recall: 84%	The study does not include multiclasification	Broader classification will be performed	2023

Table 2 Literature review results—part II

Reference	Dataset	Sample numbers	Methods	Results	Deficiencies	Future contributions	Publication year
[32]	HAM 10000	3000 samples (training set: 2250, test set: 750)	SVM, softmax regression	SVM accuracy: 68.3%; softmax regression accuracy: 54.7%; specificity:-; recall:-	Deep learning was not used, and the data utilized was incomplete	Increasing sample size and balancing lesion classes may improve success	2022
[33]	Kaggle-MNST HAM 10000	10015 samples (MEL: 1113, BKL: 1099, BCC: 514, AK: 327, dermatofibrom: 115, MN: 6705, VL: 142)	CNN, MLP-Mixer, VIT	CNN accuracy: 86.22%; MLP-mixer accuracy: 84.96%; VIT accuracy: 83.87%	The error rate may increase due to the insufficient number of samples in the current dataset	Data augmentation can balance classes and improve model performance	2022
[22]	ISIC2018	2841 samples (benign: 1216, malignant lesion: 1627)	KNN, SVM, RF	Accuracy: 82%	No data augmentation has been done	To increase the improvement rate, the accuracy rate will be increased by expanding the dataset	2022
[34]	ISIC 2018	3533 samples (benign and malignant)	CNN, ResNet50, InceptionV3	CNN accuracy: 83.18%; ResNet50 accuracy: 83.64%; InceptionV3 accuracy: 85.76%	Data augmentation techniques have not been applied	It is recommended to conduct tests with a broader range of cancer types and larger datasets	2022
[16]	ISIC 2017	628 samples (Seboreik Keratoz: 254, melonama: 374)	CNN, RNN	CNN accuracy: 96%; RNN accuracy:93%; specificity:-; recall:-	Only two classification categories were considered, and the entire dataset was not fully utilized	The results indicate that CNN may be the most suitable model for further research	2021

(continued)

Table 2 (continued)

Reference	Dataset	Sample numbers	Methods	Results	Deficiencies	Future contributions	Publication year
[10]	HAM 10000	25673 samples (benign: 11495, malignant lesion: 14178)	CNN	Accuracy: 87.51%	Noise removal has not been effectively achieved	Noise in images can be automatically segmented to help clinicians better visualize the relevant regions	2021
[35]	ISIC 2017	2550 samples (training set: 2000, validation set: 150, test set: 600)	CNN	Accuracy: 93.47%	Study limited to three classes without transfer learning	Proposed architecture may serve as a hybrid model reference	2021
[36]	HAM 10000	60 samples (MEL: 30, MN: 30)	FNN, DT, RF	Accuracy: 83.3%; specificity: 71.7%; recall: 78.33%	Other classes and samples were not evaluated	Using more ML and DL methods may improve performance	2021
[37]	HAM10000	3297 samples (benign: 1800, malignant lesion: 1497)	MobileNetV2, RD, SVM, ResNet-50	Accuracy: 88.35%; specificity: 88%; recall: 86%	Lack of from-scratch deep learning caused performance drop	Comparisons with other datasets will evaluate performance	2021
[38]	ISIC 2018	2637 samples (benign:1440, malignant lesion: 1197)	CNN, SqueezeNet, ShufleNet, DarkNet-19, DarkNet-53	Accuracy: 89.89%	No data preprocessing has been performed specifically for low-contrast images	Future work will focus on increasing the accuracy rate by applying data preprocessing techniques	2021

Table 3 Literature review results—part III

[39]	HAM10000	10015 samples (MEL: 1113, BKL: 1099, BCC: 514, AK: 327, dermatofibrom: 115, MN: 6705, VL: 142)	KNN, DT, SVM	Accuracy: 76%	Hyperparameter tuning has not been performed with sufficient precision	Hyperparameter and batch size settings should be carefully reviewed and optimized to achieve higher accuracy	2021
[40]	ISIC 2019	26985 samples (training set: 25684, test set: 1301)	ResNet50, DL-CAD	Accuracy: 70.1%; specificity:-; recall: 67.59%	Image filtering has not effectively improved classification and needs refinement	A more comprehensive algorithm is needed to improve metrics and model reliability	2021
[41]	HAM10000	10015 samples (MEL: 1113, BK: 1099, BCC: 514, AK: 327, dermatofibrom: 115, MN: 6705, VL: 142)	VGG19, InceptionV3, InceptionV2, Resnet50, Xception, MobileNet	Accuracy: 90%	The details regarding proper hyperparameter tuning are incomplete	Transfer learning algorithms will be finetuned with the aim of improving the accuracy rate	2021
[19]	ISBI 2016	900 samples (training set: 630, test set: 270)	CNN	Accuracy: 93.46%; specificity: 93.22%; recall: 87.88%	Comparison with other architectural methods has not been performed	It is possible to examine the effect of encoder depth and different color channels on segmentation	2020
[42]	ImageNet	10.015 samples (training set: 80%, validation set: 20%)	DenseNet201, ResNet152, InceptionV4	Accuracy: 86.37%; recall: 96.42%; sensitivity: 86.53%	Data augmentation techniques have not been applied	Additional data will be collected from individuals with darker skin tones, and the results will be reevaluated accordingly	2020

(continued)

Table 3 (continued)

Reference	Dataset	Sample numbers	Methods	Results	Deficiencies	Future contributions	Publication year
[43]	PH2	200 samples (MEL: 40, other lesions: 160)	SVM	Accuracy: 98%	The deep learning method was not utilized	Different methods can be explored to improve performance	2020
[44]	HAM10000	10015 samples (benign: 8389, malignant lesion: 1626)	AlexNET, CNN	Accuracy: 93%	No detailed analysis was provided for the low performance of full transfer learning	Adversarial attacks will be simulated to test model security and develop countermeasures	2020
[45]	National Cancer Center Hospital data	4732 samples (MEL: 1279, BCC: 344, MN: 2302, SK: 606, SL: 62, H/H: 139)	FRCNN, BCD, TRN	Accuracy: 91.5%; specificity: 94.5%; recall: 83.3%	Advanced and popular methods were not compared	Improvements for higher accuracy will be explored	2020
[46]	ISIC 2018	2594 samples (training set: 70%, validation set: 30%)	U-Net	Accuracy: 93%; specificity: 91%; recall: 97%	Entire dataset was not taken into account	RGB models can be combined into one segmentation map	2019
[47]	HAM 10000	10015 samples (benign: 8389, malignant lesion: 1626)	CNN	Accuracy: 85.62%	No noise cleaning or data augmentation applied	K-fold can be used to build a well-validated model	2019

2.1 Common Findings

In recent years, DL and ML techniques have been extensively employed in skin cancer diagnosis, with CNNs and transfer learning architectures standing out prominently. Studies by Goreke [16], Dogan et al. [33], and others have frequently utilized datasets such as ISIC or HAM10000, where data augmentation techniques—including rotation, flipping, and scaling—have been widely applied. Segmentation-focused research has gained significant importance in studies like those by Hasan [46] and Sahin et al. [19], where architectures such as U-Net and SegNet have been used to eliminate artifacts like hair or ruler markings from dermoscopic images. Furthermore, innovative contributions to the field include hyperparameter optimization methods (e.g., particle swarm optimization (PSO)) and the proposal of novel network architectures such as C4Net, LinkNet-RCB7, and FCN-ResAlexNet, as demonstrated in the work of Ozbay et al. [28]. Many studies have compared classical ML algorithms—such as support vector machine (SVM), random forest (RF), and decision tree (DT)—to DL methods and have explored transfer learning approaches, as seen in the works of Ergun et al., and Dogan et al. These collective efforts have primarily focused on improving model accuracy, addressing class imbalance, and developing robust CAD systems. Moreover, DL-based approaches for skin cancer detection have been extensively investigated, with architectures like ResNet, DenseNet, EfficientNet, VGGNet, MobileNet, and Inception frequently highlighted in studies by Dedeturk et al. [22], Kacmaz et al. [12], Fofanah et al. [29], Demir [37], Jinnai et al. [45], and Jain et al. [41]. Transfer learning has been commonly utilized across these works. The majority of studies have relied on the ISIC or HAM10000 datasets, with images typically normalized to a resolution of approximately 224×224 pixels. Data augmentation has often involved traditional techniques such as rotation, flipping, and zooming, as well as more advanced methods like generative adversarial networks (GANs), as exemplified by the work of Firildak et al. [44], aiming to mitigate overfitting and enhance generalizability. While segmentation has been explored, many studies have instead focused on classifying entire images without prior segmentation, as observed in the works of Soylu et al. [38]. Additionally, numerous studies have sought to compare different CNN architectures to identify the models with the highest performance. For instance, Jain et al. evaluated six transfer learning architectures. While binary classification (benign vs. malignant) is commonly used, studies like Jinnai et al. and Jain et al. have also explored multiclass problems. Success rates usually range from 80 to 90%, though clinical applicability remains limited.

2.2 Literature Review—Discussion

Nonetheless, significant differences and several limitations can be observed across these studies. For example, Akyel et al. differentiated their work by categorizing data into four classes; however, they encountered issues such as low performance in detecting fine hair and the need for manual masking. Goreke introduced a different approach by working with numerical data but conducted only binary classification and used a small dataset. Sendel et al. [32] focused on classical machine learning methods but achieved a lower accuracy of 68.3%, trailing behind deep learning approaches. Ozbay et al. achieved high performance (99.33%) through PSO optimization but reduced the image size to 28×28 pixels, resulting in significant loss of detail.

Hasan performed only segmentation without integrating classification, while Kaya et al. conducted hyperparameter tuning on EfficientNet-B3 but reported a moderate accuracy of 82.34%. Kadiroglu et al. reported a high accuracy of 98% using the very small PH2 dataset, raising concerns about generalizability. Although Barin [35] proposed the FCN-ResAlexNet architecture, the study did not present clear performance metrics. Cevik et al. [47] achieved seven-class classification but fell short of high-end CNN models with an accuracy of 85.62%. Ozturk et al. [36] experimented with classical methods based on statistical features, but did not test modern DL architectures. Dogan et al. tested innovative architectures such as ViT and MLP-Mixer; however, with an accuracy of 86.22%, their results lagged behind strong CNN-based studies. Similarly, Dedeturk et al. focused solely on ResNet50 and explored different preprocessing scenarios, yet their accuracy remained between 80 and 82%, and they did not implement segmentation. Kacmaz et al. compared DenseNet201, DarkNet19, and EfficientNet in terms of filter sizes, but their exclusive focus on binary classification and the use of a low number of epochs limited model learning. Fofanah et al. [29] proposed a low-parameter model, but achieved only 84.8% accuracy, trailing behind more advanced models in the literature. Demir extracted features from MobileNetV2 and performed classification using classical machine learning algorithms but was limited to an accuracy of 88.35% and did not apply segmentation. Firildak et al. increased accuracy to 93% through GAN-based data generation; however, the GAN training process was time-consuming, and it remained unclear whether the generated images had received clinical validation. Soylu et al. tested four lightweight architectures but did not perform segmentation or provide multiclass classification results. Kaya et al. compared the VGGNet family for binary classification but achieved only 83% accuracy, falling behind newer CNN architectures in the literature. Cengil et al. [39] evaluated hybrid classifiers and achieved 76% accuracy in seven-class classification with their proposed H7 method but fell short of newer CNN models. Yalcin et al. [40] demonstrated the contribution of preprocessing on ResNet50; however, their study was limited by the lack of segmentation and lower performance in the SCC class. Cetiner [27] modified the DenseNet201 architecture and reported a remarkable accuracy of 99.51%, yet concerns about overfitting and the absence of testing on external datasets were highlighted. Kara et al. experimented with CNN and long short-term memory (LSTM) for skin type classification but diverged from the primary focus of skin cancer detection. Gauda et al. contributed to the literature by applying ESRGAN for image enhancement but limited their study to binary classification and lacked external dataset validation, which constrained the model's generalizability. Jinnai et al. achieved 91.5% accuracy with the FRCNN model, rivaling dermatologists, but did not test its clinical integration. Similarly, Jain et al. reported 90% accuracy with Xception Net in multiclass classification but faced criticism for not implementing segmentation and lacking clinical validation.

Moreover, recent studies conducted by Aruk et al. [24] and Ozyildiz et al. [25] have provided valuable contributions to skin cancer classification using deep learning approaches. Aruk et al. utilized the ISIC 2017 dataset comprising 2,000 images categorized into three classes and tested 21 different CNN architectures, achieving an accuracy of 84.00% with the EfficientNet-b0 model. However, the methodology remains limited due to its reliance on a single dataset, class imbalance issues, and the absence of hybrid or ensemble methods, leaving generalizability uncertain. On the other hand, Ozyildiz et al. performed binary classification on the ISIC dataset containing 3,297 images, employing models such as ConvNeXt-Large, InceptionV3, and EfficientNetV2-S, and attained an accuracy of 88.49%. Despite utilizing modern architectures and transfer learning, this study is constrained by its focus on binary rather than multiclass classification, its exclusive dependence on a single dataset, and the lack of hybrid methods, thereby highlighting opportunities for future research.

While all these studies offer significant innovations, they share common limitations, including gaps in clinical applicability, the absence of segmentation integration, and insufficient generalization testing. Nevertheless, despite these advances, there remains substantial room for further research to enhance the generalizability and clinical integration of AI-driven skin lesion classification systems.

3 Method

3.1 Dataset

3.1.1 Data Source

In this study, the publicly available ISIC2019 dataset, widely used in skin lesion classification research, was utilized. This dataset includes melanoma and other types of skin lesion images, which are analyzed by experts and released through annual challenges. Figure 3 shows example images from its subsets: HAM10000 [48], BCN20000 [49], and MSK [50]. All images were retrieved from the official ISIC archive and are licensed under the Creative Commons Attribution Non-commercial (CC BY-NC) license.

3.1.2 Data Types

The ISIC2019 dataset contains MEL, BCC, AKIEC, BKL (Benign Keratosis-like lesions), DF (dermatofibroma), VASC (vascular lesions), SCC, and NV (melanocytic nevi).

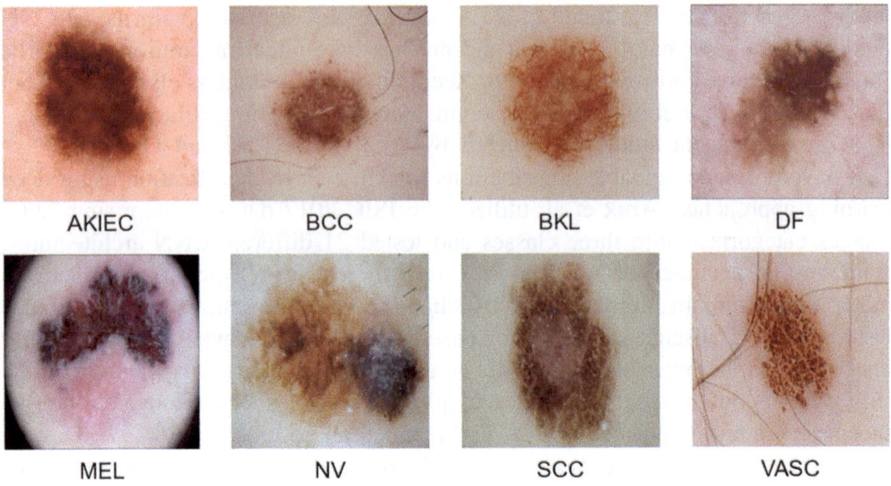

Fig. 3 Sample lesion images from the ISIC2019 dataset, including classes such as AKIEC, BCC, BKL, DF, MEL, NV, SCC, and VASC. The example images shown were manually compiled by the authors for illustrative purposes, in accordance with the dataset's license

3.1.3 Dataset Description

The dataset used in this study comprises a total of 33,126 samples. Among these, 25,331 images are used for training, while the remaining samples are allocated for validation and testing purposes. The distribution of samples across the classes is as follows: MEL -4,522, BCC -3,323, AKIEC -867, BKL -2,624, DF -239, VASC -253, SCC -628, and NV -12,875.

3.2 Feature Extraction

Feature extraction plays a crucial role in image-based classification tasks. In this study, the VGG16 and ResNet-50 architectures, both CNN-based, are utilized due to their proven high performance in disease diagnosis and effective feature extraction from skin lesion images.

In this study, feature extraction was separately performed using VGG16 and ResNet-50, and the resulting features were combined to obtain a richer and more comprehensive representation. This approach leveraged the distinct learning mechanisms and strengths of both architectures, enhancing the model's ability to accurately distinguish various lesion types in the ISIC2019 dataset. Although rare in the literature, the integration of features from VGG16 and ResNet-50 significantly improved performance. After combining, a single MinMaxScaler was applied to standardize the feature vectors, ensuring healthier model training. These combined features were directly used for classification in machine learning models. In the hybrid model, however, the features were fed into newly designed dense layers, which were retrained to learn more complex feature relationships—a key distinction from classical ML models. DL models, conversely, learn features automatically from images within their layers.

3.2.1 VGG16

VGG16 is a DL architecture pretrained on the ImageNet dataset, which comprises 1.2 million labeled images [51]. This pretraining has significantly contributed to advancements in visual recognition tasks. Compared to VGG16, the VGG19 architecture was developed to extract deeper features; however, increasing the number of layers led to gradient-related issues such as vanishing gradients [52]. The architecture of VGG16 consists of five convolutional blocks, where the output of each block serves as the input for the next. Filters within the layers are optimized using backpropagation, enabling the extraction of meaningful features from images for effective representation in classification tasks [16].

Sharing similar characteristics with VGG19, VGG16 has proven effective in accurately representing complex patterns found in skin lesion images due to its depth and structured layer architecture, making it a preferred choice in this study. Its homogeneous and consistent design provides stability during model training and ensures a more predictable and reliable feature extraction process. Therefore, VGG16 was considered suitable for use in this study to improve the classification performance of different lesion types within the ISIC2019 dataset.

3.2.2 ResNet-50

The ResNet-50 architecture, like VGG16, is based on pretraining with the ImageNet dataset. However, it is distinguished by its use of residual blocks, which allow the learning process to continue effectively even in the presence of training challenges such as vanishing gradients [51, 53]. These residual connections enable the network to learn deeper and more complex features without the degradation of performance often seen in very deep architectures. This capability is particularly valuable when handling the complex patterns present in the ISIC2019 dataset, as it allows for the extraction of highly discriminative features and contributes to stable and efficient model training. Therefore, ResNet-50 was chosen in this study to enhance feature extraction and improve classification performance for various types of skin lesions.

3.3 Data Preprocessing

Data preprocessing plays a crucial role in feature selection and extraction, enhancing the model's speed of processing, efficiency, and contributing to the overall optimization of the process [54]. To ensure more accurate classification of the data, specific preprocessing steps are implemented. In this study, the primary preprocessing steps are discussed and detailed under the following headings:

3.3.1 Data Cleaning

Data cleaning involves detecting and eliminating missing, defective, imbalanced, or inconsistent data elements that could negatively affect classification performance, and such inconsistencies are often referred to as noise [55]. Specific cleaning steps applied in this study are detailed in Sect. 3.3.5.

3.3.2 Scaling

Scaling has two primary meanings: The first relates to developing a measurement tool, while the second involves transforming data from the classification level to an equal-interval scale [56]. Ultimately, scaling refers to converting data into a specific range or standard [57]. In this study, ImageNet normalization is employed to avoid performance loss and enable more accurate and efficient learning, especially for complex datasets. This method is particularly important when using architectures pretrained on the ImageNet dataset [58]. The formula for ImageNet normalization is provided below.

$$X_{\text{norm}, c} = \frac{X_c - \mu_c}{\sigma_c}. \tag{1}$$

Here:

- X_c denotes the pixel value in the input image for channel c, where $c \in \{R, G, B\}$.
- μ_c denotes the mean value of the ImageNet dataset for channel c:

$$\mu_R = 0.485, \quad \mu_G = 0.456, \quad \mu_B = 0.406.$$

- σ_c denotes the standard deviation of the ImageNet dataset for channel c:

$$\sigma_R = 0.229, \quad \sigma_G = 0.224, \quad \sigma_B = 0.225.$$

Therefore, the normalization for each channel is computed as

$$X_{\text{norm}, R} = \frac{X_R - 0.485}{0.229}, \tag{2}$$

$$X_{\text{norm}, G} = \frac{X_G - 0.456}{0.224}, \tag{3}$$

$$X_{\text{norm}, B} = \frac{X_B - 0.406}{0.225}. \tag{4}$$

3.3.3 Image Resizing

Since the pretrained layers of the model are utilized, input images must be resized to 224×224×3 (width, height, depth (RGB)). If the input size differs from the expected dimensions required by the VGG16 and ResNet-50 architectures, the model may fail to operate properly. Therefore, all images are resized to ensure compatibility with these architectures. Other deep learning models were prepared using input dimensions tailored to their specific architectural requirements.

3.3.4 Data Splitting

This step is critical for effective model training and evaluation. Data is usually split into training, validation, and test sets, all of which must be properly used for reliable classification [59]. In preliminary experiments of this study, both K-fold and stratified K-fold cross-validation methods were tested for data partitioning. However, due to its superior ability to handle class imbalance, stratified K-fold cross-validation with K=5 was ultimately selected for reporting the final results. In this method, the dataset is split into equal parts defined by the k parameters, with each fold used in turn for training and testing. Approximately, 80% of the data in each fold was used for training, while the remaining 20% was allocated for testing. This approach ensures a more robust assessment of the model's accuracy and reliability.

K-Fold Cross-Validation K-fold cross-validation is a commonly used method in DL studies for data partitioning. In this method, the dataset is divided into k equally sized subsets. The model is trained and tested k times, each time using a different subset for testing and the remaining k–1 subsets for training. The average performance across the k iterations provides the overall classification accuracy [60].

Stratified K-Fold Cross-Validation Stratified K-fold cross-validation operates similarly to standard K-fold but ensures that each fold maintains the original class distribution, addressing class imbalance in datasets [61]. Unlike standard K-fold, which may overlook this imbalance, the stratified method preserves class proportions across all folds. In this study, $K = 5$ is used to account for class imbalance during evaluation.

3.3.5 Dataset Subsampling and Class Balance Control

In the initial preprocessing steps, all image files were listed, and only valid formats were retained. Subsequently, the ground-truth CSV file was read and cleaned to ensure accurate mapping between file names and labels. Categorical labels were converted into numerical values suitable for model training, and the overall class distribution was analyzed to monitor class imbalance. No samples were removed to address class imbalance before applying data augmentation or SMOTE; instead, the class distribution was analyzed to inform subsequent balancing techniques.

Although the original dataset contains a total of 25,132 images, a subset comprising the first 40% (10,132 images) was selected to manage computational load effectively. In determining this final subset, both random sampling and sequential selection of the first 10,132 samples were tested. It was observed that random sampling slightly increased the proportion of majority classes (e.g., NV), whereas selecting the first 10,132 samples maintained a relatively higher proportion of minority classes (e.g., VASC). Therefore, the first 10,132 samples were chosen to achieve a more balanced representation of minority classes and to ensure the reproducibility of the study.

Labels were transformed into numerical format, and class distribution was examined. To reconcile differences in column structures between model predictions and true labels, the get_dummies() and reindex() functions from the pandas library were used, ensuring consistency in metric calculations. In managing class imbalance, data augmentation techniques (such as flipping, rotation, and brightness adjustments) and the SMOTE algorithm were applied to enhance the representation of minority classes. Altogether, this comprehensive preprocessing and balancing strategy facilitated overcoming hardware constraints and enabled the model to operate reliably, with good generalization capability and high performance.

3.4 Feature Selection

Feature selection is a crucial step for improving model performance. Its goal is to identify the most relevant information in the dataset, while eliminating irrelevant details and selecting the most significant features [62]. As a result, it also helps to lower computational costs. In this study, principal component analysis (PCA) and linear discriminant analysis (LDA) are employed for feature selection.

PCA Introduced by Karl Pearson in 1901, PCA is a statistical technique widely applied in areas such as classification, compression, face recognition, and motion detection [63]. Its primary goal is dimensionality reduction, enabling the compression of high-dimensional data and reducing redundancy in datasets. PCA transforms the original variables into a smaller set of new variables, known as principal components, which are linear combinations of the originals and are mutually independent, thereby eliminating dependencies among features [64]. It is commonly used for 2D or 3D visualizations, where the first component captures the greatest variance, and the second, orthogonal to the first, captures the next highest variance [65]. The method also helps reduce training time. The five-step process for PCA is summarized below, with an optional sixth step.

Step 1: Subtracting the Mean of the Data

$$\mu_j = \frac{1}{n}\sum_{i=1}^{n} X_{ij}. \tag{5}$$

- X_{ij}: The value of the jth feature of the ith example
- μ_j: Mean of the jth feature across all samples
- n: Number of samples

The data is centralized by subtracting the mean from each attribute:

$$X_{ij}^{\text{centered}} = X_{ij} - \mu_j. \tag{6}$$

Here:

- X_{ij}^{centered}: Each element of the mean-centered data

Step 2: Computing the Covariance Matrix

$$\Sigma = \frac{1}{n-1}\left(X^{\text{centered}}\right)^T X^{\text{centered}}. \tag{7}$$

Here:

- Σ: Covariance matrix
- X^{centered}: Mean-centered data matrix

Step 3: Computing Eigenvalues and Eigenvectors

$$\Sigma\, v = \lambda\, v. \tag{8}$$

Here:

- v: Eigenvector
- λ: Eigenvalue

Step 4: Selecting Principal Components

The eigenvalues are sorted in descending order, and the top k eigenvectors are selected to form the projection matrix. The new principal components of the data are obtained by projecting the mean-centered data onto the selected eigenvectors:

$$X_{\text{new}} = X^{\text{centered}} V_k. \tag{9}$$

Here:

- X_{new}: New reduced data matrix
- V_k: Matrix consisting of the top k eigenvectors

Optional Step: Whitening Process

The whitening process normalizes the data so that the variance of each principal component becomes 1. It is computed as

$$X_{\text{whitened}} = X_{\text{new}}\, \Lambda_k^{-1/2}. \tag{10}$$

Here:

- Λ_k: Diagonal matrix of the top k eigenvalues
- $\Lambda_k^{-1/2}$: The inverse square root of Λ_k

Alternatively, whitening can also be expressed as

$$X_{\text{whitened}} = V_k \, \Lambda_k^{-1/2} \, V_k^T \, X^{\text{centered}}. \tag{11}$$

Each of the above steps forms the mathematical basis of PCA and is used to reduce the dimensionality of the dataset.

LDA LDA allows variables in a dataset to be divided into two or more distinct groups. Its primary goal is to minimize within-class similarity and maximize between-class differences [66]. LDA constructs functions, either linear or nonlinear, known as discriminant functions, to identify groups by capturing shared characteristics. The features used for separation are called discriminant variables. In essence, LDA highlights differences between groups using these variables [67]. The key difference between LDA and PCA is that LDA is used for classification and requires labeled data, whereas PCA focuses on dimensionality reduction and visualization and does not require labels. The formulation for LDA is provided below [68].

The interclass scatter matrix S_B is expressed as follows:

$$S_B = \sum_{i=1}^{C} \sum_{j=1}^{N_i} \left(x_{i,j} - \mu_i\right) \left(x_{i,j} - \mu_i\right)^T. \tag{12}$$

Here:

- $x_{i,j}$: Feature vector of the jth sample in the ith class
- μ_i: Mean vector of the ith class
- N_i: Number of samples in the ith class
- C: Total number of classes

After computing the interclass scatter matrix S_B and the intraclass scatter matrix S_W, the following generalized eigenvalue problem is solved:

$$S_B \, a = \lambda \, S_W \, a. \tag{13}$$

Here:

- λ: eigenvalue
- a: eigenvector
- S_W: intraclass scatter matrix

This is the solution to the generalized eigenvalue problem. The r largest eigenvectors corresponding to the largest eigenvalues are selected to construct the transformation matrix P. This matrix projects the data onto a lower-dimensional space that maximizes class separability.

3.5 Model Selection

3.5.1 ML Algorithms

The manual analysis of large datasets quickly and accurately is not feasible. In this context, ML introduces methods that aim to identify the most suitable solutions for new data by leveraging past experiences and patterns [69]. The ML techniques employed in this study are outlined below.

K-Nearest Neighbors (KNNs) When examining the working principle of this model, it can be observed that the dataset is first divided into training and test sets. Based on the predetermined k parameter, the nearest neighbors are identified to classify the sample into the group with the highest frequency. Choosing an odd k value is crucial to avoid ties, which could reduce model efficiency [70]. In this study, the KNN algorithm was chosen because it is a simple yet effective method for distinguishing visually similar classes, such as skin lesions, and it produces stable results even with small sample sizes.

- **Distance Measurement:** The first step is to calculate the distance between the test sample and all training samples. The most commonly used distance measure is the Euclidean distance:

$$d(x_{\text{test}}, x_{\text{train}}) = \sqrt{\sum_{i=1}^{n} \left(x_{\text{test},\, i} - x_{\text{train},\, i}\right)^2}. \tag{14}$$

  Here:

  - $x_{\text{test}} = (x_{\text{test},\,1}, x_{\text{test},\,2}, \ldots, x_{\text{test},\,n})$: Feature vector of the test data sample
  - $x_{\text{train}} = (x_{\text{train},\,1}, x_{\text{train},\,2}, \ldots, x_{\text{train},\,n})$: Feature vector of a training data sample
  - n: Number of features

- **Selection of K-Nearest Neighbors:** After computing the distances between the test sample and all training samples, the k closest samples are selected as neighbors. These neighbors are sorted in ascending order of their distances to the test sample.
- **Class Prediction:** The majority class among the selected k neighbors is assigned as the predicted class of the test sample:

  - **Majority Voting:** The predicted class is determined by the majority vote of the class labels of the k neighbors.
  - **Weighted Voting:** Alternatively, a weighted voting scheme can be applied where closer neighbors contribute more to the classification decision. For example, the weight assigned to neighbor j can be computed as

$$w_j = \frac{1}{d(x_{\text{test}}, x_{\text{train}}^{(j)})}. \tag{15}$$

  The predicted class is determined based on the sum of weighted votes.

SVM SVM are an algorithm based on inductive reasoning and structural risk minimization (SRM), making them well-suited for handling complex data structures. They create classification boundaries that effectively separate data points, leveraging kernel functions for flexible modeling of nonlinear relationships [71]. In this study, SVM was chosen for its ability to achieve high accuracy even on small and complex datasets, as well as its widespread use in the literature. Especially in skin lesion images where class imbalance and high visual similarity exist between classes, SVM's kernel functions allow it to model nonlinear decision boundaries, providing significant advantages in distinguishing between different lesion types. These capabilities make it a promising method for identifying rare lesion categories.

DT DT is widely used for classification and prediction tasks due to its interpretability and simplicity, as reported in several studies [72]. The model works by constructing a tree structure based on inductive reasoning, where decisions are made through a series of branches representing feature-based splits. Its graphical representation helps domain experts understand how decisions are formed and compare model outputs with their own expertise. Given these advantages and its frequent use in studies involving datasets like ISIC2019, DT was selected for this study:

- ***Root***: The first node of the tree where the initial decision is made
- ***Nodes***: Points in the tree where a condition on a feature is evaluated
- ***Edges***: Paths that connect nodes, representing the outcome of a decision
- ***Leaves***: End nodes that represent final outcomes or decisions

The fundamental formulas used in the decision tree model are as follows:

1. Gini Index

The Gini index measures how heterogeneous the data is in a given node. It is computed as

$$Gini(t) = 1 - \sum_{i=1}^{c} p_i^2. \tag{16}$$

Here:

- t: Data subset (node) being evaluated in the decision tree
- c: Number of classes
- p_i: Probability of the ith class in node t

2. Entropy

Entropy is another metric that quantifies the level of uncertainty or impurity within a node. It is calculated as

$$H(t) = -\sum_{i=1}^{c} p_i \log_2 p_i. \tag{17}$$

Here:

- t: Data subset (node) being evaluated in the decision tree
- c: Number of classes
- p_i: Probability of the ith class in node t.

Artificial Neural Networks (ANNs) The ANN model, inspired by the human brain, mathematically simulates the learning process and is also known as a parallel, distributed, and neuromorphic network. ANN is commonly used for tasks such as prediction, classification, pattern recognition, data association, and noise reduction [73]. Although ANN architectures can capture complex, nonlinear relationships, their efficient operation often requires parallel computing capabilities, while most current computer systems process information serially, posing limitations in some applications [74]. In this study, ANN was chosen because its multilayer and flexible structure helps overcome significant class imbalances in the ISIC2019 dataset, where traditional methods often struggle. ANN can effectively learn hidden patterns, capture nonlinear relationships, and handle variations in color and texture, thus enhancing generalization and classification performance for skin lesion analysis. ANN possesses several fundamental characteristics, including the following [73]:

- ***Nonlinearity and Generalization***: Artificial neural networks are capable of modeling nonlinear relationships and can learn and generalize complex patterns present in data.
- ***Parallel Processing and Flexibility***: Artificial neural networks can perform parallel processing, allowing them to handle large datasets efficiently, and they can adapt to various problems thanks to their flexible architecture.
- ***Learning and Error Tolerance***: By learning from training data, neural networks develop robustness and can tolerate certain errors or noise in the data due to their fault-tolerant nature.
- ***Handling Incomplete Data and Adaptability***: Artificial neural networks demonstrate resilience to missing or incomplete data and can adapt dynamically to changes in the environment.
- ***Utilizing Multiple Variables and Parameters***: Artificial neural networks can tackle complex, high-dimensional problems by working with numerous input variables and a large set of model parameters.

RF RF is a method widely applied across various industries and comprises an ensemble of decision trees combined with random feature selection. Introduced by Leo Breiman in 1997 and inspired by the work of Amit and Geman, it was developed as an alternative to Boosting. RF is often preferred because it offers fast training and prediction, requires fewer regularization parameters, and mitigates overfitting by increasing diversity among trees [75]. In this study, RF was selected for its robust performance on high-dimensional datasets such as skin lesion classification. Its flexible hyperparameter tuning and inherent ability to reduce overfitting make it suitable for complex data. Given the structure of the dataset used, RF's ensemble strategy enables more balanced and stable decisions. This capability

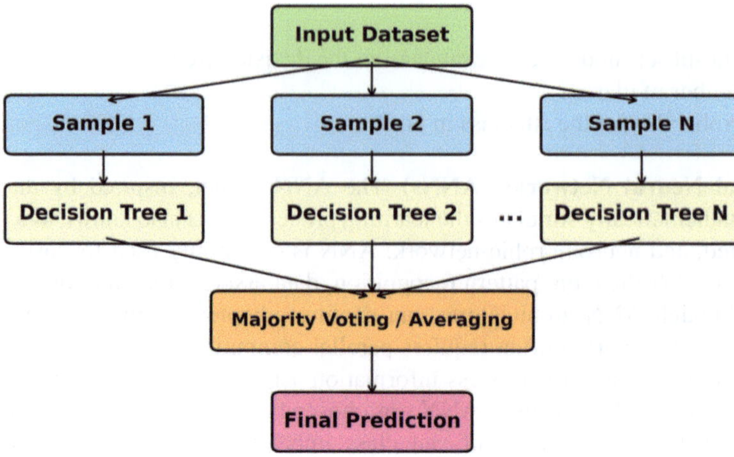

Fig. 4 Fundamental operating principles of the RF algorithm, illustrated by the authors

assists in identifying significant features, enhancing the model's effectiveness in distinguishing between different lesion types, thus contributing valuable insights to the literature. As shown in Fig. 4, a schematic representation of the RF model illustrates the process from data input to final prediction via majority voting.

3.5.2 DL Algorithms

DL, a subfield of ML, has emerged as a powerful approach for complex image classification tasks, including medical imaging and skin lesion analysis [76]. In this study, Inception-V3, U-Net, recurrent neural network (RNN), VGG19, and CNN architectures were employed due to their proven effectiveness in extracting meaningful features and enhancing classification performance.

Inception-V3 Introduced by Szegedy et al. in 2015, Inception-v3 is a convolutional neural network trained on over one million images, achieving over 78.1% accuracy on the ImageNet dataset [77]. The architecture uses symmetric and asymmetric modules, including convolutions, pooling layers, and fully connected layers, resulting in a network depth of 48 layers capable of classifying images into 1000 object categories. It processes input images of size 299×299 pixels and has learned rich feature representations across diverse images [78]. In this study, the Inception-v3 architecture was chosen for its high capacity to distinguish complex visual patterns, offering strong accuracy potential and the ability to extract multiscale, deep visual features, which is particularly valuable for detailed image classification tasks.

U-Net The U-Net architecture, developed by Ronneberger et al., is a convolutional neural network composed of repetitive convolutional blocks and designed primarily for segmentation tasks [79]. Its characteristic "U" shape enables precise pixel-level classification. The encoder comprises repeated 3×3 convolutions followed by ReLU activations and 2×2 max pooling, reducing spatial dimensions while preserving critical features. The decoder mirrors this structure but integrates skip connections from the encoder, enhancing spatial detail recovery. The final layer employs a 1×1 convolution with a sigmoid activation to produce a segmentation mask [79]. In this study, U-Net is chosen due to its proven success in achieving high performance, even with limited data, making it well-suited for segmenting and classifying skin lesions in the ISIC2019 dataset. Its encoder-decoder structure with skip connections is particularly effective for preserving fine visual details and delineating precise boundaries in skin lesions. Furthermore, U-Net's ability to generate detailed feature maps supports robust classification despite variations in lesion color, size, and shape, underscoring its relevance and contribution to the literature in this domain.

The U-Net architecture typically comprises between 11 and 15 layers, although the exact number can vary depending on the complexity and requirements of the specific application:

- The encoder generally consists of four to five convolutional blocks, each composed of convolutional layers followed by pooling operations.
- The bottleneck layer usually consists of a single convolutional block that connects the encoder and decoder paths.
- The decoder typically contains the same number of transposed convolutional (or upsampling) blocks as the encoder, enabling precise reconstruction of spatial dimensions.

RNN This architecture utilizes internal memory and recurrent connections to process sequential data. Memory cells are linked in a chain, performing identical operations on each element in the input sequence. Its strength lies in learning direct input-output mappings, enhancing performance. However, RNNs face challenges like vanishing or exploding gradients, for which LSTM networks are often recommended [80]. RNNs can be single-layered or multilayered, allowing flexibility based on specific applications. In this study, the RNN architecture is chosen for its ability to capture sequential patterns in color and texture transitions between adjacent pixels in skin lesion images from the ISIC2019 dataset. This capability helps in accurately detecting lesion boundaries and understanding contextual relationships with surrounding tissues, thereby contributing significantly to classification performance.

VGG19 VGG19 was developed as an extension of the earlier VGG16 architecture and takes input images sized 224×224×3. It achieved 88% accuracy on the ImageNet dataset [51]. The model consists of 24 layers: 16 convolutional, 5 pooling, and three fully connected layers, with about 138 million parameters [51]. Despite its depth, VGG19 maintains training stability due to its regular layer structure, allowing it to effectively learn complex visual patterns. To manage computational cost, it uses 3×3 convolutional filters [81]. VGG19, with its deep architecture and regular layer arrangement, provided stability during the training process and made parameter tuning more predictable. Due to these features, it was preferred and used in this study for classification tasks involving datasets requiring complex and precise visual analysis, such as skin lesion images.

CNN This architecture stands out for its ability to automatically analyze and infer deep relationships between objects, mirroring human cognitive processes. For example, it can deduce that a person wearing sports attire near a basketball and a hoop is playing basketball. Comprising five layers, CNN captures hierarchical features from low-level edges and corners to high-level shapes and object integrity [82]. In this study, CNN was chosen because challenges such as background noise, reflections, and other environmental factors in the ISIC2019 dataset hinder high-accuracy classification using traditional methods. Its multilayered structure enables hierarchical feature extraction, which enhances classification performance and makes it well-suited for this research.

Below, the functions of the core layer types commonly used in deep learning models are described [82]:

Below, the functions of the core layer types commonly used in convolutional neural networks (CNNs) are described [82]:

- ***Convolutional Layer***:
  - Responsible for detecting and extracting local features from the input data by applying learnable filters across the spatial dimensions of the input.
- ***Nonlinear Activation Layer***:
  - Introduces nonlinearity into the model by applying activation functions such as ReLU, Sigmoid, or Tanh, enabling the network to learn complex patterns.
- ***Pooling Layer***:
  - Reduces the spatial dimensions of the feature maps, thereby decreasing the number of parameters and computational complexity. It also helps to make the model more robust to small translations in the input.
- ***Flatten Layer***:
  - Converts multidimensional feature maps into a one-dimensional vector, preparing the data for processing by fully connected layers.
- ***Fully Connected Layer***:
  - Serves as the final stage in the network, where the learned features are used for classification or regression tasks. All neurons in this layer are connected to all activations in the previous layer.

The hybrid algorithm approach employed in this study aimed to enhance classification performance by integrating transfer learning, the SMOTE, Optuna, AdamW, and GPU acceleration. Transfer learning was applied exclusively to the convolutional layers of the VGG16 and ResNet50 architectures, while the dense and flatten layers were completely replaced. New dense layers were introduced to adapt the model specifically for skin lesion classification. The dataset included several small and imbalanced classes, notably the melanoma class, which contained a limited number of samples that negatively impacted classification performance. To mitigate this issue, SMOTE was applied, with the sampling_strategy parameter adjusted according to the dataset's characteristics. Subsequently, feature extraction was performed using both VGG16 and ResNet50, and the extracted features were combined to construct a new neural network model. Although applying these techniques increased training time, GPU acceleration helped reduce computational costs. For weight optimization, AdamW was utilized, and for hyperparameter tuning, Optuna provided a systematic approach to exploring the parameter space. Additionally, class_weight was used to assign greater importance to underrepresented classes. By combining these advanced techniques, this study aimed to improve the model's classification performance.

Transfer Learning This technique is employed in both ML and DL contexts. In traditional ML, models are typically effective only within the specific domain or class they were trained on. However, DL approaches have demonstrated broader generalization capabilities. Transfer learning refers to leveraging knowledge, such as learned weights and feature representations, from pretrained models to improve performance or extract new insights in different but related tasks [83].

SMOTE This model, commonly applied to address class imbalance, generates synthetic samples by considering the nearest k neighbors of the examined instances, rather than simply duplicating the minority class data, which can help improve the accuracy of underperforming minority classes [84]:

1. **Step 1**: Identify the k-nearest neighbors for each observation belonging to the minority class.
2. **Step 2**: For a given minority class observation x_i and one of its k-nearest neighbors x_j, compute the difference vector as

$$\Delta x = x_j - x_i. \tag{18}$$

3. **Step 3**: Select a random number α uniformly distributed in the interval (0, 1). Multiply the difference vector obtained in Step 2 by this random number:

$$\Delta x_\alpha = \Delta x \times \alpha. \tag{19}$$

4. **Step 4**: Generate a new synthetic observation x_{new} using the following formula:

$$x_{\text{new}} = x_i + \Delta x_\alpha. \tag{20}$$

5. **Step 5**: Repeat Steps 1–4 until the desired number of synthetic minority class observations is created.

GPU GPUs feature an architecture optimized for large-scale parallel computations, making them highly suitable for executing complex mathematical operations, particularly those involving graphical data. Compared to central processing units (CPUs), GPUs are preferred due to their superior capability to handle high volumes of data simultaneously, which enhances computational efficiency and performance. Their parallel processing structure accelerates both data analysis and the execution of intricate algorithms, contributing significantly to tasks such as image processing and DL applications [85]. GPUs were used in the experimental studies to train the models.

3.5.3 Novelty and Contributions of the Proposed Hybrid Method

The proposed hybrid algorithm uniquely and systematically integrates several advanced techniques to address critical challenges in skin lesion analysis, including class imbalance, feature representation, and reliable model evaluation. The primary innovative aspects and contributions of the proposed method are as follows:

1. Hybrid Feature Extraction Through Selective Transfer Learning and Multimodel Feature Integration While many previous studies have relied either entirely on pretrained networks or on training networks from scratch, this study employs only the convolutional layers of the VGG16 and ResNet-50 architectures for feature extraction. The original dense and flatten layers were completely removed, and new dense layers specifically designed for skin lesion classification were introduced. Thus, the model captures strong and diverse features, while adapting them to the specific problem. Features extracted from both VGG16 and ResNet-50 were combined and fed into newly constructed dense layers. These layers were tailored for skin lesion classification and updated during training to learn complex interrelations among the combined features. This approach enhances the diversity and richness of the feature set, significantly improving the model's ability to distinguish visually similar skin lesions.

2. Comprehensive Handling of Class Imbalance Unlike many previous studies that either overlook class imbalance or apply only basic balancing methods, the SMOTE technique is utilized for minority classes, with the sampling_strategy parameter adjusted according to the dataset's characteristics. Additionally, during model training, the class_weight method is employed to assign higher importance to underrepresented classes. This approach aims to improve the representation of rare classes such as MEL.

3. Integration of Modern Optimization Techniques In this study, Optuna for automated hyperparameter tuning uses the AdamW optimizer for weight updates. The combined use of advanced optimization techniques with hybrid feature integration is relatively rare in the literature. Particularly in hybrid models that involve complex processes such as transfer learning and high-dimensional feature vectors, hyperparameter optimization plays a critical role. Accordingly, the use of modern techniques like Optuna and AdamW in this study significantly contributed to achieving superior performance compared to traditional approaches.

4. Stratified K-Fold Cross-Validation, Dimensionality Reduction Methods, and Multi-metric Evaluation Among the methodologies employed in this study are K-fold cross-validation, dimensionality reduction techniques such as PCA and LDA, and the use of multiple performance metrics. Although these methods are widely used in ML and DL models, they have been systematically applied in the hybrid model proposed in this study as well. The key novelty of the hybrid model lies not only in extracting features from different pretrained architectures (VGG16 and ResNet-50) but also in uniquely combining these features and learning their complex interactions in newly designed dense layers. Consequently, the hybrid model not only achieves high classification accuracy but also improves its ability to distinguish visually similar skin lesions and enhances generalizability through consistent performance across different data partitions. Furthermore, this approach offers a comprehensive evaluation based on multiple performance metrics, particularly for detecting rare classes, thus providing a more explainable and practical solution suitable for clinical applications. The innovative feature extraction and integration capabilities of the proposed hybrid model, combined with robust validation and evaluation processes, contribute significant and unique value to the literature.

A review of existing literature reveals that many studies have not utilized K-fold or stratified K-fold cross-validation (e.g., [7, 16]). In contrast, this study systematically applies stratified K-fold cross-validation to ensure reliable model evaluation, thereby improving consistency across different data partitions and enhancing the model's generalizability. This methodological distinction further strengthens the scientific contribution of this research and offers valuable advances in the field of skin lesion analysis.

3.6 Model Training

During the model training process, several hyperparameters needed to be defined, as they played a critical role in influencing the model's performance. The specific hyperparameters employed in this study are described below.

Batch Size This hyperparameter defines the number of data samples processed by the model during each step. In other words, it describes the use of small batches of training data instead of processing the entire dataset at once. In artificial intelligence studies, processing all data simultaneously is highly demanding in terms of memory and time. This is because during training, backpropagation and gradient calculations are performed in each iteration to update the model's weights and minimize the error. The larger the dataset, the longer these operations require. Therefore, selecting an optimal value for this hyperparameter is crucial for efficient model training [86].

Epoch Number Each iteration of the training process is called an epoch. Having too few epochs may result in insufficient training, while an excessive number of epochs can reduce model performance and cause overfitting. These factors are critical considerations during model training. If not properly managed, they can prevent the artificial neural network from functioning correctly. Therefore, selecting the optimal number of epochs is essential for achieving reliable performance [87].

Learning Rate This hyperparameter defines the step size for updating the model's weights. The learning rate is a positive scalar value that determines how large each update step is. It is often manually tuned during training to achieve high accuracy, although it can also be implemented as a dynamic parameter that changes based on model performance over time. Typically, values between 0.0001 and 0.001 are used, and they may be adjusted depending on performance results [88].

Dropout Rate Dropout serves as a regularization technique in deep learning to reduce overfitting. It works by randomly deactivating neurons during each training step, which improves the model's ability to generalize. While a dropout rate of 0.5 is commonly applied, this value can vary depending on the dataset and problem. Dropout rates can also differ across layers instead of being uniformly set. Additionally, random neuron elimination introduces sparsity, and the dropout threshold is defined within the range of [0, 1] [89].

Details about the training mode implemented in this study were presented.

For hyperparameter tuning, the initial epoch value was set to 20. However, if accuracy had shown significant improvement during training, the number of epochs was planned to be increased to further enhance the model's performance, considering the large-scale dataset used in this study. Ultimately, an optimal epoch value was determined. Since a GPU was utilized, it was essential to select an appropriate batch size to avoid memory bottlenecks. Therefore, to maintain balance and ensure efficient GPU memory usage, the batch size was chosen between 32 and 64. Regarding the learning rate hyperparameter, a balanced value of 0.0002 was selected to prevent excessive slowdowns while ensuring stable training. If model performance had deteriorated, adjustments would have been made to optimize this parameter, allowing a more cautious approach. Another critical hyperparameter considered was the dropout rate. Given the use of SMOTE and transfer learning, careful selection of this value was deemed necessary. Setting it neither too high nor too low was aimed at maintaining the model's stability and reliability. Therefore, the initial dropout rate was set to 0.35 to mitigate the risk of overfitting without introducing unnecessary complexity. Further fine-tuning of this value was planned through experimental analysis to determine the most suitable setting. For general hyperparameter optimization, a hybrid algorithm and optimization techniques specific to each model were applied. Additionally, k-fold cross-validation was implemented, with k set to 5. In this study, confusion matrix calculations were performed as part of the experimental evaluation.

In some cases, two issues can arise that negatively impact a model's performance: overfitting and underfitting.

Overfitting When overfitting occurs, the model becomes overly tailored to the training data, which undermines its performance and leads to poor results. The model learns the noise in the training set too well and loses its ability to generalize. In short, it performs well on the training data but fails to adapt effectively to the test data [90].

Underfitting Underfitting, on the other hand, shows the opposite behavior of overfitting. In other words, the model performs poorly on both the training and test data. Essentially, it means that the model fails to learn the patterns within the dataset, which limits its ability to generalize effectively [91].

In this study, several precautions were taken to avoid encountering these two issues. If no negative outcomes had been observed with the initial epoch value, the number of epochs was gradually increased. In imbalanced datasets, underfitting could occur. Since the dataset used in this study was imbalanced, the SMOTE technique was applied to address the underfitting issue. By providing more training data, particularly for the minority class, this technique was expected to reduce underfitting in the dataset. Additionally, the dropout hyperparameter was employed to maintain a balance between these two issues and to mitigate the likelihood of their occurrence.

3.7 Evaluation Metrics

In evaluating model performance, several metrics are commonly used. Among them, the confusion matrix serves as a fundamental tool for assessing classification results by comparing predicted and actual classes. Figure 5 presents the basic structure of a confusion matrix for explanatory purposes.

3.7.1 Confusion Matrix

Confusion matrices serve as essential tools for evaluating the performance of classification models. These matrices display the number of examples that a model correctly or incorrectly classifies. Unlike other evaluation metrics, confusion matrices highlight how different factors contribute to the overall performance of a model. Each class in a confusion matrix includes four key values: true positive (TP), false positive (FP), true negative (TN), and false negative (FN) [92].

TP represents the metric indicating instances where the model correctly predicts the positive class. When the actual class is positive, the model also outputs a positive prediction [92].

TN represents the metric indicating instances where the model correctly predicts the negative class. When the actual class is negative, the model also outputs a negative prediction [92].

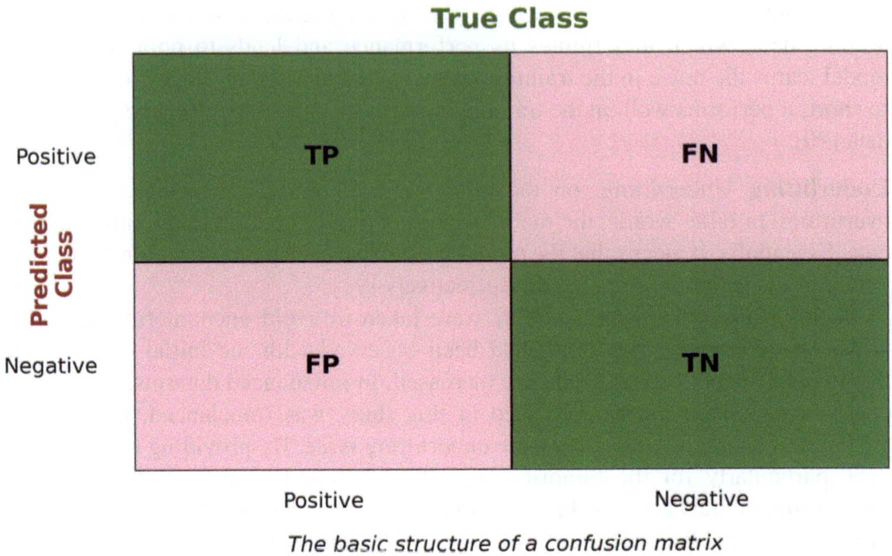

Fig. 5 Basic structure of a confusion matrix illustrating the relationship between predicted and actual class labels (illustrated by the authors)

FP is a metric that highlights instances where the model predicts a positive class, but the true class is actually negative. This situation is commonly referred to as a type I error [92].

FN is a metric that reveals examples where the model predicts a negative class, but the true class is actually positive. This situation is sometimes referred to as a type II error [92]. Many metrics can be calculated using confusion matrices. The main metrics used are as follows:

Accuracy Accuracy alone is often insufficient for disease classification tasks, as the consequences of misclassifying a positive instance as negative, or vice versa, can vary significantly in the medical field. Misclassifying a patient as healthy when they are actually sick may lead to critical errors and adverse health outcomes. Therefore, it is essential to also consider other performance metrics, such as precision, recall, and the F1 score, which provide a more comprehensive evaluation of model performance [77].

Accuracy measures the proportion of correct predictions out of the total number of predictions made by the model [92]. It is calculated using the following formula:

$$\text{Accuracy} = \frac{\text{Number of correct predictions}}{\text{Total number of predictions}} = \frac{TP + TN}{TP + TN + FP + FN}. \tag{21}$$

Recall Recall measures the proportion of instances that are truly positive (e.g., diseased) and are correctly identified as positive by the model [77].

$$\text{Recall} = \frac{TP}{TP + FN}. \tag{22}$$

Specificity Specificity refers to the proportion of actual negative instances that are correctly identified as negative by the model [92].

$$\text{Specificity} = \frac{TN}{TN + FP}. \tag{23}$$

Precision Precision measures the proportion of instances that the model predicts as positive (or diseased) which are actually positive in the true class [77]. It is calculated as

$$\text{Precision} = \frac{TP}{TP + FP}. \tag{24}$$

F Score The F score represents the harmonic mean of precision and recall, providing a single metric that balances both measures [93]. Calculating the F score is particularly important in situations where both false negatives (FN) and false positives (FP) have significant consequences, as it helps evaluate the trade-off between precision and recall [77].

$$F1 = 2 \cdot \frac{\text{Precision} \times \text{Recall}}{\text{Precision} + \text{Recall}}. \tag{25}$$

AUC-ROC (Area Under the Receiver Operating Characteristic Curve) AUC-ROC is a metric used to evaluate the performance of a classification model. The ROC curve visually represents the trade-off between the true positive rate (TPR) and the false positive rate (FPR) at various threshold values of the model. TPR reflects the model's ability to correctly identify positive instances, while FPR indicates the proportion of negative instances that are incorrectly classified as positive. The ROC curve is typically plotted with TPR on the y-axis and FPR on the x-axis. AUC denotes the area under this curve [94]. The AUC value ranges from 0 to 1 and quantifies the model's ability to distinguish between positive and negative classes. It can be interpreted as follows:

- AUC $=$ 1: The model has perfect discrimination capability; all classes are correctly predicted.
- AUC $=$ 0.5: The model cannot distinguish between positive and negative classes and performs no better than random guessing.
- AUC $<$ 0.5: The model's predictions are inversely related to the true classes, indicating that the model systematically misclassifies instances.

The AUC is a robust measure for evaluating the overall performance of a classification model, as it summarizes model accuracy across all possible threshold values. A higher AUC value indicates a greater ability of the model to differentiate between classes, contributing to more reliable predictive performance [94].

The true positive rate (TPR) and false positive rate (FPR) used to construct the ROC curve are calculated as follows:

$$\text{TPR} = \frac{TP}{TP + FN}, \quad \text{FPR} = \frac{FP}{FP + TN}. \tag{26}$$

The AUC value is then computed as the area under the ROC curve:

$$AUC = \int_0^1 \text{TPR}(FPR)\, dFPR \tag{27}$$

$$\text{Confusion Matrix} = \begin{pmatrix} TP & FP \\ FN & TN \end{pmatrix}. \tag{28}$$

4 Experimental Results

This section presented the experimental results of classifying skin lesions using ML and DL techniques. The custom hybrid algorithm, which combined feature extraction with VGG16 and ResNet-50, utilized transfer learning on convolutional layers, and applied SMOTE for class imbalance and AdamW for optimization, was also evaluated. Data preprocessing steps, including resizing, splitting, and feature selection, were completed as outlined in the methodology. Feature extraction results from VGG16 and ResNet-50 were combined and classified using ML models such as KNN, SVM, DT, RF, and ANN. DL architectures such as VGG19, Inception-V3, U-Net, CNN, and RNN performed feature extraction within their own layers. Experimental evaluations were conducted using Python PyCharm due to its extensive AI library support. The main results are summarized in tables, and key differences between methods are discussed. In this experimental study, the ISIC2019 dataset, comprising 10,132 images, was utilized, and classification was performed across eight classes. Detailed explanations of the performance results for each applied model were provided. Following the preprocessing steps outlined in the methodology section, the dataset was divided into $k = 5$ folds. Approximately 80% of the data in each fold was used for training, while the remaining 20% was allocated for testing. Results for the training and test sets were presented in separate tables. Detailed explanations of this process are provided under the respective headings.

4.1 Model Performance and Evaluation

4.1.1 Performance Metrics

Performance metrics quantitatively measure the success and efficiency of the studied system. In this work, the accuracy, recall, specificity, precision, F score, and AUC-

Table 4 Model performance metric results: LDA test set

Model name	LDA status	Accuracy	Recall	Specificity	Precision	F score	AUC-ROC
KNN	LDA-OFF	0.7072	0.7177	0.8063	0.7193	0.7042	0.7717
	LDA-ON	0.7347	0.7916	0.8364	0.7717	0.7604	0.8126
SVM	LDA-OFF	0.7140	0.7234	0.7578	0.7467	0.7089	0.7118
	LDA-ON	**0.8183**	**0.8453**	**0.8642**	**0.8282**	0.8222	0.8858
DT	LDA-OFF	**0.6842**	**0.6728**	**0.6476**	**0.6637**	0.7239	0.6525
	LDA-ON	**0.7201**	**0.7542**	**0.7015**	**0.8033**	0.7678	0.7329
RF	LDA-OFF	**0.7129**	**0.7388**	**0.7249**	**0.7491**	0.7216	0.7424
	LDA-ON	**0.7619**	**0.7626**	**0.8018**	**0.7929**	0.7517	0.7849
ANN	LDA-OFF	0.7806	0.7988	0.7821	0.7214	0.7270	0.8325
	LDA-ON	0.7761	0.7601	0.8045	0.7779	0.7768	0.7906
Hybrid algorithm	LDA-OFF	**0.8364**	**0.8461**	**0.8953**	**0.8705**	0.8661	0.8992
	LDA-ON	**0.8805**	**0.8909**	**0.9387**	**0.9155**	0.9237	0.9326
VGG19	LDA-OFF	**0.7277**	**0.7356**	**0.8999**	**0.7523**	0.7418	0.7716
	LDA-ON	**0.8054**	**0.8216**	**0.8870**	**0.8341**	0.8270	0.8004
Inception-V3	LDA-OFF	**0.7415**	**0.7221**	**0.8121**	**0.7749**	0.7328	0.7417
	LDA-ON	**0.8010**	**0.7948**	**0.8036**	**0.8119**	0.8290	0.8631
U-Net	LDA-OFF	**0.7389**	**0.7620**	**0.8151**	**0.7932**	0.7961	0.8218
	LDA-ON	**0.8201**	**0.8129**	**0.8644**	**0.8732**	0.8262	0.8450
CNN	LDA-OFF	**0.7819**	**0.7850**	**0.7767**	**0.7831**	0.7870	0.8134
	LDA-ON	0.7811	0.7690	0.8319	0.8023	0.7721	0.8171
RNN	LDA-OFF	**0.7321**	**0.7482**	**0.7640**	**0.6837**	0.7199	0.7374
	LDA-ON	**0.7865**	**0.8223**	**0.8613**	**0.8078**	0.7940	0.8021

ROC results of the models are compared and presented in tables for LDA ON-OFF conditions (Tables 4 and 5) and PCA ON-OFF conditions (Tables 6 and 7).

4.1.2 The Effect of PCA on Model Performance

In this study, PCA and LDA were separately applied to the training and test sets for feature selection. Examining the results in the tables reveals that PCA positively influenced the performance of some models, while negatively impacting others. This variation is attributed to factors such as dataset imbalance, the reduced interpretability of the model caused by PCA's complexity, and excessive dimensionality reduction applied by PCA.

4.1.3 The Effect of LDA on Model Performance

Similar to PCA, the results presented in the tables show that LDA did not improve the performance of all models. This can be attributed to factors such as class imbalance and the presence of highly similar classes.

Table 5 Model performance metric results: LDA training set

Model name	LDA status	Accuracy	Recall	Specificity	Precision	F score	AUC-ROC
KNN	LDA-OFF	0.8361	0.8540	0.8768	0.8961	0.8454	0.8994
	LDA-ON	0.7543	0.8121	0.8705	0.8246	0.8196	0.8581
SVM	LDA-OFF	0.7767	0.7640	0.7789	0.7917	0.7367	0.7579
	LDA-ON	**0.8623**	**0.8598**	**0.8786**	**0.8265**	0.8626	0.8967
DT	LDA-OFF	**0.8856**	**0.8862**	**0.8886**	**0.8762**	0.8758	0.8609
	LDA-ON	**0.7921**	**0.8068**	**0.7391**	**0.8214**	0.8352	0.7899
RF	LDA-OFF	**0.7712**	**0.7721**	**0.7411**	**0.7702**	0.7853	0.7619
	LDA-ON	**0.8190**	**0.8099**	**0.8441**	**0.8254**	0.7817	0.8027
ANN	LDA-OFF	0.8105	0.8302	0.8441	0.7971	0.7814	0.8444
	LDA-ON	0.8226	0.8401	0.8590	0.8130	0.8227	0.8593
Hybrid algorithm	LDA-OFF	**0.8670**	**0.8868**	**0.9344**	**0.9101**	0.9089	0.9332
	LDA-ON	**0.9061**	**0.9560**	**0.9366**	**0.9489**	0.9459	0.9588
VGG19	LDA-OFF	**0.7567**	**0.7414**	**0.9138**	**0.7867**	0.7631	0.7981
	LDA-ON	**0.8401**	**0.8516**	**0.9106**	**0.8720**	0.8871	0.8498
Inception-V3	LDA-OFF	**0.7677**	**0.7829**	**0.8576**	**0.8116**	0.7910	0.7899
	LDA-ON	**0.8421**	**0.8303**	**0.8514**	**0.8518**	0.8727	0.9138
U-Net	LDA-OFF	**0.7940**	**0.8254**	**0.8610**	**0.8416**	0.8441	0.8603
	LDA-ON	**0.8739**	**0.8890**	**0.9186**	**0.9276**	0.8683	0.8819
CNN	LDA-OFF	**0.8010**	**0.8201**	**0.8180**	**0.8350**	0.8450	0.8578
	LDA-ON	0.8143	0.8351	0.8805	0.8546	0.8396	0.8681
RNN	LDA-OFF	**0.7746**	**0.7829**	**0.8050**	**0.7084**	0.7679	0.7588
	LDA-ON	**0.8126**	**0.8511**	**0.8988**	**0.8636**	0.8528	0.8358

4.1.4 Comparison

The table presents the performance comparison results of the hybrid algorithm evaluated in this study alongside various ML and DL models. While training set accuracies were generally higher—indicating potential overfitting in some models—no significant overfitting was detected across all models, demonstrating the robustness of the approaches.

Based on the analyses of raw data (PCA-OFF and LDA-OFF), among the ML models, the ANN achieved the highest accuracy rate of 78.06%, owing to its effective capability to learn variations in color, texture, and shape present in medical images. The model optimization was conducted using the ADAM algorithm, and the data were normalized via the StandardScaler() method. Other ML models demonstrated competitive and closely matched performance; however, signs of overfitting were observed in the KNN and DT models, limiting their suitability for this dataset. The hybrid model, with its distinctive architecture, outperformed both ML and DL models by achieving an accuracy of 83.64%. Among DL architectures, CNN and Inception-V3 exhibited superior performance compared to others, attaining accuracy rates of 78.19% and 74.15%, respectively, with enhanced performance facilitated by the application of modern optimization techniques.

Table 6 Model performance metric results: PCA test set

Model name	PCA status	Accuracy	Recall	Specificity	Precision	F score	AUC-ROC
KNN	LDA-OFF	0.7072	0.7177	0.8063	0.7193	0.7042	0.7717
	PCA-ON	0.7093	0.7381	0.8013	0.7504	0.7393	0.7586
SVM	PCA-OFF	0.7140	0.7234	0.7578	0.7467	0.7089	0.7118
	PCA-ON	**0.7822**	**0.8108**	**0.7756**	**0.8032**	0.8122	0.7941
DT	PCA-OFF	**0.6842**	**0.6728**	**0.6476**	**0.6637**	0.7239	0.6525
	PCA-ON	**0.7412**	**0.7028**	**0.7990**	**0.7542**	0.7625	0.7818
RF	PCA-OFF	**0.7129**	**0.7388**	**0.7249**	**0.7491**	0.7216	0.7424
	PCA-ON	**0.7713**	**0.7836**	**0.7112**	**0.7921**	0.7503	0.7819
ANN	PCA-OFF	0.7806	0.7988	0.7821	0.7214	0.7270	0.8325
	PCA-ON	0.7605	0.7503	0.7910	0.8092	0.8461	0.8102
Hybrid algorithm	PCA-OFF	**0.8364**	**0.8461**	**0.8953**	**0.8705**	0.8661	0.8992
	PCA-ON	**0.8648**	**0.8519**	**0.8296**	**0.8787**	0.8790	0.8962
VGG19	PCA-OFF	**0.7277**	**0.7356**	**0.8999**	**0.7418**	0.7418	0.7716
	PCA-ON	**0.7592**	**0.7721**	**0.8209**	**0.7491**	0.7246	0.7599
Inception-V3	PCA-OFF	**0.7415**	**0.7221**	**0.8121**	**0.7749**	0.7328	0.7417
	PCA-ON	**0.8070**	**0.7719**	**0.8329**	**0.7644**	0.7948	0.8050
U-Net	PCA-OFF	**0.7389**	**0.7620**	**0.8151**	**0.7932**	0.7961	0.8218
	PCA-ON	**0.7009**	**0.7218**	**0.8144**	**0.7257**	0.7265	0.7639
CNN	PCA-OFF	**0.7819**	**0.7850**	**0.7767**	**0.7831**	0.7870	0.8134
	PCA-ON	0.8345	0.8036	0.8342	0.8286	0.8494	0.9130
RNN	PCA-OFF	**0.7321**	**0.7482**	**0.7640**	**0.6837**	0.7199	0.7374
	PCA-ON	**0.7213**	**0.7461**	**0.8446**	**0.7554**	0.7323	0.7698

When examining the test set results for the LDA-ON condition, it was observed that among the ML algorithms, SVM and ANN demonstrated superior performance compared to other models. The SVM algorithm achieved an accuracy of 81.83%, while ANN reached 77.61%, reflecting strong performance. To mitigate class imbalance issues in ANN, class weight and early stopping techniques were applied, whereas optimal parameter tuning for SVM was conducted using the GridSearch method. Additionally, due to the efficient performance of SVM on the CPU, GPU acceleration was not utilized. Although other ML algorithms were optimized, they did not achieve results comparable to SVM and ANN. The hybrid model exhibited the highest performance with an accuracy of 88.05%, identifying it as the most suitable model for the dataset. Among DL algorithms, U-Net, VGG19, and Inception-V3 demonstrated similar and high performances, with accuracy rates of 82.01%, 80.54%, and 80.10%, respectively. The performances of all models were obtained within the scope of experimental studies, following the preprocessing and optimization steps outlined in the methodology section.

In the evaluations conducted for the PCA-ON condition, SVM and RF demonstrated higher accuracy rates compared to other models, achieving 78.22% and 77.13%, respectively, thus emerging as the most suitable models for the given

Table 7 Model performance metric results: PCA training set

Model name	PCA status	Accuracy	Recall	Specificity	Precision	F score	AUC-ROC
KNN	PCA-OFF	0.8361	0.8540	0.8768	0.8961	0.8454	0.8994
	PCA-ON	0.7642	0.7756	0.8245	0.7811	0.7856	0.8013
SVM	PCA-OFF	0.7767	0.7640	0.7789	0.7917	0.7367	0.7579
	PCA-ON	**0.8397**	**0.8591**	**0.8329**	**0.8330**	0.8501	0.8356
DT	PCA-OFF	**0.8856**	**0.8862**	**0.8886**	**0.8762**	0.8758	0.8609
	PCA-ON	**0.7818**	**0.7588**	**0.8324**	**0.7920**	0.8019	0.8401
RF	PCA-OFF	**0.7712**	**0.7721**	**0.7411**	**0.7702**	0.7853	0.7619
	PCA-ON	**0.8271**	**0.8440**	**0.7719**	**0.8410**	0.8146	0.8331
ANN	PCA-OFF	0.8105	0.8302	0.8441	0.7971	0.7814	0.8444
	PCA-ON	0.8175	0.8055	0.8109	0.8446	0.8877	0.8553
Hybrid algorithm	PCA-OFF	**0.8670**	**0.8868**	**0.9344**	**0.9101**	0.9089	0.9332
	PCA-ON	**0.9064**	**0.8801**	**0.8658**	**0.9161**	0.9281	0.9028
VGG19	PCA-OFF	**0.7567**	**0.7414**	**0.9138**	**0.7867**	0.7631	0.7981
	PCA-ON	**0.7741**	**0.7910**	**0.8676**	**0.7799**	0.7696	0.7938
Inception-V3	PCA-OFF	**0.7677**	**0.7839**	**0.8576**	**0.8116**	0.7910	0.7899
	PCA-ON	**0.8484**	**0.8120**	**0.8801**	**0.8120**	0.8311	0.8491
U-Net	PCA-OFF	**0.7940**	**0.8254**	**0.8610**	**0.8416**	0.8441	0.8603
	PCA-ON	**0.7621**	**0.7712**	**0.8516**	**0.7570**	0.7492	0.7850
CNN	PCA-OFF	**0.8010**	**0.8201**	**0.8180**	**0.8350**	0.8450	0.8578
	PCA-ON	0.8776	0.8479	0.8677	0.8673	0.8894	0.9394
RNN	PCA-OFF	**0.7746**	**0.7829**	**0.8050**	**0.7084**	0.7679	0.7588
	PCA-ON	**0.7456**	**0.7601**	**0.8942**	**0.8032**	0.7730	0.8132

dataset. Modern optimization techniques were applied to both models. The KNN algorithm, with an accuracy of 70.93%, performed poorly compared to other models, similar to its performance in the PCA-OFF condition, indicating its unsuitability for this dataset. The hybrid algorithm proved to be the ideal model for classification, with an accuracy of 86.48% and superior performance across all other metrics. DL models generally outperformed ML algorithms, with CNN and Inception-V3 showing notable accuracies of 83.45% and 80.70%, respectively. The U-Net model, however, showed a significant decrease in accuracy to 70.09%, compared to previous results, suggesting that the PCA-ON condition is not suitable for this dataset.

4.1.5 Error Analysis

Error analysis is essential for identifying model weaknesses such as overfitting and underfitting. The confusion matrix provides key insights into misclassification patterns. The lower performance of KNN and DT in PCA-OFF and LDA-OFF test scenarios stems from their limited adaptation to hyperparameter tuning and scaling. Test results show that models using optimization techniques have fewer misclassifications. Additionally, dataset imbalance increases the risk of reduced performance. The proposed algorithm achieves lower error rates than other models by applying techniques like SMOTE, transfer learning, and essential methodological improvements.

4.2 Training and Test Performance Evaluation

4.2.1 Comparison of Training and Test Accuracy

The usability of the proposed model is assessed by comparing the performance metrics of the training and test datasets, with results presented separately for detailed evaluation. As shown, most models perform better on the training data, likely due to data distribution differences and the model's iterative weight updates based on training errors. This highlights the need to address potential overfitting or generalization issues.

4.2.2 Comparison of Training and Test Accuracy: Use of PCA

The table provides a comparative evaluation of model performance under PCA-ON and PCA-OFF conditions. While some algorithms exhibit a decline in performance when PCA is applied, the overall use of PCA offers a performance advantage. The training dataset under the PCA-ON condition shows higher results compared to the test dataset. This improvement is primarily attributed to PCA's ability to reduce high-dimensional data into lower dimensions, effectively filtering out noise and low-scale features, thereby minimizing data loss. However, the reduced performance of certain algorithms under the PCA-ON condition suggests that these models may not be well-suited to the transformed data produced by PCA.

4.2.3 Comparison of Training and Test Accuracy: Use of LDA

The analysis of the relevant table reveals a notable difference in metric results between cases where LDA-ON is applied and where it is not (LDA-OFF). The primary reason for the improved performance observed in models utilizing LDA is its ability to maximize class separation while reducing data dimensionality. This process effectively minimizes unwanted noise, thereby enhancing classification accuracy.

4.2.4 Overfitting and Underfitting Cases

Examining the training set tables, the overall model performance under PCA-OFF, LDA-OFF, PCA-ON, and LDA-ON conditions showed no significant difference between training and test sets, indicating no evident overfitting. However, overfitting was detected in the KNN and DT algorithms when both PCA and LDA were off. To address this, the n_neighbors parameter in KNN was optimally tuned using Optuna, and similar corrective actions were taken for DT. Throughout the experiments, no underfitting was observed in any model.

4.3 Evaluation of Time and Resource Utilization

4.3.1 Training and Testing Time Evaluation

Performance results should not be limited to training and test set metric performances but also consider computational efficiency, which provides a more comprehensive evaluation. The analysis revealed notable differences in training and testing durations across models, reflecting variations in model complexity, hyperparameter tuning, and optimization strategies. Models with longer training times typically involve more parameters or intensive data processing to enhance accuracy. Conversely, some models with minimal training times may suffer from issues like overfitting, as evidenced by the DT algorithm's extremely short durations coupled with overfitting signs. Thus, computational efficiency alongside accuracy metrics is crucial for a holistic assessment of model performance.

4.3.2 Training and Testing Time: Use of PCA

When evaluating the use of PCA with the training and test sets, it is observed that, as shown in Fig. 6, the duration values obtained under the PCA-ON condition show a significant improvement compared to the PCA-OFF and LDA-OFF conditions (Fig. 7). The primary reason for this improvement is that the reduction in data dimensionality enables the models to undergo faster learning processes.

4.3.3 Training and Testing Time: Use of LDA

As illustrated in Fig. 8, the use of LDA demonstrates that both the performance results and the durations of the training and test sets are more advantageous compared to the situation where LDA is not applied. The primary reason for this advantage is that LDA reduces data dimensionality, making the process more efficient. This optimization, particularly in DL models, significantly contributes to reducing processing time.

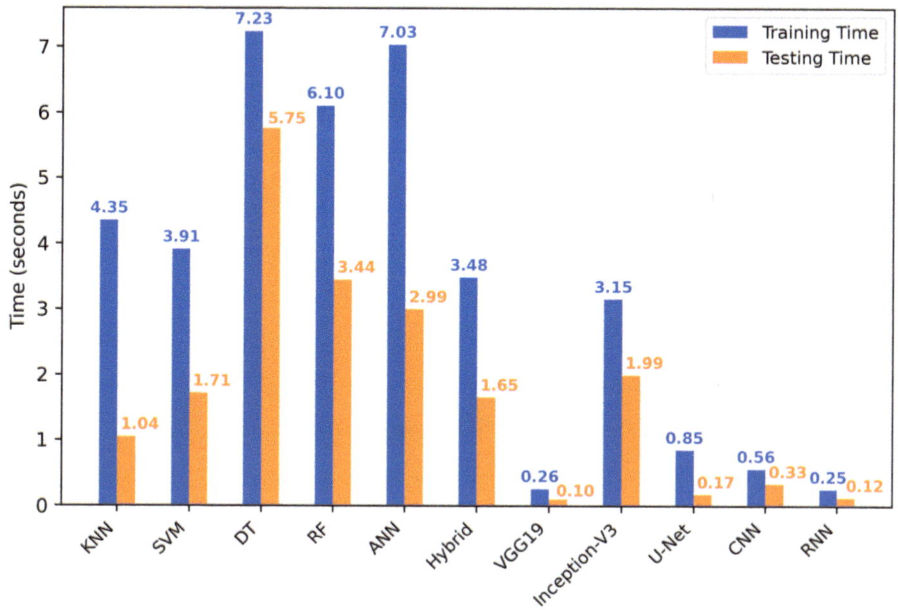

Fig. 6 Training and testing time evaluation: PCA ON, illustrated by the authors

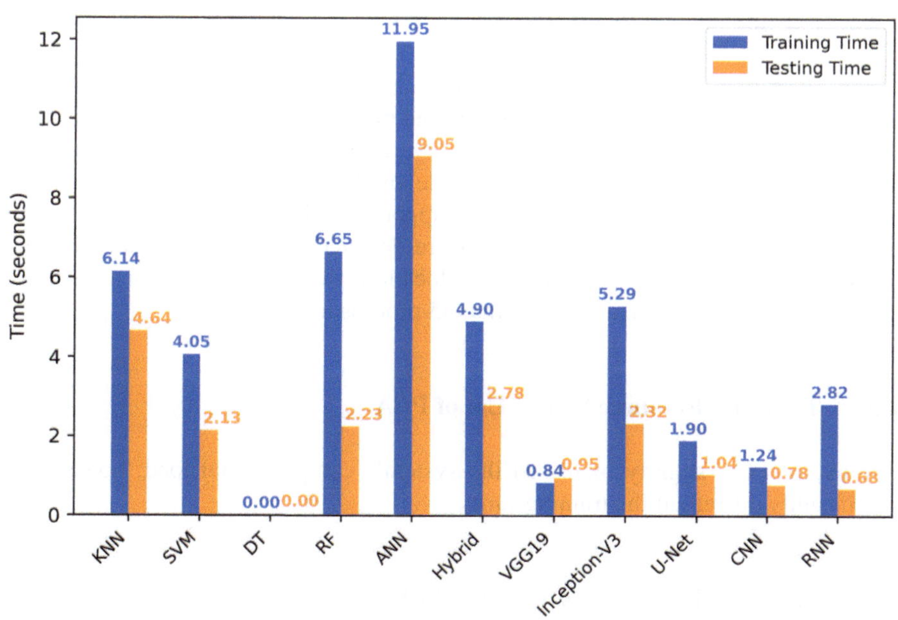

Fig. 7 Training and testing time evaluation: raw data, illustrated by the authors

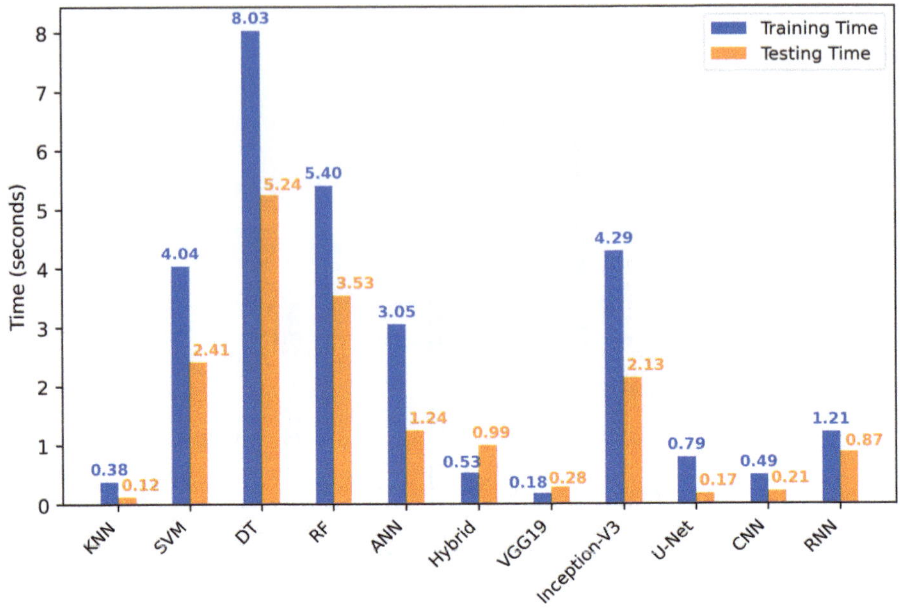

Fig. 8 Training and testing time evaluation: LDA ON, illustrated by the authors

4.3.4 Use of Computational Resources

When examining the memory usage of each model, it was found that RAM limitations occurred due to the dataset size and model complexity used in this study. DL models, owing to their higher complexity, required significantly more memory. Moreover, hybrid algorithms that combine multiple methods further increased memory demands. Consequently, GPU support was implemented for almost all models. No significant memory issues were detected for ML algorithms. During model training, dynamic GPU memory allocation was applied to manage memory efficiently. The CPU utilized was an Intel i5 processor.

4.3.5 Time and Resource Usage: Use of PCA

The use of PCA slightly increased the system's computational load; however, it significantly decreased the training time.

4.3.6 Time and Resource Usage: Use of LDA

With the use of LDA, a slowdown in computer performance was observed, independent of the training time. Although the result retrieval time increased significantly, the training and testing times were completed in shorter durations.

4.4 Model Generalization Ability

A model's generalization goes beyond fitting training data and includes accurate predictions on real-world cases. In image tasks, factors like resolution, lighting, and angles can impact its performance. Thus, evaluating the model on new datasets reveals its true robustness. The models used in this study have demonstrated strong generalization in this respect.

4.5 Data Augmentation

Data augmentation is a technique used to expand the existing dataset by generating additional training samples through various methods. This helps the model to see more data, which enhances its ability to generalize better and prevents overfitting. In this study, SMOTE has been utilized for the hybrid algorithm, while ADASYN has been applied for other models.

4.5.1 SMOTE

In line with the reviewed literature, data augmentation was initially performed on the raw dataset to enhance the model's generalization capacity and to capture greater variability reflective of real-world images. During this stage, transformations such as rotation ($\pm 25°$), horizontal flipping, zooming (zoom range = 0.2), and brightness adjustments (brightness range = 0.9–1.2) were applied in a manner that would not overly complicate the learning process for medical images. These operations increased the diversity of the dataset.

Following augmentation, the augmented images were transferred to the architectures for feature extraction prior to the application of SMOTE to address class imbalance. Subsequently, feature extraction was carried out on the augmented images. In this process, all images were resized to dimensions of (224, 224, 3), and VGG16 and ResNet50 models were employed solely for feature extraction purposes, with the include_top=False parameter set. The images were processed in batches via the FeatureExtractor class, and the resulting feature vectors were combined using the np.vstack() function. The high-dimensional tensors obtained were then reshaped into vectors using the reshape(X_train.shape[0], -1) command, as the SMOTE algorithm operates only on two-dimensional inputs.

In the final step, the SMOTE algorithm was applied to mitigate class imbalance. For this operation, the parameters sampling_strategy='not majority', random_state=42, and k_neighbors=5 were used. This ensured that only the minority classes were oversampled, preserving the natural structure of the dataset and reducing the risk of overfitting. As a result of this process, the dataset, which initially contained 10,132 samples, was expanded to 35,544 samples, creating a more balanced learning environment for the hybrid model.

The effectiveness of SMOTE was evaluated indirectly by comparing metrics such as accuracy, F1 score, and AUC-ROC on the test set before and after the application of SMOTE. If the synthetic examples generated by SMOTE had negatively impacted the model's generalization ability, a decline in performance metrics would have been expected. However, the results indicated that SMOTE contributed positively to the dataset and to the overall model performance.

4.5.2 ADASYN

In this study, ADASYN was applied to address the class imbalance problem specifically in ML and DL models, whereas SMOTE was exclusively used for the hybrid model. Unlike SMOTE, ADASYN adaptively generates synthetic samples by focusing on minority class regions with lower data density, thereby improving the learning of complex decision boundaries. As a result of applying ADASYN, the dataset size increased from 10,132 to 36,948 samples.

4.6 Hyperparameter Settings and Model Performance

Hyperparameter tuning performed during model training significantly enhances the learning process and has a direct impact on overall performance. By carefully adjusting hyperparameters, models can better capture complex patterns within the data, thereby improving both accuracy and computational efficiency.

4.6.1 Batch Size

In this study, initial experiments tested batch size values of 32, 64, and 128, as commonly recommended in the literature. The results indicated that, for ML models, a batch size of 32 was generally more suitable, whereas for DL models, either 32 or 64 performed better. These choices were guided by considerations of training performance, memory utilization, and accuracy metrics. For the hybrid model, a batch size of 64 was selected due to the combined complexity of techniques such as transfer learning, SMOTE, and Optuna. This value proved efficient in terms of GPU memory usage and balanced the training duration, while enhancing the model's accuracy. Thus, although a broad range of batch sizes was tested, 64 was ultimately identified as the optimal setting for the hybrid architecture.

4.6.2 The Number of Epochs

In this study, an initial range of 20 to 50 epochs, as recommended in the literature, was tested. However, based on preliminary experimental analyses conducted for both ML and DL models, 20 epochs was determined to be the most suitable value in terms of balancing model accuracy and training duration. For the hybrid algorithm, the maximum number of epochs was set to 30 in the model.fit() function, but an early stopping mechanism was implemented, terminating the training process if no improvement was observed for 15 consecutive epochs. This approach effectively mitigated the risk of overfitting, while optimizing training time. Thus, although a broad range of epoch values was explored, 20 epochs was ultimately chosen as the optimal setting for most models.

4.6.3 The Learning Rate

In this study, an initial learning rate range between 0.0001 and 0.001, as recommended in the literature, was evaluated. However, preliminary experimental analyses revealed that learning rates of 0.0001 and 0.0002 enhanced model accuracy and contributed to more stable training performance on the ISIC2019 dataset. Therefore, these values were preferred. For the hybrid algorithm, considering its complex structure and the integration of techniques such as transfer learning and SMOTE, an initial learning rate of 0.0001 was selected. This choice helped mitigate the risk of overfitting and enabled more precise weight updates during training.

4.6.4 The Dropout Rate

In this study, the dropout rate was carefully determined to mitigate the risk of overfitting and to enhance the model's generalization performance. While values between 20% and 50% are commonly recommended in the literature, preliminary experimental analyses indicated that a rate of 35% yielded optimal results on the ISIC2019 dataset for both ML and DL models. Particularly in datasets rich in visual details, such as skin lesion images, excessively high dropout rates can result in significant loss of crucial features, whereas rates that are too low may lead to overfitting. Consequently, a dropout rate of 35% was selected to improve generalization capacity, while preserving essential feature information.

For the hybrid algorithm, considering its complex structure and the integration of techniques such as transfer learning and SMOTE, an initial dropout rate of 35% was applied in the early layers. Additionally, a dynamic approach was employed using the Optuna optimization framework, allowing the dropout rate to be fine-tuned between 0.1 and 0.5 on a layer-specific basis. This strategy aimed to maximize both the flexibility and performance of the hybrid model.

4.7 Optimize

Various optimization algorithms and hyperparameter tuning methods were employed in this study for training DL, ML, and hybrid models. Among these algorithms and methods are Adam, SGD, AdamW, RMSprop, RandomizedSearchCV, Optuna, and GridSearch.

4.7.1 SGD Algorithm

In the literature, this algorithm is commonly referred to as "Gradient Descent." However, stochastic gradient descent (SGD) differs from traditional gradient descent because it updates the model's weights using randomly selected minibatches of data rather than the entire dataset in each iteration [95]. This method improves memory efficiency and offers significant advantages for training DL models on large datasets. In this study, the SGD algorithm was used to train models such as CNN, RNN, and Inception-V3.

4.7.2 RMSprop

This algorithm is an optimization technique designed to improve the efficiency of the standard gradient descent method. Specifically, it dynamically adjusts the learning rate for each parameter during training, allowing the model to learn more effectively and converge faster. As a result, the training process becomes more stable, facilitating a smoother and more reliable path toward the optimal solution [95]. In this study, this optimization method was applied to the U-Net architecture.

4.7.3 ADAM Algorithm

The Adam algorithm is an optimization method that combines the principles of RMSprop and momentum. It dynamically adjusts the learning rate during training, enabling models to learn more efficiently and converge faster [95]. Due to its strong performance in reaching optimal solutions, it has been preferred in this study for training both DL models and ML pipelines where applicable.

4.7.4 Adamw

AdamW is a variant of the Adam optimizer that applies weight decay more precisely at each optimization step. This technique helps prevent overfitting, particularly in deep learning models. Unlike the original Adam algorithm, AdamW decouples weight decay from gradient updates, leading to better generalization and improved regularization [96]. Therefore, AdamW was selected as the optimizer for the hybrid algorithm in this study to enhance performance and control overfitting.

4.7.5 RandomizedSearchCV

Unlike GridSearchCV, which systematically tests all possible parameter combinations, RandomizedSearchCV randomly samples a predefined number of parameter settings from specified distributions, allowing efficient exploration of a wide hyperparameter space with fewer iterations [97]. In this study, RandomizedSearchCV was employed for hyperparameter tuning in both ML and DL algorithms.

4.7.6 GridSearch

Grid Search is a hyperparameter optimization method commonly used in machine learning. It systematically explores all possible combinations of predefined hyperparameter values to identify the best model configuration. Although Grid Search can be computationally intensive due to the exhaustive nature of its search, it is highly effective at finding optimal parameters [98]. In this study, Grid Search was applied to the RF algorithm under both PCA-OFF and LDA-OFF conditions.

4.7.7 Optuna

Optuna is an advanced optimization framework designed for automated hyperparameter tuning in machine learning models. It efficiently searches for the most optimal hyperparameter configurations using techniques such as tree-structured Parzen estimators (TPE) [99]. In this study, Optuna was implemented for hyperparameter tuning in the hybrid algorithm to improve performance and stability.

5 Discussion

In this section, the results obtained from experimental studies will be discussed.

Experimental results showed moderate to high success for both ML and DL algorithms. On the PCA test set, SVM, RF, and ANN were the best-performing ML models, while KNN and DT, despite optimizations, achieved lower accuracy. Overall, DL models performed better and are preferred for better dataset adaptation. Similar patterns were observed in the LDA test set, where SVM and ANN excelled among ML models, and U-Net delivered the highest performance among DL models.

The hybrid algorithm outperformed both DL and ML models, demonstrating a better fit for the dataset. Its multifaceted approach combined SMOTE for addressing class imbalance, feature extraction via transfer learning on the convolutional layers of pretrained VGG16 and ResNet-50 models, and optimization using the AdamW algorithm. This strategy led to strong results, achieving an accuracy of *83.64%* on the raw data and, in PCA and LDA OFF-ON scenarios, accuracies of *86.48%* and *88.05%*, respectively, which surpassed other models. Data imbalance contributed to lower-than-expected results in individual models. ANN struggled due to limited data size, while KNN performed poorly on complex patterns. DT was sensitive to data complexity, affecting outcomes in PCA-OFF and LDA-OFF conditions. Despite higher resource demands, SVM achieved better overall results. DL models exhibited unique complexities influencing performance. Overall, metric scores ranged from moderate to high, and training times remained reasonable despite model complexity.

The dataset used in this study influenced model performance differently across algorithms. While some models achieved strong results, others, as shown in the table, were moderately affected. With 10,132 images, the dataset faced challenges due to limited size and class imbalance, leading to reduced performance. To address these issues, SMOTE was applied in the hybrid model, while ADASYN was used for the other models, effectively reducing data limitations and enhancing overall performance.

The data preprocessing steps applied to the models, combined with feature extraction using VGG16 and ResNet-50, and independent feature selection methods, clearly demonstrate their impact on model performance. Although both K-fold and stratified K-fold cross-validation were explored in preliminary experiments, the final results were obtained using stratified K-fold cross-validation, which offered reliable insights into training and testing durations.

The choice of metrics for evaluating model performance depends on the specific context and the model's intended outcomes. These metrics are interconnected and should be interpreted collectively. In this study, six metrics were assessed. Notably, given the imbalance in the dataset, the F score stands out as a particularly important measure.

Due to the complexity and imbalance of the dataset, as observed in existing literature, DL algorithms are often preferred. In this study, they demonstrated higher accuracy across six metrics. Considering time and resource consumption, models with shorter training and testing durations generally achieved moderate to high performance. Among ML algorithms, ANN and SVM required longer training and testing times but delivered better results. The hybrid algorithm yielded the optimal performance, with a balanced duration relative to its outcomes. Nevertheless, models with higher accuracy typically demanded greater computational resources.

In the evaluation of the model, similar to the study by Charan et al. [100] (2022), which employed a 10-fold cross-validation approach on the ISIC2019 dataset, the same dataset was used in this study, but with stratified 5-fold cross-validation. This facilitated systematic and reliable assessment across different data splits. Charan et al. developed two CNN architectures: a single-path model and a dual-path model that combined the original image with the segmentation mask. To address class imbalance, they applied data augmentation techniques such as rotation, flipping, and zooming. In their findings, the single-path CNN achieved an accuracy of up to 58.3% when segmentation and augmentation were combined, while the dual-path architecture reached 88.6%, indicating that preprocessing techniques substantially improved model performance. In comparison, the proposed hybrid method attained an accuracy of 83.64% on raw data and even higher results of 86.48% and 88.05% when using PCA and LDA representations, respectively. This performance can be attributed to advanced feature extraction through transfer learning, integration of features from VGG16 and ResNet-50, and optimization strategies including SMOTE, AdamW, and Optuna. Despite the more complex dual-path architecture and extensive data augmentation used by Charan et al., the hybrid method demonstrated competitive results. Minor differences in outcomes may stem from the different cross-validation strategies, as Charan et al. utilized 10-fold cross-validation, whereas stratified 5-fold cross-validation was employed in this study. This comparison highlights the competitive performance of the proposed hybrid approach even when evaluated against more complex architectures and different validation strategies. Overall, the proposed hybrid model shows strong and competitive performance on the ISIC2019 dataset, underscoring its potential to rival state-of-the-art methods reported in the literature.

When examining the innovative contributions of the proposed algorithm in comparison to existing methods, it is evident that no model has previously incorporated both SMOTE and transfer learning. Additionally, the proposed algorithm utilizes AdamW and Optuna for hyperparameter tuning and model optimization. To further enhance the hybrid algorithm, additional techniques could be developed and integrated.

Both ML and DL models in this study were processed using GPU memory, highlighting the computational resources required for model training and inference. Notably, it was observed that longer computation times did not always translate into higher performance, indicating that model efficiency and resource utilization are not directly proportional to accuracy outcomes.

In future studies, further experimentation and exploration will focus on determining the most optimal and efficient optimization methods for each model, laying the groundwork for applying these techniques to various datasets. Moreover, the models will be tested across different platforms using suitable algorithms to achieve even higher performance. Additionally, incorporating advanced segmentation techniques could further enhance classification accuracy, particularly in cases involving complex lesions.

The limitations of this study include the limited number of image samples and varying levels of success in handling class imbalance across different models. Therefore, future research should aim to develop solutions that specifically address these limitations using appropriate methodologies. By overcoming these challenges, it will be possible to further enhance the current performance results. Additionally, further improvements could be achieved by customizing algorithms and model architectures to fit specific requirements. As an important first step, addressing class imbalance in complex and highly imbalanced datasets, such as ISIC-2019, remains crucial, as it has a significant impact on overall performance outcomes.

6 Result

In this study, the classification of skin lesions, which can be fatal in certain cases, into eight distinct types as either benign or malignant was performed. During the classification process, both DL and ML algorithms were employed. Initially, feature extraction was carried out using VGG16 and ResNet-50, and the extracted features were subsequently combined for further processing. Furthermore, data cleaning procedures were applied to enhance accuracy, and scaling and resizing operations were performed to meet the input requirements of the models. For data partitioning, the K-fold validation method with a parameter of $k = 5$ was selected, and the impact of this parameter on model performance was analyzed. Finally, LDA and PCA were sequentially applied, and classification results were evaluated on both the training and test datasets.

When examining the accuracy values of ML algorithms for the PCA-ON test set, the results were as follows: KNN achieved 70.93%, SVM 78.22%, DT 74.12%, RF 77.13%, and ANN 76.05%. The hybrid algorithm outperformed these methods, reaching an accuracy of 86.48%. Regarding DL algorithms, VGG19 achieved 75.92%, Inception-V3 80.70%, U-Net 70.09%, CNN 83.45%, and RNN 72.13%. For the LDA-ON test set, the ML results were: KNN 73.47%, SVM 81.83%, DT 72.01%, RF 76.19%, and ANN 77.61%, while the hybrid algorithm reached 88.05% accuracy. Among DL models, VGG19 achieved 80.54%, Inception-V3 80.10%, U-Net 82.01%, CNN 78.11%, and RNN 78.65%.

During the hyperparameter tuning process of the hybrid model, the epoch value was set to 30, which was found sufficient for effective optimization with AdamW. Additionally, the early stopping epoch value was determined as 15, ensuring that these two parameters operated complementarily. The batch size was defined as 64, and a learning rate of 0.0001 was selected to fine-tune the transfer learning models, followed by further optimization with AdamW. Importantly, integrating these settings with feature extraction from VGG16 and ResNet50 achieved a good balance between convergence speed and stability. Moreover, setting the dropout rate at 0.35 contributed significantly to the model's successful performance. On the PCA-ON test set, the hybrid algorithm achieved the following metric values: accuracy 86.48%, sensitivity 85.19%, specificity 82.96%, precision 87.87%, F score 87.90%, and AUC-ROC 89.62%. On the LDA-ON test set, the hybrid algorithm also outperformed the other models, achieving metric values of accuracy 88.05%, sensitivity 89.09%, specificity 93.87%, precision 91.55%, F score 92.37%, and AUC-ROC 93.26%.

The classification performed using the ISIC2019 dataset achieved the most reliable results with the hybrid algorithm, CNN, VGG19, and certain ML architectures, particularly SVM and ANN models. The dataset is a comprehensive resource for analyzing dermatological images, where each image is labeled with a predefined class. The classification task was conducted across eight distinct classes within the dataset. This extensive dataset, encompassing various types of skin lesions, serves as a valuable foundation for developing models capable of accurately diagnosing dermatological conditions, thereby supporting early detection and treatment planning in clinical practice.

Future research in skin lesion classification may focus on integrating larger datasets and exploring diverse algorithmic approaches. For example, the HAM10000 dataset, which includes over 10,000 skin lesion samples, serves as a valuable resource for enhancing model generalization. Combining this dataset with other large-scale datasets could further improve the models' ability to deliver comprehensive and robust results. In scenarios where data remains limited, data augmentation techniques can be utilized to significantly enhance model accuracy. Regarding algorithm selection, hybrid models may be prioritized to achieve superior outcomes. In particular, combining DL architectures such as CNN and VGG19 holds potential for improving classification performance, potentially leading to higher success rates in this domain.

According to the findings of this study, high mortality rates associated with delayed diagnosis and treatment are particularly pronounced in skin lesion types such as MEL. Early diagnosis and precise treatment are crucial in managing these life-threatening conditions, highlighting the importance of achieving high classification accuracy for clinical applications. With the growing integration of technology in healthcare, physicians are increasingly supported by diagnostic tools designed to aid disease detection. However, despite these technological advancements, diagnostic decisions ultimately rest with the physician, and the possibility of human error remains. Nonetheless, these innovations provide valuable guidance, contributing to more accurate diagnoses and improved patient management outcomes.

Acknowledgments The authors used language editing support tools, including large language models, to assist with grammar correction and clarity improvements during manuscript preparation. All scientific content and interpretations were developed and critically reviewed by the authors.

Competing Interests The authors have no competing interests to declare that are relevant to the content of this chapter.

Ethics Approval This chapter is based on publicly available secondary data and does not involve any direct experimentation on human participants or animals. Hence, ethical approval was not required.

References

1. R. Bütüner, M.H. Calp, Makine öğrenmesi yöntemleri kullanılarak melanom cilt kanserinin tahmin edilmesi. Gazi Mühendislik Bilimleri Dergisi **10**(1), 141–154 (2024)
2. E. Acer, H.K. Erdoğan, Sık görülen deri kanserlerinin epidemiyolojisi, in *Eskişehir Türk Dünyası Uygulama ve Araştırma Merkezi Halk Sağlığı Dergisi* (2019)
3. A. uysal, S.A. Özsoy, Ş. Ergül, Öğrencilerin cilt kanseri risklerinin ve güneş ışınlarından korunmaya yönelik uygulamalarının değerlendirilmesi. Ege Tıp Dergisi **43**(2), 95–99 (2004)

4. E.N.H. Kırğıl, C.B. Erdaş, Skin cancer diagnosis using deep learning techniques feed by dermoscopic images, in *2023 Medical Technologies Congress (TIPTEKNO)* (IEEE, New York, 2023), pp. 1–4
5. S.M.A. Hurmuzi, Evrişimsel sinir ağları kullanarak cilt kanseri risk değerlendirmesi. M.s. thesis (Selçuk Üniversitesi Fen Bilimleri Enstitüsü, 2019)
6. S. Kasap, M.L. Pektas, Y. Dere, M. Altiparmak, Muğla'daki cilt kanseri olgularının retrospektif değerlendirilmesi. Muğla Sıtkı Koçman Üniversitesi Dergisi **2**(3), 34–37 (2015)
7. C. Akyel, N. Arıcı, Cilt kanserinde kıl temizliğii ve lezyon bölütlemesinde yeni bir yaklaşım. Politeknik Dergisi **23**(3), 821–828 (2020)
8. S. Allinson, Skin cancer: more people die from types that aren't melanoma—surprise new finding, Oct 2023. https://theconversation.com. Accessed: Jul. 27, 2025
9. H. Aksoy, D.D. Uyan, K. Dağcıoğlu, M. Durmuş, E. Sarı, İ. Fidancı, D.A. Başer, M. Cankurtaran, Tıp fakültesi dönem 5 ve 6 öğrencilerinin melanom hakkında farkındalığı: Tanımlayıcı bir çalışma. Turkish Journal of Family Practice **26**(1), 6–11 (2022)
10. E. Ergün, K. Kılıç, Derin öğrenme ile artırılmış görüntü seti üzerinden cilt kanseri tespiti. Black Sea Journal of Engineering and Science **4**(4), 192–200 (2021)
11. D. Buckley, Cancer and pre-cancer of the skin, in *Textbook of Primary Care Dermatology* (Springer, Berlin, 2021), pp. 397–428
12. R.N. Kaçmaz, R.S. Doğan, Dermatolojik görüntü analizi için derin öğrenme modellerinin karşılaştırılması: Efficientnet zirvede. Erciyes Universitesi Fen Bilimleri Enstitusu Fen Bilimleri Dergisi **40**(2), 383–393 (2024)
13. O. Baykara, Kanser tedavisinde güncel yaklaşımlar. Balıkesir Sağlık Bilimleri Dergisi **5**(3), 154–165 (2016)
14. A. Furkan, B. Akalın, Onkoloji alanında yapay zeka yöntemleri. Gevher Nesibe Journal of Medical and Health Sciences **7**(18), 81–92 (2022)
15. Z. Yazıcı, K. kemoterapisi, in *Temel ve Klinik Farmakoloji*, ed. by B.G. Katzung, S.B. Masters, A.J. Trevor, 12 edn. (Nobel Tip Kitapevleri, Istanbul, 2014), pp. 949–975
16. V. Göreke, Cilt lezyonlarının sınıflandırılmasında derin öğrenme tabanlı bir yöntem. Türk Doğa ve Fen Dergisi **10**(1), 30–36 (2021)
17. T. Doğanay, O. Yıldız, Beyin tümör tespiti için derin öğrenme temelli bilgisayar destekli tanı sistemi. Duzce University Journal of Science and Technology **10**(4), 1748–1762 (2022)
18. O. Polat, M.S. Kartal, Derin öğrenme ile pencere ayarlı görüntüler kullanılarak beyin inme segmentasyon performansının geliştirilmesi. Gümüşhane Üniversitesi Fen Bilimleri Dergisi **13**(4), 1094–1109 (2023)
19. N. Şahin, N. Alpaslan, Segnet mimarisi kullanılarak cilt lezyon bölütleme performansının iyileştirilmesi. Avrupa Bilim ve Teknoloji Dergisi (2020), pp. 40–45
20. O. Yıldız, Derin öğrenme yöntemleriyle dermoskopi görüntülerinden melanom tespiti: Kapsamlı bir çalışma. Gazi Universitesi Muhendislik Mimarlik Fakultesi Dergisi **34**(4), 2241–2260 (2019)
21. T. Uzun, Yapay zeka ve sağlık uygulamaları. İzmir Katip Çelebi Üniversitesi İktisadi ve İdari Bilimler Fakültesi Dergisi **3**(1), 80–92 (2020)
22. B.A. Dedetürk, K. Taşdemir, B. Bakır-güngör, Cilt kanseri görüntü sınıflandırması için görüntü ön işlemenin evrimsel sinir ağları performansı üzerindeki etkileri. Erciyes Üniversitesi Fen Bilimleri Enstitüsü Fen Bilimleri Dergisi **38**(2), 190–200 (2022)
23. M. Çiftçi, Derin öğrenme metodu kullanarak bt görüntülerinden akciğer kanseri teşhisi. Dokuz Eylül Üniversitesi Mühendislik Fakültesi Fen ve Muhendislik Dergisi **24**(71), 487–500 (2022)
24. I. Aruk, A.N. Toprak, Cilt kanseri tanısı için farklı evrişimsel sinir ağı modellerinin karşılaştırılması. J. Instr. Sci. Technol. **15**(1), 25–38 (2025)
25. H. Özyıldız, G. Sonugür, Skin cancer diagnosis using deep learning architectures, in *International Scientific Research and Innovation Congress-II* (Adana, Türkiye, 2025). Conference held in Dec 2024; publication uploaded Jan 2025

26. A.B. Karlı, B. Kaya, Cilt kanseri görüntüleri kullanılarak eğitilen efficientnet-b3 mimarisinde hiperparametre seçiminin sınıflandırma performansına etkisinin incelenmesi. Fırat Üniversitesi Mühendislik Bilimleri Dergisi **36**(1), 499–507 (2024)
27. H. Çetiner, Skin lesions identification and analysis with deep learning model using transfer learning. Osmaniye Korkut Ata Üniversitesi Fen Bilimleri Enstitüsü Dergisi **7**(3), 1030–1045 (2024)
28. E. Özbay, F.A. Özbay, Parçacık sürüsü optimizasyon algoritması ile optimize edilmiş evrişimsel sinir ağı kullanılarak dermoskopik görüntülerden cilt kanserinin sınıflandırılması. Fırat Üniversitesi Mühendislik Bilimleri Dergisi **35**(1), 261–273 (2023)
29. A.B. Fofanah, E. Özbilge, Y. Kırsal, Skin cancer recognition using compact deep convolutional neural network. Çukurova Üniversitesi Mühendislik Fakültesi Dergisi **38**(3), 787–797 (2023)
30. F.B. Kara, R. Kara, S.S. Çelik, Skin type detection with deep learning: A comparative analysis. Duzce University Journal of Science and Technology **11**(2), 729–742 (2023)
31. V. Kaya, İ. Akgül, Classification of skin cancer using VGGNet model structures. Gümüşhane Üniversitesi Fen Bilimleri Dergisi **13**(1), 190–198 (2022)
32. E. Sendel, I. Yıldırım, Makine öğrenmesi ile cilt lezyonu sınıflandırması: Skin lesion classification with machine learning, in *Proceedings of the ELECO 2022 Conference on Electrical, Electronics and Biomedical Engineering* (Bursa, Turkey, 2022)
33. Y. Doğan, B. A. Soysal, F. Tunçer, M. Akçakaya, Derin öğrenme yöntemleriyle cilt lezyonlarının sınıflandırması: Cnn, mlp-mixer ve vit, in *3rd International Siirt Scientific Research Congress* (Siirt, Türkiye, 2022)
34. W. Gouda, M. Khalil, A. Soliman, A.A. Abd El-Latif, H.A. Elsalamony, S. El-Rabaie, R. Tolba, Detection of skin cancer based on skin lesion images using deep learning. Healthcare **10**(7), 1230 (2022)
35. S. Barın, Deri lezyonlarının derin öğrenme yöntemleri ile segmentasyonu. Master's thesis, Erciyes Üniversitesi, Fen Bilimleri Enstitüsü, Biyomedikal Mühendisliği Ana Bilim Dalı (2021)
36. E. Öztürk, S. İçer, Classification of dermoscopy images with feed forward neural network, decision trees and random forest. Int. J. Multidisciplinary Studies and Innov. Technol. **5**(2), 129–135 (2021)
37. F. Demir, Derin öğrenme tabanlı yaklaşımla kötü huylu deri kanserinin dermatoskopik görüntülerden saptanması. Fırat Üniversitesi Mühendislik Bilimleri Dergisi **33**(2), 617–624 (2021)
38. E. Soylu, R. Demir, Development and comparison of skin cancer diagnosis models. Avrupa Bilim ve Teknoloji Dergisi **28**, 1217–1221 (2021)
39. E. Cengil, A. Çınar, M. Yıldırım, Hybrid convolutional neural network architectures for skin cancer classification. Avrupa Bilim ve Teknoloji Dergisi **28**, 694–701 (2021)
40. T. Yalçın, A.T. Gürsel, Improving digital image quality for convolution neural network based computer-aided diagnosis (CNN-CAD) of skin cancer. Çukurova Üniversitesi Mühendislik Fakültesi Dergisi **36**(4), 1099–1110 (2021)
41. S. Jain, U. Singhania, B. Tripathy, E.A. Nasr, M.K. Aboudaif, A.K. Kamrani, Deep learning-based transfer learning for classification of skin cancer. Sensors **21**(23), 8142 (2021)
42. R. Manne, S. Kantheti, S. Kantheti, Classification of skin cancer using deep learning, convolutional neural networks—opportunities and vulnerabilities—a systematic review. Int. J. Mod. Trends Sci. Technol. **6**(11), 101–108 (2020)
43. Z. Kadiroğlu, B.N. Akılotu, A. Şengür, M. Kayaoğlu, Derin öznitelikler ve renk kullanılarak dermoskopik görüntülerin sınıflandırılması: Classification of dermoscopic images using deep features and color (2020). Presented at IESS 2019 Conference
44. K. Fırıldak, M.F. Talu, G. Çelik, Transfer öğrenme ve çekişmeli üretici ağ yaklaşımlarını kullanarak cilt lezyonu sınıflandırma doğruluğunun iyileştirilmesi. Fırat Üniversitesi Mühendislik Bilimleri Dergisi **32**(2), 491–498 (2020)

45. S. Jinnai, Y. Yamamoto, A. Sugawara, K. Yamashita, T. Fujisawa, K. Fujita, The development of a skin cancer classification system for pigmented skin lesions using deep learning. Biomolecules **10**(8), 1123 (2020)
46. S.N. Hasan, Derin öğrenme yöntemleri ile cilt lezyon bölütlemesi. Master's thesis, İstanbul Üniversitesi, Fen Bilimleri Enstitüsü, Enformatik Anabilim Dalı (2019). https://nek.istanbul.edu.tr/ekos/TEZ/ET001149.pdf
47. E. Çevik, K. Zengin, Classification of skin lesions in dermatoscopic images with deep convolution network, in *Avrupa Bilim ve Teknoloji Dergisi, Özel Sayı* (2019), pp. 309–318
48. P. Tschandl, C. Rosendahl, H. Kittler, The HAM10000 dataset, a large collection of multi-source dermatoscopic images of common pigmented skin lesions. Sci. Data **5**, 180161 (2018)
49. N.C.F. Codella, D. Gutman, M.E. Celebi, B. Helba, M.A. Marchetti, S.W. Dusza, A. Kalloo, K. Liopyris, N. Mishra, H. Kittler, A. Halpern, Skin lesion analysis toward melanoma detection: a challenge at the 2017 International Symposium on Biomedical Imaging (ISBI), hosted by the International Skin Imaging Collaboration (ISIC). arXiv preprint arXiv:1710.05006 (2017)
50. C. Hernández-Pérez, M. Combalia, S. Podlipnik, N.C. Codella, V. Rotemberg, A.C. Halpern, O. Reiter, C. Carrera, A. Barreiro, B. Helba, S. Puig, V. Vilaplana, J. Malvehy, BCN20000: Dermoscopic lesions in the wild. Sci. Data **11**(1), 641 (2024)
51. B. Karadağ, A. Arı, M. Karadağ, Derin Öğrenme modellerinin sinirsel stil aktarımı performanslarının karşılaştırılması. J. Polytechnic **25**(6), 1611–1622 (2021)
52. H. Üzen, M. Altın, I.B. Çiçek, Bal arı hastalıklarının sınıflandırılması için convmixer, vgg16 ve resnet101 tabanlı topluluk Öğrenme yaklaşımı. Fırat Üniversitesi Mühendislik Bilimleri Dergisi **36**(1), 133–145 (2024)
53. B. Taşçı, Ön eğitimli evrişimsel sinir ağı modellerinde öznitelik seçim algoritmasını kullanarak cilt lezyon görüntülerinin sınıflandırılması. Fırat Üniversitesi Mühendislik Bilimleri Dergisi **34**(2), 541–552 (2022)
54. O.F. Göçgün, A. Onan, Amazon ürün değerlendirmeleri üzerinde derin öğrenme/makine öğrenmesi tabanlı duygu analizi yapılması. Avrupa Bilim ve Teknoloji Dergisi **24**, 445–448 (2021)
55. E. Coşlu, Veri madenciliği. Akademik Bilişim **23**(5) (2013)
56. M.A. Güvendir, Y. Özer Özkan, İki ölçekleme yönteminin karşılaştırılması: İkili karşılaştırma ve sıralama yargıları. Eğitim Bilimleri Araştırmaları Dergisi **3**(1), 105–119 (2013)
57. S. Gündüz, Uzaklık fonksiyonlarının çok boyutlu ölçekleme algoritmalarındaki etkinliğinin incelenmesi ve uygulamalar, in *Yüksek lisans tezi, Fen Bilimleri Enstitüsü, İstatistik Anabilim Dalı* (2011)
58. A. Kızrak, Ölçeklendirme ile cnn modelinin doğruluk ve verimliliğini artırma: Efficientnet (2019). Erişim tarihi: 12 Aralık 2019
59. A. Alan, M. Karabatak, Veri seti-sınıflandırma ilişkisinde performansa etki eden faktörlerin değerlendirilmesi. Fırat Üniversitesi Mühendislik Bilimleri Dergisi **32**(2), 531–540 (2020)
60. O. Çetin, F. Temurtaş, Görsel uyaranlara ilişkin manyetoensefalografi sinyallerinin genelleştirilmiş regresyon sinir ağı ile sınıflandırılması. Dicle Med. J. **46**(1), 19–25 (2019)
61. S. Prusty, S. Patnaik, S.K. Dash, SKCV: stratified K-fold cross-validation on ml classifiers for predicting cervical cancer. Front. Nanotechnol. **4**, 972421 (2022)
62. I. Kuş, S.B. Keser, E. Yolaçan, Saldırı tespit sistemlerinde topluluk öğrenme yöntemlerinin kıyaslanması. Avrupa Bilim ve Teknoloji Dergisi **31**, 725–734 (2021)
63. M. Sarıkoç, M. Çelik, Boyut İndirgeme teknikleri ve lstm derin Öğrenme ağı İle bist100 endeksi fiyat tahmini. Avrupa Bilim ve Teknoloji Dergisi **34**, 519–524 (2022)
64. Ş.M. Ersungur, A. Kızıltan, O. Polat, Türkiye'de bölgelerin sosyo-ekonomik gelişmişlik sıralaması: temel bileşenler analizi. Atatürk Üniversitesi İktisadi ve İdari Bilimler Dergisi **21**(2), 55–66 (2007)
65. K. Yıldız, Y. Çamurcu, B. Doğan, Veri madenciliğinde temel bileşenler analizi ve negatifsiz matris çarpanlarına ayırma tekniklerinin karşılaştırmalı analizi, in *Akademik Bilişim 2010* (2010), p. 248

66. S. Sevindik, G.Ü. Şiray, Diskriminant analizi ve bazı alternatif regresyon analizleri. Çukurova Üniversitesi Fen ve Mühendislik Bilimleri Dergisi **35**(9), (2018)
67. O. Cangül, Diskriminant analizi ve bir uygulama denemesi. Master's thesis (Bursa Uludağ University, Bursa, 2006). ProQuest Dissertations & Theses, No. 28741495
68. E. Yıldız, Y. Sevim, Sınıflandırma yöntemleri üzerinde lineer boyut indirgeme yöntemlerinin karşılaştırılması, in *Proceedings of the International Conference on Electrical and Electronics Engineering, Bursa, Turkey* (2016), pp. 161–164
69. B. Diri, Makine öğrenmesine giriş. Online lecture notes (2014). https://www.ce.yildiz.edu.tr/personal/banud/file/2634/Makine+Ogrenmesi-ML-10.pdf
70. B.Ö. Başer, M. Yangın, E.S. Sarıdaş, Makine öğrenmesi teknikleriyle diyabet hastalığının sınıflandırılması. Süleyman Demirel Üniversitesi Fen Bilimleri Enstitüsü Dergisi **25**(1), 112–120 (2021)
71. I. Özcan, B. Taşar, A.B. Tatar, O. Yakut, Destek vektör makinası algoritması ile kalp hastalıklarının tahmini. Comput. Sci. **4**(2), 74–79 (2019)
72. F. Tümincin, A. Aytekin, A. Ayaz,Veri madenciliğinde karar ağacı algoritması, in *Proceedings of the SADAB 5th International Conference on Social Researches and Behavioral Sciences,* Tbilisi, Georgia (2019)
73. K. Öztürk, M.E. Şahin, Yapay sinir ağları ve yapay zekâ'ya genel bir bakış. Takvim-i Vekayi **6**(2), 25–36 (2018)
74. M.O. Öğücü, Yapay sinir ağları ile sistem tanıma. Yüksek lisans tezi, İstanbul Teknik Üniversitesi, İstanbul, Türkiye (2006)
75. S. Çelik, D. Özdemir, Rastgele orman regresyon algoritmasi ile bitcoin fiyat tahmini. J. Sci. Reports-B **008**, 55–64 (2023)
76. I. Dalkıran, M. Ozan, Derin öğrenme teknikleri kullanılarak borsadaki hisse değerlerinin tahmin edilmesi. Avrupa Bilim ve Teknoloji Dergisi **39**, 143–148 (2022)
77. N.H. Güldemir, A. Alkan, Derin öğrenme ile optik koherens tomografi görüntülerinin sınıflandırılması. Fırat Üniversitesi Mühendislik Bilimleri Dergisi **33**(2), 607–615 (2021)
78. N. Zakiroğlu, Yapay zeka teknikleri kullanarak kemik yaşı tespiti üzerinde bir uygulama, in *Yüksek lisans tezi, İstanbul Aydın Üniversitesi, Fen Bilimleri Enstitüsü, İstanbul* (2019). Bilgisayar Mühendisliği Ana Bilim Dalı
79. D. Arıkan, F. Yıldız, Göktürk-1 uydu görüntülerinden u-net modeli kullanılarak binaların segmentasyonu. Turkish J. Remote Sens. **5**(1), 50–58 (2023)
80. M. Akın, Ş. Sağıroğlu, Yoğunluk tabanlı kümeleme yöntemiyle karakteristiği oluşturulan yollar için rnn yöntemi ile kısa zamanlı trafik hız tahmini. Gazi Üniversitesi Mühendislik Mimarlık Fakültesi Dergisi **37**(2), 581–594 (2022)
81. A. Şener, B. Ergen, Beyin mr görüntüleri Üzerinde tümör tespitinde vgg-19 model tabanlı yeni bir yaklaşım, in *Proceedings of the 6th International Artificial Intelligence and Data Processing Symposium, Malatya, Turkey* (2022)
82. E. Öztad, Meme kanseri tespitinde sınıflandırma ve sinir ağları yöntemlerinin karşılaştırılması. İleri Mühendislik Çalışmaları ve Teknolojileri Dergisi **1**(1), 49–54 (2020)
83. K. Fırıldak, M.F. Talu, Evrişimsel sinir ağlarında kullanılan transfer öğrenme yaklaşımlarının incelenmesi. Comput. Sci. **4**(2), 88–95 (2019)
84. M. Yavaş, A. Güran, M. Uysal, Covid-19 veri kümesinin smote tabanlı örnekleme yöntemi uygulanarak sınıflandırılması, in *Avrupa Bilim ve Teknoloji Dergisi, Ejosat Özel Sayı 2020 (HORA)* (2020), pp. 258–264
85. S. Aydın, R. Samet, O.F. Bay, Gpu programlamada cuda platformu kullanılan paralel görüntü işleme çalışmalarının incelenmesi. Politeknik Dergisi **23**(3), 737–754 (2020)
86. F. Atlan, E. Hançer, I. Pençe, U-net ile çekirdek segmentasyonunda hiper parametre optimizasyonu etkisinin değerlendirilmesi, in *Avrupa Bilim ve Teknoloji Dergisi, Ejosat Special Issue 2020 (ISMSIT)* (2020), pp. 60–69
87. A. Değirmenciler, B. Cengiz, K. İleri, Covid-19'un yayılmasını önlemek için cnn ile yüz maskesi tespiti. Mühendislik Bilimleri ve Araştırmaları Dergisi **4**(2), 259–265 (2022)
88. S. Altun, M.F. Talu, Derin sinir ağları için hiperparametre metodlarının ve kitlerinin incelenmesi. Dicle Üniversitesi Mühendislik Fakültesi Mühendislik Dergisi **12**(2), 187–199 (2021)

89. N. Çarkacı, Derin öğrenme uygulamalarında en sık kullanılan hiper-parametreler (2018). https://medium.com/deep-learning-turkiye/derin-ogrenme-uygulamalarinda-en-sik-kullanilan-hiper-parametreler-ece8e9125c4 (Accessed: Jul. 27, 2025)
90. E. Seyyarer, T. Uçkan, C. Hark, F. Ayata, M. İnan, A. Karcı, Applications and comparisons of optimization algorithms used in convolutional neural networks, in *2019 International Artificial Intelligence and Data Processing Symposium (IDAP)*, Malatya, Turkey (IEEE, New York, 2019)
91. Devreyakan, Aşırı öğrenme (overfitting) ve az öğrenme (underfitting) (2021). https://devreyakan.com
92. J. Murel, E. Kavlakoğlu, What is a confusion matrix? (2023). https://www.ibm.com/think/topics/confusion-matrix
93. D. Chicco, G. Jurman, The advantages of the Matthews correlation coefficient (MCC) over F1 score and accuracy in binary classification evaluation. BMC Genomics **21**(1), 6 (2020)
94. T. Fawcett, Introduction to ROC analysis. Pattern Recognit. Lett. **27**(8), 861–874 (2006)
95. E. Seyyarer, F. Ayata, T. Uçkan, A. Karcı, Derin öğrenmede kullanılan optimizasyon algoritmalarinin uygulanması ve kıyaslanması. Comput. Sci. **5**(2), 90–98 (2020)
96. I. Loshchilov, F. Hutter, Decoupled weight decay regularization. arXiv preprint arXiv:1711.05101 (2017). Last revised: Jan. 4, 2019. https://doi.org/10.48550/arXiv.1711.05101
97. G. Gürgen, S. Serttaş, Kalp yetmezliği hastalığının erken teşhisinde makine öğrenimi algoritmalarının performans karşılaştırması. Euroasia J. Math. Eng. Nat. Med. Sci. **10**(28), 165–174 (2023)
98. N.V. Otten, Practical guide to grid search (2023). https://medium.com/@neri.vvo/practical-guide-to-grid-search-6552856c4c5f
99. V. Sinap, Optuna tabanlı hiperparametre optimizasyonu ile konut fiyat tahminlemede makine öğrenmesi tekniklerinin karşılaştırmalı analizi. Gazi Üniversitesi Fen Bilimleri Dergisi Part C: Tasarım ve Teknoloji **13**(1), 10–28 (2025)
100. D.S. Charan, H. Nadipineni, S. Sahayam, U. Jayaraman, Method to classify skin lesions using dermoscopic images. arXiv preprint arXiv:2008.09418 (2020). Last revised: Dec. 20, 2022. https://doi.org/10.48550/arXiv.2008.09418

Next-Gen Diagnostics: Utilizing AI Classification Algorithms for Enhanced Obesity Detection and Intervention

Yunus Emre Hos and Gulay Cicek

Abstract Analyzing obesity-related factors and classifying individuals based on their risk status are critical for improving the effectiveness of health policies. This study aimed to predict individuals' predisposition to obesity using classification algorithms. The dataset, obtained from an open-access data source, contains 22,869 records and 16 attributes, including demographic information, physical activities, and dietary habits. Various preprocessing steps were performed on the data to improve model accuracy and reliability by improving data quality. This preprocessing phase included removing missing data, scaling data, and processing outliers. Principal component analysis and linear discriminant analysis were used to identify the most useful attributes by removing irrelevant attributes from the data. After identifying useful features in the dataset, a hybrid model was developed to classify individuals' obesity levels by leveraging the strengths of various machine learning (support vector machines, decision trees, gradient boosting, random forest, and logistic regression) and deep learning algorithms (autoencoders, convolutional neural networks, and recurrent neural networks), as well as individual classification algorithms. In order to achieve higher classification performance, a hybrid model was developed. K-Fold cross-validation was performed to evaluate the performance of this model alone. The hybrid model demonstrated the highest classification performance among all individual models, with an accuracy rate of 90%. Considering the global impact of obesity, the findings of this study will make significant contributions to many areas such as early diagnosis and risk assessment, development of health policies, reduction of health expenditures, efficient use of resources, and development of personalized intervention strategies.

Y. E. Hos
Faculty of Engineering and Architecture, Department of Software Engineering, Istanbul Beykent University, Istanbul, Türkiye
e-mail: 2203013089@student.beykent.edu.tr

G. Cicek (✉)
Faculty of Engineering and Architecture, Department of Biomedical Engineering, Istanbul Beykent University, Istanbul, Türkiye
e-mail: gulaycicek@beykent.edu.tr

N. E. M. Khalifa, M. H. N. Taha (eds.), *Next-Gen Healthcare*,
https://doi.org/10.1007/978-3-032-07267-2_14

Keywords Classification · Obesity · Machine learning · Neural network · Hybrid model

List of Abbreviations

DNN	Deep neural network
DT	Decision tree
RF	Random forest
SVM	Support vector machine
GB	Gradient boosting
LassoReg	Lasso regularized logistic regression
EBM	Explainable boosting machine
XGB	Extreme gradient boosting
NB	Naïve Bayes
KNN	K-nearest neighbors
ANN	Artificial neural networks
LSTM	Long short-term memory
LGB	Light gradient boosting
LGBM	Light gradient boosting machine
GBT	Gradient boosting tree
MLP	Multilayer perceptron
LR	Logistic regression
HGB	Histogram-based gradient boosting
AB	Adaptive boosting
RBF	Radial basis function
J48	Decision tree variation
GNB	Gaussian Naive Bayes
NN	Neural network
BNB	Bernoulli Naive Bayes
HCNN	Haar cascade classifier
RR	Ridge regression
GBDT	Gradient boosting decision tree
RC	Ridge classifier
LASSO	Least absolute shrinkage and selection operator
BPNN	Backpropagation neural network
RS	Random subspace
SKM	Simple K-means
CART	Classification and regression trees
ACC	Accuracy
AUC	Area under curve
REC	Recall

1 Introduction

Nutrition is the process of acquiring and utilizing the nutrients necessary for an organism's survival. Proper nutrition supports an individual's physical and mental health, improving their quality of life, strengthening their resistance to disease, maintaining a balanced energy level, promoting growth, development, and healthy aging, reducing the risk of chronic diseases such as obesity and diabetes, and contributing positively to daily functions such as sleep patterns, mood, and focus. Proper and balanced nutrition is achieved by meeting the body's needs with macronutrients such as protein, fat, and carbohydrates, as well as micronutrients such as vitamins and minerals. Conversely, inadequate and unbalanced nutrition leads to various health problems, negatively impacting an individual's physical and mental health, weakening the immune system, reducing learning capacity, and contributing to the development of metabolic disorders, thus reducing quality of life [1, 2].

1.1 Health Issues Caused by Insufficient and Irregular Nutrition

Inadequate and unbalanced nutrition can weaken the immune system, increasing susceptibility to infection. It also increases the risk of cardiovascular disease, hypertension, obesity, diabetes, and some types of cancer; negatively impacts mental performance and concentration, reducing learning capacity; disrupts the digestive system, leading to conditions such as constipation, bloating, and stomach problems; and negatively impacts growth, development, and healthy aging.

Macronutrients (carbohydrates, protein, and fat) can cause serious health problems in the body. Protein deficiency can lead to muscle loss, weakened immune systems, and slowed healing processes, while carbohydrate insufficiency can lead to energy loss, fatigue, dizziness, and mental focus problems. Fat deficiency can lead to hormonal imbalances, impaired absorption of fat-soluble vitamins, and dry skin [3].

Vitamin and mineral deficiencies negatively impact the body's ability to maintain basic functions, leading to numerous health problems, including a weakened immune system, low energy levels and fatigue, growth and developmental disorders, poor bone and dental health, and skin, hair, and nail problems. For example, iron, B12, and folic acid deficiencies can lead to low energy levels, while vitamin D, calcium, and phosphorus deficiencies can lead to conditions like osteoporosis and rickets. Furthermore, vitamin and mineral deficiencies can impair nervous system function, hinder metabolic efficiency, and reduce the body's overall resilience. For example, vitamin C deficiency weakens the immune system and slows the healing process [4, 5].

1.2 Obesity

Obesity, caused by excessive caloric intake, is a chronic condition resulting from long-term energy surplus, leading to excess fat accumulation with associated structural and physiological complications [6]. This condition is associated with cardiovascular disease, type 2 diabetes, respiratory problems, joint problems, 13 different types of cancer, and metabolic syndromes [7–9].

Irregular and high-calorie eating habits, lack of physical activity, lifestyle changes associated with urbanization, long-term use of certain medications, genetic predisposition, and endocrine disorders are among the factors that influence the development of obesity [10]. Obesity negatively impacts individuals' daily activities, such as loss of employment, early retirement, and reduced productivity, exacerbating the economic impact of obesity. Furthermore, it leads to increased healthcare costs at both the individual and societal levels, and treating this disorder places a significant economic burden on the healthcare system [11].

Obesity can negatively impact an individual's participation in the workforce. The increased health problems caused by obesity lead to a decrease in the working population and increased rates of mandatory early retirement, threatening the sustainability of social security systems. Furthermore, obesity-related labor inefficiency leads to lower productivity in the economy and can narrow the tax base [12–14].

The negative impacts of obesity on the workforce are also evident. Health problems associated with obesity result in workforce losses and situations such as forced early retirement, which are believed to add further strain to social security systems. It is anticipated that the decline in productivity due to obesity indirectly affects the economy, potentially leading to reduced productivity and a decrease in tax revenues.

1.3 Obesity Classification

Obesity is determined by the body mass index (BMI), which is calculated based on an individual's weight and height. As shown in Fig. 1, individuals with a BMI below 18.50 are considered underweight, those between 18.50 and 24.99 are considered normal weight, those between 25.00 and 29.00 are considered overweight, those between 30.00 and 34.99 are considered obese, and those above 35.00 are considered severely obese [15]. However, BMI alone is not a sufficient indicator for obesity classification because it does not directly provide information on body fat percentage and body composition, nor does it consider individual differences such as age, gender, and muscle mass [16, 17]. Obesity is a health problem directly related to an individual's lifestyle [18]. Therefore, for an accurate and comprehensive diagnosis of obesity, various factors such as age, gender, energy balance, activity level, dietary habits, genetic predisposition, and hormonal status must be analyzed together [19, 20].

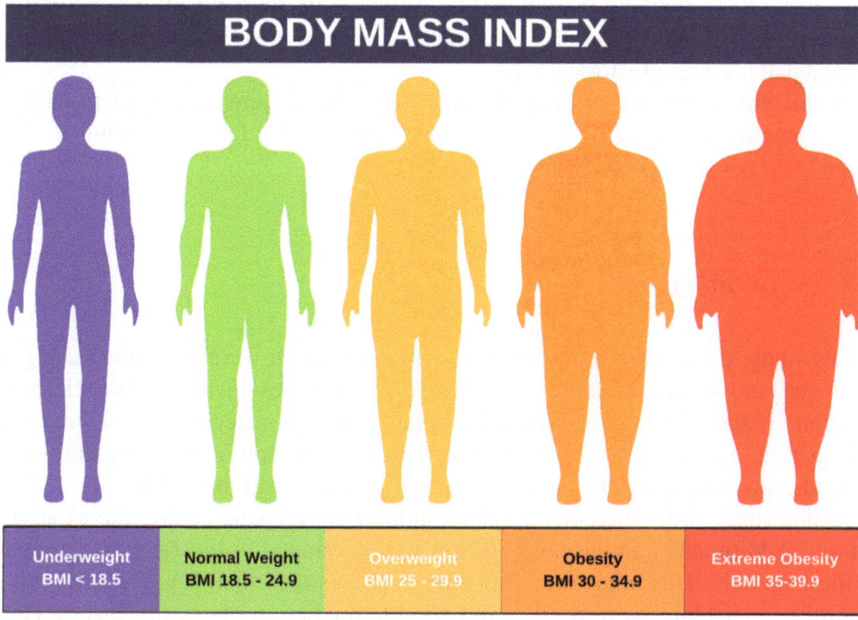

Fig. 1 Body mass index

1.4 The Importance of Early Diagnosis in Obesity and the Use of Artificial Intelligence

Early diagnosis of obesity helps prevent the development of many chronic diseases, demonstrating positive long-term effects on reducing healthcare costs, improving quality of life, and improving workforce performance. The number of fat cells can increase throughout an individual's life, but weight loss only reduces their volume, not their number. Therefore, obese individuals may gain fat more quickly if they consume more energy. Early diagnosis helps individuals manage their weight more easily and develop healthy habits [21–23].

In clinical practice, obesity is typically determined through physical measurements such as body fat percentage and skinfold thickness, which requires time-consuming assessments of individuals. However, obesity is a complex condition that requires consideration of numerous variables, including lifestyle, habits, and environmental factors. Therefore, technology-based approaches that integrate lifestyle data offer innovative and effective alternatives to traditional diagnostic methods.

Artificial intelligence (AI) techniques can rapidly analyze multidimensional data containing numerous variables—such as individuals' lifestyles, health records, and demographic characteristics—enabling early and accurate diagnosis of obesity. These techniques provide healthcare professionals with preliminary insights about their patients and allow individuals to assess their own health status swiftly. Furthermore, AI can deliver effective analyses even in novel situations by utilizing learned patterns from historical data.

In this study, various machine learning algorithms were employed to analyze these complex, interrelated factors and to classify individuals according to their obesity levels.

1.5 Originality of the Study

In this study, classification models for obesity detection were developed using an expanded and balanced dataset. Data mining processes included data cleaning, integration, and selection. The dataset, which contained categorical and numerical information, was converted into digital format using appropriate transformation methods, paving the way for the development of classification models.

In this study, individual classification models were created using the expanded dataset. Additionally, an ensemble model was developed to leverage the strengths of these models. This innovative approach improves the efficiency of classification algorithms, enabling more precise and reliable prediction of obesity levels. Thus, the study aims to make a valuable contribution to the literature [24, 25].

Although an increase in sample size does not directly guarantee higher classification performance, increasing both the number of samples and the diversity of features—especially the inclusion of frequently used parameters related to demographic information, dietary habits, and physical activity—makes a significant contribution to increasing the reliability of the model for obesity detection.

The dataset underwent a rigorous preprocessing process that included the detection and removal of outliers and the standardization (normalization) of the features. Inconsistencies in the data entry, particularly for some attributes such as weight (e.g., some values were integers such as 89 kg, while others contained unnecessary decimal places such as 89.797), were corrected. Data integrity was ensured by converting such values into a standard format (e.g., limited to two decimal places). Furthermore, meaningless and repetitive features were removed from the dataset. These preprocessing steps increased the consistency and reliability of the dataset, contributing to the classification models producing more robust results.

Although the hybrid model consists of only two core algorithms (random forest and gradient boosting), it offers flexibility and room for improvement. This hybrid model performed better in terms of accuracy than either of these two algorithms alone. Furthermore, it was observed that further improvements could be achieved by optimizing the model's parameters or extending it with additional algorithms. This approach can serve as a guide for researchers who want to work on more complex ensemble models in the future.

The proposed models have the potential to be integrated into various digital health tools. While not intended to replace professional medical assessment, these models can support healthcare providers in their prescreening processes and assist individuals seeking personal health information. This demonstrates their potential for use in early diagnosis support, personalized healthcare, and public health planning.

Contributions of the Study to the Literature

- By comparing the performance of the hybrid model and various algorithms, the conditions under which these algorithms perform and the outcomes they produce or may produce have been reported.
- Through the use of an expanded and balanced dataset, a unique study has been presented that differs from the frequently used datasets in the literature.
- Potential for Integration into Health Technologies: The study highlights the potential for the proposed models to be integrated into early diagnosis, personalized healthcare services, and public health programs.

The literature review section of the article evaluates a total of 29 studies on obesity detection using machine learning algorithms. Each study is summarized in a comprehensive table (Table 1) that includes information on participants, machine learning algorithms used, best-performing algorithm, performance metrics, and publication year. Following this table, the analysis highlights the contributions of our study to the existing literature. The Methodology section provides detailed information on the methods and techniques used to construct the classification models developed for obesity detection. The Experimental Results section analyzes the performance of these models using commonly applied evaluation metrics such as accuracy, sensitivity, specificity, and the F-measure [26]. The Discussion section addresses potential areas for model improvement and outlines possible future contributions, while the Conclusion section offers a comprehensive and holistic assessment summarizing the key findings and contributions of the study.

2 Literature Review

Obesity classification has been a frequently discussed topic in recent years. Numerous artificial-intelligence-based methods have been developed to improve classification accuracy. This section presents a synthesis of existing studies in the literature, including the datasets used, sample sizes, methods applied, and performance results obtained. Furthermore, key trends, limitations, and methodological gaps related to the current study are identified, clearly highlighting how this study differs from similar studies in the literature.

Table 1 Recent obesity detection studies

Ref.	Participants	Machine learning algorithms	Best Best	Performance metrics	Publication year
[27]	2111	DT, RF, SVM	RF	%96.00 ACC, 0.95 F1	2024
[30]	2971	EBM, GBT, LASSOReg	EBM	%86.00 ACC, 0.73 AUC	2024
[32]	89	XGB, RF	RF & XGB	%78.00 AUC	2024
[33]	46057	RF, DT, GBDT	GBDT	%78.00 AUC	2024
[28]	1678	KNN, XGB, GBT, LGB, DT, SVM, MLP, RF	XGB	%95.00 ACC, 0.95 AUC	2024
[34]	1610	RF, SVM, KNN	RF	%87.82 ACC 0.90 AUC	2024
[35]	1179	GB, RF, LR, AB, HCNN, DT, GNB, BNB	HCNN	%80.00 ACC, %89 REC	2024
[36]	2111	DNN	DNN	%96.46 ACC	2023
[37]	160	LG, DT, RF, SVM, RF, GB, AB	RF	%80.00 ACC, 0.79 F1	2023
[38]	72	RF	RF	%87.00 ACC	2023
[39]	1185	LASSO, LR	LR	%74.00 ACC, 0.82 AUC	2023
[40]	5000	DT, RF, SVM, NB, LR, XGB, KNN, ANN	XGB	%93.00 ACC, 0.81 AUC	2023
[41]	117	SVM, RC, LR	SVM	%90.25 ACC	2023
[42]	21100	RF, SVM, LR, MLP, LGBM	MLP	%78.00 ACC, 0.78 AUC	2023
[43]	90	XGB, CART	XGB	%71.00 ACC, 0.83 AUC	2023
[44]	2111	NN	NN	%93.06 ACC, 0.90 F1	2023
[45]	2111	HGB, RF, SVM, DT	HGB	%98.00 ACC, 0.90 F1	2022
[29]	6614	LSTM	LSTM	%0.98 MAE	2022
[31]	1879	SVM, RF, KNN, LR, GBDT, RR	SVM	%70.80 ACC, 0.48 R^2	2022
[46]	1110	KNN, SVM, NB, LR, DT, RF, MLP, AB, GBM	LR	%97.09 ACC	2021
[47]	7162	NB, RBF, KNN, CVR, RS, J48, MLP, RF	RF	%70.01 ACC, 0.63 AUC	2021
[48]	2111	DT, SVM, KNN, GNB, MLP, RF, GB	RF	%77.69 ACC, 0.78 F1	2021
[49]	618898	LR, NB	LR	%72.00 ACC, 0.79 AUC	2021
[50]	27203	LR, SVM, NN, XGB, GNB, BNB, DT	XGB	%66.14 ACC, 0.81 AUC	2021
[51]	+12K	SVM, NB, DT, RF, KNN, LR	SVM	%95.00 ACC, 0.95 R^2	2020
[52]	+34M	SVM, RF, GBM, ANN, NB	SVM	%87.00 ACC	2020
[53]	178	DT, SVM, SKM	DT	%97.20 ACC, 0.98 AUC	2020
[54]	1053	LR, NB, DT, RF, KNN, AB	RF	%100.0 ACC, 100 AUC	2019
[55]	7200	J48	J48	%92.00 ACC	2019

2.1 Common Findings

In recent years, a total of 29 AI-based classification models have been developed for obesity detection. An examination of the methodologies, challenges, and results of these studies reveals that some consistent modeling approaches stand out. Findings in the literature reveal that numerous variables must be considered in the assessment of obesity. Most studies consider lifestyle factors such as poor eating habits and physical inactivity as the primary risk category. The most frequently used attributes include lifestyle variables, demographic information, genetic predispositions, and socioeconomic indicators.

A review of the literature reveals that ensemble methods—particularly random forest and gradient boosting (XGBoost) algorithms—achieve higher accuracy rates compared to other models. These algorithms have stood out, demonstrating accuracy between 80% and 96% in various studies [27, 28]. Despite producing competitive results on large datasets, deep-learning-based models are criticized for their lack of interpretability, which limits their widespread adoption in clinical practice [29]). Additionally, 17 studies in the literature were found to be excessively reliant on the same dataset of 2,111 participants. This points to significant methodological issues, such as inadequate dataset diversity and class imbalance. To overcome these limitations, many studies have employed synthetic data augmentation techniques. Finally, next-generation data collection methods, such as wearable technologies [30] and microbiome analyses [31], have the potential to advance obesity research beyond traditional lifestyle surveys, providing more in-depth, multilayered, and rich data structures. In this respect, these approaches offer significant opportunities for future research.

2.2 Literature Review and Discussion

The literature review section analyzes the datasets and methods used in existing obesity detection studies, their performance results, their future contributions, and identified shortcomings, positioning the original and unique aspects of our study within this context. A significant portion of existing research either relies on a limited number of real-world datasets (e.g., 160 participants in the [37] study) or repeatedly uses the same dataset of 2,111 participants, a common feature in the literature. This severely limits the generalizability of the developed models.

In contrast, this study utilized a comprehensive synthetic dataset consisting of 22,869 samples, providing a holistic solution to these limitations. This dataset significantly increases the sample size and variable diversity, while preserving the underlying patterns of the original data, thus enabling the development of more robust and generalizable predictive models.

Previous studies have generally focused on algorithm selection and parameter optimization, often neglecting critical aspects such as data quality and representativeness. To address this shortcoming, synthetic data generation techniques using the SMOTE method were applied in our study, reducing both the class imbalance problem and improving overall model performance. The 90.09% accuracy rate achieved with the hybrid RF-GB model reflects not only an algorithmic success but also a success based on the high quality and representativeness of the dataset architecture. In terms of clinical applicability, while many studies report high accuracy rates, practical benefit is limited due to uninterpretable model structures called "black boxes." In our study, this challenge was overcome by integrating SHAP values and feature importance analysis, providing both high predictive ability and explainability, making a valuable contribution to clinical use. Furthermore, the performance degradation observed during the application of dimensionality reduction techniques such as PCA and LDA once again demonstrated the importance of preserving all variables in modeling the multidimensional structure of obesity. The findings from this study contribute to the literature in the following ways:

- Creating a synthetic yet comprehensive and original dataset that addresses the widespread lack of data diversity in the literature
- Designing a hybrid classification architecture after preprocessing steps to improve data quality
- Increasing clinical applicability with explainable artificial intelligence techniques

This holistic approach provides a robust methodological and practical framework for future studies on the early detection and prevention of obesity.

3 Method

This section presents all the stages of the modeling process developed for obesity detection in detail. The dataset used, the preprocessing steps applied, the feature selection methods, the preferred classification algorithms, and the metrics used to evaluate model performance are systematically explained.

3.1 Dataset

This study used two different publicly available datasets. The first dataset, [56], contains information on the dietary habits and physical activity levels of participants in Mexico, Peru, and Colombia. Approximately 23% of this dataset consists of real data obtained from online sources, while the remaining 77% consists of synthetic data generated using the synthetic minority oversampling technique (SMOTE) method for data augmentation. The first dataset, [56], contains data from a total of 2,111 participants, each with 16 attributes (Table 2). The second dataset, [57], was obtained from the Kaggle platform and consists of synthetic data generated using deep learning algorithms based on the first dataset, [56]. Both datasets are consistent in their features and were combined to create a large and balanced training dataset of 22,869 participants. The dataset contains seven different classes: "underweight," "normal weight," "level 1 overweight," "level 2 overweight," "level 1 obesity," "level 2 obesity," and "level 3 obesity." This classification was maintained across all datasets. Features were determined based on dietary behaviors and physical activity levels highlighted in the literature. The first and second datasets were combined to create a new dataset with the features detailed in Table 3. The training dataset included 22,869 participants with 16 features per participant. The test dataset consisted of 6,860 participants assigned to one of the seven classes in Table 4: underweight, normal weight, overweight level 1, overweight level 2, obesity level 1, obesity level 2, and obesity level 3. These classes were consistent across all datasets. Feature selection was based on dietary habits and physical activity status, as outlined in the literature review.

3.1.1 Limitations of Synthetic Data and SMOTE: Implications for Generalizability

While SMOTE effectively balances classes, it has known limitations. By interpolating between minority class samples, SMOTE may produce artificial patterns that do not exist in real populations. This can lead to model overfitting, especially when the majority of the training data is synthetic. Moreover, SMOTE assumes linearity between feature vectors and does not account for the distribution of the majority class, which may cause class overlap and misclassification.

Although real data is present in the original dataset, the extensive use of synthetic augmentation raises questions about generalizability. Models trained on such data might struggle to perform reliably on unseen, real-world datasets. Therefore, cross-validation and rigorous evaluation metrics were employed to mitigate these concerns. Nonetheless, external validation with independent real-world data remains essential for ensuring robustness and clinical applicability.

3.2 Justification of Feature Selection

The dataset used in this study consists of 16 attributes that have been shown in the literature to be associated with obesity. These attributes include demographic information such as age and gender, anthropometric data such as height and weight, as well as lifestyle indicators such as cigarette and alcohol use, daily water consumption, duration of technology use, and preferred mode of transportation. Numerous studies have consistently demonstrated that these attributes are strong predictors of obesity and metabolic health outcomes [27, 36, 45]. For example, the consumption of high-calorie foods (calorie intake patterns), time spent using technological devices, and physical activity levels are frequently reported as key factors contributing to the development of obesity. Additionally, factors such as

Table 2 Attribute table

Attribute	Values	Quantity or range
Gender	1 = Male	11403
	2 = Female	11446
Age	Integer	14–61 (age range)
Height	Integer (centimeters)	140–197 (height range)
Weight	Integer (kilograms)	39–165 (weight range)
Overweight family member	0 = Yes	18739
	1 = No	4129
Frequent consumption of high-calorie foods (FAVC)	0 = Yes	20847
	1 = No	2021
Vegetable consumption frequency (FCVC)	1	1611
	2	12948
	3	8310
Number of main meals (NCP)	1	3380
	2	2117
	3	16638
	4	784
Consumption of food between meals (CAEC)	4 = Always	419
	3 = Often	2713
	2 = Sometimes	19293
	1 = No	329
Smoking (SMOKE)	0 = Yes	290
	1 = No	22580
Daily water consumption (CH2O)	1	6905
	2	14231
	3	1733
Calorie consumption tracking (SCC)	0 = Yes	783
	1 = No	22086
Frequency of physical activity (FAF)	0	5455
	1	9313
	2	3674
	3	1169
	4	270
	5	350
	6	477
	7	467
	8	680
	9	1014

(continued)

Table 2 (continued)

Time spent on technological devices (TUE)	0	7123
	1	7696
	2	2067
	3	476
	4	780
	5	817
	6	854
	7	941
	8	909
	9	1206
Alcohol consumption (CALC)	4 = Always	1
	3 = Often	599
	2 = Sometimes	16467
	1 = No	5802
Transportation type (MTRANS)	1 = Car	3991
	2 = Bicycle	38
	3 = Motorcycle	48
	4 = Public transport	18266
	5 = Walking	521

Table 3 Class table

Class	Values	Quantity or range
Obesity level (NObeyesdad)	1 = Underweight	2795
	2 = Normal weight	3368
	3 = Overweight level 1	2716
	4 = Overweight level 2	2717
	5 = Obesity level 1	3360
	6 = Obesity level 2	3544
	7 = Obesity level 3	4369

Table 4 Machine learning algorithms training performances

Model	Accuracy	Precision	Recall	F1 score	AUC-ROC
SVM	89.35%	89.29%	89.35%	89.31%	98.79%
Decision tree	99.83%	99.83%	99.83%	99.83%	99.99%
Gradient boosting	90.02%	89.97%	90.02%	89.97%	98.86%
Random forest	99.83%	99.83%	99.83%	99.83%	99.99%
Logistic regression	86.01%	85.75%	86.01%	85.85%	97.95%

genetic predisposition (family history) and individuals' self-monitoring behaviors are also known to influence weight status and health awareness.

3.3 Data Preprocessing

Data preprocessing requires performing various operations on raw data to make it suitable for analysis. During this process, irregularities in the data were resolved, and a structure that can be utilized for modeling was established.

The dataset used for obesity detection was made suitable for analysis by undergoing the following preprocessing steps:

- Missing Data Handling: Missing or erroneous data in the dataset were filled in using relevant statistical methods or removed without compromising the analysis quality. Additionally, categorical variables were converted into numerical format using methods such as labeling or one-hot coding, ensuring a more robust analysis process. This step is critical for maintaining data integrity.
- Outlier Detection and Handling: Outliers in the dataset were identified, and the impact of such noisy data was reduced. This prevented any negative impact on the model's learning process.
- Scaling (Normalization and Standardization): Features at different scales were brought within a specific range, ensuring comparability of the data. The mathematical formulas of the applied techniques are detailed in the Eqs. (1) and (2) sections:
  - **Min-Max Scaling (Normalization):** Features are scaled between a minimum and maximum value (typically [0, 1]).

$$x' = \frac{x - \min(x)}{\max(x) - \min(x)}. \tag{1}$$

  - **Z-Score Standardization:** It is a method of rescaling data so that its mean is zero and its standard deviation is one, in order to bring the data to the same scale.

$$z = \frac{x - \mu}{\sigma}. \tag{2}$$

  μ: Mean of the feature
  σ: Standard deviation of the feature

- Feature extraction and selection: In order to reduce model complexity, shorten the training process, and create more robust and reliable models, repetitive features that do not contribute to the analysis were removed from the dataset, and important features supported by literature were selected.

3.4 Data Splitting and Cross-Validation

Various data splitting strategies were applied to evaluate model performance and increase generalization ability. In this study, 70% of the dataset was allocated as training and 30% as test set. The performance of the trained model was evaluated on the test data [58]. The validation set, which is typically used for hyperparameter tuning and overfitting control, was not included in this study. The training results of the models are detailed in Table 4.

K-Fold Cross-Validation: This is a common method that aims to obtain more reliable and stable results by evaluating the model on different sub-datasets. This method is used to reduce the risks of overfitting and underfitting, especially when the dataset is limited. In this study, the K-fold cross-validation method was preferred to evaluate the performance of the hybrid model [59].

3.5 Feature Selection Methods

In classification algorithms, feature selection is crucial to increase model accuracy, reduce unnecessary processing load, prevent overfitting, and obtain more robust results by finding effective features.

Linear Discriminant Analysis (LDA) Linear discriminant analysis (LDA) is an effective dimensionality reduction technique that improves the accuracy and generalization ability of classification algorithms by drawing clearer boundaries between classes. The primary goal of LDA is to create a new, optimized subspace that maximizes separation between classes in a dataset. To this end, interclass variance is increased, while intraclass variance is minimized. This allows for clearer separation of data and contributes positively to classification performance. LDA can be effectively applied not only to small datasets but also to multidimensional and complex data structures. It is widely used in fields with high-dimensional data, such as text classification, medical diagnosis, and bioinformatics, as it provides meaningful data representation and high classification accuracy. Unlike other feature selection algorithms, LDA actively incorporates class information into calculations. This has made it a more preferred method for classification problems. Its efficiency and computational efficiency facilitate class separation in large datasets and increase model performance:

- These are widely preferred approaches in feature selection processes in high-dimensional datasets. These methods select the most significant ones by determining the statistical relationship of each feature with the target variable. The relationship of each feature to the class is evaluated using statistical tests such as chi-square tests, ANOVA, and correlation coefficients. One of the greatest advantages of these methods is their ability to operate independently of the model. Feature selection can be performed without the need for a machine learning algorithm. Furthermore, because they are computationally fast, they offer a practical solution when working with large datasets. However, because the relationships between features are not considered, some disadvantages such as excluding some meaningful feature combinations and negatively impacting model performance are also present.

- **Wrapper Methods:** Wrapper methods adopt a model-based approach to feature selection, testing different feature combinations and evaluating the impact of each combination on the model. The greatest advantage of these methods is that they select by considering the interactions between features. This allows for high accuracy and strong generalization. However, testing all combinations can lead to high computational costs. Therefore, wrapper methods are generally preferred in small feature spaces or environments with high processing power.
- **Embedded Methods:** Embedded methods are approaches that perform feature selection in an integrated manner with the model's training process. The model determines which features are most effective during training and is trained using only the meaningful features accordingly. This way, feature selection occurs as a natural part of model training, not as a separate step. By eliminating unnecessary or low-impact features, the risk of overfitting is reduced, and the model's performance on new data is improved. Embedded methods are widely preferred in fields such as healthcare, finance, and natural language processing. Furthermore, selecting meaningful features increases the interpretability of the model.
- **Principal Component Analysis (PCA):** PCA is a statistical dimensionality reduction technique used to reduce the number of features in high-dimensional datasets. This method creates new components representing the highest variance in the data, allowing the original features to be represented with fewer components. This minimizes information loss and simplifies the data. PCA is particularly effective in analyzing high-dimensional, noisy, or correlated data. It is frequently applied in image processing, face recognition, genetic data analysis, and machine learning preprocessing processes. Dimensionality reduction reduces modeling time and reduces the risk of overfitting. However, PCA only considers linear relationships, and the resulting new components may not be directly interpretable with the original features, which can be a disadvantage in terms of interpretability:
  - **PCA Steps:**
    - Zero-centering the dataset (removing the mean)
    - Calculating the covariance matrix
    - Deriving the eigenvectors and eigenvalues from the covariance matrix
    - Sorting the eigenvectors according to their magnitude
    - Selecting the components corresponding to the largest eigenvectors

PCA is crucial for dimensionality reduction and mitigating overfitting. However, PCA may result in the loss of the original meanings of features. Therefore, it should not be confused with feature selection; PCA transforms features into a new space, whereas feature selection identifies a subset of existing features [60].

3.6 *Model Selection*

- Machine Learning Algorithm:
  - **Support Vector Machine (SVM)**: SVM is a supervised learning algorithm used for classification and regression. Its primary aim is to find the best hyperplane that separates data classes. This hyperplane is designed to maximize the margin, which is the gap between the hyperplane and the closest data points, known as support vectors. For data that is linearly separable, the hyperplane acts as a straight boundary. If the data is not linearly separable, kernel functions (e.g., RBF, polynomial) map the data into a higher-dimensional space to enable separation. SVM is effective for high-dimensional data and reduces the risk of overfitting. However, it may require significant computation for large datasets, and careful kernel selection and parameter tuning are critical. Due to its margin optimization and strong generalization, SVM is widely used in various fields [61].
  - **Decision Tree (DT)**
    Decision trees, a supervised learning method, are employed to address both classification and regression tasks. The algorithm organizes data into a hierarchical tree structure, formulating decision rules that facilitate classification or prediction. Feature importance is evaluated to identify the optimal splits within the dataset, with decision rules generated at each node. Common splitting criteria include the Gini index, entropy, or variance reduction. The terminal nodes, or leaf nodes, represent class labels or predicted outcomes. Decision trees are highly interpretable due to their straightforward structure, making them easy to understand. However, excessively deep trees can result in overfitting and diminished generalization capacity. To mitigate this, techniques such as limiting tree depth or pruning are often applied. Known for their speed and robust performance on complex datasets, decision trees remain popular for their generalization capability and adaptability. Despite these strengths, model accuracy can be influenced by dataset imbalances. Nevertheless, decision trees are a preferred choice for solving a wide range of problems. The core logic of the algorithm—recursive binary splitting based on impurity reduction—is schematically illustrated in Fig. 2, where each internal node represents a decision rule and each leaf node corresponds to a predicted outcome. The model's performance metrics are detailed in Table 5 [62].
  - **Gradient Boosting (GB)**
    Gradient boosting is a powerful technique for constructing highly accurate models by sequentially combining simple base models, typically decision trees. In this iterative process, each new model is trained to correct the

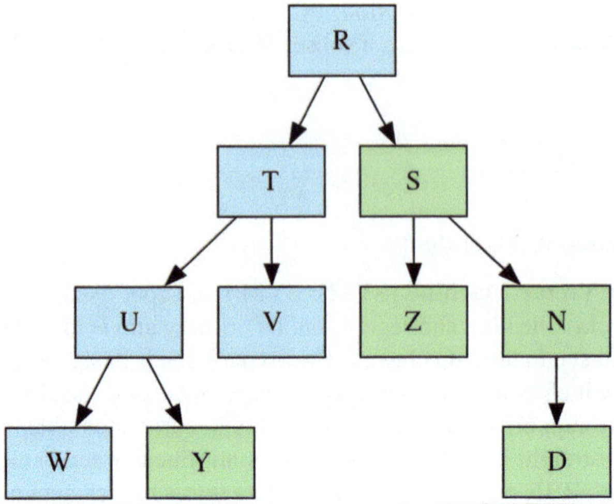

Fig. 2 Decision tree

residual errors of the previous models, minimizing the overall error rate. This optimization is achieved through the gradient descent method, which adjusts the loss function at each step. By iteratively refining the model, gradient boosting effectively manages complexity and reduces the risk of overfitting. Key hyperparameters such as the learning rate, tree depth, and the number of iterations require careful tuning, as improper configurations can negatively affect performance. Gradient boosting consistently delivers high-accuracy results, making it suitable for both classification and regression tasks. However, the algorithm's iterative nature can lead to prolonged training times and significant computational demands, especially with large datasets. Despite these challenges, gradient boosting is widely preferred for complex problems due to its strong generalization ability. The model's performance metrics are provided in Table 5 [63].

- **Random Forest Algorithm (RF)**
  Random forest is a versatile and robust machine learning technique that operates by aggregating the predictions of multiple decision trees. For classification tasks, it employs majority voting, while for regression problems, it averages the predictions. The algorithm introduces randomness by selecting a random subset of the training data and features for each tree, which helps reduce the risk of overfitting inherent to single decision trees and enhances generalization performance. Moreover, random forest contributes to data analysis by offering feature importance rankings. This algorithm is particularly effective on high-dimensional and complex datasets, demonstrating resilience against noisy data. However, its reliance on a large number of trees can lead to high computational costs, necessitating substantial resources for large datasets. Despite this, random forest remains a popular choice in both

classification and regression tasks due to its accuracy and flexibility. The model's performance metrics are detailed in Table 5 [64].

- **Logistic Regression (LR)**
  Logistic regression is a statistical technique primarily employed for classification tasks. It predicts the probability of an event occurring based on a set of independent variables, producing an output value as a probability between 0 and 1.
  The algorithm applies the sigmoid function to transform the linear model's output into a probability, defined as follows:

$$f(x) = \frac{1}{1 + e^{-z}} \tag{3}$$

$$z = w_1x_1 + w_2x_2 + \cdots + w_nx_n + b. \tag{4}$$

  Here, z represents a linear combination of the independent variables.
  To determine the decision boundary, logistic regression employs the maximum likelihood estimation method, ensuring linear separability for classification tasks. The model assesses the influence of independent variables on the target variable and calculates regression coefficients to quantify these effects. Widely utilized for binary classification problems, logistic regression can also be extended to handle multiple classes. It is valued for its simplicity, interpretability, and capacity for generalization. However, its performance diminishes in scenarios involving nonlinear relationships or complex decision boundaries, where more advanced algorithms may be required [65]. The performance metrics are detailed in Table 5.
- **Artificial Neural Networks (ANNs)** ANNs are computational algorithms designed to replicate the functioning of neural networks in the human brain to uncover patterns and relationships in data. They are extensively applied in classification and regression tasks. The architecture of an ANN comprises an input layer, one or more hidden layers, and an output layer. Within the hidden layers, data undergo both linear and nonlinear transformations, enabling the network to learn and model complex patterns effectively. By capturing intricate relationships among various types of data, ANNs achieve high levels of accuracy. Moreover, their structure can be easily optimized according to the model's requirements, making them highly adaptable to a wide range of applications [66].

– Deep Learning Algorithms: The selected models were chosen because they are compatible with the dataset.
  Deep learning, a branch of artificial intelligence, facilitates data analysis and addresses complex problems using artificial neural networks modeled after the human brain's structure and function. This approach excels in processing large datasets, enabling automatic feature extraction and hierarchical information

Table 5 Test performances of machine learning algorithms

Model	Accuracy	Precision	Recall	F1 score	Specificity	AUC-ROC
SVM	85.42%	85.45%	85.42%	85.42%	97.60%	98.01%
SVM (PCA: on)	56.04%	56.43%	56.04%	51.83%	92.65%	85.53%
SVM (LDA: on)	81.35%	81.28%	81.35%	81.26%	96.93%	96.63%
Decision tree	83.62%	83.72%	83.62%	83.66%	97.31%	89.82%
Decision tree (PCA: on)	67.41%	67.56%	67.41%	67.46%	94.63%	79.73%
Decision tree (LDA: on)	74.10%	74.02%	74.10%	74.05%	95.73%	83.75%
Gradient boosting	88.25%	88.24%	88.25%	88.23%	98.07%	98.39%
Gradient boosting (PCA: on)	69.90%	69.07%	69.90%	69.23%	95.02%	92.75%
Gradient boosting (LDA: on)	81.91%	81.85%	81.91%	81.86%	97.02%	96.79%
Random forest	88.60%	88.65%	88.60%	88.60%	98.12%	98.42%
Random forest (PCA: on)	74.74%	74.68%	74.74%	74.62%	95.83%	94.67%
Random forest (LDA: on)	79.84%	79.72%	79.84%	79.77%	96.68%	95.64%
Logistic regression	85.57%	85.39%	85.57%	85.46%	97.62%	97.75%
Logistic regression (PCA: on)	64.60%	63.30%	64.60%	63.36%	94.14%	90.86%
Logistic regression (LDA: on)	81.80%	81.75%	81.80%	81.73%	97.01%	96.86%

representation. The multiple layers within neural networks represent data at varying levels of abstraction, progressively learning more intricate features at each layer. During the training phase, patterns are extracted from the data, leading to high accuracy rates across diverse applications, including image recognition and natural language processing [67].

- **Convolutional Neural Networks (CNNs)** CNNs are specialized algorithms predominantly applied to image data, excelling in feature extraction and pattern recognition. They demonstrate strong performance, particularly on large datasets. Convolutional layers learn local relationships within the data, while pooling layers reduce data dimensionality and extract more meaningful features [68].
- **Recurrent Neural Networks (RNNs)**
  RNNs are algorithms designed to work with time series and sequential data. They are particularly useful in situations where the prediction of a data point is related to previous data points. Each cell stores information from previous steps, enabling the learning of patterns in sequential data. This structure allows for the modeling of temporal relationships. RNNs exhibit strong performance in learning temporal changes and modeling long-term dependencies. Additionally, they offer a specialized structure for sequential data analysis [69].
- **Deep Belief Networks (DBNs)**
  Deep belief networks are algorithms that process data in a multilayered structure to extract abstract representations. They are particularly effective in dealing with complex and large datasets. DBNs contain multiple hidden layers, with each layer using information learned from lower layers to create

higher-level representations. This algorithm abstracts significant information from high-dimensional data, thereby enhancing classification accuracy [70].

- **Autoencoders (AEs)**
  Autoencoders are specialized algorithms designed to reduce data dimensionality and extract essential features. They are widely utilized in applications such as anomaly detection and noise reduction. The architecture of an autoencoder consists of two primary components: an encoder and a decoder. The encoder compresses input data into a lower-dimensional representation, while the decoder reconstructs the original data from this compressed form. By reducing dimensionality, autoencoders decrease processing times and accelerate the learning process. At the same time, the elimination of redundant information enhances overall model performance [71].

Hybrid Model

The hybrid model combines gradient boosting and random forest algorithms. The model takes the probabilities predicted by each algorithm and averages them to make the final classification. Confusion matrix is detailed in Fig. 7. The training and testing splits of the hybrid model are provided in Table 8.

3.7 Rationale for Algorithm Selection

Since the goal of this study is to classify individuals into discrete obesity levels, the problem is inherently a multiclass classification task. Accordingly, the selected algorithms were chosen for their strong performance in structured classification problems.

Among the machine learning models, random forest and gradient boosting are known for their ability to capture complex nonlinear relationships and reduce overfitting through ensemble learning. Support vector machines are effective in high-dimensional spaces and perform well with margin-based separation. Decision trees provide rule-based transparency, while logistic regression offers a reliable probabilistic baseline [72].

On the deep learning side, models like ANN, CNN, and RNN were used to evaluate the capacity of deep architectures to learn hierarchical and temporal patterns in lifestyle-related data. Autoencoders and DBNs were included for their representation learning abilities, which can uncover latent structures relevant to obesity status [73].

Using a diverse set of models allowed for a comprehensive evaluation of classification performance and generalization, tailored to the characteristics of this problem and dataset.

3.8 Model Training

In the training process conducted on a dataset consisting of 22,869 samples, each with 16 features, the concepts of batch and epoch were used as the foundation for configuration. A batch represents a small portion of the dataset, while an epoch signifies the processing of the entire dataset by the model once. For this training, the batch size was set to 50, chosen to efficiently utilize hardware capacity and balance the training process. Each epoch consisted of 457 steps. The initial number of epochs was set to 50, and early stopping was applied to prevent overfitting. Smaller batch sizes increased sensitivity during learning, while larger batch sizes negatively affected learning stability. Consequently, a batch size of 50 was determined to be ideal for achieving balance. During the training process, validation loss and accuracy metrics were monitored to optimize the number of epochs. As a result, the batch size and number of epochs were found to be effective in optimizing the model's performance [74].

3.8.1 Hyperparameter Selection and Optimization Strategy

The selection of hyperparameters—such as batch size, the number of epochs, and learning rate—was based on empirical evaluation and best practices from the literature to ensure optimal model performance and training stability:

- **Batch Size:** A batch size of 50 was chosen after testing different values (32, 50, 64, 128). This value provided a balance between computational efficiency and learning stability. Smaller batch sizes increased training noise, while larger sizes caused slow convergence and memory issues. Batch size = 50 allowed sufficient gradient updates without overburdening system memory.
- **Epochs:** The number of epochs was initially set to 50. However, to avoid overfitting, an early stopping mechanism was applied by monitoring the validation loss during training. The model was stopped once the validation loss ceased to improve. This strategy helped determine the effective number of epochs dynamically, often stabilizing around the 30–40 range.
- **Learning Rate:** For deep learning models, an initial learning rate of 0.001 was used, consistent with common practice in similar classification tasks. Adaptive learning rate schedulers (e.g., ReduceLROnPlateau) were employed to decrease the learning rate upon performance stagnation, enhancing convergence.
- **Validation Strategy:** Although a dedicated validation set was not used, performance tuning was guided by validation metrics monitored during the training process. For the hybrid model, a 5-fold cross-validation approach ensured robust evaluation and helped mitigate overfitting risks.

  This optimization strategy contributed significantly to the stability and generalizability of the models, while maintaining computational efficiency.

3.9 Performance Results

- **True Positive (TP):** The count of instances correctly predicted as positive, which also belong to the positive category
- **True Negative (TN):** The count of instances correctly classified and predicted as negative
- **False Positive (FP):** The count of instances incorrectly predicted as positive, while actually belonging to the negative category
- **False Negative (FN):** The count of instances incorrectly predicted as negative, while actually belonging to the positive category [75]

A variety of metrics are employed to evaluate the performance of artificial intelligence models. In this study, the effectiveness of the AI models was measured using widely utilized metrics, including precision, recall, specificity, F-measure, and accuracy. These metrics are calculated based on the binary confusion matrix and provide a comprehensive representation of the classification performance of the models [76]:

- **Accuracy (ACC):** Represents the proportion of correctly classified instances relative to the total number of instances, providing a percentage that reflects the overall success of the model.

$$\text{Accuracy} = \frac{\text{TP} + \text{TN}}{\text{TP} + \text{FP} + \text{FN} + \text{TN}} \times 100. \tag{5}$$

- **Precision (PRC):** Calculates the proportion of correctly classified positive instances out of all instances predicted as positive. This metric reflects the ACC of the model's positive predictions.

$$\text{Precision} = \frac{\text{TP}}{\text{TP} + \text{FP}}. \tag{6}$$

- **Recall (RCL):** The proportion of actual positive instances correctly predicted as positive is measured. This metric indicates the correct classification rate of positive instances.

$$\text{Recall} = \frac{\text{TP}}{\text{TP} + \text{FN}}. \tag{7}$$

- **Specificity:** The proportion of negative instances correctly predicted as negative is calculated. This metric represents the success of negative classification.

$$\text{Specificity} = \frac{\text{TN}}{\text{TN} + \text{FP}}. \tag{8}$$

- **F-Measure (F1S):** The harmonic mean of precision and recall is calculated. This metric highlights the balance between the two metrics when evaluating model performance.

$$\text{F-Measure} = \frac{2 \times \text{Accuracy} \times \text{Recall}}{\text{Accuracy} + \text{Recall}}. \tag{9}$$

  These metrics comprehensively evaluate the model's performance [77].
- **AUC (Area Under the Curve):** The area under the curve (AUC) represents the total area under the ROC curve, offering a unified metric for assessing a classification model's performance. It evaluates how effectively the model distinguishes between positive and negative classes. The AUC score ranges from 0.5 to 1, with values closer to 1 signifying superior discriminatory ability. AUC is widely used to compare different classifiers. Together, the ROC curve and AUC are vital tools for analyzing the precision and reliability of classification models [78].

4 Experimental Results

In this section, an analysis is conducted on determining obesity levels using a dataset based on individuals' lifestyle habits. The study examines the role and effectiveness of artificial intelligence methods in obesity prediction. The dataset used includes features such as demographic information, physical activities, and dietary habits, and preprocessing steps such as handling missing values, outlier processing, data scaling, feature extraction, and selection have been applied. For classification, machine learning algorithms such as support vector machine, decision tree, gradient boosting, random forest, and logistic regression, as well as deep learning methods like artificial neural networks, convolutional neural networks, recurrent neural networks, deep belief networks, and autoencoders, have been used. Additionally, a hybrid model combining gradient boosting and random forest algorithms has been developed.

This section provides a detailed examination of the performance of the algorithms, comparing their accuracy rates. The analysis aims to demonstrate the potential of artificial intelligence methods in detecting obesity.

4.1 Model Performance and Evaluation

Metrics for evaluating the performance of classification models are essential for assessing the accuracy and reliability of the models. Accuracy indicates the overall classification success, while recall and specificity assess the correct prediction rates for positive and negative classes, respectively. Precision and F1 score measure the

ACC of positive predictions and the balance between recall and precision. The AUC-ROC curve provides a visual representation of the model's performance across various threshold values, offering a comprehensive evaluation. Together, these metrics form a robust framework for analyzing a model's strengths and limitations.

4.1.1 Effect of PCA on Model Performance

In this study, PCA with 10 components was applied to reduce data dimensionality. However, analyses revealed that PCA decreased model performance, particularly in terms of accuracy and other metrics. This decline is attributed to the information loss caused by PCA. These results highlight the importance of carefully selecting the suitability of PCA for the dataset and determining the appropriate number of components.

4.1.2 Effect of LDA on Model Performance

In this study, LDA with two components was applied to reduce dimensionality and enhance class separation. While LDA produced more successful results compared to PCA, it did not improve the model's raw performance and even caused a slight decline. This outcome is attributed to LDA's inability to completely prevent information loss in the dataset. The findings emphasize the need for careful evaluation of dimensionality reduction methods.

4.1.3 Comparison

Tables 5, 6, and 7 summarize the performance of all tested models, including five machine learning (ML), five deep learning (DL) algorithms, and the proposed hybrid model. Among these, the hybrid model, which integrates the predictions of random forest and gradient boosting classifiers, achieved the highest accuracy at 90.09%, outperforming both its individual ML constituents (RF: 88.60%, GB: 88.25%) and the top DL models (e.g., AE: 86.85%, RNN: 86.05%).

In addition to accuracy, the hybrid model demonstrated superior results in other key metrics such as F1 score (89.14%) and AUC-ROC (98.87%), indicating strong overall classification performance and high discriminative capability. One notable advantage of the hybrid approach was a reduction in false positives, which is especially valuable in health-related classification tasks where minimizing misclassification is important. Compared to lower-performing models such as deep belief networks (47.43% accuracy), the hybrid approach maintained robust performance even with imbalanced and high-dimensional data.

While the hybrid model required slightly longer training time (49.46 seconds) than individual models, this trade-off was acceptable considering the gains in classification precision. All models were trained using CPU resources only, without

Table 6 Deep learning algorithms test performances

Model	Accuracy	Precision	Recall	F1 score	Specificity	AUC-ROC
Artificial neural networks	85.57%	84.43%	83.95%	83.95%	84.43%	98.00%
Artificial neural networks (PCA: on)	74.93%	72.69%	72.12%	72.08%	72.69%	94.78%
Artificial neural networks (LDA: on)	81.78%	79.66%	80.08%	79.77%	79.66%	96.89%
Convolutional neural networks	83.54%	81.95%	82.04%	81.80%	81.95%	97.54%
Convolutional neural networks (PCA: on)	68.52%	66.72%	64.55%	63.67%	66.72%	92.58%
Convolutional neural networks (LDA: on)	82.06%	80.03%	80.24%	80.10%	80.03%	96.93%
Recurrent neural networks	84.48%	82.95%	83.10%	82.79%	82.95%	97.84%
Recurrent neural networks (PCA: on)	86.05%	84.90%	84.69%	84.75%	84.90%	98.13%
Recurrent neural networks (LDA: on)	81.77%	79.86%	79.79%	79.74%	79.86%	96.92%
Deep belief networks	47.43%	46.95%	42.44%	36.58%	46.95%	66.74%
Deep belief networks (PCA: on)	74.04%	73.04%	70.94%	71.17%	73.04%	94.70%
Deep belief networks (LDA: on)	81.65%	79.58%	79.54%	79.45%	79.58%	96.87%
Autoencoders	86.85%	85.55%	85.57%	85.55%	85.55%	91.70%
Autoencoders (PCA: on)	72.99%	70.09%	70.24%	70.07%	70.09%	82.89%
Autoencoders (LDA: on)	81.90%	80.03%	80.14%	80.06%	80.03%	88.58%

Table 7 Hybrid model performance results

Model	Accuracy	Precision	Recall	F1 score	Specificity	AUC-ROC
Hybrid model	90.09%	89.17%	89.16%	89.14%	89.17%	98.87%
Hybrid model (PCA: on)	75.58%	73.29%	73.19%	73.11%	73.29%	94.97%
Hybrid model (LDA: on)	81.48%	79.54%	79.74%	79.62%	79.54%	96.82%

GPU acceleration, indicating that the hybrid model's performance gain is attainable even under modest hardware constraints.

Feature selection methods such as PCA and LDA were also tested across models. Although they improved certain underperforming algorithms, they generally led to performance degradation in already well-performing models. For the hybrid model, PCA and LDA preprocessing reduced accuracy to 75.58% and 81.48%, respectively, reinforcing the effectiveness of using the original feature set for complex ensemble architectures.

The performance comparison underscores that combining ensemble ML architectures with appropriate feature engineering and rigorous evaluation can outperform both standalone ML and DL models in obesity classification tasks.

4.1.4 Error Analysis

In this section, an analysis of models' misclassification cases (false positive and false negative) has been conducted. Confusion matrices were utilized to evaluate each model's classification performance in greater detail. This analysis plays a critical role in identifying the strengths and weaknesses of the models and revealing areas for improvement.

Confusion matrices explicitly display each model's true positive, true negative, false positive, and false negative classifications. This allowed for an examination of the reasons behind misclassifications and an analysis of the factors influencing classification performance. Our unique hybrid model demonstrated superior performance, particularly in reducing false positive and false negative rates compared to other models. However, it was observed that models incorporating dimensionality reduction methods (PCA and LDA) experienced an increase in misclassification rates.

Confusion matrices detailing the misclassifications for the lowest-performing SVM model with PCA applied, the SVM models without PCA/LDA, the highest- and lowest-performing deep learning algorithms, and the hybrid model are presented.

In all models, the rows in the confusion matrices represent the true values, while the columns represent the predicted values.

According to the confusion matrix, the SVM algorithm demonstrated a high ratio of correct classifications, although the false positive and false negative rates could not be reduced to zero (see Fig. 3). In the PCA-applied version, due to information loss, the false classification rates increased significantly (see Fig. 4). The LDA-applied version performed better compared to PCA, but was still less successful than the model operating with raw data (see Fig. 3).

The confusion matrix of the ANN algorithm shows high accuracy rates (see Fig. 5). However, in the PCA-applied version, the number of misclassifications increased significantly, indicating that PCA caused information loss. The LDA-applied version slightly reduced the misclassification rates compared to PCA but still fell short of the performance achieved with the raw data (see Fig. 5).

The raw version of the DBN algorithm exhibited the highest misclassification rates among all models, according to the confusion matrix (see Fig. 6). This highlights the model's limited capacity to handle the complexity of the dataset. The PCA- and LDA-applied versions reduced the misclassification rates and significantly improved the model's performance. This suggests that DBN benefitted positively from dimensionality reduction methods. In particular, the LDA-applied version considerably lowered the misclassification rates and delivered performance improvements.

The hybrid model demonstrated the lowest error rates among all models, as seen in its confusion matrix (see Fig. 7). The low false positive and false negative rates illustrate the effectiveness of combining the strengths of gradient boosting and random forest algorithms to deliver superior classification performance. However, the hybrid model experienced performance degradation when PCA and LDA

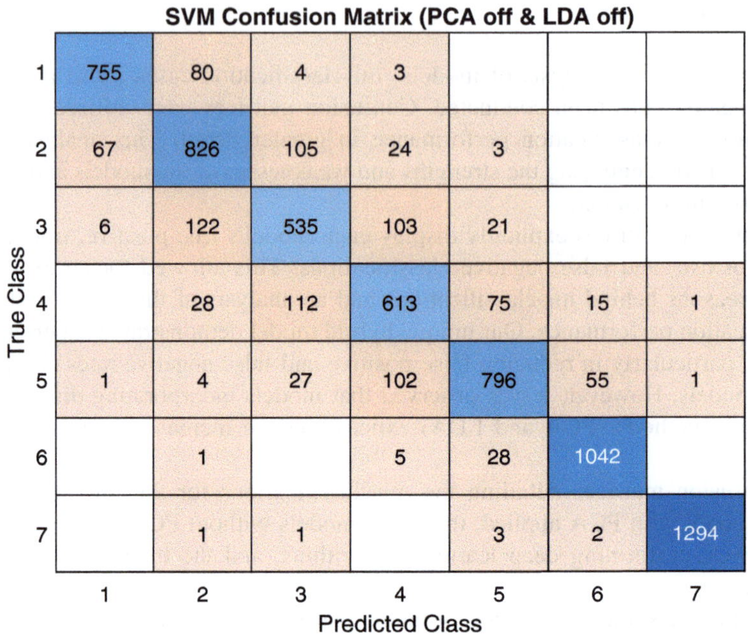

Fig. 3 Confusion matrix of SVM model without PCA and LDA

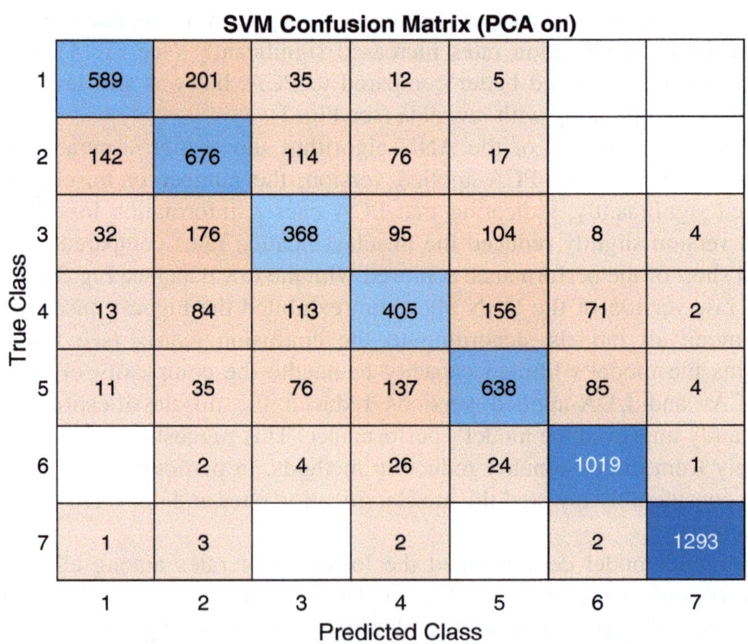

Fig. 4 Confusion matrix of SVM model with PCA applied

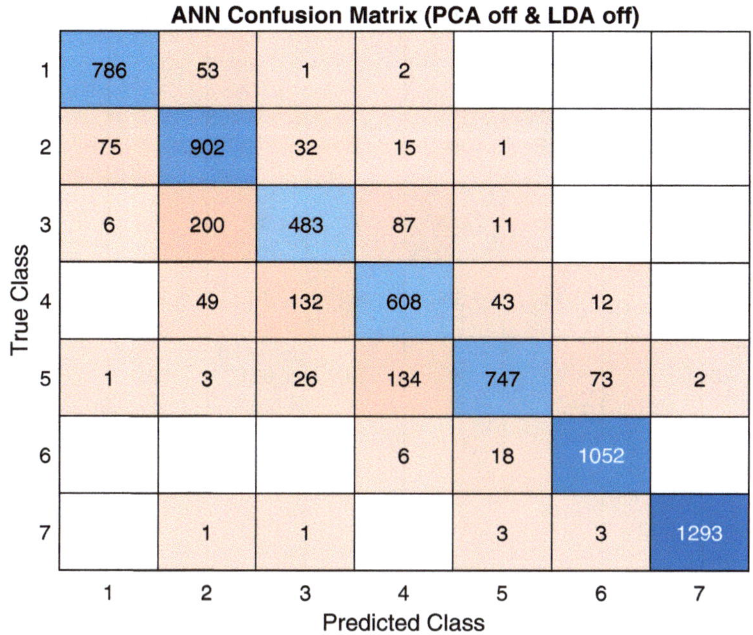

Fig. 5 Confusion matrix of ANN model without PCA and LDA

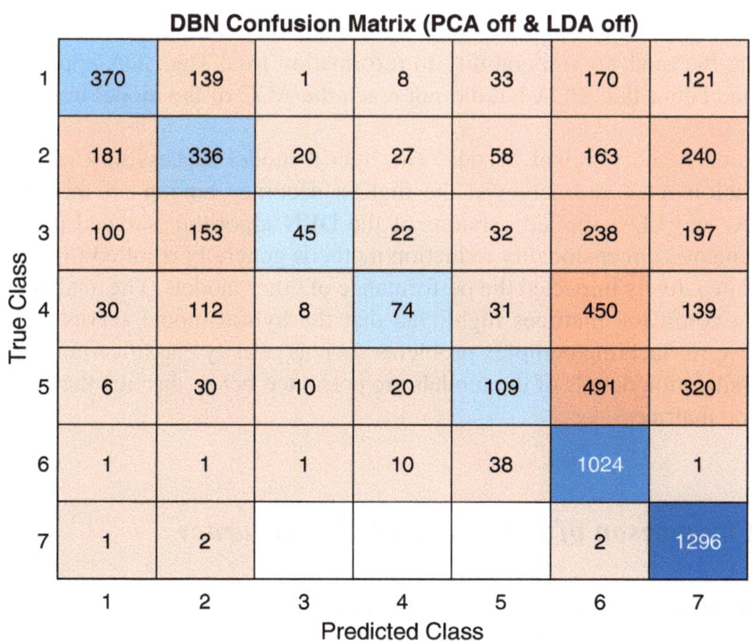

Fig. 6 Confusion matrix of DBN model without PCA and LDA

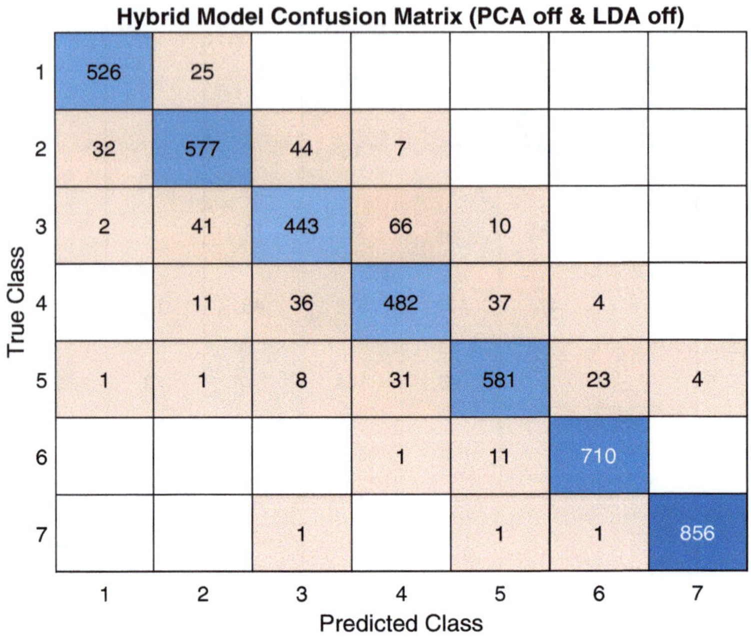

Fig. 7 Confusion matrix of hybrid model without PCA and LDA

were applied. The PCA-applied version exhibited increased misclassification rates, reflecting the model's vulnerability to information loss. The LDA-applied version performed better than PCA but did not reach the ACC of the model trained on raw data.

Success of the Original Model: The hybrid model successfully reduced misclassification rates and achieved the highest accuracy among all models. While the PCA- and LDA-applied versions of the DBN algorithm showed performance improvements, dimensionality reduction methods generally resulted in information loss and negatively impacted the performance of other models. The analysis derived from the confusion matrices highlights that the hybrid model serves as a robust alternative for tackling complex problems such as obesity classification. The errors and classification details of the models are presented below through their respective confusion matrices.

4.2 Comparison of Training and Test Accuracy

The comparison between training and test datasets is crucial for assessing a model's learning and generalization capabilities. The training dataset facilitates the model's learning process, while the test dataset evaluates its ability to perform on new

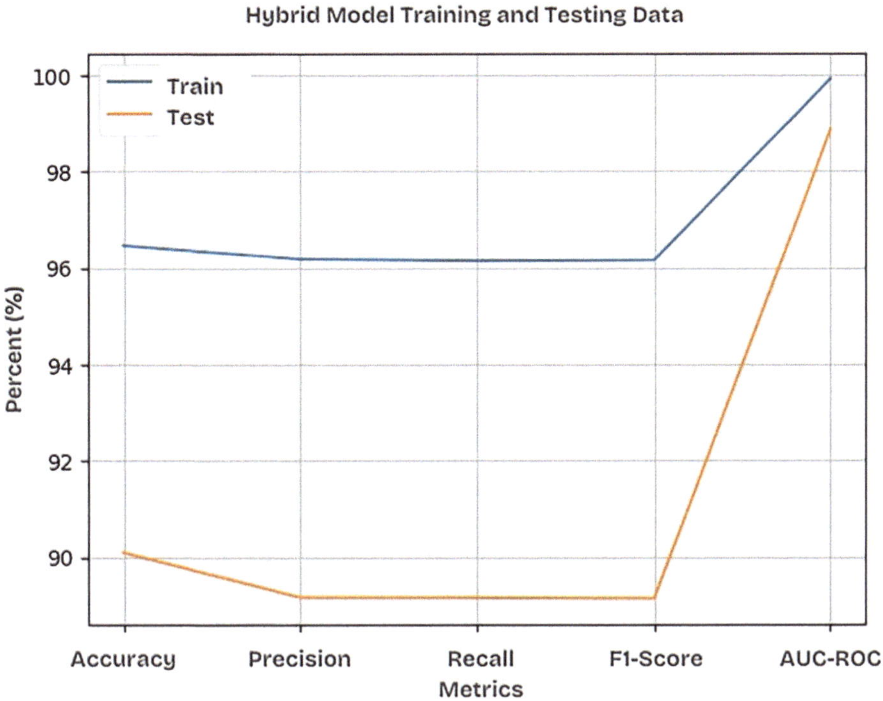

Fig. 8 Training/test line graph

Table 8 Hybrid model training and test data

Dataset	Accuracy (%)	Precision (%)	Recall (%)	F1 score (%)	AUC-ROC (%)
Train	96.469	96.182	96.146	96.161	99.923
Test	90.091	89.166	89.160	89.143	98.870

and unseen data. This comparison aids in identifying overfitting or underfitting scenarios, ensuring the model's balance and applicability in real-world contexts. Performance details of machine learning models are provided in Table 4, while information related to deep learning models is presented in Table 11. When analyzing the performance of the hybrid model on training and test datasets, the following results were observed (also shown in Fig. 8): On the training dataset, the model achieved 96.469% accuracy, 96.182% precision, 96.146% recall, 96.161% F1 score, and 99.923% AUC-ROC. On the test dataset, these metrics were calculated as 90.091% accuracy, 89.166% precision, 89.160% recall, 89.143% F1 score, and 98.870% AUC-ROC (Table 8).

These results indicate that the model demonstrates consistent performance across both datasets. Despite achieving high accuracy on the training dataset, the slight decline in performance on the test dataset is not considered a sign of overfitting.

The high metrics on the test dataset reflect the model's successful generalization capacity. Furthermore, the AUC-ROC values are very close between the training and test datasets, calculated as 99.923% and 98.870%, respectively. This confirms that the model exhibits strong classification capability in both datasets and does not suffer from significant generalization loss. Based on this analysis, it can be concluded that the hybrid model effectively avoids overfitting.

4.3 Training and Testing Durations

The evaluation of training and testing times plays a crucial role in determining the efficiency of models in terms of time and resource utilization. For machine learning models, training and testing times have been considered separately, and total durations have been calculated. However, for deep learning models, training and testing times have been recorded as a combined total runtime and could not be analyzed separately. This limitation arises due to the high computational requirements and cost associated with deep learning algorithms (Table 9). These comparisons not only assess the performance of models but also provide insights into their resource efficiency, playing a critical role in determining which model is more suitable in terms of time efficiency (Table 10).

There are significant differences in the training and testing times of machine learning and deep learning algorithms. The use of dimensionality reduction methods such as PCA and LDA has significantly increased training times, particularly for deep learning models. However, LDA generally executed operations in shorter times compared to PCA. Among machine learning models, the decision tree algorithm demonstrated the shortest processing times for both training and testing. For instance, decision tree training took only 0.06 seconds, while applying PCA increased this time to 0.28 seconds. The SVM algorithm required longer times compared to others, with a training duration of 35.16 seconds. However, notable reductions in processing times were observed with PCA and LDA. In the gradient boosting algorithm, applying PCA significantly increased the processing time (22.73 seconds), demonstrating the computational overhead introduced by PCA.

For deep learning models, total processing times were much higher compared to machine learning models. For example, the artificial neural network (ANN) algorithm's runtime with raw data was 110.18 seconds, while PCA reduced this to 107.76 seconds, and LDA further decreased it to 107.83 seconds. The convolutional neural network (CNN) algorithm had the longest runtime, completing tasks in 141.71 seconds with raw data. PCA reduced this to 136.76 seconds, while LDA further reduced it to 131.18 seconds. The deep belief network (DBN) algorithm demonstrated a significant reduction in processing time when LDA was applied compared to PCA. For example, PCA increased the runtime to 146.17 seconds, whereas LDA reduced it to 47.36 seconds, indicating LDA's efficiency in reducing computational overhead for certain algorithms.

Table 9 Models' runtimes part 1

Model	Runtime (second)
SVM train	35.16
SVM	3.53
SVM (PCA)	3.85
SVM (LDA)	1.49
DT train	0.06
DT	0.06
DT (PCA)	0.28
DT (LDA)	0.06
GB train	6.79
GB	6.49
GB (PCA)	22.73
GB (LDA)	7.16
RF train	2.57
RF	2.10
RF (PCA)	6.16
RF (LDA)	2.66
LR train	12.41
LR	11.96
LR (PCA)	11.88
LR (LDA)	0.49
ANN	110.18
ANN (PCA)	107.76
ANN (LDA)	107.83
CNN	141.71
CNN (PCA)	136.76
CNN (LDA)	131.18
RNN	140.21
RNN (PCA)	143.88
RNN (LDA)	140.55
DBN	47.36
DBN (PCA)	146.17
DBN (LDA)	139.48
AE	98.01
AE (PCA)	97.32
AE (LDA)	97.73
Hybrid	49.46
Hybrid (PCA)	268.24
Hybrid (LDA)	67.19

The hybrid model exhibited higher processing times compared to other models but was still lower than most deep learning models. The runtime with raw data was calculated as 49.46 seconds. However, applying PCA increased the time significantly to 268.24 seconds, illustrating PCA's impact on processing times. With

Table 10 Models runtimes part 2

Model	Runtimes (seconds)
LR train	12.41
LR	11.96
LR (PCA)	11.88
LR (LDA)	0.49
ANN	110.18
ANN (PCA)	107.76
ANN (LDA)	107.83
CNN	141.71
CNN (PCA)	136.76
CNN (LDA)	131.18
RNN	140.21
RNN (PCA)	143.88
RNN (LDA)	140.55
DBN	47.36
DBN (PCA)	146.17
DBN (LDA)	139.48
AE	98.01
AE (PCA)	97.32
AE (LDA)	97.73
Hybrid	49.46
Hybrid (PCA)	268.24
Hybrid (LDA)	67.19

LDA, the runtime decreased to 67.19 seconds, highlighting LDA's efficiency in managing computational load.

All operations were performed using only the CPU without GPU acceleration, resulting in longer processing times, especially for deep learning models. Comparisons between CPU and GPU were not made, as the hardware used did not support GPU acceleration. Detailed timing information can be found in Table 9.

4.4 Generalization Ability of the Model

In this study, the k-fold cross-validation method was utilized to evaluate the generalization capability of the model. The value of k was set to 5, dividing the dataset into five equal subsets. During each iteration, one subset was designated as the test dataset, while the remaining four subsets were used for training. This process was repeated five times, ensuring that each subset served as the test dataset exactly once. The overall performance of the model was determined by averaging the results obtained from all iterations.

This method was applied to assess the model's consistency across various data subsets and its ability to generalize to unseen data. By employing k-fold cross-

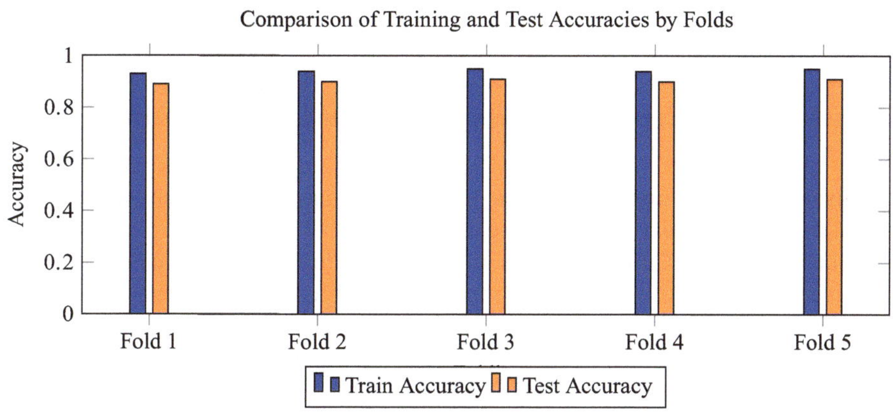

Fig. 9 Comparison of training and test accuracies of the hybrid model across folds

validation, a more reliable estimate of the model's performance was achieved, reducing the influence of data partitioning on evaluation outcomes. According to the k-fold cross-validation results, the model maintained a consistent balance between training and test accuracies. Training accuracy ranged between %93 and %95 for each fold, while test accuracy remained within the range of %89 to %91. These results demonstrate that the model exhibited high performance across different subsets of data, highlighting its strong generalization capability. The small gap between training and test accuracies indicates that the model avoided overfitting and was able to generalize effectively across different datasets. Comparison of training and test accuracies of the hybrid model across folds can be found in bar chart form in Fig. 9.

4.5 Hyperparameter Tuning and Model Performance

Hyperparameters play a critical role in the learning process and have a direct impact on the model's performance and comparability. The batch size parameter allows the model to process the dataset in smaller groups. In this study, a batch size of 10 was selected for all models, enabling the model to process and update weights for 10 data points in each iteration. A small batch size facilitated more frequent updates but increased computation time.

This configuration struck a balance between achieving effective weight updates and managing the computational resources efficiently, contributing to the overall stability and reliability of the models.

The number of epochs refers to how many times the model processes the entire dataset. In this study, the number of epochs was set to 50 for all models. This value was kept constant to ensure that each model undergoes sufficient training and to maintain comparability across all models. Selecting the same values for both the batch size and the number of epochs is important for enabling a fair comparison during the training processes of different algorithms. These hyperparameter settings aim to strike a balance between model performance and computational time, thereby enhancing the generalization capability.

Analysis of Epoch and Batch Size Values The number of epochs defines how many times the model processes the entire dataset.

Increased Epoch Count: Extending the training duration can enhance accuracy; however, it also increases processing time and resource usage. Smaller Batch Size: Allows for more frequent weight updates, potentially improving model accuracy but prolonging processing time. A line graph illustrating this relationship is shown in Fig. 10. Larger Batch Size: May reduce computational time but could lead to a decrease in generalization capacity. In this study, the number of epochs was set to 50 for all models. This value was chosen to ensure sufficient learning, while maintaining comparability across all models. Keeping the batch size and epoch values consistent is crucial for making fair comparisons between the training processes of different algorithms.

These hyperparameter settings aimed to strike a balance between model performance and computational efficiency, enhancing the model's generalization ability. By standardizing these parameters, the study ensured that the evaluation of model performance was both reliable and equitable across various algorithms:

- *Artificial Neural Network (ANN):* The ANN model achieved a training accuracy of 87.00%, indicating sufficient learning of patterns in the training data. Test accuracy was recorded at 85.57%, which is close to the training accuracy, reflecting strong generalization capability. Training loss was 35.06%, and test loss was 40.77%. The closeness of these losses indicates that the model avoided overfitting:
    - **PCA and LDA Applications:** With PCA applied, training accuracy dropped to 76.31% and test accuracy to 74.93%. LDA improved performance, yielding a training accuracy of 81.30% and a test accuracy of 81.78%, outperforming PCA.
- *Convolutional Neural Network (CNN):* The CNN model achieved a training accuracy of 84.90%. Test accuracy was calculated at 83.56%, indicating reasonable generalization from training to test data. Training loss was 37.28%, and test loss was 43.25%, suggesting a slight decline in generalization performance:
    - **PCA and LDA Applications:** With PCA, training accuracy dropped to 82.02% and test accuracy to 80.22%. With LDA, training accuracy was 82.20%, and test accuracy was 80.20%, showing similar results to PCA.
- *Recurrent Neural Network (RNN):* The RNN model achieved a training accuracy of 86.93%. Test accuracy was recorded at 86.12%, showcasing successful generalization. Training loss was 34.40%, and test loss was 38.45%:

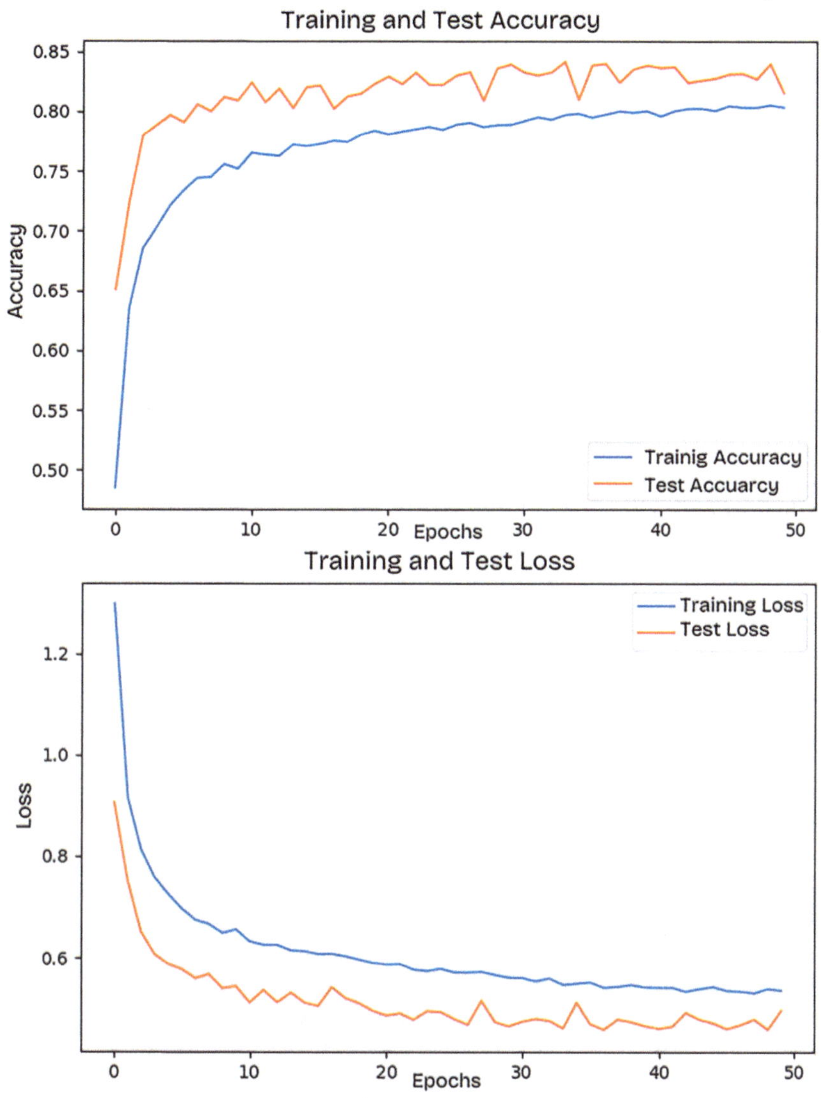

Fig. 10 Deep learning epoch mean change

- **PCA and LDA Applications:** With PCA, training accuracy was 85.10%, and test accuracy was 84.06%. With LDA, training accuracy was 85.30%, and test accuracy was 84.03%.

– *Deep Belief Network (DBN):* The DBN model achieved a training accuracy of 80.11%, showing comparatively lower performance. Test accuracy was measured at 78.04%. Training loss was 62.02%, and test loss was 66.20%, indicating limitations in generalization capacity:

- **PCA and LDA Applications:** With PCA, training accuracy was 75.11%, and test accuracy was 74.06%. With LDA, training accuracy improved to 78.45%, and test accuracy to 77.94%, outperforming PCA.

– *Autoencoders:* The autoencoder model achieved the highest training accuracy at 87.06%. Test accuracy was recorded at 86.76%, making it the best generalizing model. Training loss was 33.51%, and test loss was 35.44%:

- **PCA and LDA Applications:** With PCA, training accuracy dropped to 84.63%, and test accuracy to 84.06%. With LDA, training accuracy was 82.63%, and test accuracy was 81.90%.

4.6 Different Combinations of Hyperparameter Settings

The data presented in the tables and graphs illustrate the potential effects of altering the values of epoch count and batch size. Details are provided in Table 11. In this study, the epoch setting of 50 and batch size of 10 provided a reasonable balance between the models' generalization capabilities and processing time. While the accuracy rates and loss values indicate room for optimization of hyperparameters for

Table 11 Deep learning algorithms training and test performance

Model	Number of epochs	Batch size	Training accuracy	Test accuracy	Training loss	Test loss
ANN	50	5	87.37%	85.59%	36.16%	41.93%
ANN	50	10	87.00%	85.57%	35.06%	40.77%
ANN (PCA: on)	50	10	76.31%	74.93%	59.92%	65.44%
ANN (LDA: on)	50	10	81.80%	81.78%	47.48%	49.13%
CNN	50	5	84.42%	83.43%	43.73%	47.31%
CNN	50	10	84.93%	83.54%	41.99%	46.45%
CNN (PCA: on)	50	10	70.08%	68.52%	75.20%	78.98%
CNN (LDA: on)	50	10	82.20%	82.06%	47.58%	49.25%
RNN	50	5	86.54%	85.50%	35.78%	41.03%
RNN	50	10	85.30%	84.48%	38.28%	42.66%
RNN (PCA: on)	50	10	87.93%	86.05%	34.04%	38.54%
RNN (LDA: on)	50	10	81.93%	81.77%	47.66%	49.50%
DBN	50	5	46.94%	66.55%	24.59%	24.59%
DBN	50	10	46.94%	66.55%	24.59%	24.59%
DBN (PCA: on)	50	10	75.11%	74.04%	62.26%	66.70%
DBN (LDA: on)	50	10	81.78%	81.65%	48.04%	49.89%
AE	50	5	88.53%	86.85%	61.83%	62.60%
AE	50	10	88.53%	87.07%	61.83%	62.60%
AE (PCA: on)	50	10	74.68%	72.98%	83.65%	85.39%
AE (LDA: on)	50	10	82.05%	81.90%	63.51%	63.57%

potentially better results, the current settings delivered satisfactory outcomes. However, experimenting with different combinations of learning rates, epoch counts, and batch sizes could further enhance the models' performance. This highlights the critical importance of hyperparameter optimization.

4.7 *Reasons Behind the Obtained Performance Results*

The reasons behind the achieved performance metrics lie in the effectiveness of the modeling process and the enhancement steps applied to the dataset. Specifically, during the data preprocessing phase, completing missing data, correcting outliers, and scaling the data significantly contributed to the accuracy and reliability of the results. Additionally, identifying and integrating critical features directly affecting the model's success during the feature selection process played a crucial role in improving the metrics. In similar studies, varying success rates using the same algorithms are often attributed to the dataset characteristics, the diversity of features, and the parameter settings of the algorithms. For instance, studies using more limited or imbalanced datasets have reported lower accuracy rates with the same algorithms. Conversely, analyses conducted with much larger and more balanced datasets have demonstrated increased success rates. This observation highlights that the comprehensiveness of the dataset and the meticulous selection of features in this study positively impacted the model's performance. Furthermore, effective hyperparameter optimization and the application of methods like cross-validation enhanced the consistency and reliability of the results. These differences underscore that the outcomes depend not only on the algorithm itself but also on the ACC of decisions made during dataset preparation and the modeling process.

5 Discussion

In this section, the findings derived from the experimental results are examined from a broader perspective, and the strengths and weaknesses of the employed methods are discussed in detail. Additionally, the limitations of the study and suggestions for future research are provided.

5.1 *Performance of Classification Algorithms*

Most of the algorithms achieved evaluation results ranging between 81.00% and 89.00% in their raw forms for the classification tasks. Among the machine learning algorithms, random forest stood out for its performance. Among deep learning algorithms, autoencoders demonstrated superior results compared to other models.

However, the hybrid model surpassed both approaches by achieving better results through the combination of gradient boosting and random forest algorithms, offering an effective classification approach.

5.2 Comparison of Algorithms Using Evaluation Metrics

The models were assessed using essential performance metrics, including accuracy, precision, recall, F1 score, and AUC-ROC. Among the machine learning algorithms, random forest demonstrated strong performance in terms of generalization ability and accuracy. Among the deep learning algorithms, autoencoders excelled in data compression and reconstruction tasks. However, their classification performance lagged behind the machine learning algorithms in this study. The hybrid model combined the strengths of machine learning algorithms, offering higher accuracy and generalization capacity. Its ability to deliver consistent results across different data segments was a notable advantage.

5.3 Training and Testing Ratios

For training and testing splits, 70% of the data was allocated for training and 30% for testing in both machine learning and deep learning algorithms. For the hybrid model, the k-fold cross-validation method was applied with k set to 5, enabling a more comprehensive evaluation of the model across various data subsets.

5.4 Impact of Dataset Characteristics and Preprocessing

The dataset used in this study positively influenced the algorithms' performance, providing a well-suited structure. All data were converted into numerical format, with the dataset consisting of 22,869 samples and 16 features. Preprocessing steps played a significant role in enhancing performance, including handling outliers and scaling data. The generally balanced distribution among classes contributed to the models' favorable results. However, achieving complete balance in the "NObeyesdad" class could further improve model performance. If insufficient data were available for this class, models might exhibit lower overall performance due to class imbalance. This underscores the importance of dataset size and distribution in determining model success.

5.5 Feature Selection and Performance of Deep Learning Models

In deep learning models, except for the PCA-applied recurrent neural network, feature selection algorithms did not significantly enhance performance. PCA and LDA were used as feature selection methods in this study, but the results revealed that improperly tuned applications of these algorithms could reduce success. In most cases, PCA and LDA had a negative impact on performance under identical settings.

In a dataset with 16 features, reductions through feature or data selection resulted in performance declines, highlighting the need to evaluate obesity comprehensively through all lifestyle factors. This finding underscores the critical importance of considering individuals' demographic characteristics, physical activities, and dietary habits collectively to achieve accurate and effective classification results.

5.6 Comparison of Algorithm Time and Resource Usage

The time and resource usage of the models used in this study demonstrated significant differences between machine learning and deep learning algorithms. All models were run exclusively on a CPU, and GPU usage could have significantly reduced processing times. In terms of time efficiency, machine learning algorithms operated faster than deep learning algorithms, making them more efficient in this regard. However, this does not imply that machine learning algorithms are superior in all cases; the dataset and algorithm configurations significantly impact performance. Among machine learning algorithms, the fastest model was the decision tree, completing its tasks in only 0.06 seconds. However, it also had the lowest performance among machine learning models. On the other hand, the gradient boosting algorithm with PCA had the longest runtime of 22.73 seconds, yet it did not achieve the best results. The most successful machine learning algorithm, random forest, operated in just 2.10 seconds and stood out with high performance metrics. This highlights that focusing solely on runtime when selecting an algorithm can be misleading. In deep learning algorithms, the shortest runtime was achieved by the deep belief network (DBN) model at 47.36 seconds. However, this model delivered the lowest performance results among deep learning algorithms. The longest runtime was observed with the PCA-applied deep belief network at 146.17 seconds, and this algorithm also did not achieve high performance. Among deep learning models, the most successful algorithm, autoencoders, reached high accuracy, precision, recall, F1 score, and specificity values with a runtime of 98.01 seconds. The hybrid model, which combined machine learning and deep learning methods, stood out with its raw version achieving the best results in just 49.46 seconds. This demonstrates that the hybrid model provides a balanced solution between performance and runtime. In conclusion, selecting an algorithm based solely on runtime or performance may not be the most appropriate approach. With better optimization and adjustments, deep learning algorithms have the potential to achieve higher successes in shorter runtimes.

5.7 The Role of Metrics in Classification Performance

Performance metrics in classification problems acquire importance depending on the specific characteristics and requirements of the problem. Accuracy is an effective measure of a model's overall success when class distribution is balanced; however, it may be misleading in cases of class imbalance. Precision evaluates the correctness of positive predictions and is particularly valuable in scenarios where minimizing false positives is critical. Recall becomes essential in situations where missing positive cases must be avoided. The F1 score, which harmonizes precision and recall, is particularly suited for datasets with class imbalances. Specificity is highlighted in contexts where accurately identifying negative classes is a priority. AUC-ROC provides a robust assessment of class separation, offering a general evaluation of the model's performance and generalization ability. These metrics were selected to ensure a comprehensive evaluation of the models' performance.

5.8 Classification Success and Potential of the Hybrid Model

The hybrid model offered a novel approach in this study by combining the strengths of gradient boosting and random forest algorithms. This combination aimed to enhance classification performance by leveraging the generalization capability and detailed learning capacity of both algorithms. The hybrid model demonstrated higher accuracy and generalization capacity compared to traditional methods, highlighting its innovative solution to classification problems. The model's performance could be further improved through various parameter optimizations or by exploring alternative model combinations. However, the hybrid model's more complex structure may lead to increased processing time and resource consumption. These limitations can be mitigated through methods that improve the algorithm's resource efficiency.

5.9 Factors Influencing Model Performance and Optimization Suggestions

Some models achieved very high accuracy rates on the training datasets. For example, decision tree and random forest models demonstrated impressive results on training data; however, while random forest maintained consistent performance on test data, the decision tree failed to sustain expected performance levels. This discrepancy suggests that the decision tree model may have overfitted the training data. In such cases, employing regularization techniques, reducing model complexity, or utilizing a larger and more balanced dataset could resolve the issue. On the other hand, the deep belief network (DBN) exhibited the lowest performance among all models in test results. This may stem from suboptimal configuration settings or the model's inability to adequately learn complex relationships within the dataset. To address this, optimizing hyperparameters, selecting features from the dataset more effectively, or reconstructing the model using a different architecture could be recommended. Additionally, increasing the amount of training data may significantly enhance the model's generalization capacity and overall performance.

5.10 The Impact of Dataset Size on Model Performance

The size of the dataset has a significant impact on both training time and accuracy rates of the models. A larger number of samples does not always guarantee better model performance. Instead, using a balanced dataset is far more critical for enhancing the model's generalization ability and classification success. In the literature, there are studies where larger datasets failed to achieve the success rates obtained in this study, or smaller datasets surpassed these results. This demonstrates that the quality of the dataset is more decisive than its size. As the dataset size increases, there is a notable rise in training time, and the risk of overfitting also grows. Conversely, a smaller dataset can lead to underfitting, negatively affecting the model's generalization capability. Therefore, the dataset's size should be optimized and balanced, with a focus on maintaining a high-quality and well-distributed composition to improve model performance. To balance training time and model performance effectively, careful preprocessing of the dataset and the application of necessary data preparation steps are essential.

5.11 Future Directions and Applications for Further Research

Future studies could focus on testing the consistency of these models by applying them to datasets expanded with features such as different age groups, geographic regions, and lifestyle habits. Additionally, examining the performance of the hybrid model on more complex and dynamic datasets could reveal its versatility. The use of classification algorithms in the healthcare sector, particularly for personalized recommendations aimed at improving individuals' lifestyles, holds significant potential for future research. Specifically, testing the model's ability to work with real-time data would be valuable for improving its performance and understanding how its outcomes can be optimized for practical applications. Such studies could evaluate the limitations of current algorithms from a broader perspective and pave the way for innovative solutions in this field.

5.12 Limitations and Areas for Improvement

The limitations of this study include the characteristics and size of the dataset used, which may constrain its broader generalization capacity. While the dataset represents a specific demographic group, testing the models with data from diverse regions or lifestyles could expand the applicability of the results. Additionally, further optimization of the hyperparameter settings of the algorithms used is an area that could be addressed in future research to enhance model performance. Future studies could explore the adaptability of the model to real-time data streams, enabling the development of more effective applications in healthcare services. Specifically, adapting such algorithms to systems that provide personalized health recommendations based on individuals' lifestyles could become a significant area of research.

6 Conclusion

This study aimed to detect individuals' obesity levels using classification algorithms. The dataset used comprised 22,869 samples and 16 features, with preprocessing steps such as imputing missing values, handling outliers, and scaling applied to the data. The overall performance of the models was evaluated using key metrics such as accuracy, precision, recall, F1 score, and specificity. Notably, several models achieved success rates between 80% and 89% without applying feature selection methods.

Among machine learning algorithms, the random forest demonstrated strong performance with accuracy, precision, recall, F1 score, and specificity metrics of 88.60%, 88.65%, 88.60%, 88.60%, and 98.12%, respectively. Among deep learning algorithms, autoencoders stood out with an ACC of 86.85% and a PRC of 85.55%, performing best among deep learning models. However, the hybrid model achieved the highest results, with an ACC of 90.09% and outperforming random forest in all performance metrics except specificity. The success of the hybrid model can be attributed to its combination of the strengths of machine learning and deep learning methods. Nevertheless, random forest surpassed the hybrid model in the specificity metric.

In the study, it was observed that feature selection methods reduced performance rather than enhancing it with the current settings. This finding suggests that all features in the dataset are significant for detecting obesity levels, and inappropriate or unnecessary data processing steps can harm the model. Therefore, future studies should carefully optimize feature selection and data processing steps.

High-performing algorithms can be applied in various areas, such as early detection of individuals' obesity risk, providing personalized health recommendations, and identifying risk groups in public health programs. Additionally, further studies can explore the integration of these models with mobile health applications and their use in providing clinical decision support for healthcare professionals. These approaches could enable the algorithms to create a broader impact in real-world applications.

In future studies, it is crucial to address key gaps—notably limited dataset generalizability, suboptimal hybrid model tuning, and insufficient evaluation under real-world conditions—by pursuing both data-centric and technological enhancements. From a data perspective, expanding and diversifying the dataset is essential for improving generalizability, as models trained on a single demographic group may not perform well across broader populations. This includes collecting more representative samples and incorporating additional relevant features that were not captured in the current dataset, which could further enhance the model's predictive accuracy and comprehensiveness. On the modeling front, the high-performing hybrid classifiers should be further optimized through careful hyperparameter tuning and ensemble calibration, since current optimization methods (such as PSO-based tuning) have shown convergence issues and high computational costs. Addressing these challenges and rigorously validating the system under real-world conditions is important to ensure the models maintain their accuracy and efficiency when deployed in practical settings, where they must generalize to new, diverse patient cohorts [79].

Acknowledgments The authors used language editing support tools, including large language models, to assist with grammar correction and clarity improvements during manuscript preparation. All scientific content and interpretations were developed and critically reviewed by the authors.

Competing Interests The authors have no competing interests to declare that are relevant to the content of this chapter.

Ethics Approval This chapter is based on publicly available secondary data and does not involve any direct experimentation on human participants or animals. Hence, ethical approval was not required.

References

1. N. Adak, Tüketim kültüründe beslenme: sağlıklı/sağlıksız yiyecekler. İstanbul Univ. J. Sociology **40**(1), 197–218 (2020)
2. P.C. Calder, Nutrition and immunity: lessons for covid-19. Nutr. Diabetes **11**(1), 19 (2021)
3. A. Eckart, T. Struja, A. Kutz, A. Baumgartner, T. Baumgartner, S. Zurfluh, O. Neeser, A. Huber, Z. Stanga, B. Mueller, et al., Relationship of nutritional status, inflammation, and serum albumin levels during acute illness: a prospective study. Am. J. Med. **133**(6), 713–722 (2020)

4. S.M. Nur, S. Rath, V. Ahmad, A. Ahmad, B. Ateeq, M.I. Khan, Nutritive vitamins as epidrugs. CRC Crit. Rev. Food Sci. Nutr. **61**(1), 1–13 (2021)
5. N.E. Marshall, B. Abrams, L.A. Barbour, P. Catalano, P. Christian, J.E. Friedman, W.W. Hay Jr, T.L. Hernandez, N.F. Krebs, E. Oken, et al. The importance of nutrition in pregnancy and lactation: lifelong consequences. Am. J. Obstet. Gynecol. **226**(5), 607–632 (2022)
6. M. Luli, G. Yeo, E. Farrell, J. Ogden, H. Parretti, E. Frew, S. Bevan, A. Brown, J. Logue, V. Menon, et al., The implications of defining obesity as a disease: a report from the association for the study of obesity 2021 annual conference, in *EClinicalMedicine*, vol. 58 (2023)
7. M.A. Jones, D.S. Allen, Psychological impact of obesity: a focus on depression and anxiety. Psychiatry Res. **58**(6), 611–619 (2019)
8. T. Turan, Optimize edilmiş denetimli öğrenme algoritmaları ile obezite analizi ve tahmini. Mehmet Akif Ersoy Üniversitesi Fen Bilimleri Enstitüsü Dergisi **14**(2), 301–312 (2023)
9. E. Yavuz, F. Özyürek, M. Pehlivan, Obezite enfeksiyon hastalığı mıdır? ERÜ Sağlık Bilimleri Fakültesi Dergisi **10**(1), 56–65 (2023)
10. C.D. Kassotis, L.N. Vandenberg, B.A. Demeneix, M. Porta, R. Slama, L. Trasande, Endocrine-disrupting chemicals: economic, regulatory, and policy implications. Lancet Diabetes Endocrinol. **8**(8), 719–730 (2020)
11. A. Okunogbe, R. Nugent, G. Spencer, J. Ralston, J. Wilding, Economic impacts of overweight and obesity: current and future estimates for eight countries. BMJ Glob. Health **6**(10), e006351 (2021)
12. U. Sandalc,ı, G. Tuncer, Obezitenin doğrudan ve dolaylı maliyetlerine ilişkin bir değerlendirme. Aksaray Üniversitesi İktisadi ve İdari Bilimler Fakültesi Dergisi **12**(2), 29–44 (2020)
13. M. d'Errico, M. Pavlova, F. Spandonaro, The economic burden of obesity in Italy: a cost-of-illness study. Eur. J. Health Econ. **23**(2), 1–16 (2022)
14. S. Mohan, C. Thirumalai, G. Srivastava, Effective heart disease prediction using hybrid machine learning techniques. IEEE Access **7**, 81542–81554 (2019)
15. K. Sweatt, W.T. Garvey, C. Martins, Strengths and limitations of BMI in the diagnosis of obesity: what is the path forward? Curr. Obes. Rep. **13**(3), 584–595 (2024)
16. I. Sommer, B. Teufer, M. Szelag, B. Nussbaumer-Streit, The performance of anthropometric tools to determine obesity: a systematic review and meta-analysis. Sci. Rep. **10**, 12699 (2020)
17. D. Sizoo, L.J.M. de Heide, M. Emous, T. van Zutphen, Intra-abdominal adipose tissue quantification by alternative versus reference methods: a systematic review and meta-analysis. Obes. Surg. **31**, 425–435 (2021)
18. S.A. Jebb, P. Aveyard, 'willpower' is not enough: time for a new approach to public health policy to prevent obesity. BMC Med. **21**(1), 89 (2023)
19. E.A. Sundararajan, M. Driss, W. Boulila M., Safaei, Review on obesity: understanding the causes & consequences of obesity and reviewing various machine learning approaches used to predict obesity. Computers in Biology and Medicine **136**, 104754 (2021)
20. M. Safaei, E.A. Sundararajan, M. Driss, W. Boulila, A. Shapi'i, A systematic literature review on obesity: Understanding the causes & consequences of obesity and reviewing various machine learning approaches used to predict obesity. Comput. Biol. Med. **136**, 104754 (2021)
21. S.B. Güneş, G.K. Aytuturldu, B. Akıncı, Obesity awareness-insight is inversely associated with body composition and physical activity behaviour in women with obesity at the admission to a lifestyle modification program. J. Public Health **33**, 1–7 (2024)
22. F. Hui, Y. Zhang, T. Ren, X. Li, M. Zhao, Q. Zhao, Role of metformin in overweight and obese people without diabetes: a systematic review and network meta-analysis. Eur. J. Clin. Pharmacol. **75**, 437–450 (2019)
23. T. Hollstein, P. Piaggi, Metabolic factors determining the susceptibility to weight gain: current evidence. Curr. Obes. Rep. **9**, 121–135 (2020)
24. C. Edlund, T.R. Jackson, N. Khalid, N. Bevan, T. Dale, A. Dengel, S. Ahmed, J. Trygg, R. Sjögren, Livecell—a large-scale dataset for label-free live cell segmentation. Nat. Methods **18**(9), 1038–1045 (2021)
25. B. Battal, B. Yıldırım, Ö.F. Dinçaslan, G. Cicek, Fake news detection with machine learning algorithms. Celal Bayar Univ. J. Sci. **20**(3), 65–83 (2024)

26. L. Li, Y. Huang, X. Cui, X. Cheng, X. Liu, On testing and evaluation of artificial intelligence models, in *2023 IEEE International Conference on Sensors, Electronics and Computer Engineering (ICSECE)* (IEEE, New York, 2023), pp. 92–97
27. R.R. Dutta, I. Mukherjee, C. Chakraborty, Obesity disease risk prediction using machine learning, in *International Journal of Data Science and Analytics* (2024), pp. 1–10
28. J. Du, S. Yang, Y. Zeng, C. Ye, X. Chang, S. Wu, Visualization obesity risk prediction system based on machine learning. Sci. Rep. **14**(1), 22424 (2024)
29. E.R. Cheng, R. Steinhardt, Z. Ben Miled, Predicting childhood obesity using machine learning: practical considerations. BioMedInformatics **2**(1), 184–203 (2022)
30. O. Kiss, F.C. Baker, R. Palovics, E.E. Dooley, K. Pettee Gabriel, J.M. Nagata, Using explainable machine learning and fitbit data to investigate predictors of adolescent obesity. Sci. Rep. **14**(1), 12563 (2024)
31. W. Liu, X. Fang, Y. Zhou, L. Dou, T. Dou, Machine learning-based investigation of the relationship between gut microbiome and obesity status. Microbes Infect. **24**(2), 104892 (2022)
32. Y. Wang, H. Wang, X. Yu, Q. Wu, X. Lv, X. Zhou, Y. Chen, S. Geng, Identification of metabolism related biomarkers in obesity based on adipose bioinformatics and machine learning. J. Transl. Med. **22**(1), 986 (2024)
33. Z. Sun, Y. Yuan, V. Farrahi, F. Herold, Z. Xia, X. Xiong, Z. Qiao, Y. Shi, Y. Yang, K. Qi, et al., Using interpretable machine learning methods to identify the relative importance of lifestyle factors for overweight and obesity in adults: pooled evidence from CHNS and NHANES. BMC Public Health **24**(1), 3034 (2024)
34. N. Koklu, S.A. Sulak, Using artificial intelligence techniques for the analysis of obesity status according to the individuals' social and physical activities. Sinop Üniversitesi Fen Bilimleri Dergisi **9**(1), 217–239 (2024)
35. A. Gutiérrez-Gallego, J.J. Zamorano-León, D. Parra-Rodríguez, K. Zekri-Nechar, J.M. Velasco, Ó. Garnica, R. Jiménez-García, A. López-de Andrés, N. Cuadrado-Corrales, D. Carabantes-Alarcón, et al., Combination of machine learning techniques to predict overweight/obesity in adults. J. Personalized Med. **14**(8), 816 (2024)
36. P.H.P. de Lucena, L.M.L. de Campos, Classification of obesity level using deep neural networks, in *International Conference on Intelligent Systems Design and Applications* (Springer, Berlin, 2023), pp. 99–107
37. S. Jeon, M. Kim, J. Yoon, S. Lee, S. Youm, Machine learning-based obesity classification considering 3d body scanner measurements. Sci. Rep. **13**(1), 3299 (2023)
38. R. Toderean, O. Geman, Emotional disturbances and obesity: a machine learning approach to predictive modeling, in *International Conference on e-Health and Bioengineering* (Springer, Berlin, 2023), pp. 502–510
39. H. Lim, H. Lee, J. Kim, A prediction model for childhood obesity risk using the machine learning method: a panel study on Korean children. Sci. Rep. **13**(1), 10122 (2023)
40. A. Ferreras, S. Sumalla-Cano, R. Martínez-Licort, I. Elío, K. Tutusaus, T. Prola, J.L. Vidal-Mazón, B. Sahelices, I. de la Torre Díez, Systematic review of machine learning applied to the prediction of obesity and overweight. J. Med. Syst. **47**(1), 8 (2023)
41. V. Osadchiy, R. Bal, E.A. Mayer, R. Kunapuli, T. Dong, P. Vora, D. Petrasek, C. Liu, J. Stains, A. Gupta, Machine learning model to predict obesity using gut metabolite and brain microstructure data. Sci. Rep. **13**(1), 5488 (2023)
42. J. Jeon, S. Lee, C. Oh, Age-specific risk factors for the prediction of obesity using a machine learning approach. Front. Public Health **10**, 998782 (2023)
43. Á. Torres-Martos, M. Bustos-Aibar, A. Ramírez-Mena, S. Cámara-Sánchez, A. Anguita-Ruiz, R. Alcalá, C.M. Aguilera, J. Alcalá-Fdez, Omics data preprocessing for machine learning: A case study in childhood obesity. Genes **14**(2), 248 (2023)
44. F.H. Yagin, M. Gülü, Y. Gormez, A. Castañeda-Babarro, C. Colak, G. Greco, F. Fischetti, S. Cataldi, Estimation of obesity levels with a trained neural network approach optimized by the Bayesian technique. Appl. Sci. **13**(6), 3875 (2023)

45. R. Archana, B. Rajathilagam, Comparative analysis of obesity level estimation based on lifestyle using machine learning, in *Intelligent Sustainable Systems*, ed. by J.S. Raj, Y. Shi, D. Pelusi, V.E. Balas (Springer Nature Singapore, Singapore, 2022), pp. 101–114
46. F. Ferdowsy, K.S.A. Rahi, M.I. Jabiullah, M.T. Habib, A machine learning approach for obesity risk prediction. Curr. Res. Behav. Sci. **2**, 100053 (2021)
47. X. Cheng, S.-y. Lin, J. Liu, S. Liu, J. Zhang, P. Nie, B.F. Fuemmeler, Y. Wang, H. Xue, Does physical activity predict obesity—a machine learning and statistical method-based analysis. Int. J. Environ. Res. Public Health **18**(8), 3966 (2021)
48. E. Rodríguez, E. Rodríguez, L. Nascimento, A.F. da Silva, F.A.S. Marins, Machine learning techniques to predict overweight or obesity, in *IDDM* (2021), pp. 190–204
49. S.A. Thamrin, D.S. Arsyad, H. Kuswanto, A. Lawi, S. Nasir, Predicting obesity in adults using machine learning techniques: an analysis of Indonesian basic health research 2018. Front. Nutr. **8**, 669155 (2021)
50. X. Pang, C.B. Forrest, F. Lê-Scherban, A.J. Masino, Prediction of early childhood obesity with machine learning and electronic health record data. Int. J. Med. Inform. **150**, 104454 (2021)
51. A. Chatterjee, M.W. Gerdes, S.G. Martinez, Identification of risk factors associated with obesity and overweight—a machine learning overview. Sensors **20**(9), 2734 (2020)
52. G. Colmenarejo, Machine learning models to predict childhood and adolescent obesity: a review. Nutrients **12**(8), 2466 (2020)
53. R.C. Cervantes, U.M. Palacio, Estimation of obesity levels based on computational intelligence. Inf. Med. Unlocked **21**, 100472 (2020)
54. N.C. Pereira, J. D'souza, P. Rana, S. Solaskar, Obesity related disease prediction from healthcare communities using machine learning, in *2019 10th International Conference on Computing, Communication and Networking Technologies (ICCCNT)* (IEEE, New York, 2019), pp. 1–7
55. I. Machorro-Cano, G. Alor-Hernández, M.A. Paredes-Valverde, U. Ramos-Deonati, J.L. Sánchez-Cervantes, L. Rodríguez-Mazahua, PISIoT: a machine learning and IoT-based smart health platform for overweight and obesity control. Appl. Sci. **9**(15), 3037 (2019)
56. UCI Machine Learning Repository, Estimation of obesity levels based on eating habits and physical condition. https://archive.ics.uci.edu/dataset/544/. Erişim Tarihi: 1 Aralık (2024)
57. Kaggle, Playground series—season 4, episode 2 dataset. https://www.kaggle.com/competitions/playground-series-s4e2/data. Erişim Tarihi: 1 Aralık (2024)
58. I. Muraina, Ideal dataset splitting ratios in machine learning algorithms: general concerns for data scientists and data analysts, in *7th International Mardin Artuklu Scientific Research Conference* (2022), pp. 496–504
59. Chacón, A.M.P., Ramírez, I.S., Márquez, F.P.G., K-nearest neighbour and k-fold cross-validation used in wind turbines for false alarm detection. Sustainable Futures **6**, 100132 (2023)
60. M.P. Uddin, M.A. Mamun, M.A. Hossain, PCA-based feature reduction for hyperspectral remote sensing image classification. IETE Tech. Rev. **38**(4), 377–396 (2021)
61. A.A. Khan, A.A. Laghari, A.M. Baqasah, R. Bacarra, R. Alroobaea, M. Alsafyani, J.A.J. Alsayaydeh, BDLT-IoMT—a novel architecture: SVM machine learning for robust and secure data processing in internet of medical things with blockchain cybersecurity. J. Supercomput. **81**(1), 271 (2025)
62. G.K. Walia, M. Kumar, Computational offloading and resource allocation for IoT applications using decision tree based reinforcement learning. Ad Hoc Netw. **170**, 103751 (2025)
63. C. Bentéjac, A. Csörgő, G. Martínez-Muñoz, A comparative analysis of gradient boosting algorithms. Artif. Intell. Rev. **54**, 1937–1967 (2021)
64. M. Sheykhmousa, M. Mahdianpari, H. Ghanbari, F. Mohammadimanesh, P. Ghamisi, S. Homayouni, Support vector machine versus random forest for remote sensing image classification: a meta-analysis and systematic review. IEEE J. Sel. Top. Appl. Earth Obs. Remote Sens. **13**, 6308–6325 (2020)
65. A. Ahmed, A. Jalal, K. Kim, A novel statistical method for scene classification based on multi-object categorization and logistic regression. Sensors **20**(14), 3871 (2020)

66. M.G.M. Abdolrasol, S.M.S. Hussain, T.S. Ustun, M.R. Sarker, M.A. Hannan, R. Mohamed, J.A. Ali, S. Mekhilef, A. Milad, Artificial neural networks based optimization techniques: a review. Electronics **10**(21), 2689 (2021)
67. L. Li, S. Zhang, B. Wang, Plant disease detection and classification by deep learning—a review. IEEE Access **9**, 56683–56698 (2021)
68. T. Kattenborn, J. Leitloff, F. Schiefer, S. Hinz, Review on convolutional neural networks (CNN) in vegetation remote sensing. ISPRS J. Photogramm. Remote Sens. **173**, 24–49 (2021)
69. J. Zhu, Q. Jiang, Y. Shen, C. Qian, F. Xu, Q. Zhu, Application of recurrent neural network to mechanical fault diagnosis: a review. J. Mech. Sci. Technol. **36**(2), 527–542 (2022)
70. I. Sohn, Deep belief network based intrusion detection techniques: A survey. Expert Syst. Appl. **167**, 114170 (2021)
71. A. Essien, C. Giannetti, A deep learning model for smart manufacturing using convolutional LSTM neural network autoencoders. IEEE Trans. Industr. Inform. **16**(9), 6069–6078 (2020)
72. X. Chen, X. Hu, Y. Huang, H. Jiang, W. Ji, Y. Jiang, Y. Jiang, B. Liu, H. Liu, X. Li, et al., Deep learning-based software engineering: progress, challenges, and opportunities. Sci. China Inf. Sci. **68**(1), 111102 (2025)
73. I. Price, A. Sanchez-Gonzalez, F. Alet, T.R. Andersson, A. El-Kadi, D. Masters, T. Ewalds, J. Stott, S. Mohamed, P. Battaglia, et al., Probabilistic weather forecasting with machine learning. Nature **637**(8044), 84–90 (2025)
74. I. Kandel, M. Castelli, The effect of batch size on the generalizability of the convolutional neural networks on a histopathology dataset. ICT Express **6**(4), 312–315 (2020)
75. M. Heydarian, T.E. Doyle, R. Samavi, MLCM: multi-label confusion matrix. IEEE Access **10**, 19083–19095 (2022)
76. S.A. Hicks, I. Strümke, V. Thambawita, M. Hammou, M.A. Riegler, P. Halvorsen, S. Parasa, On evaluation metrics for medical applications of artificial intelligence. Sci. Rep. **12**(1), 5979 (2022)
77. M.Z. Naser, A.H. Alavi, Error metrics and performance fitness indicators for artificial intelligence and machine learning in engineering and sciences. Archit. Struct. Constr. **3**(4), 499–517 (2023)
78. A.M. Carrington, D.G. Manuel, P.W. Fieguth, T. Ramsay, V. Osmani, B. Wernly, C. Bennett, S. Hawken, O. Magwood, Y. Sheikh, et al., Deep ROC analysis and AUC as balanced average accuracy, for improved classifier selection, audit and explanation. IEEE Trans. Pattern Anal. Mach. Intell. **45**(1), 329–341 (2022)
79. R.U. Arslan, I.S. Yapici, A novel hybrid approach to enhancing obesity prediction, in *The European Physical Journal Special Topics* (2025), pp. 1–19

Using Explainable AI for Assessment of Depression: A Systematic Literature Review

Andrew Macaulay, Fareed Ud Din, Phuong Anh Nguyen, Raymond Chiong, and Phillip J. Tully

Abstract Depression is a common mental health disorder worldwide, where heterogeneous presentations, high psychiatric comorbidity, and the episodic nature of this disorder compound clinical diagnosis difficulty. Social stigma combined with difficulty accessing mental health professionals further compounds this issue. This review investigates the potential of using explainable AI (xAI) as a diagnostic tool to help increase the quality-of-service delivery to patients. Through a structured literature extraction process via five prominent electronic databases, and following the Preferred Reporting Items for Systematic Reviews and Meta-Analyses (PRISMA) guidelines, we screened a total of 62 scientific papers, resulting in 17 eligible articles for an in-depth analysis. A detailed thematic analysis presents the main areas of *trust*, *model choice*, *model training*, *data utilisation*, and *personalisation*, along with the key metrics/techniques used in the latest research. We found transformer-based models using textual data such as user-generated content in a journal or social media format offer robust categorisation performance of a user's mental health status. xAI techniques are well developed for feature engineering and interpretation. However, further work is required to develop robust user explainability and understandability as well as in terms of presentation in a clinically relevant manner.

Keywords Depression · Mental health · Explainable artificial intelligence (xAI) · PRIMSA · Systematic literature review

A. Macaulay · F. U. Din (✉) · P. A. Nguyen
School of Science and Technology, University of New England, Armidale, NSW, Australia
e-mail: fuddin@une.edu.au

R. Chiong
School of Science and Technology, University of New England, Parramatta, NSW, Australia

School of Medicine and Public Health, University of Newcastle, Callaghan, NSW, Australia

P. J. Tully
Centre for Men's Wellbeing, University of Adelaide, Adelaide, SA, Australia

School of Psychology, Deakin University, Burwood, VIC, Australia

N. E. M. Khalifa, M. H. N. Taha (eds.), *Next-Gen Healthcare*,
https://doi.org/10.1007/978-3-032-07267-2_15

Abbreviations

ACM	Association of computing machinery
AI	Artificial intelligence
CNN	Convolutional neural network
DT	Decision tree
EMA	Ecological momentary assessment
JBI	Joanna Briggs Institute
LIME	Local interpretable model-agnostic explanations
LR	Logistics regression
LSTM	Long short-term memory
ML	Machine learning
PHQ	Patient Health Questionnaire
PRISMA	Preferred reporting items for systematic reviews and meta-analyses
RF	Random forest
RNN	Recurrent neural network
RQs	Research questions
SHAP	Shapley additive exPlanations
SVM	Support vector machine
xAI	Explainable AI

1 Introduction

Australian mental health statistics [1] provide for sobering reading—1 in 5 Australians will experience depression in their lifetime, and 1 in 3 Australians will experience anxiety, with 51.1% of women seeking help versus only 36.4% of men. While counseling service access difficulty and limited numbers of practising psychologists contribute to the lack of help-seeking behavior, so does the perceived social stigma and negatives of mental health treatment. Sarkar et al. [2] showed similar findings in high-income countries, with 1.6 million U.K. residents on waiting lists for professional mental health help and 1 in 5 Americans experiencing depression in their lifetime. The number of people experiencing depression has also increased by as much as 18% between 2005 and 2015 [3].

A major depression episode is characterised by near-daily experience of depressed mood and/or anhedonia over a 2-week period in addition to 4 or more symptoms from among weight change, sleep change, psychomotor change, fatigue/loss of energy, feelings of worthlessness or guilt, difficulty concentrating, and suicidality that cause distress or impairment in daily functioning [4]. Individuals with depression also experience difficulty in decision-making, which often results in poor quality of daily life [5]. Among recent developments in mental health assessment, digital phenotyping has gained interest from professionals to monitor human behaviors (e.g., sociability, physical activity), habits (e.g., mobility, sleep) and other information of interest (e.g., environmental context, mood, vocal cues)

[6]. The unique combination of symptoms necessitates a binary classification of polythetic disorders [7]. Accurate clinical diagnosis and referral are difficult within the limited capacity of primary care and rely on accurate reporting by patients of their symptoms. Misdiagnosis of mental health can be as high as 55 ~ 76%, with false positives detrimental to a person's wellbeing [8].

With the application of artificial intelligence (AI) in psychiatry, it could become easier for patients to share their symptoms with doctors without the fear of being judged, reporting biases, stigma or low mental health literacy [9]. Furthermore, AI can perform well without being unencumbered by human factors such as inconsistency, confirmation bias, stress, fatigue, and low job satisfaction levels among others. While AI may lead to improved treatment outcomes [10], the reduced administrative burden on primary care and other mental health professionals could also lead to healthcare cost savings.

Despite the advantages of technology, the use of advanced machine learning algorithms for depression detection [11–13] typically results in black-box models, where it is difficult to understand how decisions are made by the AI system. That leads to ethical concerns and hesitation among the public; thus, explainable AI (xAI) is an essential component of translating AI into healthcare settings—xAI methods are helpful tools to build trust in users, as they can be leveraged to describe how a model reaches its prediction including potential biases and expected impact [14, 15]. Despite the growing use of xAI, no systematic review has comprehensively analysed its role in depression diagnosis. Existing reviews (e.g., [8, 15, 16]) either lack a systematic approach or focus broadly on xAI in healthcare without specific emphasis on depression. This review fills this gap by systematically evaluating xAI methods used in depression classification, identifying challenges, and proposing future research directions. To achieve this, we structured the review around the following research questions (RQs):

- RQ1: What xAI methods have been applied for depression detection, and how do they enhance transparency and trust?
- RQ2: What types of data inputs and preprocessing techniques are used in xAI-based models for depression assessment?
- RQ3: How can xAI outputs be made clinically actionable and integrated into real-world mental health workflows?

The rest of this chapter is organised as follows: Sect. 2 and Sect. 3 discuss the research scope, RQs, and application survey; Sect. 4 presents the results of the review; Sect. 5 includes discussions of the review; and Sect. 6 concludes our study.

2 Related Work

To identify relevant articles in this field, and to ensure comprehensive coverage of relevant literature, a systematic search was conducted in prominent electronic databases including the ACM Digital Library, Scopus, ProQuest, EBSCOhost,

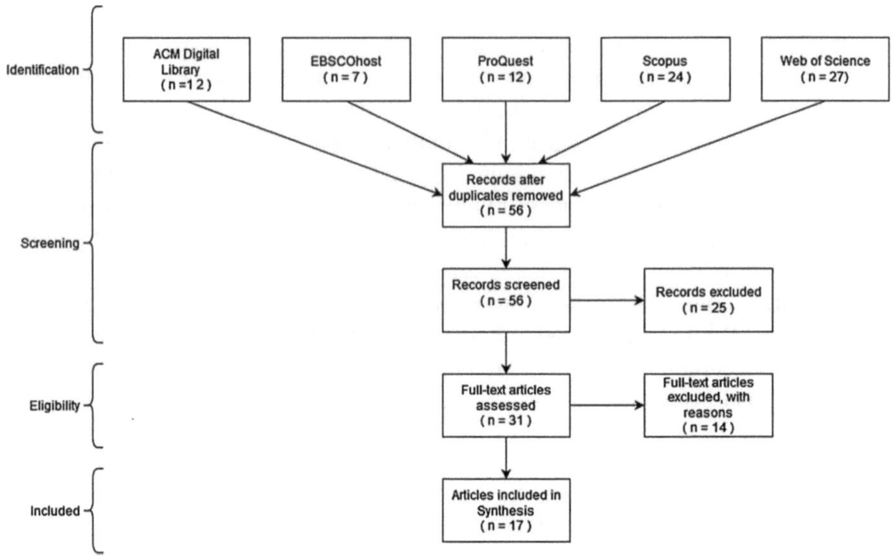

Fig. 1 PRISMA overview of the literature inclusion process

and Web of Science from the period 2017 to 2024 along with an additional supplementary ad hoc search via Google Scholar to broaden the search, which yielded only three review papers in this domain [8, 15, 16]. Of these review papers, Oyebode et al. [15] did not focus on xAI, while Joyce et al. [16] and Byeon [8] were not systematic reviews—Joyce et al. [16] focused on clarifying xAI definitions and concepts, leading to a framework being established; Byeon provided a narrative summary of six studies published between 2021 and 2022 that used xAI to discriminate high-risk depression groups. Our study here investigates the potential of using xAI as a diagnostic tool to help increase the quality-of-service delivery to depression-related patients, and we have covered many studies published in 2023 and 2024, as can be seen in Fig. 1.

3 Methodology

This study follows the guidelines outlined by the PRISMA (Preferred Reporting Items for Systematic Reviews and Meta-Analyses) framework and the approach of systematic literature reviews in computer science [17]. We aim to review the existing literature to analyse the potential of using xAI as a diagnostic tool for the assessment of depression by focusing on key RQs. Following PRISMA guidelines, this review addresses the following RQs:

- RQ1: What xAI methods have been applied for depression detection, and how do they enhance transparency and trust?

- RQ2: What types of data inputs and preprocessing techniques are used in xAI-based models for depression assessment?
- RQ3: How can xAI outputs be made clinically actionable and integrated into real-world mental health workflows?

The methodology involved a comprehensive search, selection, and synthesis of relevant studies to identify current trends, gaps, and future research directions in this area.

3.1 Search and Selection Strategy

A comprehensive systematic search was conducted of the Scopus, ACM Digital Library, EBSCOhost, ProQuest and Web of Science online databases. In order to refine the scope, the search was limited to journal articles or conference papers, published from January 2017 to November 2024, using the search terms "Explainable AI" and "Mental Health or Depression," searching only article abstracts to ensure the focus was on these keywords. Search queries were formulated using combinations of the key terms (Boolean logic method, e.g., using 'AND' and 'OR' operators) from the different domains, adapting them to each database's specific syntax and requirements. The search terms were designed to capture both xAI methodologies and mental health applications. Although several potentially high-value preprints were identified, they and other article types were excluded. Other related keywords were also considered, such as the concepts related to "Mental Health" including mental illness, mental disorder, stress, anxiety, suicidality, mood, and depression. Similarly, keywords related to "Explainable AI" were also considered, such as artificial intelligence or AI, machine learning or ML, algorithms, and xAI. Table 1 details the article inclusion criteria utilised to ensure the desired period, language, type, accessibility, and keywords.

Additionally, it is important to assess the quality of the included studies in order to support the inclusion/exclusion process and to perform comparative analysis. There are no universal quality metrics to perform systematic literature reviews as they have their own specific criteria. In this review, the quality of the selected studies was assessed using a predefined checklist as utilised by Hilton [18], which included questions related to the clarity of research objectives, applicability of

Table 1 Inclusion/exclusion criteria

No.	Criteria	Inclusion	Exclusion
1	Period	2017–2024	Otherwise
2	Language	English	Otherwise
3	Type	Journal articles, conference proceedings	Otherwise
4	Accessibility	Articles accessible via UNE library	Not accessible
5	Keyword	Includes selected keywords only	Otherwise

xAI approaches and mental health, appropriateness of study design, and relevance of findings to the RQs. Given the subjectivity in assessing the quality, each paper was independently reviewed based on research clarity, reproducibility, and methodological rigor. Disagreements were resolved through discussion.

3.2 Risk of Bias Assessment

In order to avoid the risk of bias, two independent reviewers were assigned to manually evaluate the chosen literature. We adhered to the standards specified by Hilton, M., in the Joanna Briggs Institute (JBI) Critical Appraisal Checklist [18] in order to guarantee methodological rigour. The evaluation considered biases in reporting (e.g., selective outcome reporting), performance (e.g., applicable technologies), detection (e.g., outcome assessment), and selection (e.g., inclusion criteria). A third reviewer was consulted for consensus and to settle disagreements amongst the reviewers.

3.3 Data Extraction

The first two authors independently participated in the screening process, following supervision and oversight from the rest of the research team. After a comprehensive review of the article titles, those found irrelevant to the RQs were excluded from further consideration. For articles lacking a clear title or abstract, the authors reviewed the full text to determine their relevance for inclusion. The authors achieved a 100% agreement rate after discussion of results, resulting in 17 articles for synthesis. Figure 1 details the process undertaken as per PRIMSA guidelines.

4 Results from the Systematic Literature Review

Figure 2 shows the number of articles published between 2017 and 2024, excluding duplicate articles. It suggests that research in the application of xAI methods in mental health is only in its early stages. However, the growing trend in research on xAI can be attributed to the increasing need to address public concerns regarding the trustworthiness and transparency of AI systems. Despite the numerous benefits that AI offers, many individuals remain hesitant and distrustful of using AI in critical decision-making scenarios, as demonstrated by Jones-Jang and Park [19]. xAI has become a potential solution to this challenge, offering insights into AI decision-making processes and improving user trust and acceptance.

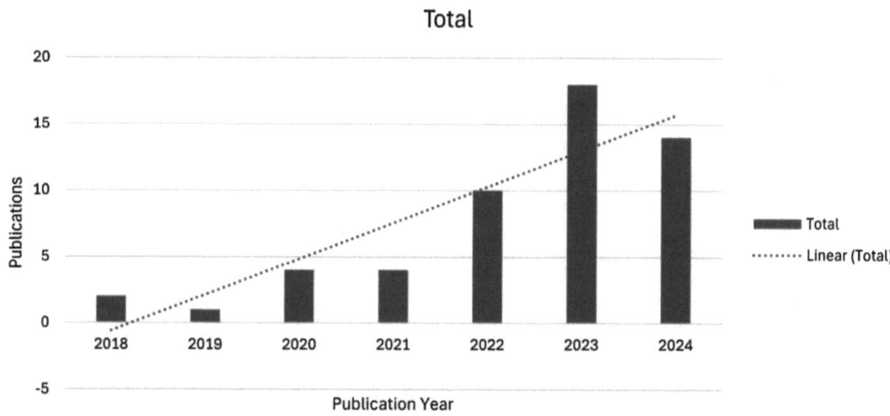

Fig. 2 Summary of potential literature returned by search, excluding duplicates

Table 2 Key themes and subthemes from eligible articles

Theme	Subthemes	References
Trust	Explainability, understandability, safety, xAI techniques • Local interpretable model-agnostic explanations (LIME) • Shapley additive exPlanations (SHAP) • ANCHORS and other uncommon methods	[2, 3, 8, 16, 20–25]
Model choice	Classical models (SVM/RF/DT/LR), deep learning (RNN/CNN/LSTM), transformer (BERT, RoBERTa and MentalBERT)	[3, 8, 15, 21–26]
Model training	Training production application,pretrained, suitable training data availability, imbalanced data	[3, 15, 21, 23–26]
Data utilisation	Origin, preprocessing, feature extraction, user-generated content (informal text), ecological momentary assessment (EMA), NLP encoding (one hot/TF-IDF), passive data	[3, 8, 15, 21–26]
Personalisation	Idiographic, nomothetic	[15, 21, 22]

4.1 Thematic Analysis

The analysis followed six steps of familiarisation with data, initial code generation, thematic search, thematic review, defining and naming themes, and reporting. During the data analysis, all authors agreed on key themes frequently available in the final selected pool of studies, namely trust, model choice, model training, data utilisation, and personalisation. Table 2 presents a summary of these key identified themes, with their subthemes and related studies.

Trust As Joyce et al. [16] pointed out, while there is a growing body of research about xAI methods and a corresponding growing consensus of the terms explainability, trust, understandability and safety, there is no clarity around how one might use xAI methods such as SHAP and LIME in an intuitive manner in a real-world application. Furthermore, they demonstrated clinical reasoning such as inductive and abductive in terms of undertaking a diagnosis and how presenting information in this manner is consistent with good clinical practice. Sarkar et al. [2] noted the emerging concept of user-level explainability as opposed to system level explainability (SHAP, LIME, ANCHORS) to differentiate these two concepts. Techniques such as SHAP, LIME, and ANCHORS help identify features that influence the model outcome; however, those features may not translate well in a clinical setting. For the reviewed papers SHAP and LIME were clearly the predominant xAI methods utilised with equal mentions. Jaber et al., [20] investigated the need for preparation of a clinically compatible report and explored how one might be derived from the SHAP method. In the context of mental health, safety is a critical aspect with Sarkar et al. [2] showing that existing mental health focused chatbots, such as wysa or woebot, can have interactions with users that do not conform to PHQ-9 clinical guidelines. The researchers introduced the concepts of knowledge-infused learning and knowledge graphs to incorporate domain knowledge in large language models (LLMs) to provide conversations that adhere to the clinical guidelines found in the DSM-5 and PHQ-9 practice manuals.

Model Choice Deep learning models (LSTM/BERT) were consistently shown to outperform classical models (RF/LR/SVM/DT) in studies by Pandit et al. [26], Oyebode et al. [15], Chatterjee et al. [21], Byeon [8], Aalbers et al. [22], Zia et al. [3], Kerz et al. [23], Thushari et al. [24], and Malhotra & Jindal [25]. However, it was noted that classical models featured an element of inherent explainability, for example, logistic regression provides a simple clear link between input features and their relationship with the classification output. Byeon [8] and Thushari et al. [24] showed how the xAI methods SHAP and LIME could address this issue. Models using user-generated textual data, (e.g., social media posts or journaling entries) achieved the highest accuracy. Zia et al. [3] obtained >0.96 F1-score across different test data sets using careful feature design and LSTM training. Open-source transformer-based models such as BERT offer the convenience of pretrained models with reduced input preprocessing. Malhotra and Jindal [25] investigated the performance of multiple BERT models across four datasets and found the BERT model pretrained in the mental health domain, MentalBERT, achieved F1-scores of 0.885, 0.966, 0.975, and 0.624 across four different datasets. In the context of App development, this model offers a low-effort, performant implementation option. It also highlights the sensitivity of model performance to input data quality.

Model Training Oyebode et al. [15] highlighted the challenges of obtaining quality data for training in this domain due to patient information being subject to more stringent access requirements, inconsistency in self-reported symptoms or inconsistency in the generation of written textual content by the patient. The researchers also noted that textual data was expensive, challenging for experts to correctly label, and subject to different annotations by different experts. Thushari et al. [24] and Oyebode et al. [15] discussed the data imbalance problem where the imbalance between class distributions leads to model underperformance. Techniques such as undersampling and class weights helped ensure the model received sufficient exposure to the minority class and improved classification performance.

Data Utilisation Oyebode et al. [15] discussed multimodal and data fusion, but these approaches did not appear to improve classification outcomes over less complex approaches. The preponderance for utilising textual data corresponds to the observation that models using such data performed better than models using nontextual data, which can use an interface between primary, secondary, and tertiary healthcare systems [27]. Malhotra and Jindal [25] detailed a common textual data preprocessing pipeline that was relatively consistent with other papers utilising textual data. The exception was Zia et al. [3] who applied a novel one-hot process rather than standard natural language processing (NLP) techniques such as term frequency-inverse document frequency (TF-IDF) using a carefully labeled lexicon to generate features for the model to consume. This model achieved extremely high accuracy $\geq$0.96. Models such as BERT or MentalBERT were able to consume textual information directly (once tokenised) allowing removal of the text preprocessing phase. Kerz et al. [23] detailed the use of general linguistic features (GLFs) and lexicon-based features (LBFs) for training an LSTM model. They compared this with a MentalRoBERTa model, which outperformed the GLF or LBF consuming model. Other types of data generated timeseries numerical measurements and standard data cleansing methods were utilised. For questionnaire-driven data, Chatterjee et al. [21] used the concept of ecological momentary measurement, a timeseries capture of short questions or survey responses from the user, and questions usually centered around the user's perception of their mood or anxiety.

Personalisation Chatterjee et al. [21] explored models trained by individuals, and found that feature influence varied by person. This is not inconsistent given that depression is a multi modal disease; however, training a model by individuals risks over-fitting and is not always practical to implement in the context of an App in the wild. Aalbers et al. [22] defined nomothetic (group level) and idiographic (by individual) and hence created models that consumed data for a single person (idiographic) or for a group (nomothetic). They compared the resultant performance and found that the nomothetic models performed better that the idiographic models.

4.2 Explainable AI (xAI)

From the reviewed relevant studies, several xAI methods are consistently employed across a variety of machine learning and deep learning models. The most widely used techniques include LIME (local interpretable model-agnostic explanations) and SHAP (SHapley additive exPlanations) (Fig. 3) [3, 8, 19, 22, 24, 25]. Other methods used include ANCHORS ALE [21], and feature attribution-based explainable (FAE) [26].

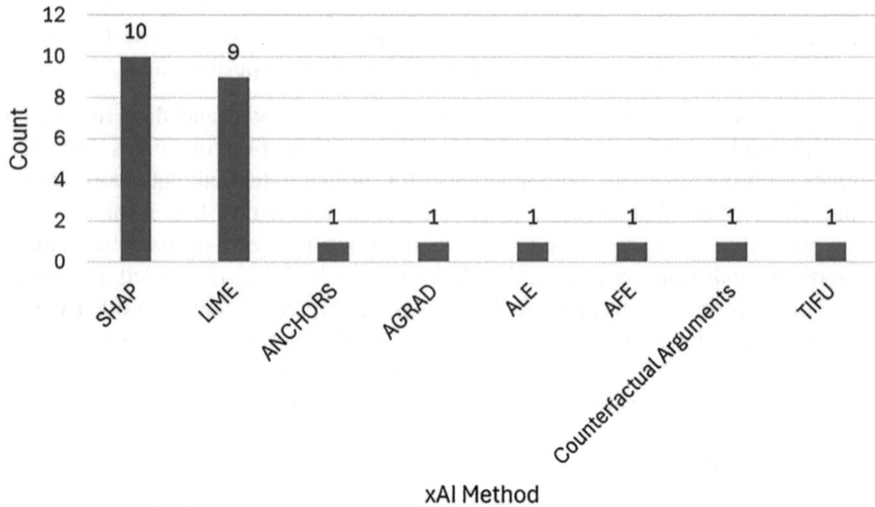

Fig. 3 xAI methods used in publications

4.3 Data Types

Figure 4 shows the frequency of data types utilised in the reviewed articles. Textual data is clearly the most popular type followed by biophysiological and behavioral. Table 3 presents the summary of the data types and the preprocessing techniques used in the final set of included articles.

5 Discussion

5.1 Explainable AI (xAI)

For xAI implementation, LIME, a model-agnostic technique that can be used with any type of model, is one of the most frequently used tools, especially for text classification tasks. Thushari et al. [24] emphasised in their study that the application of LIME not only improves model performance but also fully provides the transparency of black-box processes. For instance, they highlighted an example where a test text, "I want to turn into an alcoholic and die in 6 years," was misclassified by non-context-based models such as XGBoost and Naive Bayes; these decisions were often guided by the presence of class-representative words such as "die" rather than the full context of the post. In contrast, context-based models, such as BERT and MentalBERT, performed better in understanding the

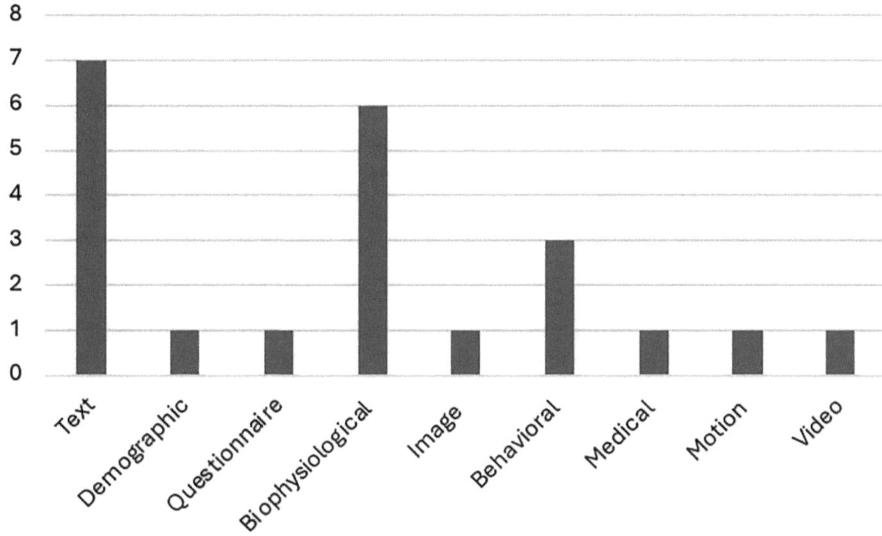

Fig. 4 Frequency of data types utilised in the reviewed articles

overall context of the text, and correctly classified the test text as "self.depression" by analysing the entire post rather than just a few critical words.

In the context of a user application, further work is required to establish user compliance with utilising a journaling approach or to quantitatively establish the availability and suitability of social media posts on a per-user basis. In a clinical or diagnostic setting, establishing trust requires further work in developing user explainability when reporting content and a format that enables providing mental health professionals a clear and understandable report explaining how the AI assessed a user's mental health state and arrived at the conclusion of that assessment. This will involve studies comparing diagnostic methods such as structured clinical interviews and screening tools (e.g., PHQ-9) against practical xAI methods. As Joyce et al. [16] noted, this so-called presentation layer needs to align with the cognitive strategies used by clinicians drawing on abductive and inductive reasoning. There exist multiple Apps in this domain, including MindDoc, Mello and Reflectly and Mood Tracker Diary, which provide insights into potential patient user flows and clinician interactions. The Mello App was subject to a pilot study, which demonstrated that even simple Apps do have usefulness in this space.

Furthermore, Maholtra and Jindal [25] pointed out the importance of LIME in understanding the impact of stop words (such as "but," "I," etc.) that can alter the actual meaning of words. Other papers also demonstrated that using xAI methods like LIME in text-based data helped bridge the gap between complex, high-performing models and their interpretability, and provided meaningful insights into the decision-making process of each algorithm. LIME's performance worked well with nontext-based datasets that were numerical and categorical [8].

Table 3 Data types and preprocessing techniques used in reviewed articles

Articles	Data types	Preprocessing techniques *(if applicable)*
Rahman et al. [28]	Text	Handling missing values, removing noise, stemming, removing stop words
Thushari et al. [24]	Text	Removing noise, removing stop words, tokenisation
Islam et al. [29]	Text	TF-IDF LIWC
Nguyen and Byeon [30]	Multimodal dataset: demographic data, biophysiological data, questionnaire	Handle missing values, rebalance variables, and encode labels
De Oliveira et al. [31]	Text	Lowercase conversion, text cleaning, removing stop words, tokenisation, stemming, TF-IDF
Hussna et al. [32]	Questionnaire	Removed data with missing information, replaced some features' names, encoded the categorical data, labeled the data
Upadhya et al. [33]	Biophysiological signals data, facial expressions data—image	Data normalisation, extracting pixel data and converting it into a numpy array
Malhotra and Jindal [25]	Text	Lowercase conversion, removal of noise, tokenisation, stop words removal
Ramon et al. [34]	Behavioral data	Data normalisation, classification task
Kharrat et al. [35]	Multimodal dataset: demographic data, medical data	Handling imbalance dataset with SMOTE
Pandit et al. [26]	Video	
Jaber et al. [20]	Multimodal dataset: biophysiological measurements, motion data	
Chatterjee et al. [21]	Multimodal dataset: biophysiological data, behavioral and cognitive data	Deletion—handling missing data Manual imputation—impute/fill data Automatic imputation—removing features where all values are constant and incorrect
Aalbers et al. [22]	Biophysiological measurements, behavioral data	Feature scaling, feature extraction
Hamed et al. [36]	Text	Feature extraction
Kerz et al. [23]	Text	Data filtering, down-sampling
Nowakowska et al. [37]	Biophysiological measurements	Random down-sampling with replacement

On the other hand, Kerz et al. [23] applied both LIME and a model-specific self-explaining method AGRAD in their study and concluded that AGRAD provided more pronounced differences between the basic Mental RoBERTa models and the information-infused models.

Unlike LIME, SHAP calculates the Shapley values for each feature to provide measurement of its influence on the model's prediction by calculating model error [38]. There are a number of studies applying SHAP to explain their models and managed to identify the contribution of each feature in the datasets [22, 35].

SHAP also was used in facial expression data. Upadhya et al. [33] emphasised that SHAP values help identify which features (in this case, pixels) are most influential for the model's predictions. The visualisation distinguishes between pixels that negatively impact the model's output (shown in darker areas) and those that positively influence it (lighter areas). This analysis reveals that the model pays particular attention to specific facial features, like the eyes and mouth. With text-based data, Maholtra and Jindal [25] concluded that SHAP visualisations allow for fine-tuning the model by highlighting the features or words that lead to incorrect classifications. For example, some models incorrectly relied on positive sentiment words for a negative prediction, providing an opportunity to adjust the model for more accurate performance.

Chatterjee et al. [21] computed the mean of absolute SHAP values to assess overall feature importance across a dataset. They used a fivefold cross-validation approach to ensure that the SHAP values are derived from distinct data instances, enhancing the robustness of the analysis. They also applied ALE (accumulated local effects) plots to illustrate how specific features influence model predictions, and suggested that clinicians can be supported with SHAP and ALE plots to find the most influential features for intervention.

There are also other papers that used attribution-based explanation (FAE) [26] or calculated feature importance to explain prediction [37]. They all successfully found out the most influential attribution/feature in the model prediction to provide the transparency of its results.

For xAI systems to be usable in real-world clinical settings, explanations must align with clinician decision-making processes. This includes integrating xAI outputs into electronic medical record dashboards as structured reports with natural language summaries, confidence scores, and risk levels (e.g., low/moderate/severe). Visual aids such as SHAP summary plots or LIME-based word importance highlights can be embedded within digital interfaces to support interpretability. For example, a MentalBERT-based application could generate a one-page summary: highlighting key phrases detected, the rationale for classification, and an associated risk score. Structured presentation formats like the PHQ-9 comparison table or DSM-5 criteria match could support direct clinical interpretation. Additionally, integrating these tools into triage or screening systems in telehealth platforms or mobile Apps could enable early flagging of at-risk patients and guide referrals or interventions.

5.2 Data Types

Textual data is the most common in the context of mental health assessment [3, 23–26, 28, 29] with preprocessing steps such as tokenisation, stemming, removal of stop words, and noise reduction being applied. Furthermore, it is commonly used with LIME methods and shows significant performance in context-based models such as MentalBERT and BERT [24].

Biophysiological measurements, as used in [19, 21, 22, 35, 37], are used with SHAP methods, which helps them to find which features in the dataset have the most impact on the model decisions. With this kind of data, handling missing values, encoding labels, and handling imbalance datasets is important in preprocessing to enhance the data and result quality.

Pandit et al. [26] used 200 muted videos in their study to assess the emotions of participants and compute feature attributions to explain the model. Their model relies heavily on action markers like "laughter," "slight laugher" for prediction. Overall, models consuming textual data consistently outperformed models consuming other types of data. The choice of xAI method is influenced by the nature of the input data. Each data type requires specific preprocessing steps and benefits from distinct xAI approaches.

5.3 Trust

Building trust in AI solutions, especially in critical areas like mental health, requires transparency and explainable decisions because they could have a significant negative impact on people's lives [8], leading to critical diseases such as Alzheimer's [39]; hence, clinical applications have high stakes [16].

Joyce et al. [16] proposed the TIFU framework (Fig. 5) for understandable AI in mental health applications, which focuses on transparency and interpretability to build trust from clinicians. They defined "understandability" as a means for clinicians to relate the model's behavior with their own diagnostic processes, even though the algorithms may be complex. One of the important components they mentioned is "presentation": the model must present input/output that is consistent with clinicians' strategies.

Ramon et al. [34] highlighted an example about the use of local explanations in decision-making of experts. Local explanations could be used to provide insights about a model's predictions, allowing psychologists and psychiatrists, among others, to validate or overrule decisions based on their domain knowledge. For instance, when a model predicts that a person may be experiencing mental health issues based on their web history, experts can use local explanations to find out which behaviors led to this conclusion. This allows them to focus on specific,

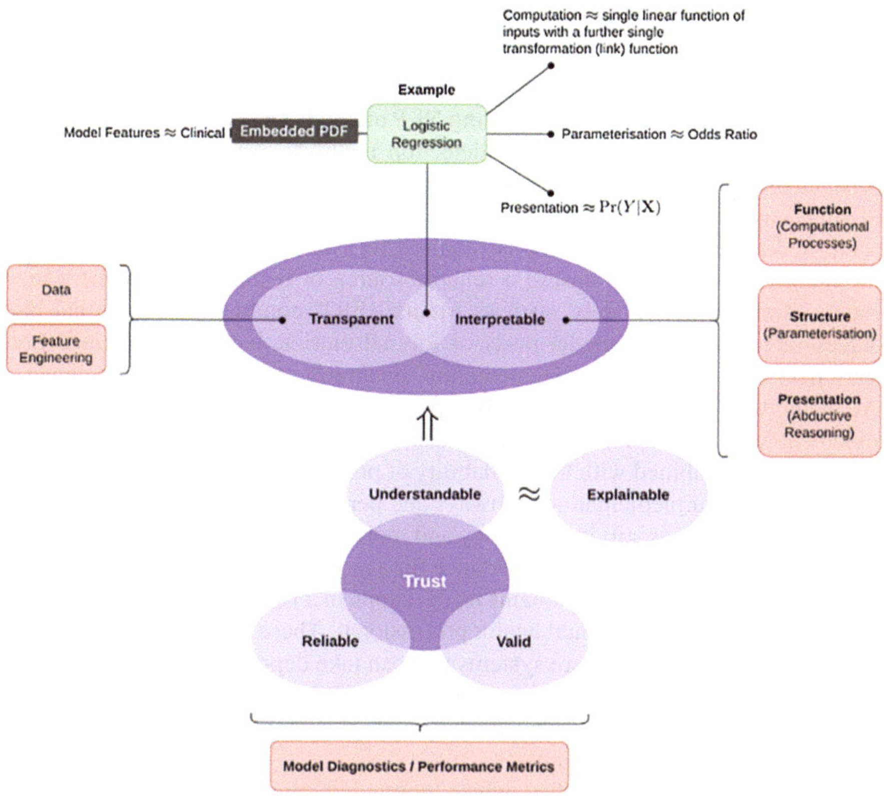

Fig. 5 TIFU framework [16]

relevant information rather than going through large amounts of data. For example, when a user is classified as "depressed" because they searched for "symptoms of depression," experts can leverage xAI methods to know why the decision was made, and they can overrule the decision when they figure out that the user actually is a psychology student and the search query is a common for them. The synthesis of the included studies generally suggests that by providing understandable and context-specific explanations, xAI solutions allow professionals and experts to assess and interact with the model's input or output. This increases transparency and interpretability, which significantly builds trust in the model among users and clinicians.

5.4 Gaps and Future Research Opportunities

While the review clearly showed that user-generated textual content such as social media posts or journaling processed using NLP methods and classified using models such as MentBERT provided robust detection methods, it was not clear whether social media posts or journaling could be relied upon to be available on a per-individual user basis. Another key element to note is that not everyone posts on social media, hence further work is required to assess user compliance in using journaling functionality to ensure a reliable source of textual data for the xAI to process. Transformer models, such as MentalBERT, combined with textual data sources including social media posts or journal entries, have demonstrated both robust detection and ease of implementation. Integrating them with well-understood xAI methods such as SHAP or LIME provides a powerful, robust, and easy-to-implement xAI solution. These models also offer the advantages of minimal text preprocessing combined with the availability of pretrained open-source models with well-understood implementation pathways and performance boundaries.

Furthermore, xAI is still in its infancy and more research is required to bridge the gap from understanding feature importance for a model (SHAP, LIME) to producing a user explainable report that explains its decisions in a format and with content that is relatable to the user or mental health professional. These xAI models provide the foundation for future healthcare systems that can take depression related symptoms are a baseline for overall strategic implementation [40]. Further developing a picture over time of the user's mental state and presenting this to the clinician is more useful than a single measurement in time.

We did not find any studies which compared clinical diagnosis with xAI diagnosis; although technically out of scope for this chapter, this would be useful in building clinical confidence.

6 Conclusion

This systematic literature review on the use of xAI for depression assessment highlighted the significant potential of AI-driven approaches in mental health diagnostics. The study synthesised findings from 17 selected articles as presented in Table 4 underscored the advantages of using transformer-based models such as BERT and MentalBERT for detecting symptoms of depression from textual data, including social media posts and journaling. It also identified key themes related to trust, model choice, data utilisation, and explainability, noting that while AI can enhance accessibility to mental health support, challenges remain in ensuring transparency, interpretability, and clinical relevance. Widely used xAI techniques such as SHAP and LIME provide insights into model decisions, but further efforts are needed to align AI-generated explanations with clinical reasoning frameworks for better adoption by mental health professionals.

Despite promising advancements, the study also identified gaps in user compliance, data availability, and the lack of direct comparisons between AI-based depression assessment and traditional clinical diagnoses. Future research should focus on refining xAI methods to enhance user and clinician trust, integrating multimodal data sources for improved prediction accuracy, and developing structured, interpretable reports that align with clinical decision-making processes. Addressing these challenges will be crucial in translating AI-based mental health diagnostics into real-world applications that are both effective and ethically sound.

Appendix (Table 4)

Table 4 Synthesised articles summary

No.	Study	Algorithm	XAI technique	Data processing methods *(if applicable)*	Dataset features	Result
1.	Rahman et al. [28]	XGBoost, decision tree, SVM, naive Bayes, simple gradient descent, stochastic gradient descent, K-nearest centroid, KNN, AdaBoost, RF, and LR	LIME	Handling missing values, removing noise, stemming, removing stop words	4472 samples Text	Accuracy: 37–71%
2.	Thushari et al. [24]	LR, RF, stochastic gradient descent, naive Bayes, XGBoost, LSTM, CNN, BERT, MentalBERT	LIME	Removing noise, removing stop words, tokenisation	46,103 instances Text	Recall: 61.40–76.59 Precision: 67.40–76.66 Accuracy: 65.29–76.70
3.	Islam et al. [29]	RF, SVM, Gaussian NB, logistic regression, K-neighbors, BERT, LSTM, BiLSTM	LIME SHAP	TF-IDF, LIWC	24,101 posts from Reddit Text	Recall: 48.28–99.22 Precision: 19.52–98.43 Accuracy: 62.78–98.58
4.	Nguyen and Byeon [30]	Deep neural network	Applied LIME	Handle missing values, rebalance variables, and encode labels	36,258 samples with 22 variables Multimodal dataset: demographic data, biophysiological data, questionnaire	Recall: 97.32 Precision: 93.55 Accuracy: 89.92
5.	De Oliveira et al. [31]	Extra trees, random forest, and SVC	Applied ELI5	Lowercase conversion, text cleaning, removing stop words, tokenisation, stemming, TF-IDF	3788 tweets from twitter Text	Recall: 74–97 Precision: 86–92 Accuracy: 90.1–90.6

6.	Hussna et al. [32] COVID-19 context	Logistic regression, random forest, XGBoost, and AdaBoost	LIME SHAP	Removed data with missing information, replaced some features' names, encoded the categorical data, labeled the data	1181 samples with 19 variables Questionnaire	Recall: 50–54 Precision: 44–63 Accuracy: 84.7–88.52
7.	Upadhya et al. [33] Stress detection	LSTM and SVM for physiological signals data CNN models: VGG16, custom CNN for facial expressions data	LIME SHAP	Data normalisation, extracting pixel data and converting it into a numpy array	288,144 samples Biophysiological signals data—numerical Facial expressions data—image	Recall: 72–83 Precision: 79–85 Accuracy: 79–86
8.	Malhotra and Jindal [25] Including suicide and depression detection	Supervised fine-tuning of various BERT-based LLMs Unsupervised topic modeling BERTopic	LIME SHAP	Lowercase conversion, removal of noise, tokenisation, stop words removal	4 datasets: 23,520 tweets from twitter 231,967 posts from Reddit 5540 posts from Reddit 1895 posts from Reddit Text	Recall: 84.6–98.5 Precision: 88.2–98.1 Accuracy: 87.3–97.4
9.	Ramon et al. [34]	Linear and logistic regression and random forest	Counterfactual rules Rule extraction		4,539,634 Financial transactions Behavioral data	Accuracy: Min = 53.13%, max = 61.82% (linear) Accuracy: Min = 53.35%, max = 63.98% (nonlinear)

(continued)

Table 4 (continued)

No.	Study	Algorithm	XAI technique	Data processing methods *(if applicable)*	Dataset features	Result
10.	Kharrat et al. [35]	Logistic regression (LR), random forest (RF), extreme gradient boosting (XGBoost), multilayer perceptron (MLP)	SHAP	Handling imbalance dataset with SMOTE	103 individuals with features Multimodal dataset: demographic data, medical data	AUC: 79–87 95–97
11.	Pandit et al. [26]	Convolutional neural network	Attribution-based explanation (FAE)		200 videos Video	CCC 31.5–62.5
12.	Jaber et al. [20]	Random forest	Tree-SHAP		15 samples Multimodal dataset: biophysiological measurements, motion data	Fourfolds. Average F1 score: 78
13.	Chatterjee et al. [21]	10 classical ML as baseline: Adaboost regressor, adaboost classifier, elasticnet regressor, gradient boosting classifier, gradient boosting regressor, Poisson regressor, random forest classifier, random forest regressor, support vector regressor, support vector classifier and support vector regressor, compared to MLP model	SHAP ALE plot Anchors	Deletion—handling missing data Manual imputation—impute/fill data Automatic imputation—removing features where all values are constant and incorrect	14 samples 43 features Multimodal dataset: biophysiological data, behavioral and cognitive data	MAE; MAPE as metric

14.	Aalbers et al. [22]	Least absolute shrinkage and selection operator (LASSO), regression, support vector regression (SVR), and random forest (RF) regression	SHAP	Feature scaling, feature extraction	224 samples 3 categories of features (8 in total) Biophysiological measurements Behavioral data	
15.	Hamed et al. [36]	RNN based on LSTM	LIME	Feature extraction	2 datasets 1–11,807 texts 21,470 texts	Accuracy: 81–91%
16.	Kerz et al. [23]	BiLSTM (bidirectional long-short-term memory), MentalRoBERTa	LIME AGRAD	Data filtering, down-sampling	4 publicly datasets obtained from media social posts Text	Recall: 57.59–81.59 Precision: 57.88–81.65 Accuracy: 57.57–82.22
17.	Nowakowska et al. [37]	RF, GBT, XGBoost, AdaBoost	Calculating features importance	Random down-sampling with replacement	224 patients Biophysiological measurements	62% (RF)

References

1. Statistics Beyond Blue (2025), https://www.beyondblue.org.au/mental-health/statistics. Retrieved 16 June 2025
2. S. Sarkar, M. Gaur, L. Chen, M. Garg, B. Srivastava, A review of the explainability and safety of conversational agents for mental health to identify avenues for improvement. Front. Artif. Intell. **6**, 1229805 (2023). https://doi.org/10.3389/frai.2023.1229805
3. U.M. Zia, K.K. Dysthe, F. Asbjørn, B.P. Bae, Deep learning for prediction of depressive symptoms in a large textual dataset. Neural Comput. Applic. **34**(1), 721–744 (2022). https://doi.org/10.1007/s00521-021-06426-4
4. DSM-5 TR, Psychiatric Association, *Diagnostic and Statistical Manual of Mental Disorders*, 5th edn. (American Psychiatric Association, Washington, 2022). https://doi.org/10.1176/appi.books.9780890425787
5. H. Jin, S.S. Nath, S. Schneider, D. Junghaenel, S. Wu, C. Kaplan, An informatics approach to examine decision-making impairments in the daily life of individuals with depression. J. Biomed. Inform. **122**, 103913 (2021). https://doi.org/10.1016/j.jbi.2021.103913
6. I. Moura, A. Teles, D. Viana, J. Marques, L. Coutinho, F. Silva, Digital phenotyping of mental health using multimodal sensing of multiple situations of interest: A systematic literature review. J. Biomed. Inform. **138**, 104278 (2023). https://doi.org/10.1016/j.jbi.2022.104278
7. R.F. Krueger, S. Bezdjian, Enhancing research and treatment of mental disorders with dimensional concepts: Toward DSM-V and ICD-11. World Psychiatry **8**(1), 3–6 (2009). https://doi.org/10.1002/j.2051-5545.2009.tb00197.x
8. H. Byeon, Advances in machine learning and explainable artificial intelligence for depression prediction. Int. J. Adv. Comput. Sci. Appl. **14**(6), 140656 (2023). https://doi.org/10.14569/ijacsa.2023.0140656
9. T.K. Houston, L.A. Cooper, D.E. Ford, Internet support groups for depression: A 1-year prospective cohort study. Am. J. Psychiatry **159**(12), 2062–2068 (2002). https://doi.org/10.1176/appi.ajp.159.12.2062
10. D.D. Luxton, Artificial intelligence in psychological practice: Current and future applications and implications. Prof. Psychol. Res. Pract. **45**(5), 332–339 (2014). https://doi.org/10.1037/a0034559
11. R. Chiong, G.S. Budhi, S. Dhakal, F. Chiong, A textual-based featuring approach for depression detection using machine learning classifiers and social media texts. Comput. Biol. Med. **135**, 104499 (2021). https://doi.org/10.1016/j.compbiomed.2021.104499
12. R. Chiong, G.S. Budhi, S. Dhakal, Combining sentiment lexicons and content-based features for depression detection. IEEE Intell. Syst. **36**(6), 99–105 (2021). https://doi.org/10.1109/MIS.2021.3093660
13. R. Chiong, G.S. Budhi, E. Cambria, Detecting signs of depression using social media texts through an ensemble of ensemble classifiers. IEEE Trans. Affect. Comput. (2025). https://doi.org/10.1109/TAFFC.2025.3571749
14. A.F. Markus, J.A. Kors, P.R. Rijnbeek, The role of explainability in creating trustworthy artificial intelligence for health care: A comprehensive survey of the terminology, design choices, and evaluation strategies. J. Biomed. Inform. **113**, 103655 (2021). https://doi.org/10.1016/j.jbi.2020.103655
15. O. Oyebode, J. Fowles, D. Steeves, R. Orji, Machine learning techniques in adaptive and personalized systems for health and wellness. Int. J. Human-Comput. Interact. **39**(9), 1938–1962 (2023). https://doi.org/10.1080/10447318.2022.2089085
16. D.W. Joyce, A. Kormilitzin, K.A. Smith, A. Cipriani, Explainable artificial intelligence for mental health through transparency and interpretability for understandability. npj Dig. Med. **6**(1), 6 (2023). https://doi.org/10.1038/s41746-023-00751-9
17. A. Carrera-Rivera, W. Ochoa, F. Larrinaga, G. Lasa, How-to conduct a systematic literature review: A quick guide for computer science research. MethodsX **9**, 101895 (2022). https://doi.org/10.1016/j.mex.2022.101895

18. M. Hilton, JBI critical appraisal checklist for systematic reviews and research syntheses. J. Can. Health Libr. Assoc. **45**(3), 180–183 (2024). https://doi.org/10.29173/jchla29801
19. S.M. Jones-Jang, Y.J. Park, How do people react to AI failure? Automation bias, algorithmic aversion, and perceived controllability. J. Comput.-Mediat. Commun. **28**(1), 29 (2022). https://doi.org/10.1093/jcmc/zmac029
20. D. Jaber, H. Hajj, F. Maalouf, W. El-Hajj, Medically-oriented design for explainable AI for stress prediction from physiological measurements. BMC Med. Inform. Decis. Mak. **22**(1), 38 (2022). https://doi.org/10.1186/s12911-022-01772-2
21. S. Chatterjee, J. Mishra, F. Sundram, P. Roop, Towards personalised mood prediction and explanation for depression from biophysical data. Sensors **24**(1), 164 (2023). https://doi.org/10.3390/s24010164
22. G. Aalbers, A.T. Hendrickson, M.M. Vanden Abeele, L. Keijsers, Smartphone-tracked digital markers of momentary subjective stress in college students: Idiographic machine learning analysis. JMIR Mhealth Uhealth **11**, e37469 (2023). https://doi.org/10.2196/37469
23. E. Kerz, S. Zanwar, Y. Qiao, D. Wiechmann, Toward explainable AI (XAI) for mental health detection based on language behavior. Front. Psych. **14**, 1219479 (2023). https://doi.org/10.3389/fpsyt.2023.1219479
24. P.D. Thushari, N. Aggarwal, V. Vajrobol, G.J. Saxena, S. Singh, A. Pundir, Identifying discernible indications of psychological well-being using ML: Explainable AI in Reddit social media interactions. Soc. Netw. Anal. Min. **13**(1), 141 (2023). https://doi.org/10.1007/s13278-023-01145-1
25. A. Malhotra, R. Jindal, XAI transformer based approach for interpreting depressed and suicidal user behavior on online social networks. Cogn. Syst. Res. **84**, 101186 (2024). https://doi.org/10.1016/j.cogsys.2023.101186
26. V. Pandit, M. Schmitt, N. Cummins, B. Schuller, I see it in your eyes: Training the shallowest-possible CNN to recognise emotions and pain from muted web-assisted in-the-wild video-chats in real-time. Inf. Process. Manag. **57**(6), 102347 (2020). https://doi.org/10.1016/j.ipm.2020.102347
27. A. Giri, F. Ud Din, Role of data as an interface between primary, secondary and tertiary care: Evidence from literature. Inf. Health **2**(1), 63–72 (2025). https://doi.org/10.1016/j.infoh.2025.01.004
28. T. Rahman, R. Shahrin, F.A. Pospu, N. Sultana, R.M. Rahman, Text-based data analysis for mental health using explainable AI and deep learning, in *Studies in Computational Intelligence*, (Springer, Cham, 2024), pp. 17–31. https://doi.org/10.1007/978-3-031-53274-0_3
29. M.R. Islam, M.K.H. Sakib, S.A. Prome, X. Wang, A. Ulhaq, C. Sanin, D. Asirvatham, *Machine Learning with Explainability for Suicide Ideation Detection from Social Media Data* (IEEE, New York, 2023). https://doi.org/10.1109/besc59560.2023.10386773
30. H.V. Nguyen, H. Byeon, Explainable deep-learning-based depression modeling of elderly community after COVID-19 pandemic. Mathematics **10**(23), 4408 (2022). https://doi.org/10.3390/math10234408
31. A.C. De Oliveira, E.J. Diniz, S. Teixeira, A.S. Teles, How can machine learning identify suicidal ideation from user's texts? Towards the explanation of the Boamente system. Proc. Comput. Sci. **206**, 141–150 (2022). https://doi.org/10.1016/j.procs.2022.09.093
32. A.U. Hussna, I.I. Trisha, I.J. Ritun, M.G.R. Alam, in COVID-19 impact on students' mental health: Explainable AI and classifiers. *2021 International Conference on Decision Aid Sciences and Application (DASA)* (2021), https://doi.org/10.1109/dasa53625.2021.9682371
33. J. Upadhya, K. Poudel, J. Ranganathan, A comprehensive approach to early detection of workplace stress with multi-modal analysis and explainable AI (2024), https://doi.org/10.1145/3632634.3655878
34. Y. Ramon, R. Farrokhnia, S.C. Matz, D. Martens, Explainable AI for psychological profiling from behavioral data: An application to big five personality predictions from financial transaction records. Inform **12**(12), 518 (2021). https://doi.org/10.3390/info12120518
35. F.G.Z. Kharrat, C. Gagne, A. Lesage, G. Gariépy, J. Pelletier, C. Brousseau-Paradis, L. Rochette, E. Pelletier, P. Lévesque, M. Mohammed, J. Wang, Explainable artificial intelligence

models for predicting risk of suicide using health administrative data in Quebec. PLoS One **19**(4), e0301117 (2024). https://doi.org/10.1371/journal.pone.0301117
36. S.H. Hamed, H. Elbakry, H. Elghareeb, S. Elhishi, Using XAI techniques to persuade text classifier results: A case study of covid-19 tweets. Indian J. Sci. Technol. **15**(30), 1484–1494 (2022)
37. K. Nowakowska, A. Sakellarios, J. Kaźmierski, D.I. Fotiadis, V.C. Pezoulas, AI-enhanced predictive modeling for identifying depression and delirium in cardiovascular patients scheduled for cardiac surgery. Diagnostics **14**(1), 67 (2023). https://doi.org/10.3390/diagnostics14010067
38. A. Nayak, *Idea Behind LIME and SHAP* (Towards Data Science, San Francisco, 2019). https://towardsdatascience.com/idea-behind-lime-and-shap-b603d35d34eb
39. S.A. Malec, S.B. Taneja, S.M. Albert, C.E. Shaaban, H.T. Karim, A.S. Levine, R.D. Boyce, Causal feature selection using a knowledge graph combining structured knowledge from the biomedical literature and ontologies: A use case studying depression as a risk factor for Alzheimer's disease. J. Biomed. Inform. **142**, 104368 (2023). https://doi.org/10.1016/j.jbi.2023.104368
40. M. Khadgi, F. Ud Din, Towards AI/ML-powered hybrid project management strategy for the healthcare sector, in *Machine Learning and Soft Computing. ICMLSC 2025. Communications in Computer and Information Science*, ed. by L. Huang, vol. 2487, (Springer, Singapore, 2025). https://doi.org/10.1007/978-981-96-6400-9_15

MIX
Papier aus verantwortungsvollen Quellen
Paper from responsible sources
FSC® C105338

If you have any concerns about our products,
you can contact us on
ProductSafety@springernature.com

In case Publisher is established outside the EU,
the EU authorized representative is:
Springer Nature Customer Service Center GmbH
Europaplatz 3, 69115 Heidelberg, Germany

Printed by Libri Plureos GmbH
in Hamburg, Germany